Infections in Hematology

Infections in Hematology

Editor: Justin Ramos

AMERICAN
MEDICAL PUBLISHERS
www.americanmedicalpublishers.com

AMERICAN
MEDICAL PUBLISHERS
www.americanmedicalpublishers.com

Cataloging-in-Publication Data

Infections in hematology / edited by Justin Ramos.
p. cm.
Includes bibliographical references and index.
ISBN 978-1-63927-225-9
1. Hematology. 2. Infection. 3. Blood--Diseases. 4. Blood--Diseases--Treatment. I. Ramos, Justin.
RC633 .I54 2022
616.075 61--dc23

American Medical Publishers,
41 Flatbush Avenue,
1st Floor, New York,
NY 11217, USA

ISBN 978-1-63927-225-9 (Hardback)

Contents

Preface

This book aims to highlight the current researches and provides a platform to further the scope of innovations in this area. This book is a product of the combined efforts of many researchers and scientists, after going through thorough studies and analysis from different parts of the world. The objective of this book is to provide the readers with the latest information of the field.

Hematology is a branch of medicine that deals with the study of causes, treatments, prognosis and prevention of blood-related diseases. It is concerned with the treatment of diseases that affect the production of blood and its constituents including blood cells, hemoglobin, platelets, bone marrow, blood proteins, spleen and blood vessels. The microbiological culture of the blood detects infections that spread through the bloodstream, such as bacteremia and sepsis. Bacteremia is an infectious disease that is caused by the presence of bacteria in the blood. It is treated with antibiotics. The reverse response of the immune system to the bacteria or other pathogens such as fungi, viruses and protozoan causes sepsis. The book presents researches and studies performed by experts across the globe. It strives to provide a fair idea about infections in hematology and to help develop a better understanding of their diagnosis and management. Those in search of information to further their knowledge will be greatly assisted by this book.

I would like to express my sincere thanks to the authors for their dedicated efforts in the completion of this book. I acknowledge the efforts of the publisher for providing constant support. Lastly, I would like to thank my family for their support in all academic endeavors.

Editor

1

Stenotrophomonas maltophilia bloodstream infection in patients with hematologic malignancies: a retrospective study and in vitro activities of antimicrobial combinations

Sung-Yeon Cho[1,2], Dong-Gun Lee[1,2,3*], Su-Mi Choi[1,2], Chulmin Park[2], Hye-Sun Chun[2], Yeon-Joon Park[4], Jae-Ki Choi[1,2], Hyo-Jin Lee[1,2], Sun Hee Park[1,2], Jung-Hyun Choi[1,2] and Jin-Hong Yoo[1,2]

Abstract

Background: *Stenotrophomonas maltophilia* causes serious infections in immunocompromised hosts. Here, we analyzed the clinical characteristics of *S. maltophilia* bloodstream infection (BSI) in patients with hematologic malignancies and evaluated in vitro synergistic effects of antimicrobial combinations.

Methods: We retrospectively reviewed all consecutive episodes of *S. maltophilia* BSIs in adult hematologic patients from June 2009 to May 2014, with in vitro susceptibility and synergy tests using high-throughput bioluminescence assay performed for available clinical isolates.

Results: Among 11,004 admissions during 5-year period, 31 cases were identified as *S. maltophilia* BSIs. The incidence rate of *S. maltophilia* BSI was 0.134 cases/1,000 patient-days. Overall and attributable mortality of *S. maltophilia* BSI was 64.5% and 38.7%, respectively. Severe neutropenia (adjusted hazard ratio [HR] 5.24, p =0.013), shock at the onset of BSI (adjusted HR 6.05, p <0.001), and pneumonia (adjusted HR 3.15, p =0.017) were independent risk factors for mortality. In vitro susceptibilities to ceftazidime, levofloxacin, ticarcillin-clavulanic acid (TIM) and trimethoprim-sulfamethoxazole (SXT) were 11.1%, 44.0%, 40.7%, and 88.9%, respectively. MIC_{50}/MIC_{90} for moxifloxacin and tigecycline were 1/4 mg/L and 4/8 mg/L. The 50% and 90% fractional inhibitory concentrations (FIC^{50}/FIC^{90}) of clinical isolates against a combination of SXT and TIM were 0.500/0.750. For SXT plus levofloxacin or moxifloxacin, FIC^{50}/FIC^{90} were 0.625/1.000 and 0.625/0.625, respectively.

Conclusion: *S. maltophilia* BSIs show high mortality, which is related to severe neutropenia, shock, and *S. maltophilia* pneumonia. Based upon drug susceptibility testing, the primary treatment of choice for *S. maltophilia* BSIs should be SXT in hematologic patients, rather than quinolones, with combination therapies including SXT serving as a feasible treatment option.

Keywords: Bacteremia, Drug combinations, Hematologic diseases, Mortality, *Stenotrophomonas maltophilia*

* Correspondence: symonlee@catholic.ac.kr
[1]Division of Infectious Diseases, Department of Internal Medicine, College of Medicine, The Catholic University of Korea, St. Mary's Hospital, 222, Banpo-daero, Seocho-gu, Seoul, Republic of Korea
[2]Vaccine Bio Research Institute, College of Medicine, The Catholic University of Korea, St. Mary's Hospital, 222, Banpo-daero, Seocho-gu, Seoul, Republic of Korea
Full list of author information is available at the end of the article

Background

Stenotrophomonas maltophilia is an emerging nosocomial pathogen in immunocompromised patients [1-3]. Although *S. maltophilia* exhibits a limited pathogenicity in immunocompetent hosts, it has been shown to cause fatal infections in patients with hematologic malignancies. The overall mortality of *S. maltophilia* bloodstream infections (BSIs) ranges from 21 to 50%, with the mortality associated with neutropenia [4-6]. Failure to administration of early susceptible antibiotics for *S. maltophilia* BSI can have clinical implications, as *S. maltophilia* is naturally resistant to many antimicrobial agents including carbapenem.

Trimethoprim-sulfamethoxazole (SXT) is the antimicrobial agent of choice for the treatment of *S. maltophilia* infections [7-9]. Levofloxacin is also a viable treatment option in cases where drug susceptibilities are known [10]. However, SXT is known to cause adverse events related to bone marrow suppression, which might delay recovery from neutropenia in patients with hematologic malignancies. Fluoroquinolone is commonly used as prophylaxis during stem cell transplantation (SCT) or chemotherapy. As recent guidelines and experts have suggested that there are concerns about potential resistance to fluoroquinolone-based prophylaxis, this prophylactic strategy can lead to a limited effectiveness of levofloxacin in *S. maltophilia* infections [7,11-13]. Data regarding the clinical characteristics and the treatment outcomes of *S. maltophilia* BSIs in hematologic patients who received quinolone prophylaxis remain insufficient.

As *S. maltophilia* BSIs are associated with a high mortality rate, and increased resistance to monotherapy, many groups have suggested the need for combination antimicrobial therapies [7,14,15]. However, the effectiveness of combination therapy for *S. maltophilia* has not yet been established. Here, we investigated the clinical characteristics and outcomes related to *S. maltophilia* BSIs in patients with hematologic malignancies. Clinical isolates from these patients were then evaluated for in vitro susceptibilities with synergistic effects of several antimicrobial combinations to identify potential therapeutic regimens that may improve clinical outcomes.

Methods

Study design and hospital setting

We retrospectively reviewed medical records of all consecutive episodes of *S. maltophilia* BSIs in adult patients with hematologic malignancies from June 2009 to May 2014 at the Catholic Blood and Marrow Transplantation Center of Seoul St. Mary's Hospital.

Clinical data collection

Eligible patients included those with hematologic malignancies older than 19 years of age, with documented blood cultures positive for *S. maltophilia*. Clinical data obtained for each patient included age, sex, underlying diseases, severity and duration of neutropenia, length of hospital stay, simplified acute physiology score II (SAPS II) at the onset of BSI, the presence of central venous catheters, organisms isolated from blood and the antimicrobial susceptibility, administered antibiotics, and survival status at 30 days after the onset of BSI. The Institutional Review Board of Seoul St. Mary's Hospital approved the research protocol and waived the requirement for informed consent (KC13SISI0163).

S. maltophilia 16S rRNA gene analysis & pulsed-field gel electrophoresis

Available clinical isolates underwent phylogenetic group determination and pulsed-field gel electrophoresis (PFGE). Clinical isolates were screened using a specific 16S rRNA gene polymerase chain reaction (PCR) assay, and sequenced to confirm taxonomic identities. PCR was performed using primers SM1f (5′-GTTGGGAAAGAAATCCAGC-3′) and SM4 (5′-TTAAGCTTGCCACGAACAG-3′) as described previously [16,17]. Sequence analysis of PCR products was conducted with MEGA version 3.1 using the maximum likelihood method. AB695350 (*S. maltophilia* strain 4APB) was used as a control [18]. *S. maltohpilia* clinical isolates were typed using PFGE with *Xba* I digestion as described previously [19]. PFGE was performed with a CHEF-DR III apparatus (Bio-Rad Korea, Seoul, Korea) using 5 to 35 s of linear ramping at 6 V/cm for 20 h at 14°C. Digital images were analyzed with Fingerprinting II Informatix software (Bio-Rad, Hercules, CA, USA) using the Dice coefficient and UPGMA with a 1% tolerance and 0.5% optimizing setting value. The results were interpreted using the criteria of Tenover et al. [20].

Antimicrobial susceptibilities and fractional inhibitory concentrations using a luciferase-based assay

An in vitro susceptibility test was performed for seven antimicrobial agents (ceftazidime, ciprofloxacin, levofloxacin, moxifloxacin, ticarcillin-clavulanic acid [TIM], tigecycline, and SXT) using the broth microdilution method according to 2013 Clinical and Laboratory Standards Institute guidelines [21]. Quality controls were assessed by using *Escherichia coli* ATCC 25922 and *Pseudomonas aeruginosa* ATCC 27853. TIM was obtained from Biovim Korea Vine & Company (Seoul, Korea). Tigecycline was obtained from Pfizer Inc. (New York, NY, USA) via a compound transfer program. Other antibiotics were obtained from Sigma-Aldrich (St. Louis, MO, USA). All susceptibility testing was performed using cation-adjusted Mueller-Hinton broth (BD, Spark, MD, USA). To identify synergistic effects between SXT and other antibiotics (levofloxacin, moxifloxacin, or TIM), a checkerboard assay was performed using 96-well

U-bottom microplates. Due to a previous report that broth microdilution endpoint for SXT are difficult to read because of trailing and bacteriostatic activity of *S. maltophilia*, a luciferase-based bacterial cell viability assay was used [22,23]. In this study, a BacTiter-Glo™ microbial cell viability kit (Promega Corp., Madison, WI, USA) was used to determine the number of viable bacterial cells in culture, based on quantification of adenosine triphosphates (ATPs). Graded concentrations of antibiotics were mixed to assess synergy test. Each well was inoculated with 5×10^4 CFU of each isolate in cation-adjusted Mueller-Hinton broth. The plates were then incubated for 24 h at 35°C in ambient air. All assays were performed in triplicate. After 24 h of incubation, a volume of BacTiter-Glo™ reagent equal to the volume of the cell culture medium was added to 100 μL of microbial broth culture in an opaque-walled multi-well plate, according to the manufacturer's instructions. Relative luminescence units (RLU) were measured using a SpectraMax L luminescence microplate reader (Molecular Devices, Sunnyvale, CA, USA). The percentage of RLUs compared to the antibiotic-free controls (%RLU) was calculated, with minimal inhibitory concentrations (MICs) defined as <10%RLU, corresponding to an inhibitory concentration of 90% (IC_{90}). Total fractional inhibitory concentrations (FIC) were calculated according to the formula: ΣFIC = FIC of agent A + FIC of agent B, where FIC of agent A or B = MIC of agent A or B in combination/MIC of agent A or B alone. ΣFIC values ≤0.5 indicate synergy, ΣFIC values of >0.5 and ≤4 indicate indifference, and ΣFIC values >4 indicate antagonism [24].

Definitions

S. maltophilia BSIs were defined as at least one *S. maltophilia*-positive blood culture in association with clinical signs or symptoms indicative of infection [6]. Polymicrobial BSIs were defined as the presence of an organism other than *S. maltophilia* in the same blood culture. The source of bacteremia was determined clinically on the basis of the presence of an active site of infection as determined by chart review or isolation of the organism from other clinical specimens coincident with the episode of bacteremia [4]. Neutropenia was defined as an absolute neutrophil count (ANC) <500/mm^3, or <1000/mm^3 with predicted falls to <500/mm^3 within 2–3 days. Severe neutropenia was defined as an ANC <100/mm^3 [11,12]. The length of hospitalization before BSI was defined as the number of days from hospital admission to the development of BSI. Previous antibiotic use was defined as the administration of antibiotics for more than 24 hours within 30 days before the onset of the *S. maltophilia* BSI [25]. Mortality was considered attributable to the *S. maltophilia* BSI in any of the following cases: (1) blood cultures positive for *S. maltophilia* at the time of death; (2) death before the resolution of signs and symptoms related to *S. maltophilia* BSI; (3) death within 7 days of the onset of *S. maltophilia* BSI and with no other identifiable cause [26]. Crude mortality was defined as mortality that occurred within a month following a BSI episode [27].

Statistical analysis

Differences in continuous variables between the survivors and non-survivors were analyzed using the Mann–Whitney *U*-test. Fisher's exact test was used to compare categorical data. We used Cox's proportional hazard model with forward stepwise selection to identify independent risk factors for death. Kaplan-Meier survival curves were used to analyze mortality trends. *P* value <0.05 was considered statistically significant. All data were analyzed using SPSS ver. 18.0 (SPSS Korea, Seoul, Korea).

Results

Clinical characteristics of *S. maltophilia* bloodstream infection

Among 11,004 of admission episodes, a total of 31 patients were treated for *S. maltophilia* BSI. The incidence rate of *S. maltophilia* BSI was 0.134 cases per 1,000 patient-days during the entire study period. All patients had received broad-spectrum antibiotics such as fluoroquinolone as prophylaxis, anti-Pseudomonal cephalosporin plus aminoglycoside, or carbapenem as empirical or targeted therapy due to neutropenic fever within 30 days before the onset of the BSIs. The most commonly identified source of BSI was pneumonia (41.9%), followed by primary BSI (22.6%), catheter-related BSI (19.4%), skin and soft tissue infection (12.9%), and intra-abdominal infection (3.2%). In catheter-related *S. maltophilia* BSIs, Hickman catheters (n = 5) or chemoport (n = 1) were removed from the patient. In addition, about one-third of the patients (35.5%) had polymicrobial BSIs with nosocomial pathogens such as methicillin-resistant *Staphylococcus aureus*, methicillin-resistant coagulase-negative *Staphylococcus*, *P. aeruginosa* or vancomycin-resistant *Enterococcus*. Although antibiotic regimens were modified to appropriate targeted therapies in 26 of 31 patients (83.9%), the overall and attributable mortality of *S. maltophilia* BSIs was 64.5% and 38.7%, respectively.

Clinical characteristics of *S. maltophilia* BSIs were compared according to overall survival status (Table 1). There were no differences in age, sex, underlying hematologic diseases, SAPS II, presence of polymicrobial BSI, or shock between the two groups. Neutropenia at the onset of BSI (43% vs. 92%, p =0.038) was significantly associated with death, in terms of both neutropenia itself and the duration of neutropenia (median 3 d vs. 40 d, p =0.016). As a source of BSI, pneumonia (0% vs. 65.0%, p =0.001) was

Table 1 Clinical characteristics of patients with *Stenotrophomonas maltophilia* bloodstream infections according to the overall survival status

Variable	Survival (n = 11)	Death (n = 20)	*P* value
Age	49 (22–65)	48 (18–78)	0.416
Male	6 (54.5%)	12 (60.0%)	0.999
Underlying disease			
Myeloid malignancies	6 (54.5%)	15 (75.0%)	0.453
Lymphoid malignancies	3 (27.3%)	3 (15%)	
Others	2 (18.2%)	2 (10.0%)	
Treatment			
Chemotherapy	8 (72.7%)	9 (45.0%)	0.089
Stem cell transplantation	3 (27.3%)	4 (20.0%)	
Palliative care	0 (0.0%)	7 (35.0%)	
Hospital stay, days	26 (0–48)	23.5 (0–120)	0.119
Duration of neutropenia[a], days	3 (0–36)	40 (1–135)	0.016
Neutropenia at the onset of BSI (<500/mm^3)	7 (63.6%)	19 (95.0%)	0.042
Severe neutropenia at the onset of BSI (<100/mm^3)	6 (54.5%)	17 (85.0%)	0.095
SAPS II	30 (26–49)	38.5 (23–70)	0.030
Source of infection			
Pneumonia	0 (0.0%)	13 (65.0%)	0.001
Catheter	6 (54.5%)	0 (0.0%)	0.001
Primary	3 (27.3%)	4 (20.0%)	0.999
SSTI	1 (9.1%)	3 (15.0%)	0.999
Abdomen	1 (9.1%)	0 (0.0%)	0.355
Polymicrobial BSI	3 (27.3%)	7 (35.0%)	0.999
Shock	2 (18.2%)	12 (60.0%)	0.057

Data are presented as n (%) or median (range).
Abbreviations: BSI, bloodstream infection; SAPS II, Simplified Acute Physiology Score II; SSTI, skin and soft tissue infection.
[a]missing data (n = 11).

more common in non-survivors, while catheter-related infections (54.5% vs. 0%, p =0.001) were more common in survivors. In patients with combined *S. maltophilia* pneumonia, 64.5% (8 of 13 patients) received mechanical ventilation, while 11.1% (2 of 18 patients) with other sources of BSI received mechanical ventilation.

The results of Cox's proportional hazard analysis of factors associated with overall mortality are shown in Table 2. Severe neutropenia at the onset of BSI (adjusted hazard ratio [HR] 5.24, 95% Confidence Interval [CI] 1.411-19.493; p =0.013) and shock (adjusted HR 3.15, 95% CI 1.231-8.032; p =0.017) at the onset of BSI, and pneumonia as a source of BSI (adjusted HR 6.05, 95% CI 2.247-16.291; p <0.001) were associated with an increase in mortality. Kaplan-Meier survival curves stratified by source of BSI were shown in Figure 1.

Pulsed-field gel electrophoresis and phylogenetic group determinations

PFGE typing of available 27 *S. maltophilia* clinical isolates demonstrated 20 distinguishable banding patterns without evidence of the clonality. These 20 strains exhibited >99.9% 16S rRNA gene sequence similarity to the *S. maltophilia* type strain AB695350.

In vitro susceptibility testing and antimicrobial combinations

Broth microdilution testing of clinical isolates revealed 88.9% susceptibility to SXT and 44.4% to levofloxacin. MIC_{50} and MIC_{90} values for moxifloxacin and tigecycline showed 1 and 4 mg/L, and 4 and 8 mg/L, respectively (Table 3). Of the 27 clinical isolates, 15 were chosen for additional synergy testing based upon their MIC values. The selected isolates were representatives of the similar MIC patterns to each antmicrobial agent. Comparison of FIC indices is shown in Table 4. Synergy between SXT and TIM was found in 9 of 15 strains (60%) tested, of which the FIC for 50 and 90% of the isolates (FIC^{50}/FIC^{90}) was 0.500/0.750, with a range of 0.254 to 1.500. In the case of SXT plus levofloxacin or moxifloxacin, FICs ranged from 0.500 to 1.000, and 0.313 to 0.750, respectively. In all of the antimicrobial

Table 2 Factors associated with mortality in patients with *Stenotrophomonas maltophilia* bloodstream infections

	Univariate analysis		Multivariate analysis	
Variable	HR (95% CI)	*P* value	Adjusted HR (95% CI)	*P* value
Neutropenia at the onset of BSI (<500/mm^3)	5.87 (0.784-44.037)	0.085		
Severe neutropenia at the onset of BSI (<100/mm^3)	3.47 (1.008-11.954)	0.048	5.24 (1.411-19.493)	0.013
Duration of neutropenia >21 days	3.29 (0.978-11.072)	0.054		
Hospital stay >30 days	1.44 (0.586-3.531)	0.428		
SAPS II >40	3.14 (1.265-7.783)	0.003		
Source of infection				
Pneumonia	4.27 (1.687-10.816)	0.002	6.05 (2.247-16.291)	<0.001
Catheter	0.03 (0.000-1.817)	0.093		
Polymicrobial BSI	1.43 (0.570-3.603)	0.444		
Shock	3.09 (1.245-7.666)	0.015	3.15 (1.231-8.032)	0.017

Abbreviations: BSI, bloodstream infection; CI, confidence interval; HR, hazard ratio; SAPS II, Simplified Acute Physiology Score II; SSTI, skin and soft tissue infection

combinations tested, based on the SXT, the FIC^{90} values were under 1.000 without antagonism.

Discussion

In this study, we examined the clinical characteristics and treatment outcomes in hematologic patients with *S. maltophilia* BSIs, as well as the effectiveness of in vitro antimicrobial combinations against *S. maltophilia* clinical isolates. *S. maltophilia* BSIs still showed high mortality, with significant correlations seen for severe neutropenia, shock, and concomitant *S. maltophilia* pneumonia. Furthermore, we discovered that in vitro synergy tests revealed favorable FIC^{50} and FIC^{90} values against *S. maltophilia* clinical isolates obtained from hematologic patients.

Our data demonstrated that the previous exposure to broad spectrum antibiotics was preceded in all of the *S. maltophilia* BSIs. Polymicrobial infections were observed in over one third of patient. Poor prognosis in patients with combined *S. maltophilia* pneumonia might be related to higher rates of mechanical ventilation, when compared to patients with other sources of BSI. In contrast, patients with catheter related BSIs exhibited 100%

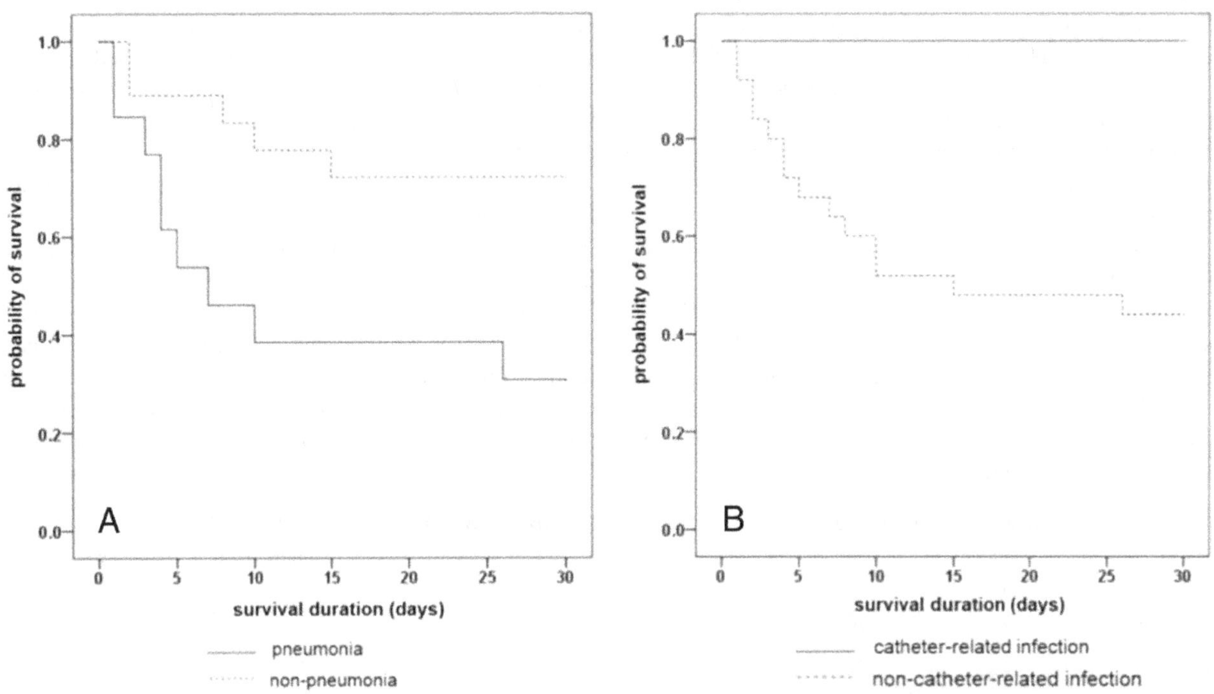

Figure 1 Kaplan-Meier curves for survival during episodes of *Stenotrophomonas maltophilia* bloodstream infections. Kaplan–Meier curves for survival stratified by pneumonia as a source of BSI **(A)**, and catheter-related BSI **(B)** (Log-rank test, *p* <0.001, and 0.003, respectively).

Table 3 In vitro activity of antimicrobial agents against *Stenotrophomonas maltophilia* isolates

Antimicrobial agent	Susceptible isolates (%)	MIC range (mg/L)	MIC_{50} (mg/L)	MIC_{90} (mg/L)
CAZ	11.11	4 ~ ≥128	32	≥128
CIP	0	4 ~ ≥ 64	32	64
LVX	44.44	0.5 ~ 16	4	8
MXF	-	0.125 ~ 8	1	4
SXT	88.89	0.25/4.75 ~ 4/76	0.25/4.75	4/76
TGC	-	1 ~ 8	4	8
TIM	40.74	0.5/2 ~ ≥512/2	32/2	128/2

Abbreviations: CAZ, ceftazidime; CIP, ciprofloxacin; LVX, levofloxacin; MXF, moxifloxacin; SXT, trimethoprim-sulfamethoxazole; TGC, tigecycline; TIM, ticarcillin-clavulanic acid

survival in this study. Favorable outcomes in these cases are likely to be associated with the removal of the catheter. A previous retrospective study found that catheter-related *S. maltophilia* BSIs were cured after removal of the catheter, even without appropriate antibiotics therapy, while a different study observed a significant correlation between mortality and retained catheters [25,28]. However, these studies were limited by the small number of patients examined, and failed to evaluate other salvage management such as antibiotics lock therapy in patients using long-term catheters.

In a worldwide study of the antimicrobial susceptibilities of 1,586 clinical *S. maltophilia* isolates, SXT and tigecycline showed susceptibilities of 96.0% and 95.5%, respectively, followed by levofloxacin with a susceptibility of 83.4% [29]. A recent study reported no difference in 30-day mortality between SXT and levofloxacin treatment for *S. maltophilia* BSIs [10]. However, in vitro susceptibility results from our study also revealed characteristics indicative of patient therapies. Decreased susceptibility to levofloxacin was associated with prophylactic fluoroquinolone use during the chemotherapy or SCT for hematologic malignancies. Taken together, levofloxacin may be an appropriate alternative treatment for *S. maltophilia* infections though careful patient selection based on the history of previous fluoroquinolone exposure will be necessary. For SXT, the susceptibility rate was 88.9% using the broth microdilution method, compared to 93.9% using an automated system (Vitek-2, bioMérieux, Hazelwood, MO, USA). This difference is likely the result of the inoculum effect and trailing. The $MIC_{50/90}$ for moxifloxacin and tigecycline also showed higher values, and thus needs further evaluation for the clinical use in this group of patients.

In vitro synergy was screened for SXT in combination with other antimicrobial agents. About 90% of *S. maltophilia* isolates were susceptible to SXT, though several reports of emerging resistance to SXT have been found [29]. We included TIM as a representative of the beta-lactam antibiotics, as a result of our in vitro susceptibility tests. Fluoroquinolone was selected for synergy test due to its widespread clinical use. Another reason to choose quinolone as a combination antibiotics was the possible activity against biofilm formation in device-related infection or in cystic fibrosis patients [30,31]. Further studies are needed to identify the biofilm activity of quinolone in hematologic patients. Our study demonstrated that SXT plus TIM exhibited the highest rates of synergy among the antibiotic combinations tested. Both SXT plus levofloxacin and SXT plus moxifloxacin revealed FIC below 1.000 against all of the clinical isolates tested. Combination therapy may, therefore, represent a viable option for *S. maltophilia* BSIs. Further studies with larger number of patients will be needed to assess whether the combination therapy has clinical impact in improving outcomes of *S. maltophilia* BSI in hematologic patients.

There are several strengths of this study. First, only BSI cases were included. In non-bacteremic *S. maltophilia* infection, it is difficult to distinguish the colonization from infection, which might influence the outcome analysis. Second, we calculated the incidence rate of *S. maltophilia* BSI in hematologic patients. Third, we used a high-throughput bioluminescence assay to assess the viability in living organisms, and a luciferase-based assay for determining the number of viable cells in culture [32]. The application of the luciferase-based assay for

Table 4 Comparison of fractional inhibitory concentration ranges for each antimicrobial combination

Antimicrobial combination	ΣFIC[a]			Synergy (%)	Indifference (%)	Antagonism (%)
	50%	90%	Range			
SXT plus TIM	0.500	0.750	0.254 to 1.500	60	40	0
SXT plus LVX	0.625	1.000	0.500 to 1.000	40	60	0
SXT plus MXF	0.625	0.625	0.313 to 0.750	40	60	0

Abbreviations: FIC, fractional inhibitory concentration; LVX, levofloxacin; MXF, moxifloxacin; SXT, trimethoprim-sulfamethoxazole; TIM, ticarcillin-clavulanic acid.
[a]50% and 90%, ΣFIC for 50% and 90% of the isolates, respectively.

the measurement of FIC indices was used to overcome difficulties in reading due to trailing endpoint by converting MIC to %RLU, equivalent to IC_{90} values.

Conclusion

In conclusion, *S. maltophilia* BSIs shows high mortality in patients with hematologic malignancies. Neutropenia, shock, and combined *S. maltophilia* pneumonia are associated with mortality. Based upon drug susceptibility testing, the primary treatment of choice in hematologic patients should be SXT, with combination therapies including SXT serving as a feasible treatment option for *S. maltophilia* BSIs.

Competing interests

This study was supported by a grant from the Korean Health Technology R&D Project, Ministry of Health & Welfare, Republic of Korea (Grant No. HI12C0756). The authors declare that they have no competing interests.

Authors' contributions

SYC conducted the hospital chart review and analysis of resulting data, interpreted data, drafted the initial study report and wrote the final report. DGL conceptualized the study and contributed to data interpretation. He revised and edited the manuscript. SMC and SHP participated in critical revision of manuscript. CP and HSC performed laboratory work and contributed to interpret the results. JKC, HJL, JHC and JHY contributed the data interpretation and editing the manuscript. YJ Park contributed the interpretation of microbiologic data. All authors read and approved the final manuscript.

Acknowledgements

Part of this study was presented at the 53rd Interscience Conference on Antimicrobial Agents and Chemotherapy in Denver, CO, USA, September 10–13, 2013 (Poster No. E612). We would like to thank Biovim Korea Vine & Company (Seoul, Korea) for providing the ticarcillin-clavulanic acid used in this study. We also like to thank Pfizer Inc. (New York, NY, USA) for providing tigecycline via a compound transfer program.

Author details

[1]Division of Infectious Diseases, Department of Internal Medicine, College of Medicine, The Catholic University of Korea, St. Mary's Hospital, 222, Banpo-daero, Seocho-gu, Seoul, Republic of Korea. [2]Vaccine Bio Research Institute, College of Medicine, The Catholic University of Korea, St. Mary's Hospital, 222, Banpo-daero, Seocho-gu, Seoul, Republic of Korea. [3]The Catholic Blood and Marrow Transplantation Center, College of Medicine, The Catholic University of Korea, St. Mary's Hospital, 222, Banpo-daero, Seocho-gu, Seoul, Republic of Korea. [4]Department of Laboratory Medicine, College of Medicine, The Catholic University of Korea, St. Mary's Hospital, 222, Banpo-daero, Seocho-gu, Seoul, Republic of Korea.

References

1. Safdar A, Rolston KV. *Stenotrophomonas maltophilia*: changing spectrum of a serious bacterial pathogen in patients with cancer. Clin Infect Dis. 2007;45:1602–9.
2. Looney WJ, Narita M, Mühlemann K. *Stenotrophomonas maltophilia*: an emerging opportunist human pathogen. Lancet Infect Dis. 2009;9:312–23.
3. Kwon JC, Kim SH, Choi JK, Cho SY, Park YJ, Park SH, et al. Epidemiology and clinical features of bloodstream infections in hematology wards: one year experience at the catholic blood and marrow transplantation center. Infect Chemother. 2013;45:51–61.
4. Araoka H, Baba M, Yoneyama A. Risk factors for mortality among patients with *Stenotrophomonas maltophilia* bacteremia in Tokyo, Japan, 1996–2009. Eur J Clin Microbiol Infect Dis. 2010;29:605–8.
5. Senol E, DesJardin J, Stark PC, Barefoot L, Snydman DR. Attributable mortality of *Stenotrophomonas maltophilia* bacteremia. Clin Infect Dis. 2002;34:1653–6.
6. Garazi M, Singer C, Tai J, Ginocchio CC. Bloodstream infections caused by *Stenotrophomonas maltophilia*: a seven-year review. J Hosp Infect. 2012;81:114–8.
7. Averbuch D, Cordonnier C, Livermore DM, Mikulska M, Orasch C, Viscoli C, et al. Targeted therapy against multi-resistant bacteria in leukemic and hematopoietic stem cell transplant recipients: guidelines of the 4th European Conference on Infections in Leukemia (ECIL-4, 2011). Haematologica. 2013;98:1836–47.
8. Falagas ME, Valkimadi PE, Huang YT, Matthaiou DK, Hsueh PR. Therapeutic options for *Stenotrophomonas maltophilia* infections beyond co-trimoxazole: a systematic review. J Antimicrob Chemother. 2008;62:889–94.
9. Lee CS, Doi Y. Therapy of infections due to carbapenem-resistant gram-negatice pathogens. Infect Chemother. 2014;46:149–64.
10. Cho SY, Kang CI, Kim J, Ha YE, Chung DR, Lee NY, et al. Can levofloxacin be a useful alternative to trimethoprim-sulfamethoxazole for treating *Stenotrophomonas maltophilia* bacteremia? Antimicrob Agents Chemother. 2014;58:581–3.
11. Freifeld AG, Bow EJ, Sepkowitz KA, Boeckh MJ, Ito JI, Mullen CA, et al. Clinical practice guideline for the use of antimicrobial agents in neutropenic patients with cancer: 2010 update by the Infectious Diseases Society of America. Clin Infect Dis. 2011;52:e56–93.
12. Lee DG, Kim SH, Kim SY, Kim CJ, Park WB, Song YG, et al. Evidence-based guidelines for empirical therapy of neutropenic fever in Korea. Korean J Intern Med. 2011;26:220–52.
13. Ito JI, Tegtmeier BR, O'Donnell MR. Antibacterial prophylaxis in patients with cancer and neutropenia. N Engl J Med. 2006;354:90–4.
14. Brooke JS. *Stenotrophomonas maltophilia*: an emerging global opportunistic pathogen. Clin Microbiol Rev. 2012;25:2–41.
15. Church D, Lloyd T, Peirano G, Pitout J. Antimicrobial susceptibility and combination testing of invasive *Stenotrophomonas maltophilia* isolates. Scand J Infect Dis. 2013;45:265–70.
16. Whitby PW, Carter KB, Burns JL, Royall JA, LiPuma JJ, Stull TL. Identification and detection of *Stenotrophomonas maltophilia* by rRNA-directed PCR. J Clin Microbiol. 2000;38:4305–9.
17. Adamek M, Overhage J, Bathe S, Winter J, Fischer R, Schwartz T. Genotyping of environmental and clinical *Stenotrophomonas maltophilia* isolates and their pathogenic potential. PLoS One. 2011;6:e27615.
18. Kumar S, Tamura K, Nei M. Mega3: Integrated software for molecular evolutionary genetics analysis and sequence alignment. Brief Bioinform. 2004;5:150–63.
19. Denton M, Todd NJ, Kerr KG, Hawkey PM, Littlewood JM. Molecular epidemiology of *Stenotrophomonas maltophilia* isolated from clinical specimens from patients with cystic fibrosis and associated environmental samples. J Clin Microbiol. 1998;36:1953–8.
20. Tenover FC, Arbeit RD, Goering RV, Mickelsen PA, Murray BE, Persing DH, et al. Interpreting chromosomal DNA restriction patterns produced by pulsed-field gel electrophoresis: criteria for bacterial strain typing. J Clin Microbiol. 1995;33:2233–9.
21. Clinical and Laboratory Standards Institute. Performance standards for antimicrobial susceptibility testing; twenty-second informational supplement. CLSI document M100-S23. Wayne, PA, USA: Clinical and Laboratory Standards Institute; 2013.
22. Poulos CD, Matsumura SO, Willey BM, Low DE, McGeer A. In vitro activities of antimicrobial combinations against *Stenotrophomonas (Xanthomonas) maltophilia*. Antimicrob Agents Chemother. 1995;39:2220–3.
23. Krueger TS, Clark EA, Nix DE. In vitro susceptibility of *Stenotrophomonas maltophilia* to various antimicrobial combinations. Diagn Microbiol Infect Dis. 2001;41:71–8.
24. Moody JA. Synergism testing: Broth microdilution checkerboard and broth macrodilution methods. In: Garcia LS, Isenberg HD, editors. Clinical microbiology procedures handbook. Washington, DC: ASM Press; 2007. p. 1–23.
25. Lai CH, Wong WW, Chin C, Huang CK, Lin HH, Chen WF, et al. Central venous catheter-related *Stenotrophomonas maltophilia* bacteraemia and associated relapsing bacteraemia in haematology and oncology patients. Clin Microbiol Infect. 2006;12:986–91.
26. Kim SH, Yoon YK, Kim MJ, Shon JW. Risk factors for and clinical implications of mixed candida/bacterial bloodstream infections. Clin Microbiol Infect. 2013;19:62–8.

27. Ortega M, Rovira M, Almela M, Marco F, de la Bellacasa JP, Martínez JA, et al. Bacterial and fungal bloodstream isolates from 796 hematopoietic stem cell transplant recipients between 1991 and 2000. Ann Hematol. 2005;84:40–6.
28. Friedman ND, Korman TM, Fairley CK, Franklin JC, Spelman DW. Bacteraemia due to *Stenotrophomonas maltophilia*: an analysis of 45 episodes. J Infect. 2002;45:47–53.
29. Farrell DJ, Sader HS, Jones RN. Antimicrobial susceptibilities of a worldwide collection of *Stenotrophomonas maltophilia* isolates tested against tigecycline and agents commonly used for *S. maltophilia* infections. Antimicrob Agents Chemother. 2010;54:2735–7.
30. Di Bonaventura G, Spedicato I, D'Antonio D, Robuffo I, Piccolomini R. Biofilm formation by *Stenotrophomonas maltophilia*: modulation by quinolones, trimethoprim-sulfamethoxazole, and ceftazidime. Antimicrob Agents Chemother. 2004;48:151–60.
31. Wu K, Yau YC, Matukas L, Waters V. Biofilm compared to conventional antimicrobial susceptibility of *Stenotrophomonas maltophilia* isolates from cystic fibrosis patients. Antimicrob Agents Chemother. 2013;57:1546–8.
32. Fan F, Wood KV. Bioluminescent assays for high-throughput screening. Assay Drug Dev Technol. 2007;5:127–36.

2

The characteristics of patients with mycobacterium tuberculosis blood stream infections in Beijing, China

Xiaoqing Liu[1,2*†], Sainan Bian[1†], Yueqiu Zhang[1], Lifan Zhang[1,2], Qiwen Yang[3], Peng Wang[3], Yingchun Xu[3], Xiaochun Shi[1], Yao Zhang[2] and Roy F. Chemaly[4]

Abstract

Background: Published information regarding the clinical characteristics, laboratory findings, and outcomes of patients with Mycobacterium tuberculosis (MTB) blood stream infection (BSI) is limited. We aimed in this study to evaluate the clinical characteristics, laboratory evaluation, and outcomes of patients with MTB BSI.

Methods: All patients diagnosed with MTB BSI at Peking Union Medical College Hospital between January 2008 and May 2014 were identified by examining the electronic database listing results of all blood cultures. Data on demographics, clinical characteristics, laboratory manifestations, management, and outcomes were abstracted from medical records.

Results: Six thousand nine hundred seventy-four patients had mycobacterial blood cultures during the study period. Of 48 patients (0.7%) with MTB BSI, 26 patients (54%) were considered to be immunocompromised (refers to a person who has a significantly impaired immune system). This was due to human immunodeficiency virus (HIV) infection ($n = 2$ of 48 tested), receiving steroids ($n = 17$, including 16 with rheumatic diseases and one with myasthenia gravis), malignancy ($n = 3$), diabetes mellitus ($n = 3$), and renal transplantation ($n = 1$). The main clinical manifestations were fever (100%, with a median of 40 °C), weight loss (48%) and cough with sputum production (46%). Most patients had one or more organs involved (81%). The median time from onset of fever to diagnosis was 8 weeks (IQR 5 ~ 14). Six patients died within 1 week after diagnosis. Of the 17 patients completing treatment, 14 patients (82%) recovered without major complications and they had a shorter time interval between onsets of symptoms to treatment compared to those died of TB.

Conclusions: In this group of patients with MTB BSI, fever and multiple organs involvement were common, the outcome was poor and timely diagnosis and treatment might favor outcome.

Keywords: Mycobacterium tuberculosis, Bacteremia, Blood stream infection

* Correspondence: liuxq@pumch.cn; liuxqpumch@126.com
†Equal contributors
[1]Department of Infectious Diseases, Peking Union Medical College Hospital, Peking Union Medical College, Chinese Academy of Medical Sciences, No.1 Shuaifuyuan, Dongcheng District, Beijing 100730, China
[2]Clinical Epidemiology Unit, International Epidemiology Network, Peking Union Medical College, No.1 Shuaifuyuan, Dongcheng District, Beijing 100730, China
Full list of author information is available at the end of the article

Background

Developing countries like China face a challenging combination of an expanding epidemic of human immunodeficiency virus (HIV) infection, cancer, and persistently high prevalence of tuberculosis (TB) [1]. These combinations may place a growing proportion of its population at risk for severe forms of Mycobacterium tuberculosis (MTB) infections, including dissemination and MTB blood stream infection (BSI) (refers to those with positive MTB blood cultures) with subsequent poor outcomes.

Hematogenous, disseminated, or miliary tuberculosis has been used exchangeably in the literature describing in most instances a lymphohematogenous spread of MTB. Miliary tuberculosis accounts for about 1–2% of all cases and about 8% of all forms of extrapulmonary TB in immunocompetent individuals [1].

Reports on MTB BSI are scarce with most published data emerging from the HIV infected patients [2, 3]. Few studies report MTB BSI among a general population [4, 5]. With the use of liquid culture methods in recent years, it became possible to isolate MTB from blood culture bottles. In a prospective cohort of 368 HIV-infected patients hospitalized with severe sepsis [3], 86 patients (23%) had MTB BSI, and the 30-day mortality of patients with or without MTB BSI was 53.2 and 30.7%, respectively. In a study enrolling 238 consecutive febrile adult patients, 173 (73%) were HIV-positive and 67 (28%) had BSI, showing that MTB ranked second at 19% as etiology of bloodstream infections [4]. In another study of 57 patients (55 were HIV positive) with MTB BSI, 42% died within 1 month of hospitalization [5].

Because of the high mortality associated with MTB BSI, we aimed in this study to better understand the clinical and laboratory manifestations and the impact of this infection among patients who were admitted to our institution, a major national referral hospital in Beijing, China.

Methods

Study population

All patients diagnosed with MTB BSI at Peking Union Medical College Hospital between January 2008 and May 2014 were identified by examining the electronic database listing results of all blood cultures. Data on demographics, clinical characteristics, underlying diseases, laboratory manifestations, management, and outcomes were abstracted from medical records.

Criteria for determining who gets mycobacterial blood culture was fever last for more than 3 weeks, temperature above 38.3 °C, and still not being diagnosed after complete history consultation, physical examination, and routine laboratory examinations for 1 week. If the patient had fever in hospital and was suspected of bacteremia, and if the patient was immunocompromised, the criteria might be a little wider which was determined by the treating clinicians.

Immunocompromised refers to a person who has a significantly impaired immune system according to the National Institute for Health and Care Excellence (NICE) guideline. For instance, this may be because of prolonged corticosteroid use, tumor necrosis factor-alpha antagonists, antirejection therapy, immunosuppression-causing medication or comorbid states that affect the immune system, for example, HIV, chronic renal disease, many haematological and solid cancers, and diabetes [6].

Laboratory diagnosis

The laboratory diagnosis of MTB BSI was based on the following: Peripheral blood cultures were collected and inoculated into a liquid culture method (Bact Alert MP, BioMerieux) between 2008 and 2010 and BD MGIT960 (BD) after 2010. Recovery of mycobacteria confirmed by acid-fast stain (Ziehl-Neelsen stain and Auramine-rhodamine stain) according to "Manual of Clinical Microbiology" [7]. And then Tuberculosis Antigen Colloidal Gold Diagnostic Kit (Kabelykit. Protocol is available at http://www.hgb.com.cn/cp1/show/id/44.html) and gene chip [8] are used to identify the type of Mycobacterium species according to the manufacturer's instructions.

The direct smear on clinical specimens is done by Auramine-rhodamine stain and Ziehl-Neelsen stain at the same time following the standard in "Manual of Clinical Microbiology" [7].

Four milliliters of peripheral blood were collected from each patient and was performed within six hours after collection by laboratory personnel blinded to patients' clinical data. In the T-SPOT.TB test, AIM-V (GIBCOT-MAIM V Medium liquid, Invitrogen, US) was used as negative control, phytohemagglutinin (PHA) as positive control, and early-secreted antigenic target 6-kDa protein (ESAT-6) and culture filtrate protein 10 (CFP-10) as specific antigens, respectively. Peripheral blood mononuclear cells (PBMCs) were separated by Ficoil-Hypaque gradient centrifugation and obtained (2.5×10^5per well) on a plate (Oxford Immunotec, Abingdon, UK) that was pre-coated with an antibody against interferon-γ. After incubation for 16 to 18 h at 37 °C in 5% carbon dioxide, wells were washed and developed with a conjugate used and an enzyme substrate against the antibody. The number of spot-forming cells (SFCs) representing an antigen-specific T cell that secreted interferon-γ were counted with an automated ELISPOT reader (AID-ispot, Strassberg, Germany). A positive result of T-SPOT.TB on PBMCs was defined as six or more SFCs in the target well and had twice the number of spots than the negative control well. In addition, the background number of spots in the negative control well should be less than ten SFCs [9].

Statistical analysis

We used Kolmogorov-Smirnov test to check if the variables followed normal distribution. Measurement data of normal distribution was expressed by mean ± standard deviation (SD), and measurement data of non-normal distribution was expressed by median and interquartile range (IQR). Enumeration data was expressed by percentage. The Pearson's Chi-square test was used to compare proportions between groups. Results with a 2-sided P value <0.05 were considered statistically significant. Statistical analysis was performed by SPSS 16.0 (SPSS Inc, Chicago, IL, USA).

Results

We searched the electronic database in the clinical microbiology laboratory at Peking Union Medical College Hospital, and found 56 reports of positive Mycobacterium species from peripheral blood samples between January 2008 and May 2014. Then we excluded eight cases of non-Mycobacterium tuberculosis (NTM), 48 patients were MTB BSI.

General conditions

Patients'characteristics are summarized in Table 1. Among the 48 patients, 25 patients (52%) were males and the median age was 44 years (IQR 26 ~ 57). In addition to the MTB BSI, 26 patients (54%) had pulmonary tuberculosis, among these patients 13 (50%) had positive sputum smear for AFB, six (23%) had positive sputum culture for MTB (four patients had smear and culture positive), and 11 (42%) had radiological findings suggestive of pulmonary tuberculosis with negative smear and cultures from sputum. Other organ(s) involvement included the central nervous system (CNS) in seven (14%) patients, serositis including pleuritis, peritonitis, and pericarditis in five (10%), liver in five (10%), osteo-articular joints in four (8%), skin and soft tissue in three (6%), lymphatic system in three (6%), intestinal tract in two (4%), and spleen in two (4%). Most of the patients (26, 54%) were immunocompromised due to their underlying conditions and/or being on immunosuppressive therapy and only two patients (4%) were positive for HIV with a CD4 count of 25/mm^3 and 60/mm^3 each (Table 1).

Clinical manifestations

The most common clinical manifestation was fever with a median time from fever to diagnosis of MTB BSI of 8 weeks (IQR 5 ~ 14). The median peak temperature was 40 °C, (IQR 39.5 ~ 40.1). Other clinical manifestations included cough with sputum production in 22 patients (46%), reported weight loss in 23 patients (48%), and night sweats in seven patients (15%). In addition, 12 patients (25%) had enlarged lymphatic nodes, 17 (35%) had hepatomegaly, and 27 (56%) had splenomegaly.

Table 1 Demographics and underlying conditions of the 48 patients with MTB BSI

Characteristic	Value (n = 48)
Gender-n.(%)	
Male	25 (52)
Female	23 (48)
Age—Year (Median, IQR)	44 (26 ~ 57)
Subgroup-year,n.(%)	
18–65	41 (85)
66–79	6 (13)
80–99	1 (2)
Immune suppression-n.(%)	26 (54)
HIV-infection	2
On Steroids	17
SLE	7
SS	2
RA	2
DM	2
MCTD	1
Undifferentiated CTD	2
Myasthenia gravis	1
Diabetes mellitus	3
Malignant tumor	3
Renal transplantation	1

HIV Human immunodeficiency virus, *SLE* Systemic lupus erythematosus, *SS* Sjogren Syndrome, *RA* Rheumatoid arthritis, *DM* Dermatomyositis, *MCTD* Mixed connective tissue diseases, *CTD* Connective tissue diseases

Laboratory examinations

The laboratory findings are depicted in Table 2. Among the 41 patients who had a T-SPOT.TB assay done, 28 (68%) were positive with a median spots counts of 556 SFC/10^{6}PBMC, (IQR 112 ~ 1704) (Table 3). The sensitivity of the T-SPOT.TB assay in patients with CD4 count > 200/mm^3 was 100% compared to 57% in patients with CD4 counts < 200/mm^3 (P = 0.018). When we looked at the absolute lymphocytes count (ALC), the sensitivity of the T-SPOT.TB assay was much higher in patients with ALC > 500/mm^3 when compared to patients with ALC < 500/mm^3 (85% vs. 52%, respectively, P = 0.025) (Table 4).

Treatment and outcome

Data on therapy was available for 39 patients as the remainder nine patients were transferred to other facilities before any therapy was initiated. All the patients received at least three out of the four drugs of the standard regimen (Isoniazid 0.3 g/d, Rifampin 0.45 g/d, Pyrazinamide 0.75 g/d, and Ethambutol

Table 2 Laboratory findings on 48 patients with MTB BSI

Characteristic	Value ($n = 48$) (n.%)
Leukocytopenia	24 (50)
Anemia	38 (79)
Low platelet count	28 (58)
High leukocyte count	17 (35)
Leukocytes, $\times 10^9$/L [median (IQR)]	4.58, (1.94 ~ 13.67)
Hemoglobin, g/L[mean ± SD]	88 ± 32
Platelets, $\times 10^9$/L[median (IQR)]	74, (25 ~ 213)
Lymphocytes, $\times 10^9$/L [median (IQR)]	0.35, (0.20 ~ 0.74)
Increased ESR	34/45(76)
Increased hsCRP	34/36 (94)
ESR, mm/h [median (IQR)]	69, (IQR 27 ~ 103)
hsCRP, mg/L [median (IQR)]	121.5, (IQR 56.4 ~ 176.5)
CD4+ count, /mm^3, [median (IQR)] ($n = 27$)	115, (IQR 77-187)
CD8+ count, /mm^3, [median (IQR)] ($n = 27$)	168, (IQR 78-246)
Time from MTB culture to a positive result, d[median (IQR)]	27, (IQR 21 ~ 33)

ESR Erythrocyte sedimentation rate, *hsCRP* Hypersensitive C reactive protein
Leukocytopenia: <4 × 10^9/L; Anemia: Male < 120 g/L and female < 110 g/L; Low platelet count: <100 × 10^9/L; High leukocyte count: >10 × 10^9/L; Increased ESR: Male > 15 mm/h and female > 20 mm/h; Increased hsCRP: >3 mg/L

0.75 g/d) and in combination with a quinolone in 27 patients (Moxifloxacin 0.4 g/d ($n = 10$), and Levofloxacin 0.5 g/d ($n = 17$)).

In total 25 patients were lost to follow-up (Nine patients were transferred to other facilities before any therapy was initiated and 16 were lost to follow-up prior to completing treatment). 14 (36%) recovered well without major complications, and one patient with tuberculous meningoencephalitis recovered but with subsequent seizures with a median duration of 12 months of treatment (range 6–30 months). The remaining eight patients (20.5%) died at a median of 2 days (range: 2 to 150 days) from diagnosis (seven died of TB, and one of gastric perforation).

Among the 26 immnocompromised patients, six patients (23%) died of TB, while among 22 immunocompetent patients, one patient (5%) died of TB ($P = 0.07$), they all had poor outcomes.

Table 3 Results of the T-SPOT.TB assay on 41 patients

T-SPOT.TB (SFC/10^{6}PBMC)	MTB
Positive results	28/41 (68%)
Total	556 (IQR 112 ~ 1704)
ESAT-6	116 (IQR 34 ~ 242)
CFP-10	100 (IQR 40 ~ 722)
Negative results	13/41 (32%)

ESAT-6: 6 kDa, specific antigens encoded in the RD1 region; CFP-10: 10 kDa, specific antigens encoded in the RD1 region

Table 4 T-SPOT.TB results stratified by CD4 counts and absolute lymphocytes count

	T-SPOT.TB positive (n, %)	T-SPOT.TB negative (n, %)
CD4 < 100/mm^3($n = 10$)	4 (40)	6 (60)
CD4 100-200/mm^3($n = 11$)	8 (73)	3 (27)
CD4 > 200/mm^3($n = 6$)	6 (100)	0 (0)
P value	0.018	
ALC < 500/mm^3($n = 21$)	11 (52)	10 (48)
ALC > 500/mm^3($n = 20$)	17 (85)	3 (15)
P value	0.025	

ALC Absolute lymphocyte count

With a comparison of the 15 patients recovered with those eight patients died, median time from onset of symptoms to receiving treatment was 30 days (IQR 17-60) and 55 days (IQR 37-96), respectively ($P = 0.023$).

Discussion

We report a large series of patients with MTB BSI. Our data showed that patients with MTB BSI usually have multiple organs involvement with varied serious complications. In addition, the time to diagnosis could be long and the outcome was generally poor. On the other hand, we found that sensitivity of T-SPOT.TB assay was high mainly in patients with CD4 count above 200/mm^3.

Tuberculosis remains one of the most challenging communicable diseases in the world. In 2013, an estimated 9.0 million individuals developed TB and 1.5 million died. China alone accounted for 11% of the total cases worldwide [10]. Although pulmonary tuberculosis is the form given the most attention for its public health relevance, other forms of TB, including MTB BSI are also important, particularly when more people are becoming immunocompromised due to cancers, or other chronic diseases. Interestingly, in one study conducted in Malawi showed that MTB ranked second at 19% as etiology of bloodstream infections [4]. MTB BSI was more likely to occur in HIV-positive than in HIV-negative patients (13/173 vs. 0/65; $P < 0.05$) [4]. MTB BSI in patients with HIV infection or other immunosuppressive diseases resulted in death in most patients [2, 3, 11]. Whether early and prompt diagnosis and treatment would have impact on the overall prognosis should be determined in future studies.

Hematogenous, disseminated, or miliary tuberculosis has been used exchangeably in the literature describing in most instances a lymphohematogenous spread of MTB. Miliary tuberculosis accounts for about 1–2% of all cases and about 8% of all forms of extrapulmonary TB in immunocompetent individuals. These forms of infections are more frequently encountered in immunocompromised patients [1, 12, 13] as seen in our study where the majority of patients (54%) had an underlying immunosuppression. We hypothesize that initial exposure occurs through the respiratory route that may or may not result in pulmonary TB at later stages dependent most probably on the inoculum effect and the virulence of MTB in addition to the immune status of the host. Dissemination could occur through the blood and seed many organs, oxygen rich organs in particular, such as the brain, bones, lungs, and spine.

Not surprisingly, the most common organ involved in patients with MTB BSI was the lungs (54%). The radiological manifestations were atypical in early stages and included, either normal findings, or ground-glass opacities, and progressed to miliary nodular patterns at later stages. A retrospective study of 2016 cases with culture-proven TB [14] showed that miliary and pneumonic radiographic patterns were risk factors for fatal outcomes. In addition, previous study [1] supported that there is an association between the occurrence of miliary MTB and a massive lymphohaematogenous dissemination of the pathogen from a pulmonary or extrapulmonary source resulting in embolization of the vascular beds of various organs. Subsequently, cerebral, hepatic or splenic involvement with MTB was most probably preceded by the hematogenous spread of this pathogen. Whether early diagnosis of MTB BSI in high endemic countries, like China, may prevent seeding of MTB in different organs with prompt therapy should be determined in future studies.

We also evaluated the performance of the T-SPOT.TB assay among patients with MTB BSI. The overall sensitivity was 68%, lower than what is reported in the literature [6, 15]. Although this assay performed well in patients with underlying immunosuppressive conditions, the combination of disseminated TB and the immunosuppressive status of some of our patients with low CD4 counts, may have contributed to this low sensitivity for the diagnosis of active TB. Similar results was found in another study that the sensitivity of the TB ELISPOT assay decreased from 97 to 81% when patients were stratified according to absolute lymphocytes count (ALC) above 1000/ml or less than 500/ml, respectively ($P = 0.007$) [16].

As the only confirmatory test available, the turnaround time for culture is long, which makes the diagnosis challenging and delayed. Median culture time of MTB was 26.6 days in our study which was similar to other report [17]. On another hand, it is recommended more than one blood specimen to be collected to increase the diagnostic yield for cultures [17]. We may apply the new method of GeneXpert MTB/RIF in the future which can detect MTB in 2 h with a good sensitivity and specificity [18]. It allows rapid laboratory confirmation of MTB and that empiric therapy is warranted pending laboratory confirmation, especially when disseminated TB is likely.

There are some limitations in our study. This is a retrospective study from a single referral tertiary care hospital caring most for complicated and serious diseases in China. And some patients were lost to follow-up. So our findings may not be generalizable to other patients in other centers.

Conclusions

In summary, MTB BSI is a serious complication even among non-immunosuppressed patients. Multiple organs involvement is common and is associated with poor outcomes. Rapid diagnosis and prompt therapy may favorably impact outcomes.

Abbreviations

AFB: Acid-fast bacilli; ALC: Absolute lymphocytes count; BSI: Blood stream infection; CFP-10: Culture filtrate protein 10; CNS: Central nervous system; ESAT-6: Early secretory antigenic target 6; HIV: Human immunodeficiency virus; MTB: Mycobacterium tuberculosis; SFCs: Spot-forming cells

Acknowledgments

We thank all the health care workers who took care of these patients.

Funding

This work was supported by grants from the National Major Science and Technology Research Projects for the Control and Prevention of Major Infectious Diseases in China, 2014ZX10003003, and Health Research &Special Projects Grant, 201402001. The funding bodies had no role in the design of the study and collection, analysis, and interpretation of data and in writing the manuscript.

Authors' contributions

Conceived and designed the study: XL. Performed the experiments: LZ YZ QY PW YX. Analyzed the data: SB LZ. Wrote the paper: SB YZ XL. Managed clinical information and diagnosis: SB XL XS. Discussed, wrote and revised the manuscript: RC. All authors read and approved the final manuscript.

Competing interests

The authors declare that they have no competing interests except: RFC has received grants and honorarium from Oxford Immunotec, USA.

Consent for publication

Not applicable.

Author details

[1]Department of Infectious Diseases, Peking Union Medical College Hospital, Peking Union Medical College, Chinese Academy of Medical Sciences, No.1 Shuaifuyuan, Dongcheng District, Beijing 100730, China. [2]Clinical Epidemiology Unit, International Epidemiology Network, Peking Union Medical College, No.1 Shuaifuyuan, Dongcheng District, Beijing 100730, China. [3]Laboratory Department, Peking Union Medical College Hospital, Peking Union Medical College, Chinese Academy of Medical Sciences, No.1 Shuaifuyuan, Dongcheng District, Beijing 100730, China. [4]Department of Infectious Diseases, Infection Control, and Employee Health, Unit 1460, The University of Texas MD Anderson Cancer Center, 1515 Holcombe Blvd, Houston, TX 77030, USA.

References

1. Sharma SK, Mohan A, Sharma A, Mitra DK. Miliary tuberculosis: new insights into an old disease. Lancet Infect Dis. 2005;5:415–30.
2. Daikos GL, Uttamchandani RB, Tuda C, et al. Disseminated Miliary Tuberculosis of the Skin in Patients with AIDS: Report of Four Cases. Clin Infect Dis. 1998;27:205–8.
3. Jacob ST, Pavlinac PB, Nakiyingi L, et al. Mycobacterium tuberculosis bacteremia in a cohort of hiv-infected patients hospitalized with severe sepsis in uganda–high frequency, low clinical suspicion [corrected] and derivation of a clinical prediction score. PLoS One. 2013;8:e70305.
4. Bell M, Archibald LK, Nwanyanwu O, et al. Seasonal variation in the etiology of bloodstream infections in a febrile inpatient population in a developing country. Int J Infect Dis. 2001;5:63–9.
5. Lewis DK, Peters RP, Schijffelen MJ, et al. Clinical indicators of mycobacteraemia in adults admitted to hospital in Blantyre, Malawi. Int J Tuberc Lung Dis. 2002;6:1067–74.
6. Tuberculosis. NICE guideline [NG33]. Last updated: May 2016. p. 81. https://www.nice.org.uk/guidance/ng33. Accessed 13 Jan 2016.
7. James H. J, Michael A. P. Manual of Clinical Microbiology, 11th edition. ASM Press, Washington, DC: 2015. p. 321-322, 548-554. ISBN 978-1-55581-738-1 e-book set.
8. Guo Y, Zhou Y, Wang C, et al. Rapid, accurate determination of multidrug resistance in M. tuberculosis isolates and sputum using a biochip system. Int J Tuberc Lung Dis. 2009;13:914–20.
9. Zhang L, Zhang Y, Liu X, et al. Utility of T-cell interferon-γ release assays for diagnosing tuberculous serositis: a prospective study in Beijing, China. PLoS One. 2014;9:e85030.
10. WHO. Global tuberculosis report, 2014. Geneva: World Health Organization; 2014. http://www.who.int/tb/publications/global_report/en/. Accessed 12 Nov 2014.
11. Alba MA, Mena-Madrazo JA, Flores-Suárez LF. Giant cell arteritis and disseminated tuberculosis: presentation of two cases. Scand J Rheumatol. 2013;42:509–12.
12. CDC. Reported tuberculosis in the United States, 2002. Tuberculosis cases by form of disease: States, 2002. http://www.cdc.gov/nchstp/tb/surv/surv2002/PDF/T23.pdf. Accessed 20 May 2004.
13. Burman WJ, Jones BE. Clinical and radiographic features of HIV-related tuberculosis. Semin Respir Infect. 2003;18:263–71.
14. Feng J, Sun X, Zhang H. Clinical analysis of 92 hematogenous disseminated tuberculosis in adults. J Clin Intern Med. 2009;26:701–3.
15. Rangaka MX, Wilkinson KA, Glynn JR, et al. Predictive value of interferon-γ release assays for incident active tuberculosis: a systematic review and meta-analysis. Lancet Infect Dis. 2012;12:45–55.
16. Komiya K, Ariga H, Nagai H, et al. Impact of peripheral lymphocyte count on the sensitivity of 2 IFN-gamma release assays, QFT-G and ELISPOT, in patients with pulmonary tuberculosis. Intern Med. 2010;49:1849–55.
17. Oplustil CP, Leite OH, Oliveira MS, et al. Detection of mycobacteria in the bloodstream of patients with acquired immunodeficiency syndrome in a university hospital in Brazil. Braz J Infect Dis. 2001;5:252–9.
18. Helb D, Jones M, Story E, et al. Rapid detection of Mycobacterium tuberculosis and rifampin resistance by use of on-demand, near-patient technology. J Clin Microbiol. 2010;48:229–37.

3

Enrichment of bacterial DNA for the diagnosis of blood stream infections

Ngo Tat Trung[1,7], Tran Thi Thu Hien[1], Tran Thi Thanh Huyen[1], Dao Thanh Quyen[1], Trinh Van Son[2,7], Phan Quoc Hoan[1], Nguyen Thi Kim Phuong[3], Tran Thi Lien[4], Mai Thanh Binh[5,7], Hoang Van Tong[6,7], Christian G. Meyer[6,7], Thirumalaisamy P. Velavan[6,7*] and Le Huu Song[1,2,7*]

Abstract

Background: Blood cultures are commonly employed to identify bacterial pathogens causing sepsis. PCR assays to diagnose septicemia require extraction of bacterial DNA from blood samples and thus, delay the initiation of appropriate antimicrobial treatment. The presence of abundant human DNA may hamper the sensitivity of PCR in the detection of bacteria.

Methods: We used serial dilutions of *E. Coli* spiked pseudo-blood-sepsis samples to develop a simple method that combines the use of a polar detergent solvent and adjustment of the basic pH to remove human DNA. A 16S rRNA gene-based screening algorithm was established to differentiate Gram-positive and Gram-negative groups of bacteria and the family of Enterobacteriaceae. A stringent validation with appropriate controls was implemented. The method of human DNA removal was then applied on 194 sepsis blood samples and 44 cerebrospinal fluid (CSF) samples by real-time PCR.

Results: This uncomplicated and straightforward approach allows to remove up to 98 % of human DNA from peripheral blood of septic patients. The inhibitory effect of human DNA is efficiently prevented and the detection limit of real-time PCR is increased to 10 *E. Coli* CFUs/ml. This sensitivity is 10 times higher compared to conventional real-time PCR assays. The classical blood culture detected 58/194 (30 %) of sepsis and 9/44 (21 %) of CSF samples. Out of the 194 blood samples tested, the conventional real-time PCR targeting 13 common sepsis causing pathogens correctly detected the bacterial DNA in 16/194 (8 %) only and 14/44 (32 %) in cerebrospinal fluid samples. Our newly established approach was able to provide correct diagnoses in 78 (40 %) of the 194 blood samples and in 14 (32 %) of the CSF samples. The combination of both blood cultures and our technique raised the rate of sepsis diagnoses to 112/194 (58 %). Of the total group tested positive, 46 (24 %) cases showed overlap with the classical methodology.

Conclusion: We report a simple optimized in-house protocol for removal of human DNA from blood sepsis samples as a pre-analytical tool to prepare DNA for subsequent PCR assays. With the detection increase of our in-house DNA removal approach, subsequent PCR assays can reach detection limits of 10 *E. coli* CFUs/ml and significantly improve the diagnostic rate in blood sepsis cases.

Keywords: Sepsis, Bloodstream infection, Human DNA removal, Molecular diagnosis, Blood culture

* Correspondence: velavan@medizin.uni-tuebingen.de; lehuusong@108-icid.com
Thirumalaisamy P. Velavan and Le Huu Song are shared senior authors.
[6]Institute of Tropical Medicine, University of Tübingen, Tübingen, Germany
[1]Department of Molecular Biology, 108 Military Central Hospital, Hanoi, Vietnam
Full list of author information is available at the end of the article

Background

Even after the development of new diagnostic and therapeutic techniques, the physiopathology of sepsis is still poorly understood; incidences and mortality are steadily increasing. Delayed diagnosis usually results in multi-organ failure and with frequent fatal outcomes [1]. Timely and appropriate diagnoses of bloodstream infections (BSI) have a significant and measurable impact on patient care and infection control in resource-limited settings [2]. Although the classical blood culture is widely accepted as a gold standard it still has various drawbacks. For instance, blood cultures are time-consuming and can only detect bacteria growing on suitable media used. A minimum volume of 30 ml of blood is required for each aerobic and anaerobic bacterial cultures [3]; such amounts are challenges particularly for old and neonatal patients. A rapid diagnostic method applicable under clinical conditions and complementing classical blood cultures is therefore essential.

The polymerase chain reaction (PCR) has provided new possibilities for rapid detection of bacterial pathogens in patients with sepsis [2]. In addition, the multiple-priming format (multiplex) PCR allows rapid detection of various microbial pathogens in a shorter period of time. Although many advancements in molecular diagnostics of bacterial pathogens have been achieved [4, 5], PCR based diagnoses of BSI are still difficult. A most critical factor is that PCR assays may fail to amplify sparse copies of pathogens in the abundance of human DNA. In addition, PCR-inhibitory compounds in human blood can considerably reduce the sensitivity of an assay. For instance, a typical BSI case has a bacterial density of 1-1000 CFU/ml in their peripheral blood [6]. An optimized PCR reaction can only amplify the 16S rRNA target if the bacterial load exceeds 1000 CFU/ml. Thus, PCR assays may be ineffectual in replicating blood culture results [7, 8]. The diversity of bacterial strains further complicates optimized conditions for multiplex PCR reactions.

During evolution, the fusion of two prokaryotic genomes (e.g., Archae and Proteobacteria) has resulted in the formation of a eukaryotic genome with sufficient horizontal gene transfer [9, 10]. This indicates that the possibility of the presence of homologous and/or conserved DNA sequences between human and bacterial genomes exists, possibly causing primer mispairing and consequently leading to false positive results. Commercial molecular diagnostic tests such as the SepsiTest (Molzym), and VYOO (SIRS Lab) apply various approaches to deplete human genomic DNA prior to the molecular diagnosis [7, 11–14]. In these molecular assays, either DNAses cleaving human DNA or methylated chromatography columns are used to remove human DNA. Larger volumes of human blood are recommended in these assays. Since such kits are costly, low-income countries can frequently not afford them.

We developed a simple in-house method that combines the use of a polar detergent solvent and adjustment of basic pH to remove human DNA. We also utilized a 16S rRNA based real-time PCR screening algorithm to differentiate Gram-positive and Gram-negative bacteria as well as the family of Enterobacteriaceae. Our newly developed procedure was validated in 194 peripheral blood samples obtained from septic patients with likely abundant human DNA and 44 samples of cerebrospinal fluid (CSF) with sparse human DNA. The diagnostic performance of i) the classical blood culture approach (arm-1), ii) conventional real-time PCR screening using total DNA extracted from patients samples (arm-2), and iii) our real-time PCR screening approach using templates depleted of human DNA (arm-3) were compared.

Methods

Ethics statement

The study was submitted for regulatory approval to the institutional review board of the 108 hospital and was approved. Following submission, the Ethical Committee of the 108 Military Central Hospital, Hanoi has provided consent and ethical approval for the study was duly obtained. Informed written consent was obtained from all study patients and/or from their parents if the study participant was under 18 years of age.

Dilution series formulation

The *E. coli* DH5 alpha strain (Invitrogen, Singapore) was inoculated into liquid LB medium for proliferation until reaching the log phase. A dilution series from 10000 CFU/mL to 1 CFU/mL until eventual negativity was done to spike the bacteria into 5 mL of human blood. The spiked bacteria in blood were then used for the procedure of human DNA depletion and subsequent isolation of bacterial DNA. DNA extracted from single colonies of *Klebsiella pneumoniae, Proteus mirabilis, Neisseria meningitidis, Salmonella spp., Pseudomonas aeruginosa, Acinetobacter baumannii, Staphylococcus aureus, S. epidermidis, Streptococcus pneumoniae, S. suis* and *Enterococcus spp.* were reconstituted in 200 μl of 25 mM Tris-EDTA at pH 8 containing 100 ng/μl human DNA extracted from full blood; 5 μl of these solutions were used as positive controls for all PCR or real-time PCR reactions.

Depletion of human DNA and bacterial DNA isolation

Several detergents including non-ionic (NP-40, Triton-X 100), ionic (CTAB, SDS) and zwitterionic (CHAPS) detergents were screened. Only Triton-X 100 was able to lyse mammalian cell membranes, but not those of *E. coli.* Triton-X 100 was, therefore, considered for further analyses. Different conditions such as variation in pH, time, and Na_2CO_2 concentrations were also optimized (Additional file 1: Table S1). Mammalian cell lysis buffers MCLB-1 was used to treat the pseudo-sepsis samples by mixing volumes of 1.2 ml blood from healthy donors (spiked with 100,000 *E. coli* cells) with 1.2 ml solvent. After solvent treatment, the suspensions were centrifuged to collect bacterial pellets for subsequent NaOH/SDS total DNA extraction. Residuals of human DNA and intactness of spiked *E. coli* genome were examined and quantified by RT-PCR (Additional file 1: Figures S1 and S2).

Overnight-grown *E. coli* were spiked in peripheral venous blood samples obtained from healthy donors to establish dilution serials of 1000 CFU/ml, 100 CFU/ml, 10 CFU/ml, 1 CFU/ml and 0 CFU/ml (negative control). The dilution serials were separated into two groups. The first group was subjected to human DNA removal by mixing thoroughly with an equal volume of mammalian cell lysis buffer (MCLB-1, containing 2 M Na_2CO_2 pH 9.8, 1 % Triton-X100) for three minutes at ambient temperature to allow for complete fragmentation of human chromatin into DNA fragments. After the incubation step an equal volume of neutralization buffer (1 M Tris–HCl, pH 4.5) was added in order to prevent further cell lysis. The samples were then centrifuged at 5000 g for 5 min. The supernatants were discarded and bacterial pellets were resuscitated in 200 µl of 1x phosphate buffered saline (PBS) and used for isolation of bacterial DNA by a conventional method using the NaOH/SDS approach [15]. The second group of the dilution serials also underwent conventional DNA extraction using the NaOH/SDS approach [15].

The integrity of spiked *E. coli* genomic DNA and the presence of residual human DNA was measured by *E. coli* specific primers/probe (Additional file 1: Tables S2 and S3) real-time PCR or SYBR green based real-time PCR using the beta globin-specific primers: BetaF: 5'-AGA AGA GCC AAG GAC AGG TAC G-3'; BetaR: 5'-TGC TAG TGA ACA CAG TTG TGT CAG A-3'.

Reagent preparation under aseptic conditions

Primers and labeled probes (Integrated DNA Technologies, Singapore) used are listed in Additional file 1: Tables S2 and S3. All primers and probes were available in stocks of 100 pmol/µl in 25 mM Tris–HCl and treated with 1 U DNase/20 µl reaction volume for 15 min at 37 °C. Subsequently, the DNAse was inactivated by heating at 95 °C for 40 min. After inactivation, the stock was aliquoted into volumes of 10 µl and stored at −20 °C [16]. For decontamination of the PCR mastermix, 8-methoxypsoralen was dissolved in dimethylsulfoxide (DMSO) (Sigma, Germany). For decontamination of PCR water and the real-time PCR mastermix reagents, 25 µg/mL of 8-methoxypsoralen (Sigma, Germany) and 10 min exposure to 366 nm UV irradiation over a distance of 3 cm were applied. The MCLB-1 buffer was also decontaminated by UV irradiation at 280 nm over a distance shorter than 5 cm [16]. Working places and all accessories and tools in our laboratory are decontaminated weekly by spraying with DNA-ExitusPlus™ solution (AppliChem, Germany).

Real-time PCR conditions

The real-time PCR assay mixtures consisted of 7.5 µl Taqman real-time PCR Master Mix (Qiagen, Hilden, Germany), 5 µl DNA template, 5 pmol of primers and 0.2 pmol of probe. The reaction was run in the Stratagene M3000p (Stratagene, USA) device with a preincubation step at 50 °C for 15 min, initial denaturation at 95 °C for 5 min, followed by 45 cycles of 95 °C for 15 s and 60 °C for 60 s. The first real-time PCR assay differentiates Gram-negative, Gram-positive and Enterobacteriacea bacteria. The second assay discriminates the distinct bacterial species using primers and Taqman probes specific for the 13 most common pathogens, namely *Staphylococus aureus, S. epidermidis, Streptococcus pneumoniae, S. suis, Enterococcus spp.* (Gram-positive bacteria) and *Escherichia coli, Klebsiella pneumoniae, Proteus mirabilis, Salmonella spp., Neisseria meningitidis, Pseudomonas aeruginos,* and *Acinetobacter baumannii* (Gram-negative bacteria).

Sepsis patients and blood sampling

A total of 194 peripheral venous blood and 44 CSF from septic patients were available at the 108 Military Central Hospital, Hanoi, Vietnam. Samples were collected between February 2014 and September 2015. Diagnoses of sepsis were confirmed by physicians, based on a body temperature above 38.3 °C or below 36 °C, heart rate >90 beats per minute, respiratory rate higher than 20 breaths per minute, an assumed or confirmed infection with at least one of the following signs and symptoms: significantly decreased urine output, abrupt change in consciousness/mental status, decreased platelet count, difficulty of breathing, abnormal heart pumping function, or abdominal pain [17]. Blood and CSF samples from all patients were preserved in heparinized tubes. Prior to the analyses specimens were stored at 4 °C.

In order to compare diagnostic techniques in the identification of pathogens causing sepsis, 10 ml of venous blood or 0.5 ml CSF were collected in duplicates from all patients and divided into equal portions for the detection of aerobic bacteria. The blood samples were subjected to automatic bacterial culture, and CSF was used for conventional bacterial cultures. In parallel, 2.4 ml blood or 1 ml of CSF were equally partitioned into one sample (1.2 ml blood or 0.5 ml CSF) that was used directly for total DNA extraction, and a second sample (1.2 ml blood or 0.5 ml CSF) which was used for MCLB-1 treatment to remove human DNA prior to extraction of bacterial DNA. DNA isolated from samples treated with MCLB-1 was used for screening to discriminate Gram-negative, Gram-positive and Enterobacteriacea bacteria. Samples positive in the screening step were then subjected to group-specific real-time PCR assays to identify and confirm infection by 13 common pathogens causing sepsis as mentioned above (Fig. 1a).

Automated bacterial culture

Twenty ml blood were collected per patient and aliquoted in 10 ml tubes for culturing in the BD BACTEC™ 9120 blood culture system at 36 °C ± 0.5 for 48 h until growth in both tubes was observed (Becton Dickinson, New Jersey, USA). After 24 h of incubation, identification of bacterial species was performed using the VITEK® 2 automated system (BioMérieux, France).

Conventional bacterial culture

To establish diagnostic techniques for the examination of CSF samples, we followed protocols provided by the Manual of Clinical Microbiology [18] and the CDC Laboratory Methods for the Diagnosis of Meningitis [19]. Briefly, 600 µl aliquots of CSF from each patient was vortexed in 600 µl PBS. The resulting suspension was streaked onto four media, namely blood agar, MacConkey agar, chocolate agar and buffered charcoal-yeast extract agar (BCYE) and incubated under aerobic conditions at 37 °C for three days. Colonial growth was asserted and confirmed by microbiologists.

Results

Efficiency of human DNA removal

Utilization of mammalian cell lysis buffer (MCLB-1) resulted in removal of 98 % human DNA, obviously without affecting bacterial DNA (Fig. 2a). Our data reveal that, at a high density of spiked bacteria (>1000 CFU/ml), human DNA does not impede the downstream PCR. However, at lower bacterial loads (<100 CFU/ml) human DNA inhibits subsequent PCR reactions (Fig. 2b, Table 1, Additional file 1: Figure S3). Efficient removal of inhibitory effects caused by human DNA increased the detection limits of the PCR to 10 CFU/ml, a detection limit which conventional PCR assays could not reach (Fig. 2, Table 1). The discrimination of Gram-positive and Gram-negative bacteria as well as Enterobacteriacea requires four hours only, with two additional hours of the real-time PCR assay to identify bacterial species (Fig. 1b).

Limit of detection

In order to determine the concentration of spiked *E. coli* at which the real-time PCR assay can detect bacterial DNA and the cut-off concentration at which the PCR cannot distinguish spiked bacterial DNA from pre-contaminated microbial DNA, we grew *E. coli* and spiked it in blood samples from healthy donors to establish 20 dilution serials of 1000 CFU/ml, 100 CFU/ml, 10 CFU/ml, 1 CFU/ml and 0 CFU/ml (negative control). These were equally divided into several aliquots to allow independent technical assistants to conduct MCLB-1-based removal of human DNA and DNA extraction. Bacterial DNA was

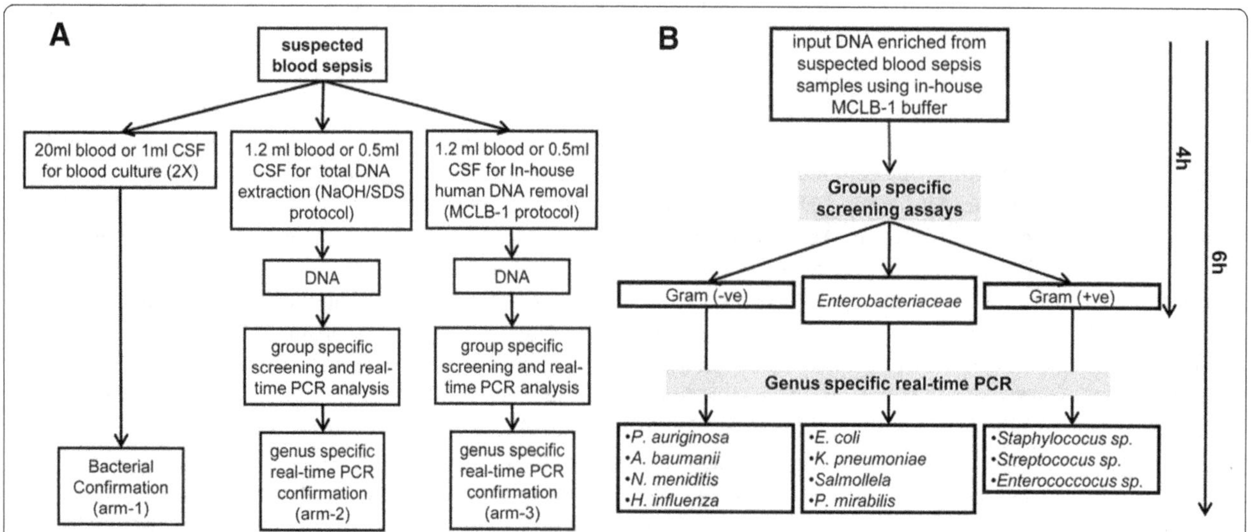

Fig. 1 Work flow of the established protocol for human DNA removal. **a** Study flowchart to compare sepsis causing pathogen diagnoses by PCR and blood culture. **b** Group-specific screening by PCR reactions targeting bacterial 16SrRNA gene to differentiate Gram-positive, Gram-negative and Enterobacteriaceae groups. Samples positive in the screening assay were subjected to genus-specific real-time PCR reactions to detect 13 most common sepsis causative pathogens

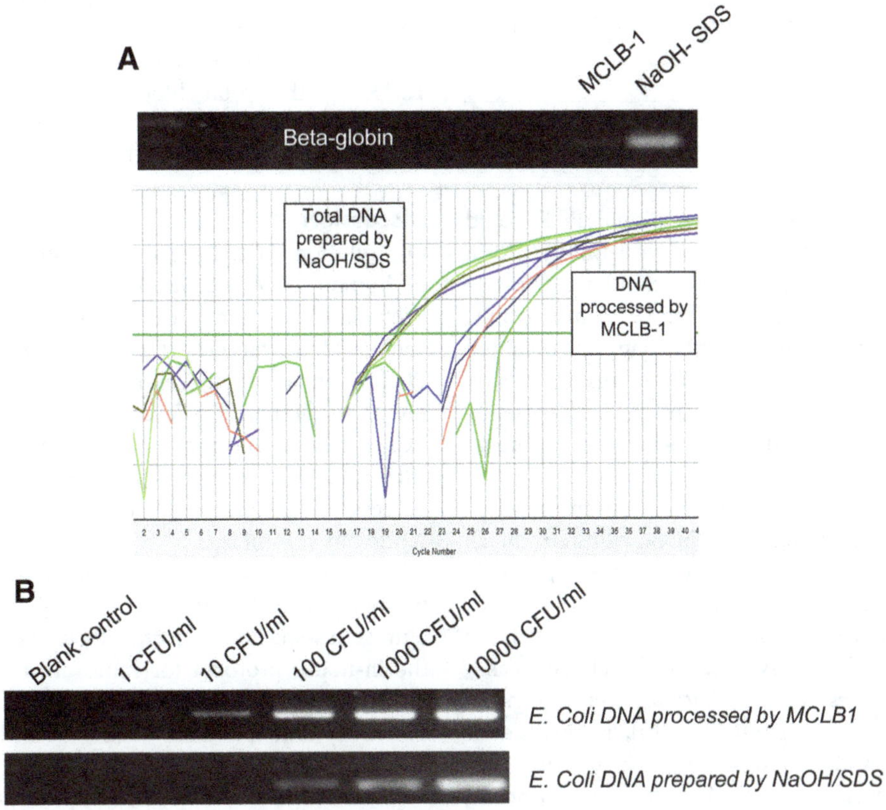

Fig. 2 Efficiency of human DNA removal and sensitivity of PCR assay. **a** Residues of human DNA after MCLB-1 treatment were monitored via beta-globin derived amplification assays. Upper panel gel based PCR assay targeting the beta-globin gene; lower panel is SYBR green based real-time PCR to quantify residual beta-globin gene fragments. **b** Detection limits of spiked *E. coli* at various densities. At high density of spiked bacteria (1000 CFU/ml or 10000 CFU/ml), removal of human DNA does not provide a significant diagnostic signal, but at low concentration (100 CFU/ml or 10 CFU), removal of human DNA enhances detection limit of the diagnostics PCR to 10 CFU/ml

used as template for real-time PCR using primers and probes specific for Enterobacteriaceae and *E. coli.* RT-PCR could detect spiked *E. coli* at concentrations of 100–1000 CFU/ml with a Ct value of 29.2 ± 0.5 at 1000 CFU/ml and of 34.5 ± 0.5 at 100 CFU/ml (Table 2, Additional file 1: Figure S4). In addition, the real-time PCR could still detect 14 out of 20 cases with Ct values of 37 ± 1 at a concentration of 10 CFU/ml. However, the real-time PCR could only detect 7 out of 20 with Ct values of 42 ± 1.3 at a concentration of 1 CFU/ml. These results indicate that our real-time PCR procedure was not able to distinguish samples with spiked bacteria at a concentration of 1 CFU/ml from pre-contaminated bacterial DNA. Therefore, for practical purposes, we set a cut-off of 10 CFU/ml, corresponding to a Ct value of 37 for all pathogens under investigation.

Comparison of blood culture versus molecular identification of pathogens

The advantage of human DNA removal prior to PCR diagnosis by treatment with MCLB-1 was validated by using 194 blood samples and 44 CSF samples from septic patients. The samples were divided into three arms, arm 1 for blood culture, arm 2 for direct NaOH/SDS DNA extraction and conventional RT-PCR analysis and arm 3 for MCLB-1 treatment and subsequent RT-PCR detection. Among 44 CSF samples, where human DNA might be present in small amounts only, conventional PCR and the PCR assays with previous MCLB-1 treatment provided identical results (14/44 positive cases). The detection rate by PCR was higher than that obtained by blood culture, which detected bacterial DNA in 9 of the 44 CSF samples only (Fig. 3). However, all

Table 1 Ct value of spiked *E. coli* dilution series upon in-house human DNA removal step

E. coli density (CFU/ml)	1000	100	10	1	0
MCLB1 processed DNA	29.2 ± 0.5	34 ± 0.5	37 ± 1	Undetectable[a]	Undetectable[a]
NaOH/SDS processed DNA	29.0 ± 0.5	37 ± 1	Undetectable[a]	Undetectable[a]	Undetectable[a]

[a]Undetectable means that the real-time PCR fluorescent signal appears later than that of cut-off assays (see the detection limits and negative control validation)

Table 2 Detection limits and frequency of detection of spiked *E. coli* dilution series upon in-house human DNA removal step

Spiked *E coli* density (CFU/ml)	1000	100	10	1	0
Average detected Ct	29.2 ± 0.5	34 ± 0.5	37 ± 1	42 ± 1.3	42 ± 1.3
Frequency of detection	20/20	20/20	14/20	7/20	6/20

positive samples identified by conventional PCR could be confirmed by MCLB-1-processed real-time PCR in the 194 blood samples (Fig. 4). Furthermore, the conventional approach could detect 16 of the 194 samples only, indicating a low power detection rate than that obtained by the MCLB-1-based approach. These results clearly show that efficient removal of human DNA from septicemic blood samples provides a considerable advantage and facilitates PCR diagnoses.

Out of the 194 blood samples obtained from septic patients, 58 (30 %) were positive by blood culture (arm 1), of which 15 (8 %) were positive for other species, namely *Enterobacter sakazaki* (1 case), *L. monocytogenes* (2 cases), *Alcaligenes. faecalis* (1 case), *Pseudomonas. fluorescens* (3 cases), *Stenotrophomonas. maltophilia* (1 case case) and *Candida albicans* (1 case), *Enterobacter. aerogenes* (1 case), *Morganella. morganii* (2 cases), *Burkholderia. pseudomallei* (1 case), *Candida. tropicalis* (1 case) and *Burkholderia. cepacia* (1 case) (Fig. 4a). The in-house real-time PCR methodology using MCLB-1-processed DNA (arm 3) detected 78 (40 %) of 194 BSI samples. The combination of blood culture with MCLB-1-based real-time PCR methods could increase the sensitivity up to 58 % (112 positive cases). We observed that 46 out of 112 positive cases (41 % of positive cases, or 24 % of the total blood samples) were correctly identified between blood culture and MCLB-1 based real-time PCR. Of the 46, 24 (21 % of the positive cases or 12 % of the total blood samples) were identified between the two methods at species level (Fig. 4a, b, Additional file 1: Figure S5).

Discussion

Our dilution series have shown a strong inhibitory effect of human DNA on subsequent PCR assays targeting bacteria. Once human DNA is removed efficiently from venous blood samples, the detection limit of real-time PCR is enhanced more than ten times. Although removal of human DNA does not improve subsequent PCR detection in samples with low human DNA content such as in CSF, it significantly enhances the diagnostic success of samples with human DNA abundance in septic blood samples.

Bacteremia accounts for a high risk of mortality, both in industrialized and in resource-limited settings [1]. Our genus-specific real-time PCR assays, together with the in-house protocol for removal of human DNA not only provides faster diagnoses, but also increases the sensitivity and specificity in the detection of pathogens compared to culture techniques.

Blood cultures are considered the gold standard for the diagnosis of bacterial or fungal BSI [2]. This method provides results after 24 – 48 h or even a longer period of time, and a tailored therapy can then be adapted based on the presumptive bacterial identification. This method is time consuming with a minimum of 24 to 48 h and treatment options may be compromised

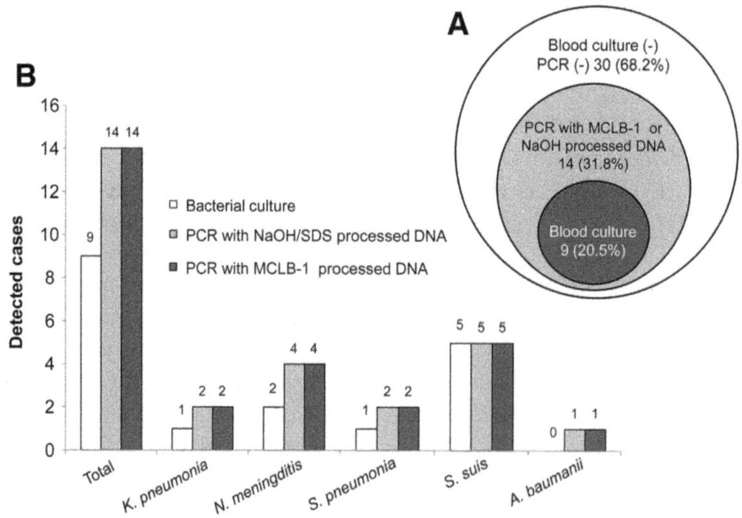

Fig. 3 Comparison of diagnostic methodologies for sepsis causing pathogens in CSF samples. **a** Venn diagram shows the diagnostic overlap of the blood culture approach (*dark gray* – arm 1), real-time PCR using conventional NaOH DNA extraction approach (*light gray* – arm 2) and real-time PCR using DNA removed DNA (*light gray* – arm 3). **b** The diagnostic performance are illustrated for classical blood culture (*gray bars*), conventional real-time PCR with total human DNA (*black bar*) and real-time PCR algorithm using MCLB1 treated samples with depleted human DNA

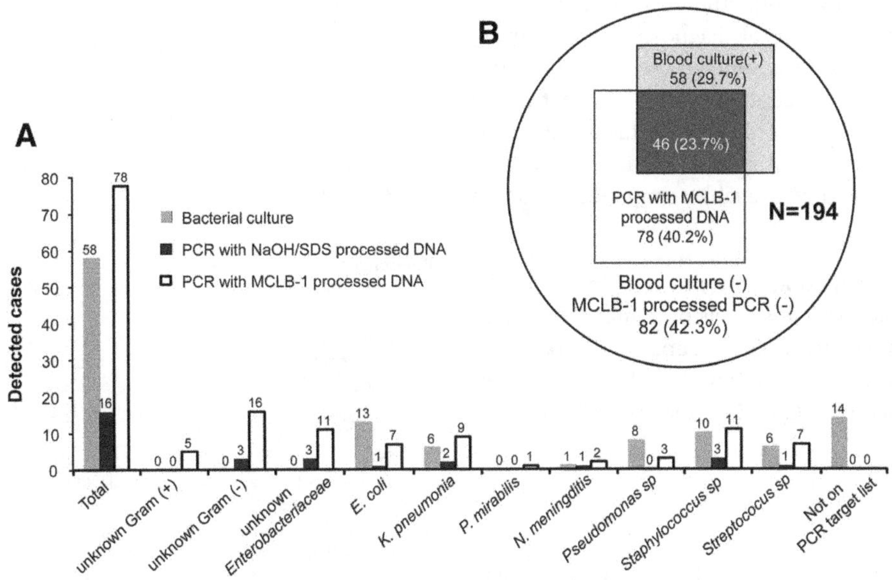

Fig. 4 Comparison of diagnostic methodologies for sepsis causative pathogens in human abundance sepsis samples. **a** Venn diagram shows the overlap between PCR using human DNA removed input samples - arm 3 and blood culture method - arm1. **b** The detailed diagnostic performance is illustrated for classical blood culture method (*gray bars*) or conventional real-time PCR approach using DNA extracted from total human blood sepsis samples (*black bar*) or real-time PCR using algorithm using MCLB-1 treated samples

severely. Early detection and adequate treatment of BSI are mandatory within the first 6–12 h [20, 21]. The development of rapid diagnostic methods for BSI is important in order to supplement conventional blood culture diagnostics [2]. Nucleic acid-based diagnostic approaches have the potential to address this need [3, 4]. However, the low amount of copies of pathogen DNA and the presence of PCR-inhibitory compounds in blood, including the presence of human DNA, remain challenges [5, 11, 22].

The combination of a mild detergent (MCLB-1, containing 2 M Na_2CO_2 pH 9.8, 1 % Triton-X100) applied for 3 min results in removal of approximately 98 % of human DNA from full blood samples. Processing of bacterial DNA prior to molecular detection requires only a short time, which does not cause significant damage of bacterial DNA. In addition, in the presence of a mild detergent, human blood cells are disrupted efficiently to release human DNA. This does not apply to bacterial and fungal cells. An elevated basic pH 9.8 Na_2CO_{3-} sodium carbonate) ensures successful degradation of human DNA. Thus, intact bacteria and fungi from blood are enriched. Nevertheless, the selective lysis reaction needs to be controlled over time as bacterial cell walls might be lysed upon prolonged exposure.

Current commercial DNA removal kits such as MolYsis Basic (MolZym GmbH & Co. KG, Bremen, Germany) and Looxster (SIRS-lab GmbH, Jena, Germany) work with high blood volumes and require methylated chromatographic columns or DNAses that are patented. Due to significant costs, these kits are commonly not available in low income communities.

Treatment of sepsis usually depends on the presumptive bacterial identification, suggested by Gram staining or/and group specificity of bacteria [23]. Our procedure is a systematic approach, with a stepwise process initiated by real-time PCR reactions to identify Gram-negative, Gram-positive and Enterobacteriacea bacteria. If a patient sample is positive for any group of pathogens, strain-specific Taqman real-time PCR assays are indicated. The diagnostic procedure can be completed within four hours, not only rapidly providing accurate results, but also significantly reducing the cost compared to individual PCR reactions for a large number of pathogens.

In our study and recommended for clinical practice we set a cut-off value of 10 CFU/ml. This limit of detection excludes positive results for patients who are infected with bacterial loads lower than 10 CFU/ml. This explains in part the fact that our molecular method could not recapitulate the positive cases revealed by blood culture. On the other hand, in patients already treated with antibiotics, blood cultures frequently do not lead to reliable diagnoses. This provides an additional explanation for the disagreement between the two methods. Our results are in line with other studies showing that the difference between two diagnostic methodologies fluctuates from 8 % to 80 %, depending on the materials used [11, 24–28]. This explains why the Septifast (Roche Diagnostics) kit is not yet recommended for clinical use in suspected sepsis [28]. Although the overlap between our method and blood cultures was 23.7 % only in our study, the combination of the two methods revealed a diagnostic sensitivity of 57.7 %. This is a significant advantage over with a positive rate of 34 % only and comparability with blood cultures of 8 % [11]. Furthermore, our procedure takes only four hours, which is significantly shorter compared to 18 h required when using any available commercial kits in market [11].

Our detection methodology does not improve the diagnoses of samples with low levels of human DNA. This applies, for example, to CSF specimens. Pretreatment provides an improved DNA template for subsequent PCR and/or real-time PCR, and reaches a sensitivity of 10 CFU/ml.

Conclusion

We established a simple optimized protocol for human DNA removal from blood sepsis samples. This method provides enriched bacterial DNA for subsequent PCR-based detection of bacterial DNA. With our established protocol, the downstream PCR assays can reach detection limits of 10 CFU/ml and, thus, enhance the positive rate of blood sepsis diagnoses.

Abbreviations

BSI, bloodstream infection; CFU, Colony-forming unit; MCLB-1, mammalian cell lysis buffer; NAT, nucleic acid testing; PCR, polymerase chain reaction

Acknowledgements

We would like to acknowledge funding from the Vietnamese Ministry of Science and Technology (Grant: KC-10.43/11-15) for this study. Dr. Velavan acknowledges financial support for MTB from DAAD-Germany. The funders have no role in study design, data collection and analysis, decision to publish, and/or preparation of the manuscript.

Author contributions

NTT, LHS and TPV designed and supervised the studies. MTB and DTQ conducted the experiments. TTTHien, TTTHuyen performed the sequencing analysis. PQH, TVS, NTKP, TTL evaluated the clinical data and provided the clinical samples. NTT, LHS, HVT and TPV analysed the data and wrote the manuscript. CGM contributed to the revision of the draft and on proof reading. All authors read and approved the manuscript.

Competing interests

The authors declare that they have no competing interests.

Consent to publish

All authors read the manuscript and have provided their consent to publish. All authors declare no conflict of interests.
consent and ethical approval for the study was duly obtained. Informed written consent was obtained from all study patients and/or from their parents if the study participant was under 18 years of age.

Author details

[1]Department of Molecular Biology, 108 Military Central Hospital, Hanoi, Vietnam. [2]Institute of Clinical Infectious Diseases, 108 Military Central Hospital, Hanoi, Vietnam. [3]Department of Clinical Microbiology, 108 Military Central Hospital, Hanoi, Vietnam. [4]Faculty of Infectious Diseases, Hai Phong Medical University, Hai Phong, Vietnam. [5]Department of Gastroenterology, 108 Military Central Hospital, Hanoi, Vietnam. [6]Institute of Tropical Medicine, University of Tübingen, Tübingen, Germany. [7]Vietnamese - German Centre for Medical Research (VG-CARE), Hanoi, Vietnam.

References

1. Angus DC, van der Poll T. Severe sepsis and septic shock. N Engl J Med. 2013;369(9):840–51.
2. Liesenfeld O, Lehman L, Hunfeld KP, Kost G. Molecular diagnosis of sepsis: new aspects and recent developments. Eur J Microbiol Immunol. 2014;4(1):1–25.
3. Mancini N, Carletti S, Ghidoli N, Cichero P, Burioni R, Clementi M. The era of molecular and other non-culture-based methods in diagnosis of sepsis. Clin Microbiol Rev. 2010;23(1):235–51.
4. Espy MJ, Uhl JR, Sloan LM, Buckwalter SP, Jones MF, Vetter EA, Yao JD, Wengenack NL, Rosenblatt JE, Cockerill 3rd FR, et al. Real-time PCR in clinical microbiology: applications for routine laboratory testing. Clin Microbiol Rev. 2006;19(1):165–256.
5. Pletz MW, Wellinghausen N, Welte T. Will polymerase chain reaction (PCR)-based diagnostics improve outcome in septic patients? A clinical view. Intensive Care Med. 2011;37(7):1069–76.
6. Yagupsky P, Nolte FS. Quantitative aspects of septicemia. Clin Microbiol Rev. 1990;3(3):269–79.
7. Hansen WL, Bruggeman CA, Wolffs PF. Evaluation of new preanalysis sample treatment tools and DNA isolation protocols to improve bacterial pathogen detection in whole blood. J Clin Microbiol. 2009;47(8):2629–31.
8. Wang HY, Kim S, Kim J, Park SD, Uh Y, Lee H. Multiplex real-time PCR assay for rapid detection of methicillin-resistant staphylococci directly from positive blood cultures. J Clin Microbiol. 2014;52(6):1911–20.
9. Simonson AB, Servin JA, Skophammer RG, Herbold CW, Rivera MC, Lake JA. Decoding the genomic tree of life. Proc Natl Acad Sci U S A. 2005;102 Suppl 1:6608–13.
10. Rivera MC, Lake JA. The ring of life provides evidence for a genome fusion origin of eukaryotes. Nature. 2004;431(7005):152–5.
11. Bloos F, Sachse S, Kortgen A, Pletz MW, Lehmann M, Straube E, Riedemann NC, Reinhart K, Bauer M. Evaluation of a polymerase chain reaction assay for pathogen detection in septic patients under routine condition: an observational study. PLoS One. 2012;7(9), e46003.
12. Peytavi R, Huletsky A, Belley-Montfort L, Martineau I. Concentration and Enrichment of Microbial Cells and Microbial Nucleic Acids from Bodily Fluids. In: Google Patents; 2011.
13. Loffler J, Hebart H, Schumacher U, Reitze H, Einsele H. Comparison of different methods for extraction of DNA of fungal pathogens from cultures and blood. J Clin Microbiol. 1997;35(12):3311–2.
14. Loonen AJ, Bos MP, van Meerbergen B, Neerken S, Catsburg A, Dobbelaer I, Penterman R, Maertens G, van de Wiel P, Savelkoul P, et al. Comparison of pathogen DNA isolation methods from large volumes of whole blood to improve molecular diagnosis of bloodstream infections. PLoS One. 2013; 8(8):e72349.
15. Ausubel FB, Kingston R, Moore D, Seidman JG, Smith J, Struhl K. Short Protocols in Molecular Biology. 3rd ed. 1995. p. 2–3.
16. Klaschik S, Lehmann LE, Raadts A, Hoeft A, Stuber F. Comparison of different decontamination methods for reagents to detect low concentrations of bacterial 16S DNA by real-time-PCR. Mol Biotechnol. 2002;22(3):231–42.
17. Dellinger RP, Levy MM, Carlet JM, Bion J, Parker MM, Jaeschke R, Reinhart K, Angus DC, Brun-Buisson C, Beale R, et al. Surviving Sepsis Campaign: international guidelines for management of severe sepsis and septic shock: 2008. Crit Care Med. 2008;36(1):296–327.
18. Murray PR, Baron EJ, Pfaller MA, Tenover FC, Yolken RH. Manual of Clinical Microbiology. Washington DC: ASM Press; 1999.
19. Laboratory Methods for the Diagnosis of Meningitism. 2nd edition. WHO Manual; 2011.
20. Morrell M, Fraser VJ, Kollef MH. Delaying the empiric treatment of candida bloodstream infection until positive blood culture results are obtained: a potential risk factor for hospital mortality. Antimicrob Agents Chemother. 2005;49(9):3640–5.

21. Ibrahim EH, Sherman G, Ward S, Fraser VJ, Kollef MH. The influence of inadequate antimicrobial treatment of bloodstream infections on patient outcomes in the ICU setting. Chest. 2000;118(1):146–55.
22. Bergthold LA. The frayed alliance: business and health care in Massachusetts. J Health Polit Policy Law. 1990;15(4):915–8.
23. Guido M, Quattrocchi M, Zizza A, Pasanisi G, Pavone V, Lobreglio G, Gabutti G, De Donno A. Molecular approaches in the diagnosis of sepsis in neutropenic patients with haematological malignances. J Prev Med Hyg. 2012;53(2):104–8.
24. Chang SS, Hsieh WH, Liu TS, Lee SH, Wang CH, Chou HC, Yeo YH, Tseng CP, Lee CC. Multiplex PCR system for rapid detection of pathogens in patients with presumed sepsis - a systemic review and meta-analysis. PLoS One. 2013;8(5), e62323.
25. Casalta JP, Gouriet F, Roux V, Thuny F, Habib G, Raoult D. Evaluation of the LightCycler SeptiFast test in the rapid etiologic diagnostic of infectious endocarditis. Eur J Clin Microbiol Infect Dis. 2009;28(6):569–73.
26. Lodes U, Bohmeier B, Lippert H, Konig B, Meyer F. PCR-based rapid sepsis diagnosis effectively guides clinical treatment in patients with new onset of SIRS. Langenbecks Arch Surg. 2012;397(3):447–55.
27. Wellinghausen N, Kochem AJ, Disque C, Muhl H, Gebert S, Winter J, Matten J, Sakka SG. Diagnosis of bacteremia in whole-blood samples by use of a commercial universal 16S rRNA gene-based PCR and sequence analysis. J Clin Microbiol. 2009;47(9):2759–65.
28. Dark P, Blackwood B, Gates S, McAuley D, Perkins GD, McMullan R, Wilson C, Graham D, Timms K, Warhurst G. Accuracy of LightCycler((R)) SeptiFast for the detection and identification of pathogens in the blood of patients with suspected sepsis: a systematic review and meta-analysis. Intensive Care Med. 2015;41(1):21–33.

4

Clinical relevance of molecular identification of microorganisms and detection of antimicrobial resistance genes in bloodstream infections of paediatric cancer patients

Fabianne Carlesse[1*], Paola Cappellano[2], Milene Gonçalves Quiles[2], Liana Carballo Menezes[2], Antonio Sérgio Petrilli[1] and Antonio Carlos Pignatari[2]

Abstract

Background: Bloodstream infections (BSIs) are the major cause of mortality in cancer patients. Molecular techniques are used for rapid diagnosis of BSI, allowing early therapy and improving survival. We aimed to establish whether real-time quantitative polymerase chain reaction (qPCR) could improve early diagnosis and therapy in paediatric cancer patients, and describe the predominant pathogens of BSI and their antimicrobial susceptibility.

Methods: Blood samples were processed by the BACTEC system and microbial identification and susceptibility tests were performed by the Phoenix system. All samples were screened by multiplex 16 s rDNA qPCR. Seventeen species were evaluated using sex-specific TaqMan probes and resistance genes *bla*SHV, *bla*TEM, *bla*CTX, *bla*KPC, *bla*IMP, *bla*SPM, *bla*VIM, *van*A, *van*B and *mec*A were screened by SYBR Green reactions. Therapeutic efficacy was evaluated at the time of positive blood culture and at final phenotypic identification and antimicrobial susceptibility results.

Results: We analyzed 69 episodes of BSI from 64 patients. Gram-positive bacteria were identified in 61 % of the samples, Gram-negative bacteria in 32 % and fungi in 7 %. There was 78.2 % of agreement between the phenotypic and molecular methods in final species identification. The *mec*A gene was detected in 81.4 % of *Staphylococcus* spp., and 91.6 % were concordant with the phenotypic method. Detection of *van*A gene was 100 % concordant. The concordance for Gram-negative susceptibilities was 71.4 % for Enterobacteriaceae and 50 % for *Pseudomonas aeruginosa*. Therapy was more frequently inadequate in patients who died, and the molecular test was concordant with the phenotypic susceptibility test in 50 %.

Conclusions: qPCR has potential indication for early identification of pathogens and antimicrobial resistance genes from BSI in paediatric cancer patients and may improve antimicrobial therapy.

Abbreviations: AML, Acute myeloid leukaemia; BC, Blood culture; BSI, Bloodstream infection; CoNS, Coagulase-negative *Staphylococcus*; CVC, Central venous catheter; ESBL, Extended spectrum β-lactamase; FN, Febrile neutropenia; ICU, Intensive care unit; MIC, Minimum inhibitory concentration; qPCR, quantitative polymerase chain reaction; VRE, Vancomycin-resistant enterococcus

* Correspondence: fabiannecarlesse@graacc.org.br
[1]Institute of Paediatric Oncology, Universidade Federal de São Paulo, Rua Botucatu 743, São Paulo 04037020, Brazil
Full list of author information is available at the end of the article

Background

Chemotherapy for childhood cancer is one of the greatest successes of modern medicine and the overall survival is now over 70 %. However myelossupression is a consequence of virtually all chemotherapy regimens and profound neutropenia (<0,5 × 10^9) is a major risk factor for overwhelming infections [1].

The relative frequency of different organisms causing bacterial infection may vary with time period and geographical location. Regardless of these variations in causative organism, and the widespread use and availability of powerful antibiotics, bacteremia/sepsis remains the most important independent prognostic marker for mortality in children with cancer who have febrile neutropenia. A diagnosis of sepsis or bacteremia increased in 10-fold increase risk of death [2].

In 40 % of children that have clinical diagnosis of sepsis and 75 % of those with high-risk FN, the microorganisms cannot be detected by currently available conventional microbiological techniques [3]. Early empirical treatment of fever in cancer patients remains the standard of care for the management of febrile neutropenia (FN).

In this context, our group developed an in-house, real-time, quantitative polymerase chain reaction (qPCR) directly from BACTEC blood culture (BC) bottles to identify the main pathogens and important resistance genes causing bloodstream infection (BSI) [4]. The aim of this study was to evaluate if this technique could anticipate and improve the diagnosis and therapy in paediatric cancer patients. The secondary objective was to describe the main pathogens of BSI and their antimicrobial susceptibilities.

Methods

Study design

Prospective study between March 2011 and March 2012 at the Institute of Paediatric Oncology, São Paulo, Brazil. Informed consent was obtained from all patients and the study was approved by the Clinical Research Ethics Committee of the Federal University of São Paulo. The samples were collected as part of standard care from patients suspected of BSI in the hospital. BSI was defined as the isolation of a bacterial or fungal pathogen from at least one BC.

All episodes of BSI were sub-classified as single agent (Gram-positive bacteria, Gram-negative bacteria, or fungi) or polymicrobial if two or more pathogens were isolated from a single BC.

We included only the BSI episodes for which BACTEC bottles were available for molecular tests without selection. We excluded polymicrobial episodes because it is not feasible to compare the conventional method with the molecular method if more than one agent grows in the same BC.

Data collection

Clinical data and bloodstream isolates were prospectively collected by local infection control practitioners.

Definitions

Neutropenia was defined as an absolute neutrophil count of <500 cells/mm^3 within 48 h after onset of bacteraemia [5]. Sepsis was defined as systemic inflammatory response syndrome in the presence of suspected or proven infection and organ dysfunction, according to international consensus guidelines. Septic shock was defined as sepsis with systolic blood pressure <90 mmHg that did not respond to adequate fluid resuscitation, and necessitated the use of a vasopressor. Severe sepsis was defined as inflammatory response syndrome triggered by a microorganism, identified or not, plus one of the following: cardiovascular organ dysfunction or acute respiratory distress syndrome; or dysfunction of two or more other organs: neurological, renal or hepatic [6].

Patients without any identifiable source of infection were classified as primary bacteraemia. Secondary BSIs were regarded as those with a clear source of bacteraemia other than a central line. Sources of secondary BSI were identified by culture of samples obtained from distant sites that yielded the same pathogen with an identical resistance pattern. Distant sites were sites other than a central line where an infection was diagnosed (e.g. pneumonia, urinary tract infection or abdominal infection). Intensive care unit (ICU) stay was defined as current stay in the ICU at onset of bacteraemia, regardless of previous history of ICU admission.

Empirical antimicrobial therapy was instituted according to the standard protocol of the institution [7] at the time of fever and suspicion of BSI after collection of blood culture. Antimicrobial therapy was analysed in two periods: Period 1: antibiotics in use when the Gram stain test of a positive bloodstream culture was available to the physician; and Period 2: antibiotics in use when the final results of microbial identification and antimicrobial susceptibility test were reported to the physician. Antimicrobial therapy was considered adequate if the treatment regimen included one or more antibiotics active in vitro against the microorganism identified by phenotypic tests.

Mortality associated with infection was defined as death within 14 days of bacteraemia and there was no other explanation for that.

Microbiological features

BCs were performed using the BACTEC 9240 instrument (Becton & Dickinson, Microbiology Systems, Cockeysville, MD, USA). Identification at the species level and susceptibility testing were performed using the automated system Phoenix 100 (Becton & Dickinson

Microbiology Systems). Minimum inhibitory concentration (MIC) determination was done by E test (AB Biodisk, Sweden) for oxacillin and carbapenems and by agar dilution for vancomycin, to confirm resistant phenotypes.

Molecular detection of microorganisms and resistance genes

Total DNA was extracted from 500 μL of positive or negative BC broth after incubation on BACTEC 9240, using the phenol–chloroform method (Brazol; LGC Biotechnologia, Cotia, Brazil) with 300-mg glass beads (0.3-mm diameter; Scientific Industries, Bohemia, NY, USA) and processed in a disruptor Genie (Scientific Industries) for 10 min to achieve cell lysis [4].

Real-time qPCR was performed as follows according to the protocols published by Menezes et al. in 2013 [4, 8]. Taqman-based multiplex detection of 16S rDNA gene with Gram-positive- and Gram-negative-specific probes; single SYBR green detection of each following resistance genes *bla*$_{SHV}$, *bla*$_{TEM}$, *bla*$_{CTX\text{-}M}$, *bla*$_{IMP}$, *bla*$_{SPM}$, *bla*$_{GIM}$, *bla*$_{SIM}$ *bla*$_{VIM}$, *bla*$_{KPC}$, *van*A, *van*B and *mec*A; and single Taqman-based detection of *Enterococcus* spp., coagulase-negative *Staphylococcus* (CoNS), *Staphylococcus aureus, Streptococcus pneumoniae, Escherichia coli, Klebsiella pneumoniae, Enterobacter cloacae, Proteus mirabilis, Salmonella* spp., *Serratia marcescens, Acinetobacter baumannii, Pseudomonas aeruginosa, Stenotrophomonas maltophilia, Mycobacterium tuberculosis, Aspergillus* spp., *Candida* spp. and *Fusarium* spp. were performed on an ABI 7500 real-time PCR System (Applied Biosystems, Foster City, CA, USA) instrument and quantified online and at the endpoint with sequence detection system software (version 2.0; Applied Biosystems) [4]. The primers were checked for specificity in a BLAST search available through the NCBI website (http://blast.ncbi.nlm.nih.gov/Blast.cgi). A primer set for the haemochromatosis gene was designed as an internal control for DNA extraction.

Resistance gene amplification by SYBR Green monoplex real-time PCR was performed in a 25-μL reaction mixture containing 12.5 μL Platinum SYBR Green qPCR SuperMix (Invitrogen, Carlsbad, CA, USA), 0.5 μM each primer, and 5 μL purified DNA extracted from samples. The real-time PCR conditions were as follows: 50 °C for 2 min and 95 °C for 10 min; 40 cycles of 95 °C for 15 s and 60 °C for 60 s; and a melting curve step (from 68 to 95 °C in increments of 0.5 °C/s). The metallo-β-lactamase amplification was performed by SYBR-based multiplex real-time PCR.

The samples with discordant antimicrobial resistance results between molecular and phenotypic analyses were submitted to a qPCR assay directly from of the isolates strains. For methicillin-resistant *Staphylococcus* strains with discordant results, we determined the MIC for oxacillin with E test (fabricante) and the diameter zone for cefoxitin with the disc diffusion method following the Clinical and Laboratory Standards Institute recommendations.

Data collection was performed using SSPS version 17.0 software (SPSS Inc., Chicago, IL, USA) and Microsoft Office Excel 2010 (Microsoft, Redmond, WA, USA).

Results

Study population and patients characteristics

We identified 168 episodes of BSI, 81 episodes were included in the study with BACTEC BC bottles and were randomly available for molecular tests. Twelve episodes with polymicrobial culture results were excluded and our final data comprised 69 episodes of BSI from 64 patients.

Patients had a mean age of 7.8 years (range 0–22 years), and 57.8 % were male. The underlying diseases were: 20 % (13/64) acute lymphoid leukaemia; 19 % (12/64) central nervous system tumour; 14 % (9/64) acute myeloid leukaemia (AML); 9 % (6/64) non Hodgkin's lymphoma; 8 % (5/64) neuroblastoma; 6 % (4/64) retinoblastoma; 5 % (3/64) osteosarcoma; 3 % (2/64) Ewing's sarcoma; 2 % (1/64) Wilms' tumour; and 20 % (13/64) others less common childhood tumours.

Among the potential factors predisposing to BSI, a central line catheter was present in 83 % (57/69), previous antimicrobial therapy was administered in 54 % (37/69), and neutropenia was present in 61 % (42/69). At onset of clinical evaluation, the use of antimicrobial therapy was observed in 85 % (59/69), sepsis was present in 68 % (47/69), septic shock occurred in 4 % (4/69), and severe sepsis in 3 % (2/69). Primary bacteraemia occurred in 91 % (63/69). Among secondary BSI caused by Gram-positive bacteria, the skin was the source in 60 %, followed by lungs and intestinal tract. In Gram-negative BSI, only one pulmonary secondary episode of BSI was identified.

Sixteen patients died during the study period, and six of these episodes occurred within 14 days and were related to BSI.

Phenotypic bacterial identification

Among 69 BSI episodes, 61 % (42/69) were caused by Gram-positive bacteria, 32 % (22/69) by Gram-negative bacteria, and 7 % (5/69) by fungi (Table 1). The three major pathogens of BSI were: CoNS in 26 % (18/69), followed by *S. aureus* in 13 % (9/69), and *P. aeruginosa* in 12 % (8/69). Five episodes were caused by fungi: *Candida tropicalis, Candida parapsilosis, Candida guillermondi, Candida lusitaniae* and *Rhodotorula* spp. (Table 1).

Comparison of molecular with phenotypic identification methods

We performed phenotypic (automated) and molecular (qPCR) method for 69 positive samples taken directly

Table 1 Rank order of bloodstream pathogens isolated from BSI in paediatric cancer patients

Agents	69 (100 %)
Gram positive	42 (61)
CoNS	18 (26)
Staphylococcus aureus	9 (13)
Viridans group *Streptococcus*	6 (9)
Streptococcus spp.	3 (4)
Corynebacterium spp.	2 (3)
Enterococcus spp.	2 (3)
Other Gram positive	2 (3)
Gram negative	22 (32)
Pseudomonas. aeruginosa	8 (12)
Escherichia coli	6 (9)
Klebisiella pneumoniae	3 (4)
Enterobacter cloacae	2 (3)
Other Gram negative	3 (4)
Fungi	5 (7)
Candida tropicalis	1 (1)
Candida parapsilosis	1 (1)
Candida guillermondi	1 (1)
Candida lusitaniae	1 (1)
Rhodotorula spp.	1 (1)

CoNS Coagulase negative *Staphylococci*

from BC bottles and compared both methods. The overall concordance was 78.2 % for final species identification.

Among 42 samples positive for Gram-positive bacteria detected by BC processing, 36 were positive by Gram-postive 16 rDNA gene probe. Of these 36, 27 were identified at specie level by qPCR, 8 were identified by DNA sequencing and 7 were not identified. Three samples were discordant; in two of them the molecular method was not able to identify any microorganism, and one BC showed *S. aureus* and CoNS by qPCR. For 22 samples with Gram-negative isolates identified by BC processing, we observed a concordance of 81.8 % (18/22) with the molecular method. In two of these samples, qPCR was not able to identify the species, and in another two samples, the methods were discordant for species identification (Table 2).

Methicillin resistance was detected in 88 % (24/27) of the 27 *Sthaphylococcus* spp. samples identified by the phenotypic method. The *mec*A gene was detected in 22/24, corresponding to 91.6 % of concordance.

Two strains were identified as *Enterococcus* spp., and one of them was resistant to vancomycin by the phenotypic method. There was 100 % of concordance with detection of *vanA* by the molecular method.

The qPCR for extended spectrum β-lactamase (ESBL) coding genes was concordant with the phenotypic

Table 2 Discordant episodes between phenotypic and molecular tests of isolates from BSI in paediatric cancer patients

Episode	Phenotypic method	Molecular method
24	*Staphylococcus warneri*	Negative
29	*Staphylococcus aureus*	Negative
47	*Staphylococcus aureus*	CoNS
5	*Escherichia coli*	Negative
59	*Pseudomonas aeruginosa*	Negative
68	*Burkholderia cepacia*	CoNS/*Ralstonia pickettii*

CoNS Coagulase negative *Staphylococci*

susceptibility profile test in 71.4 % (10/14) for Enterobacteriaceae.

Among four discordant samples, two were *E. coli* and had phenotypic detection of ESBL but no resistance gene was detected by the molecular method. One sample positive for *E. coli* with susceptibility to cephalosporins showed bla_{CTX}, which was not detected directly from the isolated colony. The last discordant sample was positive for *E. cloacae*, with resistance to cephalosporins, but no resistance gene was detected. We did not detect any Enterobacteriaceae resistant to carbapenems by the phenotypic method and by the molecular method for bla_{KPC}, bla_{IMP} and bla_{VIM} (Table 3).

Eight samples were positive for non-fermenting Gram-negative bacteria by the phenotypic method, and qPCR for resistance genes was performed in seven, we excluded the *Achromobacter* spp. sample.

Carbapenem resistance Pseudomonas aeruginosa was phenotypically detected in four samples while two samples were negative for bla_{SPM} gene. There was 50 % concordance between both methods. One of these samples had the bla_{SPM} resistance gene detected when testing the isolate strain (Table 3).

Five samples were positive for fungi, four *Candida* spp. and one *Rhodotorula* spp., and the molecular method was able to identify 80 % of the samples with *Candida*.

Antimicrobial therapy evaluation and death

Regarding antimicrobial therapy in Period 1, we observed inadequacy in 43 %. All except one episode were submitted to medical intervention at that time. In Period 2, the inadequacy remained in 12 % of episodes.

Death occurred in 16 % (11/69) of all the BSI episodes, and six of these episodes occurred within 14 days and were related to the BSI. The molecular method was concordant with phenotypic identification of the agent in 50 % of these episodes. Therapy in Period 1 was inadequate in patients whose death was related to BSI (5/6). In Period 2, three of them remained inadequate even after intervention. In these cases, we were able to identify bla_{SPM} in *P. aeruginosa* and *van*A in *Enterococcus faecium* by molecular test (Table 4).

Table 3 Resistance genes identified by molecular method and antimicrobial susceptibility for Gram-negative BSI

Episode	Phenotypic method	Resistance gene	Cefepime susceptibility	Meropenem susceptibility
1	*Klebsiella pneumoniae*	Negative	Susceptible	Susceptible
2	*Acinetobacter baumannii*	Negative	Susceptible	Susceptible
5	*Escherichia coli*	Negative	Resistant	Susceptible
6	*Escherichia coli*	Negative	Susceptible	Susceptible
8	*Serratia marcescens*	Negative	Susceptible	Susceptible
11	*Enterobacter cloacae*	Negative	Susceptible	Susceptible
16	*K. pneumoniae*	Negative	Susceptible	Susceptible
17	*Klebsiella oxytoca*	Negative	Susceptible	Susceptible
18	*Achromobacter* spp.	Negative	NT	NT
21	*Escherichia coli*	Negative	Susceptible	Susceptible
25	*Enterobacter cloacae*	Negative	Resistant	Susceptible
32	*Pseudomonas putida*	Negative	NT	NT
38	*Pseudomonas aeruginosa*	Negative	Resistant	Resistant
41	*Klebsiella pneumoniae*	bla_{TEM} bla_{CTX}	Resistant	Susceptible
43	*Escherichia coli*	bla_{CTX}	Susceptible	Susceptible
46	*Pseudomonas aeruginosa*	bla_{SPM}	Resistant	Resistant
49	*Escherichia coli*	Negative	Resistant	Susceptible
50	*Pseudomonas aeruginosa*	Negative	Resistant	Susceptible
54	*Citrobacter freundii*	bla_{CTX}	Resistant	Susceptible
59	*Pseudomonas aeruginosa*	Negative	Resistant	Resistant
65	*Escherichia coli*	Negative	Susceptible	Susceptible
68	*Burkholderia cepacia*	Negative	NT	Resistant

NT not tested

Discussion

The strategy of using empirical antibiotic therapy has greatly influenced the outcome of fever in paediatric cancer patients. Unfortunately, BC can identify pathogens in only 40 % of children with fever and can take >24 h to yield a report [3].

We evaluated 69 episodes of BSI from 64 patients. The predominant underlying disease was haematological malignancy, this group of patients constitute the group of major risk for development of invasive bacterial infections, due to aggressive chemotherapy that results in long periods of neutropenia [9].

In our study, more than half of our patients were neutropenic, which has been recognised as an important risk factor for life-threatening infection since the 1960s when Bodey et al. identified a strong inverse correlation between the degree of neutropenia and the probability of infection [10–12].

We found a predominance of Gram-positive bacteria followed by Gram-negative bacteria, and fungi. Although we only studied a small sample, our results agree with our historic series and with the literature [7, 9, 13].

Among Gram-positive bacteria, CoNS was the main agent found, followed by *Staphylococcus aureus* which

Table 4 Phenotypic susceptibility, molecular tests and antimicrobial therapy of patients with death related to BSI

Episode	Underlying disease	Method		Phenotypic susceptibility			Resistance gene	Antimicrobial therapy	
		Phenotypic	Molecular	Cefepime	Meropenen	Vancomycin		Period 1	Period 2
5	AML	*E. coli*	Negative	Resistant	Susceptible	NA	Neg	Modified	Adequate
31	Other	*C. tropicalis*	*Candida* spp.	NA	NA	NA	NA	Adequate	Adequate
46	Wilms' tumour	*P. aeruginosa*	*P. aeruginosa*	Resistant	Resistant	NA	bla_{SPM}	Modified	Inadequate
56	ALL	*C. lusitanae*	Negative	NA	NA	NA	NA	Modified	Inadequate
58	ALL	*P. aeruginosa*	Negative	Resistant	Resistant	NA	Neg	Modified	Adequate
69	RMS	*E. faecium*	*Enterococcus* spp.	NA	NA	Resistant	*vanA*	Modified	Inadequate

ALL acute lymphoid leukaemia, *RMS* Rhabdomyosarcoma, *Neg* negative, *NA* not applicable

agrees with most epidemiological studies in this setting and is related with catheter implantation [14, 15].

Complications of *S. aureus* infection have been reported in paediatric cancer patients in 10–18 % of all infections and up to 33 % of cases of bacteraemia [16]. In our study, the majority of the patients with *S. aureus* infection had central venous catheter (CVC) (66 %) and primary bacteraemia. Mortality from *S. aureus* in paediatric oncologic setting is reported at 2.3 % [16]. No patient with *S. aureus* BSI died in our study.

Viridans group Streptococcus was the third in rank order of BSI in our patients. Infections due to viridans group *Streptococcus* have been seen especially in patients with AML, corresponding to ~25 % of all BSIs in these patients [17]. The mortality rate is high as 20 % [18]. In institutions with a high prevalence of this agent, the initial empirical antibiotic therapy includes vancomycin [19].

Among Gram-negative isolates, Enterobacteriaceae were predominant, with *E. coli* followed by *K. pneumoniae* as the main agents.

Pseudomonas aeruginosa was the main agent among non-fermenting bacteria and despite improvement in recent years, the prognosis of infection due this agent in this patient population remains poor, with case fatality rates exceeding 20 % [20]. Our institution has been treating patients with FN according to risk stratification for life-threatening infections; patients considered low risk receive moxifloxacin as outpatients, and high-risk patients receive cefepime as inpatients [7, 21].

We compared 69 positive BC episodes using phenotypic and molecular methods. The overall concordance was 78.2 % for final species identification, which is similar to a study conducted by Varani et al. in 2009 who found 79.2 % concordance between the two methods [22]. Comparing the two methods only for Gram-positive pathogens, the final species concordance identification was 89.6 %.

Recent studies have observed an increase in methicillin-resistant *Staphylococcus* infections, especially in patients with haematological malignancies; 70–80 % among CoNS and 25–30 % among *S. aureus* [23]. We detected 78 % methicillin resistance in BSI caused by *S. aureus*. The molecular method was able to detect the *mec*A gene in 93 % of these cases. Two samples were discordant, and when the molecular method was applied directly to the isolated colonies, it was concordant with the phenotypic method. Samples in which the phenotypic method shows methicillin resistance and the *mecA* gene is not found must be evaluated for *mecC*, and if this is present, patients must be managed as if they have methicillin-resistant *S. aureus* [24].

Resistance to vancomycin among enterococci has emerged as a general problem and is now found in patients with FN [25]. We found that 5 % of BSIs were due to *Enterococcus* spp., and 50 % were VRE. In our study we had one patient with VRE BSI infection who died 4 days after he had a positive BC and 1 day after the final result of BC emerged, which reflects the importance of early diagnosis. The molecular method was concordant in 100 % of the cases. Early identification of VRE is important beyond the therapeutic approach because this contributes to infection control procedures to avoid the spread of these microorganisms.

Three of our four *P. aeruginosa* isolates were resistant to carbapenems by the phenotypic method, which agreed with our molecular method in 50 % of cases. In the two discordant samples, we tested for the presence of the *MBL* genes directly from the isolated colonies; one of which was positive for bla_{SPM} and one negative for *MBL* genes. This suggests that another mechanism was responsible for carbapenem resistance, such as porin loss or efflux systems.

Even though the rate of infection with carbapenem-resistant *Acinetobacter* spp. is increasing, we found only one infection due to *A. baumannii* and it was susceptible to cefepime and carbapenems.

Enterobacteriaceae were predominant among Gram-negative isolates, and the main agent was *E. coli*, followed by *K. pneumoniae*, with a high concordance in final species identification between the two methods.

The literature shows an incidence of ESBL among *E. coli* varying from 12.6 to 48.3 % [26, 27]. In our study, 60 % of *E. coli* were ESBL producers, showing 78.5 % concordance with the molecular method. Three samples were discordant. Two of those had a phenotypic profile of ESBL and no resistance genes were detected. The other sample was susceptible to cephalosporins, and we found bla_{CTX-M}, which was not confirmed in an additional test performed directly on the isolated colony. The patient received treatment with cefepime and had a good outcome.

Regarding fungal infection, our molecular method was able to identify yeasts, with the exception of one episode of *C. lusitaniae* that was responsible for one death. This is an uncommon species of *Candida* in these patients and it is important to note that it can be resistant to amphotericin B [28].

The impact of early appropriate antibiotic therapy on patient survival has been demonstrated in previous studies [1, 12, 29, 30]. In our study, we showed that only one of six patients who died within 14 days after BSI had adequate initial empirical therapy. Therapy was modified in five cases based on Gram staining of the positive BC (Period 1) and after the final results, three treatments remained inadequate. The molecular method was able to identify the microorganism and resistance gene in two of these three cases.

Early identification of the causative organism and resistance genes such as *vanA* for enterococci and *MBL* for *P. aeruginosa* is crucial for adequate antimicrobial therapy, especially in paediatric neutropenic patients. Our empirical treatment approach does not take into account the resistant microorganisms shown in our study.

A limitation of the method is that PCR is so sensitive that we could not exclude the risk of false positive from skin contamination during blood culture collection particularly for CoSN. Other molecular mechanisms of resistance could be added since our "in house" multiplex is done in an open qPCR plataform.

Conclusions

The addition of molecular tests, including qPCR, for identification of pathogens and detection of antimicrobial resistance genes to the classical phenotypic tests in BSI is particularly relevant in paediatric cancer patients.

Acknowledgements
This study was supported by a grant from Fundação de Amparo a Pesquisa do estado de São Paulo (FAPESP) Brazil.

Funding
There has been no significant financial support for this work that could have influenced its outcome.

Authors' contributions
FC carried out the data clinical acquisition, data analysis and draft the manuscript; PC; LCM and ASP participated of the design of the study, MGQ performed the PCR experiments and provided the molecular analyses; ACCP participated in the design and coordination of study. All authors read and approved the final manuscript.

Competing interests
The authors declare that they have no competing interests.

Consent for publication
Not applicable.

Author details
[1]Institute of Paediatric Oncology, Universidade Federal de São Paulo, Rua Botucatu 743, São Paulo 04037020, Brazil. [2]Infectious Diseases Division, Universidade Federal de São Paulo, São Paulo, Brazil.

References
1. Lehrnbecher T, Phillips R, Alexander S, Alvaro F, Carlesse F, Fisher B, et al. Guideline for the management of fever and neutropenia in children with cancer and/or undergoing hematopoietic stem-cell transplantation. J Clin Oncol. 2012;30:4427–38.
2. Basu SK, Fernandez ID, Fisher SG, Asselin BL, Lyman GH. Length of stay and mortality associated with febrile neutropenia among children with cancer. J Clin Oncol. 2005;23:7958–66.
3. Santolaya ME, Farfan MJ, De LM V, Cocina M, Santelices F, Alvarez AM, et al. Diagnosis of bacteremia in febrile neutropenic episodes in children with cancer: microbiologic and molecular approach. Pediatr Infect Dis J. 2011;30:957–61.
4. Menezes LC, Rocchetti TT, Bauab KC, Cappellano P, Quiles MG, Carlesse F, et al. Diagnosis by real-time polymerase chain reaction of pathogens and antimicrobial resistance genes in bone marrow transplant patients with bloodstream infections. BMC Infect Dis. 2013;13:166.
5. Freifeld AG, Bow EJ, Sepkowitz KA, Boeckh MJ, Ito JI, Mullen CA, et al. Clinical practice guideline for the use of antimicrobial agents in neutropenic patients with cancer: 2010 Update by the Infectious Diseases Society of America. Clin Infect Dis. 2011;52:427–31.
6. Goldstein B, Giroir B, Randolph A. International pediatric sepsis consensus conference: definitions for sepsis and organ dysfunction in pediatrics. Pediatr Crit Care Med. 2005;6:2–8.
7. Petrilli A, Altruda CF, Alberto Pires PC. Oral gatifloxacin in the outpatient treatment of children with cancer fever and neutropenia. Pediatr Blood Cancer. 2007;49:682–6.
8. Quiles MG, Menezes LC, Bauab KC, Gumpl EK, Rocchetti TT, Palomo FS, et al. Diagnosis of bacteremia in pediatric oncologic patients by in-house real-time PCR. BMC Infect Dis. 2015;15:283.
9. Castagnola E, Fontana V, Caviglia I, Caruso S, Faraci M, Fioredda F, et al. A prospective study on the epidemiology of febrile episodes during chemotherapy-induced neutropenia in children with cancer or after hemopoietic stem cell transplantation. Clin Infect Dis. 2007;45:1296–304.
10. Pizzo PA. Infectious complications in the child with cancer. I. Pathophysiology of the compromised host and the initial evaluation and management of the febrile cancer patient. J Pediatr. 1981;98:341–54.
11. Hakim H, Flynn PM, Srivastava DK, Knapp KM, Li C, Okuma J, et al. Risk prediction in pediatric cancer patients with fever and neutropenia. Pediatr Infect Dis J. 2010;29:53–9.
12. Bodey GP, Buckley M, Sathe YS, Freireich EJ. Quantitative relationships between circulating leukocytes and infection in patients with acute leukemia. Ann Intern Med. 1966;64:328–40.
13. Pereira CA, Marra AR, Camargo LF, Pignatari AC, Sukiennik T, Behar PR, et al. Nosocomial bloodstream infections in Brazilian pediatric patients: microbiology, epidemiology, and clinical features. PLoS One. 2013;8:e68144.
14. Cortez D, Rodriguez N, Benadof D, Zamorano A, Tordecilla J. Bacteremia in cancer patients. Experience in a pediatric hospital. Rev Chil Infectol. 2012;29:164–8.
15. Aslan S, Citak EC, Yis R, Degirmenci S, Arman D. Bacterial spectrum and antimicrobial susceptibility pattern of bloodstream infections in children with febrile neutropenia: experience of single center in southeast of Turkey. Indian J Microbiol. 2012;52:203–8.
16. McNeil JC, Hulten KG, Kaplan SL, Mahoney DH, Mason EO. Staphylococcus aureus infections in pediatric oncology patients: high rates of antimicrobial resistance, antiseptic tolerance and complications. Pediatr Infect Dis J. 2013;32:124–8.
17. Han SB, Bae EY, Lee JW, Lee DG, Chung NG, Jeong DC, et al. Clinical characteristics and antimicrobial susceptibilities of viridans streptococcal bacteremia during febrile neutropenia in patients with hematologic malignancies: a comparison between adults and children. BMC Infect Dis. 2013;13:273.
18. Gassas A, Grant R, Richardson S, Dupuis LL, Doyle J, Allen U, et al. Predictors of viridans streptococcal shock syndrome in bacteremic children with cancer and stem-cell transplant recipients. J Clin Oncol. 2004;22:1222–7.
19. Hakim H, Flynn PM, Knapp KM, Srivastava DK, Gaur AH. Etiology and clinical course of febrile neutropenia in children with cancer. J Pediatr Hematol Oncol. 2009;31:623–9.
20. Vuotto F, Berthon C, Lemaitre N, Duhamel A, Balkaran S, Le RE, et al. Risk factors, clinical features, and outcome of Pseudomonas aeruginosa bacteremia in patients with hematologic malignancies: a case-control study. Am J Infect Control. 2013;41:527–30.
21. Petrilli AS, Dantas LS, Campos MC, Tanaka C, Ginani VC, Seber A. Oral ciprofloxacin vs. intravenous ceftriaxone administered in an outpatient setting for fever and neutropenia in low-risk pediatric oncology patients: randomized prospective trial. Med Pediatr Oncol. 2000;34:87–91.
22. Varani S, Stanzani M, Paolucci M, Melchionda F, Castellani G, Nardi L, et al. Diagnosis of bloodstream infections in immunocompromised patients by real-time PCR. J Infect. 2009;58:346–51.
23. Solis Y, Alvarez AM, Fuentes D, de la Barra D, Aviles CL, Becker A, et al. Bloodstream infections in children with cancer and high risk fever and

neutropenia episodes in six hospitals of Santiago, Chile between 2004 and 2009. Rev Chil Infectol. 2012;29:156–62.
24. Shore AC, Deasy EC, Slickers P, Brennan G, O'Connell B, Monecke S, et al. Detection of staphylococcal cassette chromosome mec type XI carrying highly divergent mecA, mecI, mecR1, blaZ, and ccr genes in human clinical isolates of clonal complex 130 methicillin-resistant Staphylococcus aureus. Antimicrob Agents Chemother. 2011;55:3765–73.
25. Allendorf SD, Cortez A, Heinemann MB, Harary CM, Antunes JM, Peres MG, et al. Rabies virus distribution in tissues and molecular characterization of strains from naturally infected non-hematophagous bats. Virus Res. 2012;165:119–25.
26. Trecarichi EM, Tumbarello M, Spanu T, Caira M, Fianchi L, Chiusolo P, et al. Incidence and clinical impact of extended-spectrum-beta-lactamase (ESBL) production and fluoroquinolone resistance in bloodstream infections caused by Escherichia coli in patients with hematological malignancies. J Infect. 2009;58:299–307.
27. Gudiol C, Tubau F, Calatayud L, Garcia-Vidal C, Cisnal M, Sanchez-Ortega I, et al. Bacteraemia due to multidrug-resistant Gram-negative bacilli in cancer patients: risk factors, antibiotic therapy and outcomes. J Antimicrob Chemother. 2011;66:657–63.
28. Pfaller MA, Andes DR, Diekema DJ, Horn DL, Reboli AC, Rotstein C, et al. Epidemiology and outcomes of invasive candidiasis due to non-albicans species of Candida in 2,496 patients: data from the Prospective Antifungal Therapy (PATH) registry 2004–2008. PLoS One. 2014;9:e101510.
29. Petrilli AS, Bianchi A, Kusano E, Melaragno R, Naspitz C, Mendonca JS, et al. Fever and granulocytopenia in children with cancer: a study of 299 episodes with two treatment protocols in Brazil. Med Pediatr Oncol. 1993;21:356–61.
30. Pizzo PA, Commers J, Cotton D, Gress J, Hathorn J, Hiemenz J, et al. Approaching the controversies in antibacterial management of cancer patients. Am J Med. 1984;76:436–49.

5

Klebsiella pneumoniae bloodstream infections at a South African children's hospital 2006–2011

Heloise Buys[1,2,3*], Rudzani Muloiwa[1,2], Colleen Bamford[2,4] and Brian Eley[1,2]

Abstract

Background: *Klebsiella pneumoniae* (KP) is a significant paediatric bloodstream pathogen in children. There is little data from Africa. In this study we describe the epidemiology of multi-drug resistant *Klebsiella pneumoniae* bloodstream infection (KPBSI) at Red Cross War Memorial Children's Hospital, Cape Town, South Africa.

Methods: We conducted a retrospective cross-sectional study of KPBSI from 1 January 2006 to 31 December 2011 using conventional descriptive and inferential statistical methods.

Results: Of 410 hospitalised children with laboratory confirmed KPBSI, 339 (83 %) were caused by extended-spectrum β-lactamase (ESBL) producing isolates. The median age (IQR) was 5.0 (2–16) months, 212 (51.7 %) were male, 82 (20 %) were HIV-infected, and 241 (58.8 %) were moderately or severely underweight. The infection was hospital-acquired or healthcare-associated in 389 (95 %) children and community-acquired in 21 (5 %) children. Significant risk factors for ESBL-KPBSI included cephalosporin exposure in the 12 months prior to the KPBSI, adjusted risk ratio (aRR) 1.18 (95 % CI: 1.06–1.31); HIV infection, aRR 1.14 (1.04–1.25), and intravenous infusions for more than 3 days before the KPBSI, aRR 1.15 (95 % CI: 1.04–1.28).

A total of 109 (26.6 %) children died within 30 days of the KPBSI, their median age was four (IQR 1–11) months. The median (IQR) time between KPBSI and death was three (1–9) days. HIV-infection, aRR 2.44(95 % CI: 1.59–3.74); skin erosions at the time of KPBSI, aRR 2.15 (95 % CI: 1.54–3.00); being in PICU at the time of the KPBSI, aRR 1.64 (95 % CI: 1.03–2.61) or needing PICU admission after developing KPBSI, aRR 1.72 (95 % CI: 1.10–2.70) were significant risk factors for death.

Conclusion: ESBL-producing KP is an important cause of laboratory confirmed bloodstream infection in hospitalised children and is associated with high mortality.

Keywords: *Klebsiella pneumoniae* bloodstream infection, Children, Africa

Background

Klebsiella pneumoniae (KP) is a significant bloodstream pathogen resulting in major treatment and cost challenges for health institutions [1]. There is little data on children from Africa where the effects of socioeconomic inequalities and inadequate healthcare delivery remain challenging and influence the outcome of infectious diseases.

* Correspondence: heloise.buys@uct.ac.za
[1]Department of Paediatrics and Child Health, Red Cross War Memorial Children's Hospital, Klipfontein Road, Cape Town, Rondebosch 7700, South Africa
[2]University of Cape Town, Cape Town, South Africa

International reports show that extended-spectrum β-lactamase (ESBL) producing Gram-negative bloodstream infections (BSI) occur mainly in the setting of hospital exposure. Reported risk factors for ESBL-strain acquisition in paediatric Gram-negative BSI including KP include prior cephalosporin exposure [2–6], prior hospitalisation [3, 5], prolonged hospitalisation [7], previous corticosteroid use [2, 6], prolonged total parenteral nutrition [8], paediatric intensive care unit (PICU) admission [3], presence of a central venous pressure (CVP) line [6], neutropaenia [6], and underlying renal disease [4].

The outcome data from the limited number of paediatric studies involving Gram-negative BSI including KP portray high mortality ranging from 12.9 to 36 % [2–5, 7–10].

Over the last few years anecdotal observation suggested that ESBL-producing KP frequently caused invasive infection at our hospital. We therefore reviewed laboratory-confirmed KPBSI from 1 January 2006 to 31 December 2011 to document the extent of the problem at our hospital. The specific objectives of the study were to describe the clinical presentation of KPBSI, risk factors associated with ESBL-KPBSI, antibiotic susceptibility patterns of the KP isolates and KPBSI mortality including factors associated with in-patient mortality.

Methods

Study design and setting

This hospital based retrospective case folder review was conducted at Red Cross War Memorial Children's Hospital (RCWMCH), Cape Town, Western Cape province, South Africa. RCWMCH is a 282- bedded public children's hospital for children aged 0–13 years; it is also an academic teaching hospital of the University of Cape Town and is one of two local tertiary referral units that service 1.5 million children <14 years of age in the Western Cape. An average of 3500 new children per month (range 3000 to 6000 per month) are evaluated in its medical emergency unit, and the total number of hospital admissions peaks at 23 000 children per annum. There is a 20-bedded multidisciplinary PICU, an 18-bed burn unit, 13-bed oncology unit, 60 mixed surgical beds, 58 general paediatric beds; 29-bed cardiology and tracheostomy ward, 29 specialty medical beds, 10-bed trauma unit and 42 short stay medical beds. Dedicated newborn care is available at other hospitals in Cape Town where obstetric care is provided. Admission numbers peak during diarrhoeal seasonal months (December to April) and overcrowding commonly occurs throughout the hospital. The main entry points into the hospital are via the medical emergency or trauma units.

Study population

Most of the children admitted to RCWMCH come from homes in low socioeconomic, peri-urban settlements in the Western Cape Province. The Medical Microbiology laboratory of the National Health Laboratory Service (NHLS) identified and forwarded an electronic list of *Klebsiella pneumoniae* bloodstream isolates identified between 1 January 2006 and 31 December 2011 for children admitted to RCWMCH.

Data collection

Data were collected from paper-based medical records including patient demographics, admission diagnosis, HIV and nutrition status, age, date of current hospital admission, underlying medical condition, previous medical history, antibiotic history, site of KPBSI, potential risk factors for ESBL-KPBSI and mortality, length of hospital stay and outcome.

Laboratory procedures

All microbiology testing was conducted at the Groote Schuur National Health Laboratory Service (NHLS) microbiology laboratory. The laboratory used the BACTEC™ 9240 automated blood culture system (Becton Dickinson, Sparks, Maryland. For blood culture bottles flagging positive with mono-morphic Gram-negative bacilli seen on Gram stain, a locally validated method of direct inoculation into the automated Vitek®2 system (bioMérieux, Inc, France) was employed, [11] using Vitek® ID-GNB and AST-N133 cards for identification and susceptibility testing respectively. This direct method was supplemented, where necessary with repeat testing from bacterial colonies subcultured onto agar plates, using either Vitek, disk diffusion or E-test (bioMérieux, Marcy l'Etoile, France) methods. The following antibiotics were tested: ampicillin, co-amoxyclav, piperacillin-tazobactam, cefuroxime, cefoxitin, ceftriaxone, ceftazidime, cefepime, ertapenem, meropenem, imipenem, ciprofloxacin, gentamicin, amikacin, cotrimoxazole, tigecycline and colistin. Susceptibility results were interpreted according to the Clinical Laboratory Standards Institute (CLSI) criteria for the relevant years [12]. ESBLs were detected by the Vitek® 2 Advanced Expert system or by the double disk synergy method if using disk diffusion testing. Despite the changes to reporting of cephalosporin susceptibility in ESBL-producing organisms introduced by CLSI in 2010, the laboratory, in line with the contemporary national practice, continued to report ESBL- producing *Enterobacteriaceae* as resistant to all cephalosporins. Since ESBL production was not explicitly reported on the laboratory information system (LIS) due to limitations in the design and setup of the interface, ESBL production was assumed if *Klebsiella pneumoniae* isolates were reported to the clinicians (on the LIS) as resistant to all cephalosporins.

Definitions

Hospital-acquired Klebsiella pneumoniae Blood Stream infection (HA-KPBSI)

Klebsiella pneumoniae blood stream infection detected 48 h or more after hospital admission and not incubating at the time of hospitalisation [13].

Healthcare-associated (HCA)-KPBSI

Klebsiella pneumoniae blood stream infection detected within 48 h of hospital admission in children who have had contact with the healthcare service including admission to an intermediate care facility during the 12-month period preceding hospitalisation. An intermediate facility provides step-down care for children recovering from acute illness, for a maximum duration of 6 weeks [13].

Community-acquired (CA)-KPBSI

Klebsiella pneumoniae blood stream infection detected within 48 h of hospital admission without previous contact with the healthcare service.

ESBL-producing KP (ESBL KP)

Klebsiella pneumoniae isolates were classified as ESBL-producing if they were resistant to cefepime [13].

HIV infection

A positive HIV DNA PCR result confirmed by either a HIV RNA PCR or repeat HIV DNA PCR test, in any child < 18 months old, or 2 positive serological test results (HIV ELISA or HIV Rapitest) or a positive HIV DNA PCR result confirmed by either a HIV RNA PCR or repeat HIV DNA PCR test, in a child > 18 months old were considered HIV-infected [14].

Unknown HIV status

Any infant of child where there was no record of HIV testing at the NHLS laboratory database and whose mother's HIV status was unknown.

Severe immunosuppression

A CD4 percentage and / or an absolute CD4 count below the age defined range in an HIV-infected child, using the 2006 WHO definitions [15].

Nutritional status

Moderate and severe underweight were defined as weight-for-age z score (WAZ) between −2 and −3 standard deviations (SD) below the median World Health Organisation (WHO) growth reference standards, and a WAZ < −3 SD respectively.

Skin erosion

A burn wound or another form of skin loss (e.g. skin loss as a consequence of severe napkin dermatitis) documented in the medical or nursing notes.

Data analysis

Clinical data were extracted retrospectively from the hospital folders. Antibiotic sensitivity results were obtained from the NHLS microbiology database. The data were analysed using STATA Statistical software, release 11, (College Station, Texas, USA). Proportions were depicted as percentages. Continuous variables were tested for normality and mean and standard deviation (SD) or median and interquartile range (IQR) used to describe the data as appropriate. The Kruskal-Wallis equality of populations' rank test or Wilcoxon rank-sum tests for independent samples were used to compare all continuous variables. Factors associated with the outcome risk of ESBL- infection or mortality were explored by univariate analysis. Generalised linear models using Poisson regression with robust error variance were used to estimate risk ratios and 95 % confidence intervals after controlling for potential confounding factors. A two sided significance level of $p < 0.05$ was used in all calculations. Infection risk was calculated per 1000 hospital admissions.

Results

Risk of *Klebsiella pneumoniae* bloodstream infections

Over the 6-year study period, 410 hospitalised children had laboratory confirmed KPBSI, of whom 339 (83 %) had ESBL-KPBSI. The infection was hospital-acquired in 353, (86.1 %), healthcare-associated in 36, (8.8 %) or community-acquired in 21, (5 %). The annual risk of HA-KPBSI and ESBL-KPBSI increased from 2007, peaking in 2009 and then declining in 2011 (Fig. 1). Children hospitalised with CA-KP BSI were younger, compared to those with HA- or HCA-KPBSI, median age of 1.5 (IQR 0.7–3.8) months versus 5.5 (IQR 1.9–16.2) months, p-value = 0.01.

Characteristics of the study population

The median age was 5.0 months (IQR 2 to 16 months), 198 were male and 212 female (Table 1). Two hundred and forty one (58.8 %) children were moderately or severely underweight-for-age (UWFA).

Two hundred and six (50.2 %) children were HIV negative, 82 (20 %) were HIV-infected, and the HIV-status was unknown in 122 (29.8 %) children. There were more HIV-infected children with moderate or severe UWFA compared to uninfected children, 61/82 (74.4 %), versus 126/206 (61.2 %), $p = 0.03$. The CD4-lymphocyte counts within the 3 month period preceding KPBSI were known in 71/82 (86.6 %) of all HIV-infected children. The median absolute CD4 count was 639 cells/mm^3 (IQR 285 to 1235) and the mean CD4 percentage was 21.8 % (SD ± 12.33). Forty-two of 71 (59.2 %) HIV-infected children were severely immunosuppressed by CD4 percentage-for-age and 55/71 (77.5 %) severely immunosuppressed by absolute CD4 count-for age. Forty-one (50 %) of the eighty-two HIV-infected children were on antiretroviral therapy (ART) at the time of the KPBSI. The median time on ART before the KPBSI was 19 (IQR 8–66) days. The annual proportion of children on ART increased progressively over the study period (Fig. 2).

During the 12 month period preceding KPBSI, 40 % (155/387) of the children had received antibiotics such as 2nd – 4th generation cephalosporins, fluoroquinolones, macrolides, cotrimoxazole, aminoglycosides, piperacillin-tazobactam, and/or carbapenems. Those who acquired

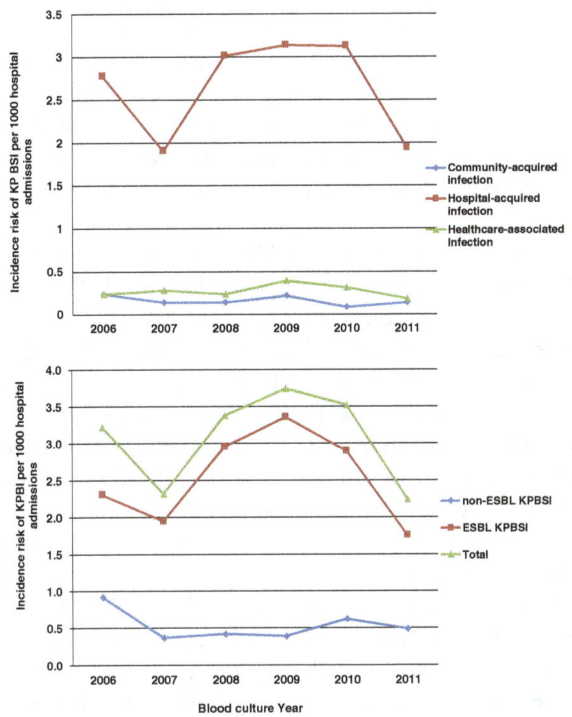

Fig. 1 Incidence risk of Klebsiella pneumoniae bloodstream infection (KPBSI) per 1000 hospital admissions at RCWMCH January 2006- December 2011. Legend: ESBL-KPBSI: extended spectrum β-lactamase producing *Klebsiella pneumoniae* bloodstream infection

ESBL-KPBSI had higher preceding antibiotic exposure (Table 1). The median time from hospitalisation to KPBSI was significantly shorter for children with non-ESBL-KPBSI compared to those who developed ESBL-KPBSI, 3 (IQR 0–7) days versus 9 (IQR 4–23) days, $p < 0.0001$.

There were 29 (6.3 %) children who had either confirmed malignancy (26/29) or aplastic anaemia (3/29). Their mean age was 69.6 months (SD ± 50.29) and 41.4 %(12/29) were male. The infection was HA-KPBSI in 26/29 (90 %) children, caused by ESBL-producing KP in all but 3 children and occurred in the neutropenic phase in 20/29 (70 %) children. At the time of the KP-BSI, their median white cell count was 0.6 × 10^9 /L (IQR 0.3–1.4).

Throughout the study period, HA-KPBSI caused by ESBL-producing isolates predominated (Table 2). Among children with CA-KPBSI, the number of ESBL-producing isolates remained low. Furthermore, there was a 47 % reduction in ESBL-KPBSI events between 2010 and 2011, from 63 to 37.

Spectrum of KP bloodstream infection

At the time of the KPBSI 70 % of children (284/405) experienced fever i.e., temperature of ≥38.0 °C. Although there was a wide range of clinical manifestations at the time of KPBSI, 80 % of the children either presented without a definable clinical focus or with pneumonia (Table 3).

Table 1 Characteristics of the children with *Klebsiella pneumoniae* bloodstream infection

Variable	All	ESBL-KP[b]	Non-ESBL-KP	*p* value
Number of children (%)	*N* = 410	*n* = 339/410 (83 %)	*n* = 71/410 (17 %)	-
Male: female	212: 198	170: 169	1.77	0.17
Median (IQR) age in months	5 (2–16)	5 (2–5)	10 (2–29)	0.12
Median weight-for-age z-score (IQR)	−2 (−4 to −1)	−2 (−4 to −1)	−1 (−3 to −1)	0.02
Moderate under-weight-for-age n/N (%)	78/410 (19.0)	66/339 (19.5)	12 /71 (16.9)	0.14
Severe underweight-for-age n/N (%)	163/410 (39.8)	143/339 (42.2)	20 /71 (28.2)	0.01
HIV-infection[a] (%)	(*n* = 288)	(*n* = 249)	(*n* = 39)	
	82 (28.5)	79 (31.7 %)	3 (7.7 %)	0.004
Exposure to a selection of antibiotics[c]	319/388 (82.2)	287/319 (90)	31/68 (46.4)	<0.0001
2nd - 4th generation Cephalosporins	205/388 (52.8)	190/205 (92.8)	15 /69 (17.8)	<0.0001
Aminoglycosides	227/388 (58.5)	206/319 (64.6)	21/69 (30.4)	<0.0001
Cotrimoxazole	96/388 (24.7)	91/319 (28.5)	5/69 (7.3)	0.001
Carbapenems	69/388 (17.8)	65/319 (20.4)	4 /69 (5.8)	0.004
Piperacillin-tazobactam	107/388 (27.6)	95/319 (29.8)	12/69 (17.4)	0.04
Fluoroquinolones	55/388 (14.2)	48/319 (15.1)	7/69 (10.1)	0.29

KP Klebsiella pneumoniae, *IQR* interquartile range, *n/N* stratum specific proportions
[a]HIV prevalence known in 288 children
[b]ESBL-KP: extended-spectrum-β-lactamase-producing *Klebsiella pneumoniae*
[c]Exposure to the following antibiotics within the last 12 months before the KP bloodstream infection: 2nd and/or 3rd and/or 4th generation cephalosporins, macrolides, fluoroquinolones, cotrimoxazole, aminoglycosides, piperacillin-tazobactam, and carbapenems

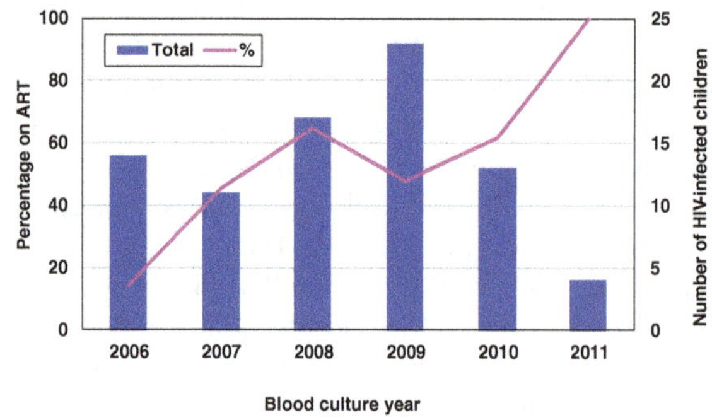

Fig. 2 The number and percentage of HIV-infected children per annum with KP BSI on ART during the study period, 2006–2011. Legend: KP BSI-*Klebsiella pneumoniae* bloodstream infection; ART-Antiretroviral therapy

Risk factors for ESBL-associated KP infection

More children with ESBL-KPBSI were moderately or severely underweight than those who had non-ESBL KPBSI, i.e., 61.7 % (209/339) versus 45.1 % (32/71); $p = 0.01$; RR 1.13 (95%CI 1.02–1.24). Univariate analysis showed that infancy, concomitant HIV infection, cephalosporin exposure during the preceding 12 month period, mechanical ventilation prior to BSI, intravenous infusion for more than 3 days before the onset of KPBSI, an indwelling urinary catheter prior to KPBSI, major surgical procedure preceding KPBSI and a KP infection in the 12 months preceding the current KPBSI were significant risk factors for ESBL-KPBSI. On multivariate analysis HIV infection, cephalosporin exposure in the 12 month period before the KPBSI and continuous intravenous infusion for more than 3 days before the KPBSI remained significant risk factors for the acquisition of ESBL-KPBSI (Table 4).

Antibiotic sensitivity profile of the isolates

All isolates, both ESBL- ($n = 339$) and non-ESBL-producing ($n = 71$) were resistant to ampicillin. Of all isolates tested, 21 % (86/409) were sensitive to gentamicin, 76.1 % (312/410) were sensitive to amikacin, 60.5 % (211/349) were sensitive to piperacillin-tazobactam, and 29.1 % (117/402] were sensitive to co-amoxyclav. All isolates were sensitive to the carbapenems imipenem (409/409 tested) and meropenem (409/409 tested), and 99.5 % [403/405) were sensitive to ertapenem. The disaggregated antibiotic sensitivity patterns of the KP isolates are shown in Table 5.

Of the 82 HIV-infected children, 38 (46.3 %) were on cotrimoxazole prophylaxis prior to the KPBSI and 96.3 % of their isolates (79/82) were ESBL-producing organisms. All (38/38) isolates of HIV-infected children on cotrimoxazole prophylaxis were resistant to cotrimoxazole as well as 37/39 (97 %) isolates of those who were not on cotrimoxazole prophylaxis. In 29 children with malignancy or aplastic anaemia, 20/29 (70 %) isolates were sensitive to piperacillin and/or amikacin.

Antibiotic therapy

Data on antibiotic therapy were available for 398 children. Antibiotic therapy was considered appropriate if the laboratory reported the organism as susceptible to the specific antibiotic and suboptimal if the organism was reported as being intermediately susceptible or resistant. Empiric antibiotic therapy was appropriate in 307/398 (77.1 %) children comprising 241/328 (73.5 %) children with ESBL KPBSI and 66/70 (94.3 %) children with non-ESBL KPBSI. Piperacillin plus amikacin was the empiric antibiotic choice in 18/29 (62 %) children with malignancy or aplastic anaemia whilst 7/29 (24 %) received a carbapenem; 25/29 (86 %) children received a carbapenem as the definitive antibiotic. Once antibiotic susceptibility results became available, antibiotic therapy was adjusted in patients in whom empiric therapy was suboptimal. This delay did not alter the 30 day mortality significantly i.e. 26.4 % (74/280) of children on appropriate empiric therapy died versus 35.3 % (30/85) on delayed optimal therapy, $p = 0.11$, RR 0.75 (95 % CI: 0.53–1.06).

Table 2 Number and percentage of non-ESBL producing and ESBL producing *Klebsiella pneumoniae* BSI within each infection category 2006–2011

Year	Community-Acquired Infection		Hospital-acquired infection		Healthcare-associated Infection		Total
	ESBL KPBSI n (%)	Non-ESBL KPBSI n (%)	ESBL KPBSI n (%)	Non-ESBL KPBSI n (%)	ESBL KPBSIN (%)	Non-ESBL KPBSI n (%)	Total KPBSI n (100 %)
2006	3 (4.3)	2 (2.9)	46 (65.7)	14 (20.0)	1 (1.4)	4 (5.7)	70 (17)
2007	0	3 (6.0)	38 (76.0)	3 (6.0)	4 (8.0)	2 (4.0)	50 (12)
2008	3 (4.1)	0	59 (80.8)	6 (8.2)	2 (2.7)	3 (4.1)	73 (18)
2009	1 (1.2)	4 (4.7)	68 (79.1)	4 (4.7)	8 (9.3)	1 (1.2)	86 (21)
2010	0	2 (2.5)	63 (78.8)	8 (10.0)	3 (3.8)	4 (5.0)	80 (20)
2011	0	3 (5.9)	37 (72.6)	7 (13.7)	3 (5.9)	1 (2.0)	51 (12)
Totals	7 (1.7)	14 (3.4)	311 (76.0)	42 (10.0)	21 (5.1)	15 (3.7)	410 (100)

ESBL KPBSI extended-spectrum-β-lactamase-producing *Klebsiella pneumoniae* bloodstream infection, *BSI* bloodstream infection

Table 3 The clinical site of infection in children with *Klebsiella pneumoniae* bloodstream infection

Clinical site of infection	All n/N (%)	ESBL n/N (%)	Non-ESBL n/N (%)	*p* value
No. with primary bloodstream infection without a definable focus	206/410 (50.5)	159/339 (46.9)	47/71 (66.2)	0.004
Common sites of infection				
Pneumonia	122 (29.8)	108 (31.9)	14 (19.7)	0.04
Vascular-catheter related	20 (4.9)	19 (5.6)	1 (1.4)	0.13
Peritonitis	20 (4.9)	16 (4.7)	4 (5.6)	0.76
UTI[a]	20 (4.9)	16 (4.7)	4 (5.6)	0.76
Septic wound and soft tissue	23 (5.7)	21 (6.2)	2 (2.8)	0.26
NEC[b]	20 (4.9)	18 (5.3)	2 (2.8)	0.37
Septic drip site (+ve[c] culture of KP)	12 (2.9)	11 (3.2)	1 (1.4)	0.4
Cholangitis	4 (1.0)	4 (1.2)	0	N/S
Dysentery	3 (0.7)	2 (0.6)	1 (1.4)	0.4
Typhilitis	3 (0.7)	3 (0.9)	0	N/S
Bacterial endocarditis	1 (0.2)	1 (0.3)	0	N/S
Necrotic tumour	1 (0.2)	1 (0.3)	0	N/S
Bowel obstruction	1 (0.2)	1 (0.3)	0	N/S

n/N stratum specific proportions, *UTI*[a] urinary tract infection, *NEC*[b], necrotising enterocolitis, *+ve*[c] positive, *ESBL* extended-spectrum-β-lactamase-producing *Klebsiella pneumoniae*

KPBSI mortality

One hundred and twenty-three of the 410 study children died over the 6 year period, giving a crude case fatality rate of 30 %. Only the children dying within 30 days of the KPBSI (109/410, 26.6 %) were included in the mortality analysis as there was higher chance of identifying factors associated with KPBSI mortality in these children. Deaths occurring beyond this time period were deemed unlikely to be related to the KPBSI. The mean time to death from KPBSI diagnosis of the 14 children who died after 30 days was 46.4 (SD ±11.2) days. Among the 109 patients dying within 30 days, the median time to death ($n = 109$) was 3 days (IQR 1–9 days) (Table 6). One hundred (91.7 %) of the deaths were associated with ESBL-KPBSI. In 37.6 % (41/109) children the deaths occurred in children with ESBL KPBSI without a definable focus and 41.3 % (45/109) occurred in children who manifested with pneumonia. The KPBSI was community acquired in four (3.7 %) children who died, two of whom had non-ESBL KP isolates. Hospital-acquired (92/109, 84.4 %) and healthcare-associated (13/109, 11.9 %) KPBSI accounted for the rest of the mortality. Of the children who died 70.6 % (77/109) had a chronic underlying medical disorder, most commonly HIV infection (37 children), congenital cardiac conditions (11 children) and gastrointestinal conditions (14 children).

Factors contributing to 30-day mortality on univariate analysis included ESBL KPBSI, HIV infection, KPBSI requiring admission to PICU, and the presence of skin erosions, while KPBSI without a source had a protective effect. On multivariate analysis HIV infection, being in the PICU at the time of the BSI, KPBSI requiring admission to PICU, and the presence of skin erosions were significant risk factors for death (Table 7).

Discussion

In this hospital based retrospective study we have described laboratory-confirmed *Klebsiella pneumoniae* bloodstream infections in children admitted to RCWMCH from 1 January 2006–31 December 2011. This is the first

Table 4 Factors associated with ESBL-*Klebsiella pneumoniae* bloodstream infection (BSI)

Risk factors for ESBL KPBSI	ESBL	Non-ESBL	Univariate analysis		Adjusted analysis ($n = 271$)	
	n/N (%)	n/N (%)	RR[a] (95 % CI)	*p*-value	RR (95 % CI)	*p*-value
Moderate or severe underweight for age	209/339 (61.7)	32/71 (45.1)	1.13 (1.02–1.24)	0.01	0.99 (0.97–1.01)	0.40
HIV-infection	79/249 (31.7)	3/39 (7.7)	1.22 (1.13–1.30)	<0.001	1.14 (1.04–1.25)	**0.01**
Patient in the PICU[b]	92/339 (27.1)	11/71 (15.5)	1.11 (1.02–1.21)	0.04	0.99 (0.88–1.12)	0.94
Cephalosporin exposure in the last 12 months pre-BSI	184/339 (54.3)	12/71 (16.9)	1.30 (1.18–1.42)	<0.001	1.18 (1.06–1.31)	**0.002**
Mechanical ventilation prior to BSI	142/335 (42.4)	13/71 (18.3)	1.19 (1.10–1.29)	<0.001	1.08 (0.93–1.24)	0.31
Continuous infusion for >3 days prior to BSI	247/334 (74.0)	30/71 (42.3)	1.31 (1.16–1.49)	<0.001	1.15 (1.04–1.28)	**0.009**
Indwelling urinary catheter prior to BSI	139/335 (41.5)	12/71 (16.9)	1.20 (1.10–1.30)	<0.001	1.09 (0.99–1.20)	0.10
Major surgical procedure prior to BSI[c]	115/336 (34.2)	16/71 (22.5)	1.10 (1.01–1.20)	0.04	1.06 (0.95–1.18)	0.33
Skin erosions	111/336 (33.0)	19/71 (26.8)	1.05 (0.96–1.15)	0.30	1.07 (0.98–1.17)	0.12
Previous KP infection within last 12 months	39/338 (11.5)	3/71 (4.2)	1.14 (1.03–1.26)	0.01	0.96 (0.84–1.11)	0.62

Multivariable model adjusted for gender, age, HIV infection, underweight-for-age, mechanical ventilation, patient in the PICU at the time of the BSI, continuous IV infusion for more than 3 days before the BSI, indwelling urinary catheter, major surgery before the BSI, Previous KP infection within last 12 months, skin erosions and cephalosporin exposure during last 12 months before the BSI. aRR adjusted risk ratio

ESBL-KP extended-spectrum-β-lactamase-producing *Klebsiella pneumoniae*, *BSI* bloodstream infection

[a]RR risk ratio; [b]PICU: paediatric intensive care unit; [c] A major surgical procedure included a laparotomy (emergency or elective), a thoracotomy, a skin graft or a craniotomy; Risk ratio 95 % confidence intervals that do not cross the null value of 1 are shown in bold

Table 5 Antibiotic susceptibility results of extended spectrum beta lactamase (ESBL) and non-ESBL *Klebsiella pneumoniae* isolates

Antibiotic	Number of resistant isolates			
	Non-ESBL KP		ESBL KP	
	n/N	(%)	n/N	(%)
Ampicillin	71/71	(100)	339/339	(100)
Co-amoxyclav	5/71	(7.1)	280/331	(84.6)
Cefotaxime	0/71	(0)	339/339	(100)
Ceftazidime	0/71	(0)	339/339	(100)
Cefepime	0/71	(0)	339/339	(100)
Ciprofloxacin	0/71	(0)	142/339	(41.9)
Cotrimoxazole	18/71	(25.4)	313/339	(92.3)
Amikacin	0/71	(0)	98/339	(28.9)
Gentamicin	4/71	(5.6)	319/338	(94.4)
Piperacillin-Tazobactam	2/67	(3.0)	136/282	(48.2)
Ertapenem	0/67	(0)	2/338	(0.6)
Imipenem	0/71	(0)	0/338	(0)
Meropenem	0/71	(0)	0/338	(0)

KP Klebsiella pneumoniae, ESBL KPBSI Extended-spectrum-beta-lactamase-producing *Klebsiella pneumoniae* bloodstream infection, *co-amoxyclav* amoxicillin-clavulanic acid co-formulation, *n/N* stratum specific proportions

comprehensive analysis of *Klebsiella pneumoniae* bloodstream infections in hospitalised children at a dedicated children's hospital in Sub-Saharan Africa. This study showed that ESBL- *Klebsiella pneumoniae* is an important cause of HA- and HCA-BSI and is associated with high mortality.

Notably 68.9 % of the children were less than 12 months old. In the only other large published paediatric case series on *KPBSI* that involved 57 American children, infancy was also the predominant age-category i.e., 68 % ($n = 38/57$) of the children were less than 12 months [10]. Young children, particularly infants, are not fully immunocompetent and more susceptible to bacterial infections including KPBSI. Young age and immunological immaturity may also contribute to the delayed diagnosis of sepsis [16]. A high prevalence of moderate and severe underweight, an indicator of malnutrition was documented. On univariate analysis moderate or severe underweight-for-age was more frequent in children with ESBL-KPBSI (209/339, 61.7 %) compared to those with non-ESBL KPBSI (32/71, 45.1 %); $p = 0.01$. Malnutrition is known to be associated with widespread micronutrient deficiencies, immune dysfunction, and susceptibility to infectious complications [17].

Table 6 Time to death in 3 time categories in study children with *Klebsiella pneumoniae* bloodstream infection

Cause of death	Time to death from KPBSI							
	≤3 days		3.1–14 days		14.1–30 days		Totals	
	n	(%)	n	(%)	n	(%)	n	(%)
Septicaemia	48	(44.0)	28	(25.7)	8	(7.3)	84	(77.1)
Pneumonia	6	(5.5)	4	(3.7)	5	(4.6)	15	(13.8)
Other	3	(2.8)	5	(4.6)	2	(1.8)	10	(9.1)
Totals	57	(52.3)	37	(33.9)	15	(13.8)	109	(100)

The study population was representative of the children living in the Western Cape region, coming mainly from peri-urban, low socio-economic sub-districts. National figures show that the incidence of under-weight-for-age (UWFA) in children <5 varied from 16/1000 (2012) to 22/1000 (2009) and that the incidence of severe acute malnutrition was 4-5/1000 (2009–2012) [18]. The 2011 national Census established that 40 % of 5 million South African children <5 years-of-age were UWFA and that there was a high incidence of stunting (26.9 %) in children <3 years-of age [19, 20]. Concomitant HIV infection is known to be a significant contributor to malnutrition and was present in 20 % of the study children.

At the time of the positive blood culture 30 % (126/410) of the study children did not experience fever and 50.2 % had no definable clinical focus. When a focus was present this was commonly in the lungs. In a parallel study on *Staphylococcus aureus* bloodstream infection at our hospital, 33 % of children had no identifiable source and, where one was identified, the lungs were the most common focus (22 %) [21]. In another paediatric study describing BSIs caused by of Gram-negative pathogens including *KP*, the absence of a clear clinical focus occurred in 68 % of the study subjects [6]. Unlike a child presenting from home with a CA-BSI where the clinical manifestations precipitate presentation to a health facility, HA-BSI may manifest with non-specific signs leading to delay in recognising active infection. Furthermore, the decision to take blood cultures were made by the caring clinicians based on clinical indications; given the retrospective study design no attempt was made to interrogate the possibility of blood culture contamination.

In the current study KPBSI was primarily a hospital-acquired infection caused by ESBL-producing isolates. Community-acquired infection was uncommon, particularly community-acquired infection caused by ESBL-producing isolates. These findings are similar to previous studies describing Gram-negative BSI in children [6, 22]. Prior cephalosporin exposure increased the risk for ESBL-KPBSI, confirming findings of previous paediatric studies [2–5]. Two additional statistically significant risk factors were identified. The risk of HIV infection probably relates to the underlying immunodeficiency, particularly as 50 % of the HIV-infected children were not on ART at the time of acquiring KPBSI. The risk of continuous intravenous infusion for more than 3 days before the BSI was diagnosed may result from poor infection control practice and / or contamination of the infused

Table 7 Factors associated with 30-day inpatient mortality in children with *Klebsiella pneumoniae* bloodstream infection

Risk factors for death	Alive	Died	Univariate analysis		Adjusted RR[a] for mortality ($n = 259$)	
	n/N (%)	n/N (%)	RR[a] (95 % CI)	*p*-value	aRR (95 % CI)	*p*-value
ESBL-KPBSI	210/267 (78.7)	100/109 (91.7)	2.36 (1.26–4.43)	0.00	1.09 (0.55–2.16)	0.80
Moderate or severe underweight-for-age	150/267 (56.2)	71/109 (65.1)	1.31 (0.94–1.83)	0.11	1.12 (0.79–1.62)	0.54
HIV-infection**	38/181 (21.0)	37/83 (44.6)	2.03 (1.44–2.85)	<0.001	2.44 (1.59–3.74)	<0.001
Patient in the PICU at time of BSI**	56/267 (21.7)	31/109 (28.4)	1.28 (0.91–1.80)	0.16	1.64 (1.03–2.61)	0.04
Patient needing to go to PICU at the time of KP bloodstream infection**	44/267 (16.5)	34/109 (31.2)	1.73 (1.26–2.38)	0.001	1.72 (1.10–2.70)	0.02
Continuous IV infusion for >3 days before the BSI	174/264 (65.9)	73/108 (67.6)	1.06 (0.75–1.48)	0.76	0.93 (0.64–1.35)	0.70
BSI without source**	145/266 (54.5)	41/108 (38.0)	0.61 (0.44–0.86)	0.004	0.82 (0.55–1.22)	0.33
Chronic underlying medical condition excluding HIV infection	124/267 (46.4)	41/109 (37.6)	0.77 (0.56–1.07)	0.12	1.30 (0.81–2.08)	0.28
Skin erosions**	70/265 (26.4)	47/108 (43.5)	1.69 (1.24–2.30)	0.001	2.15 (1.54–3.0)	<0.001

n/N stratum specific proportions; ***p*-value ≤ 0.05; *RR* risk ratio
ESBL KP BSI Extended-spectrum-beta-lactamase-producing *Klebsiella pneumoniae* bloodstream infection, *PICU* paediatric intensive care unit, *aRR* adjusted risk ratio
*:Multivariate model adjusted for age, gender, nutrition, HIV infection, ESBL, Patient in PICU, patient needing to go to PICU, continuous IV infusion for >3 days before the BSI, KPBSI without source, chronic underlying medical condition excluding HIV, and skin erosions

fluid during intravenous drug administration. Published studies have implicated these factors, but no paediatric study has previously shown a statistical relation between BSI and prior intravenous infusion on multivariate analysis [23, 24].

At the time of the study, empiric antibiotic therapy at RCWMCH for CA-BSI was ampicillin plus gentamicin and for HA- and HCA-BSI, piperacillin-tazobactam plus amikacin. These empiric regimens were also applied to children who had malignancy or aplastic anaemia. The study findings suggest that these empiric antibiotic combinations would not have been effective against 22.9 % of non-susceptible isolates, intermediate or resistant, in patients with KPBSI. Once antibiotic susceptibility results were made available to the attending clinicians these patients were started on effective antibiotic therapy, and the resultant delay did not significantly affect 30-day mortality. However, the low cover for HA- and HCA-BSI suggest that more effective empiric antibiotic therapy using a carbapenem should be considered. This suggestion concurs with previous studies [3, 5]. During the study period there was full access to all classes of appropriate antibiotics that were reported by the NHLS microbiology laboratory including ertapenem, imipenem and meropenem.

There was a notable surge and decrease in the risk of ESBL-producing KP HA-infection over 2009 and 2010. The impact of a South African measles epidemic starting in the Western Cape Province in 2009, peaking during a diarrhoeal surge season in March and April of 2010 and then abating in November of the same year was associated with severe pressure on beds and subsequent overcrowding in all wards of the hospital, this may have accounted for the surge seen. The falling trend in the risk thereafter at the hospital may well also reflect some success of the preventive strategy package driven by the hospital infection control unit e.g., increased awareness of the importance of hand hygiene, training on how to perform hand hygiene and an effort to reduce overcrowding in certain key areas of the hospital.

The impact of Gram-negative bacteraemia is significant in children with reduced immunity, including those with cancer, and access to carbapenem antibiotics is important particularly as the control of sepsis during febrile neutropenic episodes is time-critical.

The high 30-day fatality rate of 26.6 % and with 52.3 % of the deaths occurring within 3 days of the positive blood culture result were consistent with previous paediatric studies of Gram-negative BSI including *KP* where mortality ranged from 13 to 36 % [2, 3, 8–10] and a bacteraemia study in rural Kenya in which 70.5 % of deaths occurred within 3 days of positive blood culture [25]. In the present study HIV infection, being in the PICU at the time of BSI or needing PICU admission and the presence of skin erosions were significant risk factors for death. Previous paediatric studies have identified a different spectrum of independent risk factors for death including the presence of an ESBL-producing organism, shock on admission to hospital and more than 48-h delay in initiating appropriate antibiotic therapy, and in neonates infectious complications after the onset of BSI and pulmonary hypertension. In the present study, mortality was higher in children who received suboptimal empiric antibiotic therapy (35.3 % vs 26.4 %). Although this difference appeared clinically relevant, it did not achieve statistical significance, partly because the analysis was underpowered on post-hoc evaluation i.e., power of 36 % at an alpha of 0.05.

Study strengths and limitations

A strength of this study is that it is the first large African study to describe KPBSI in children, providing clinical and epidemiological information which was not previously available. Because of the retrospective study design, there were limitations in the availability and completeness of clinical and laboratory data. For example, the HIV status of 122 children was not known because there was no documentation of testing in the clinical notes or at the laboratory. Were these results available they would have influenced the risk factor analyses. One further strength of the study was that the ESBL status of the KP isolates did not influence the extraction of data from the folder review because the study team were blinded to status at the time of the data collection. The true burden of community-acquired KPBSI, particularly non-ESBL KPBSI events may have been underestimated. Before sick children are referred from primary or secondary health facilities to RCWMCH, they are often administered parenteral broad-spectrum antibiotics consistent with the World Health Organization Integrated Management of Childhood Illness guidelines that have been adapted for use in South Africa [26]. This practice frequently results in negative blood culture results. Further, due to the retrospective design the history and detail of exposure to previous hospitalisation and antibiotics was limited to what was documented in the case folders by the admitting doctors and any pharmacy prescription sheets that were available; any outpatient exposures and admissions to hospitals other than RCWMCH that were not recorded in the folders were not captured and could have led to potential under reporting as exposed to antibiotics. Because of the limitations associated with laboratory reporting, for the purposes of this study, *KP* was assumed to be an ESBL producer if it was reported to clinicians as resistant to all cephalosporins. The laboratory continued to report ESBL-producing Enterobacteriaceae as resistant to all cephalosporins, despite changes in reporting practices introduced by CLSI in 2010, hence there may have been over reporting of cephalosporin resistance in the latter years. Due to limitations in laboratory interfaces MIC data are not routinely available to clinicians.

Although the results of this study may not be generalizable to other referral hospitals or community facilities, they demonstrate that KPBSI is an important childhood infection and substantially improved infection control practice is required to reduce the burden of hospital-acquired KPBSI.

Conclusion

Multi-drug resistant *Klebsiella pneumoniae* bloodstream infection is associated with high mortality in children. Our analysis together with previous studies suggest that this infection is strongly associated with hospitalisation. Prospective studies are required to further explore the clinical and epidemiological observations documented in this study, and characterise the microbiological features and relatedness of KP isolates causing BSI in our setting.

Abbreviations

aRR: Adjusted risk ratio; ART: Antiretroviral therapy; BSI: Bloodstream infection; CA: Community-acquired; CLSI: Clinical Laboratory Standards Institute; CVP: Central venous pressure; ESBL KP: Presumed extended spectrum β-lactamase producing *Klebsiella pneumoniae*; ESBL: Extended spectrum β-lactamase; HA: Hospital-acquired; HCA: Healthcare-associated infection; HIV: Human immunodeficiency virus; IQR: Interquartile range; KP: *Klebsiella pneumoniae*; *KPBSI*: *Klebsiella pneumoniae* bloodstream infection; LIS: Laboratory information system; NEC: Necrotising enterocolitis; NHLS: National Health Laboratory Service; PICU: Paediatric intensive care unit; RCWMCH: Red Cross War Memorial Children's Hospital; SD: Standard deviation; UTI: Urinary tract infection; UWFA: Underweight-for-age; WAZ: Weight-for-age z-score; WHO: World Health Organisation

Acknowledgements

The study children who inspired this work. The dedicated nurses and doctors working at the children's hospital are acknowledged. We thank Sister Spasina King for assistance in data collection, Mr Henri Carrara of the School of Public Health and Family Medicine, Faculty of Health Sciences, University of Cape Town, Dr Katherina Kranzer of the London School of Hygiene and Tropical Medicine, UK and Dr Vash Pillay of the Department of Paediatrics and Child Health, Faculty of Health Sciences, University of Cape Town, for statistical advice.

Funding

Heloise Buys was supported in part by a Harry Crossley scholarship; the funders had no role in study design, data collection, data analysis, data interpretation, or writing of the report. The corresponding author had full access to all the data in the study and had final responsibility for the decision to submit for publication.

Authors' contributions

HB conceptualised and designed the study, acquired the data, performed the research, had full access to all of the data in the study, drafted the manuscript and approved the final manuscript as submitted and takes full responsibility for the integrity of the data and the accuracy of the data analysis. RM: Helped with the planned statistical analysis of the data, reviewed and revised the manuscript and approved the final manuscript. CB: aided in planning the study, reviewed and revised the manuscript and approved the final manuscript. BE: conceptualised and designed the study, supervised, reviewed and revised the manuscript and approved the final manuscript.

Competing interests

The authors declare that they have no competing interests.

Consent for publication

Not applicable.

Author details

[1]Department of Paediatrics and Child Health, Red Cross War Memorial Children's Hospital, Klipfontein Road, Cape Town, Rondebosch 7700, South Africa. [2]University of Cape Town, Cape Town, South Africa. [3]Ambulatory and Emergency Paediatrics, Red Cross War Memorial Children's Hospital, Klipfontein Road, Cape Town, Rondebosch 7700, South Africa. [4]National Health Laboratory Service (Groote Schuur Hospital), Cape Town, South Africa.

References

1. Pitout JD, Laupland KB. Extended-spectrum beta-lactamase-producing Enterobacteriaceae: an emerging public-health concern. Lancet Infect Dis. 2008;8(3):159–66.

2. Zaoutis TE, Goyal M, Chu JH, Coffin SE, Bell LM, Nachamkin I, McGowan KL, Bilker WB, Lautenbach E. Risk factors for and outcomes of bloodstream infection caused by extended-spectrum β-lactamase–producing Escherichia coli and Klebsiella species in children. Pediatrics. 2005;115(4):942–9.
3. Kim Y-K, Pai H, Lee H-J, Park S-E, Choi E-H, Kim J, Kim J-H, Kim E-C. Bloodstream infections by extended-spectrum β-lactamase-producing Escherichia coli and Klebsiella pneumoniae in children: epidemiology and clinical outcome. Antimicrob Agents Chemother. 2002;46(5):1481–91.
4. Tsai MH, Chu SM, Hsu JF, Lien R, Huang HR, Chiang MC, Fu RH, Lee CW, Huang YC. Risk factors and outcomes for multidrug-resistant Gram-negative bacteremia in the NICU. Pediatrics. 2014;133(2):e322–9.
5. Ariffin H, Navaratnam P, Mohamed M, Arasu A, Abdullah WA, Lee CL, Peng LH. Ceftazidime-resistant Klebsiella pneumoniae bloodstream infection in children with febrile neutropenia. Int J Infect Dis. 2000;4(1):21–5.
6. Levy I, Leibovici L, Drucker M, Samra Z, Konisberger H, Ashkenazi S. A prospective study of Gram-negative bacteremia in children. Pediatr Infect Dis J. 1996;15(2):117–22.
7. Kuo KC, Shen YH, Hwang KP. Clinical implications and risk factors of extended-spectrum beta-lactamase-producing Klebsiella pneumoniae infection in children: a case–control retrospective study in a medical center in southern Taiwan. J Microbiol Immunol Infect. 2007;40(3):248–54.
8. Samanta S, Farrer K, Breathnach A, Heath PT. Risk factors for late onset gram-negative infections: a case–control study. Arch Dis Child Fetal Neonatal Ed. 2011;96(1):F15–8.
9. Velaphi S, Wadula J, Nakwa F. Mortality rate in neonates infected with extended-spectrum beta lactamase-producing Klebsiella species and selective empirical use of meropenem. Ann Trop Paediatr. 2009;29(2):101–10.
10. Bonadio WA. Klebsiella pneumoniae bacteremia in children. Fifty-seven cases in 10 years. Am J Dis Child. 1989;143(9):1061–3.
11. Bamford C, Goodway J, Hoffmann R. Rapid identification and susceptibility testing of Gram-negative bacilli from blood cultures using the Vitek® 2 system: original research. S Afr J Epidemiol Infect. 2010;25(3):28–31.
12. Cockerill FR. Performance standards for antimicrobial susceptibility testing: twenty-first informational supplement: Clinical and Laboratory Standards Institute (CLSI); 2011.
13. Cardoso T, Almeida M, Friedman ND, Aragão I, Costa-Pereira A, Sarmento AE, Azevedo L. Classification of healthcare-associated infection: a systematic review 10 years after the first proposal. BMC med. 2014;12(1):40.
14. Schneider E, Whitmore S, Glynn K, Dominguez K, Mitsch A, McKenna MT, Control CfD, Prevention. Revised surveillance case definitions for HIV infection among adults, adolescents, and children aged < 18 months and for HIV infection and AIDS among children aged 18 months to < 13 years—United States, 2008. MMWR Recomm Rep. 2008;57(RR-10):1–12.
15. Organization WH: Antiretroviral drugs for treating pregnant women and preventing HIV infection in infants in resource-limited settings: towards universal access: recommendations for a public health approach: World Health Organization; 2006
16. Clapp DW. Developmental regulation of the immune system. Semin Perinatol. 2006;30(2):69–72.
17. Beisel WR. Nutrition and immune function: overview. J Nutr. 1996;126(10S): 2611S.
18. National Department of Health SA. Second triennial report of the Committee on Morbidity and Mortality in Children Under 5 Years (CoMMiC): 2014. In.
19. Shisana O, Labadarios D, Rehle T, Simbayi L, Zuma K, Dhansay A, Reddy P, Parker W, Hoosain E, Naidoo P, Hongoro C, Mchiza Z, Steyn NP, Dwane N, Makoae M, Maluleke T, Ramlagan S, Zungu N, Evans MG, Jacobs L, Faber M, SANHANES-1 Team. South African National Health and Nutrition Examination Survey (SANHANES-1). Cape Town: HSRC Press; 2013.
20. Statistics South Africa: Mid-year population estimates, 2011. In.; 2011.
21. Naidoo R, Nuttall J, Whitelaw A, Eley B. Epidemiology of Staphylococcus aureus bacteraemia at a tertiary children's hospital in Cape Town, South Africa. PLoS One. 2013;8(10):e78396.
22. Al-Hasan MN, Huskins WC, Lahr BD, Eckel-Passow JE, Baddour LM. Epidemiology and outcome of Gram-negative bloodstream infection in children: a population-based study. Epidemiol Infect. 2011;139(5):791–6.
23. Koerner R, Morgan S, Ford M, Orr K, McComb J, Gould F. Outbreak of Gram-negative septicaemia caused by contaminated continuous infusions prepared in a non-clinical area. J Hosp Infect. 1997;36(4):285–9.
24. Moodley P, Coovadia YM, Sturm AW. Intravenous glucose preparation as the source of an outbreak of extended-spectrum b-lactamase-producing Klebsiella pneumoniae infections in the neonatal unit of a regional hospital in KwaZulu-Natal: original article. S Afr Med J. 2005;95(11):861–4.
25. Berkley JA, Lowe BS, Mwangi I, Williams T, Bauni E, Mwarumba S, Ngetsa C, Slack MP, Njenga S, Hart CA. Bacteremia among children admitted to a rural hospital in Kenya. N Engl J Med. 2005;352(1):39–47.
26. World Health Organisation DoHSA: Integrated Management of Childhood Illness (IMCI) guidelines. 2011

6

Risk factors for bloodstream infection in patients at a Brazilian hemodialysis center

Dayana Fram[1*], Meiry Fernanda Pinto Okuno[1], Mônica Taminato[1,2], Vinicius Ponzio[3], Silvia Regina Manfredi[4], Cibele Grothe[1], Angélica Belasco[1], Ricardo Sesso[5] and Dulce Barbosa[1]

Abstract

Background: Infection is the leading cause of morbidity and the second leading cause of mortality in patients on renal replacement therapy. The rates of bloodstream infection in hemodialysis patients vary according to the type of venous access used. Gram-positive bacteria are most frequently isolated in blood cultures of hemodialysis patients. This study evaluated risk factors for the development of bloodstream infections in patients undergoing hemodialysis.

Methods: Risk factors associated with bloodstream infections in patients on hemodialysis were investigated using a case–control study conducted between January 2010 and June 2013. Chronic renal disease patients on hemodialysis who presented with positive blood cultures during the study were considered as cases. Controls were hemodialysis patients from the same institution who did not present with positive blood cultures during the study period. Data were collected from medical records. Logistic regression was used for statistical analysis.

Results: There were 162 patients included in the study (81 cases and 81 controls). Gram-positive bacteria were isolated with the highest frequency (72%). In initial logistic regression analysis, variables were hypertension, peritoneal dialysis with previous treatment, type and time of current venous access, type of previous venous access, previous use of antimicrobials, and previous hospitalization related to bloodstream infections. Multiple regression analysis showed that the patients who had a central venous catheter had an 11.2-fold (CI 95%: 5.17–24.29) increased chance of developing bloodstream infections compared with patients who had an arteriovenous fistula for vascular access. Previous hospitalization increased the chance of developing bloodstream infections 6.6-fold (CI 95%: 1.9–23.09).

Conclusions: Infection prevention measures for bloodstream infections related to central venous catheter use should be intensified, as well as judicious use of this route for vascular access for hemodialysis. Reducing exposure to the hospital environment through admission could contribute to a reduction in bloodstream infections in this population.

Keywords: Dialysis, Bacteremia, Risk factors, *Staphylococcus aureus*

Background

Infection is the leading cause of morbidity and the second leading cause of mortality among patients on renal replacement therapy [1]. Mortality from all causes in patients on dialysis treatment is 6.5–7.9 times higher than that of the general population. In patients ≥65 years of age, mortality from infection is two times higher than that in a population of the same age with a diagnosis of diabetes mellitus, neoplasms or congestive heart failure [1]. According to the US Renal Data System [1], the mortality rate at the end of the first year of hemodialysis decreased by 38% for cardiovascular causes and by 50% for infectious causes between 2000 and 2010. Among patients on hemodialysis, the mortality rate decreased by 26% between 1985 and 2000 [1]. When comparing mortality rates between the second and 12th month after initiation of hemodialysis, there was a significant reduction

* Correspondence: dayana.fram@unifesp.br

[1]School of Nursing, Paulista School of Nursing, Universidade Federal de São Paulo (Federal University of São Paulo – EPE/UNIFESP), R. Napoleão de Barros 754, São Paulo 04024-002, Brazil

in mortality from all causes, which dropped from 440 to 201 deaths per 1000 patients/year. The mortality rate from infectious causes decreased from 43 to 19.4 deaths per 1000 patients/year [1].

North American data indicate that bloodstream infection (BSI) rates in patients on hemodialysis vary between 0.5 and 27.1 per 100 patients/month depending on the type of venous access used [2]. More recent studies report a reduction in the incidence of BSI in this population between 1.09–0.89 and 2.04–0.75 per 100 patients/month after implementation of specific control measures [3,4]. This decrease was attributed to national initiatives for the reduction of healthcare-related infections [5].

The literature reports that the use of a central venous catheter (CVC), hypoalbuminemia, diabetes mellitus, anemia, female gender and colonization by *methicillin-resistant Staphylococcus aureus* (MRSA) are risk factors for the development of BSI in hemodialysis patients [6-10]. Gram-positive bacteria are the most frequently isolated agents in blood cultures from hemodialysis patients, mainly *S. aureus* [7,10,11].

According to the US Renal Data System, the principal morbidity event for hemodialysis patients is hospitalization for infections, which showed an increase of 43% between 1993 and 2011. On the other hand, hospitalizations for complications from venous access, showed a decrease of 57% [1].

Fram et al. reported that the risk factors for morbidity and mortality among patients with BSI on hemodialysis were age, isolation of *S. aureus*, and isolation of a resistant microorganism [12].

Despite the best efforts to prevent BSI specific to hemodialysis patients, BSI still has a large impact [13-16]. Therefore, the objective of this study was to evaluate risk factors for the development of BSI in patients undergoing a Brazilian hemodialysis center.

Methods

Ethical considerations

This study was conducted with the approval of the Committee on Ethics and Research at the Federal University of São Paulo.

Design, period and location of the study

This was a retrospective, case–control study conducted between January 2010 and June 2013 at the hemodialysis satellite unit at the Kidney and Hypertension Hospital of Foundation Oswaldo Ramos (HRIM/FOR) in the city of São Paulo, Brazil. The HRIM/FOR is a nephrology service, considered to be a national and international reference for teaching, research and care activities. It serves an average of 400 patients in the dialysis program/month (221 in hemodialysis). This institution follows rigorous standards for medical record keeping.

Patients with chronic renal insufficiency in a hemodialysis program, ≥18 years of age, with BSI defined according to the specific criteria of the National Healthcare Safety Network Dialysis Event Surveillance Manual (Centers for Disease Control and Prevention) [17], which defines BSI as any positive blood culture, were considered for enrollment in the study. We considered all positive blood cultures regardless of the site where blood was drawn. For common skin commensal pathogens (*Staphylococcus* coagulase negative including *Staphylococcus epidermidis*), we considered BSI when pathogens were cultured from two or more blood cultures and/or the patient was treated by a physician [17,18]. Blood cultures were processed in accordance with the recommendations of the Clinical and Laboratory Standards Institute [19].

The cases were obtained from a survey of microbiology laboratory records at the institution during the study period. For patients who had more than one positive blood culture, only the first episode was considered for this study. These patients were included in the case group. Hemodialysis patients at the same institution, ≥18 years of age, and without positive blood cultures during the study period were used as controls. Pairing criteria were: age, time on hemodialysis, and diagnosis of diabetes mellitus. The proportion of cases and controls was 1:1.

Study protocol and data collection

Data collection occurred through review of patients' medical records. For the cases group, data collection included sociodemographic characteristics, comorbidities, body mass index [20], microorganisms in blood culture, resistance profiles of antimicrobials, and previous treatment for end stage renal disease. The type, location and time of current and previous venous access, clinical complications (transfusions, number of transfusions, hospitalization because of infection, length of hospital stay, prior antimicrobial use, previous hospitalization, and number of previous hospitalizations), occurrence of death, and transfer of treatment were recorded for a period of 6 months prior to the BSI.

We defined short duration CVC as non-tunneled hemodialysis CVC. However some patients remained with this kind of catheter for a longer period due to difficult inserting other more adequate vascular access for hemodialysis. Long duration CVC was defined as tunneled hemodialysis CVC [17]. The time of current and previous venous accesses was stratified by period. This was done as in some situations they may present with similar periods.

Prior antimicrobial use was defined as every previous antimicrobial treatment for at least seven days.

Death was considered to be related to BSI when it occurred within 15 days after microbiologic diagnosis of infection [21,22].

Controls were selected from the computerized patient record system, according to the previously mentioned pairings, using the closest date of beginning dialysis in relation to the case group. Of these, the same variables described above were collected, except for the presence of BSI at the beginning of the study.

A microorganism was considered multi-resistant when it showed resistance to a pharmaceutical agent in three or more classes of antimicrobials. *Staphylococcus* was considered multi-resistant when it showed no susceptibility to *methicillin*, and *Enterococcus* was considered multi-resistant when it showed no susceptibility to vancomycin (VRE) [23-25].

Statistical analysis

A descriptive analysis of the cases and controls was conducted which examined the variables of interest. Data are presented using absolute frequencies and percentages for categorical variables, and mean ± standard deviation for continuous variables. The primary outcome was BSI. Associations between BSI and categorical variables were tested using the chi-square test, Fisher's exact test or likelihood ratio. The association between the continuous variables and the presence of BSI was examined using the student's *t*-test or Mann–Whitney test, as appropriate. Univariate logistical regression was used to investigate the relationship between each independent variable (preselected at the crossings where $p \leq 0.05$) and the dependent variable, BSI. To compare the outcomes of patients that developed BSI and the patients that did not developed BSI we used only the univariate logistical regression.

Multiple logistic regression analysis was conducted to determine the independent variables that continued to be associated with BSI after inclusion in the model of significant variables in univariate analysis. To include the variables in the regression model, the forward stepwise method was used. Odds ratios were calculated with respective confidence intervals of 95%. SPSS version 19.0 (Chicago, IL, USA) was used for statistical analyses.

Results

The total number of patients in the dialysis program for the study period was 353, of which 221 (62%) were on hemodialysis and 132 (38%) were on peritoneal dialysis. Ninety-three patients (42.1%) met inclusion criteria. Twelve patients were excluded because they were unable to be paired with a control. The final study population included 162 patients (81 cases and 81 controls). For nine cases, a control of the same age was not available, and for three cases, a control with the same time on hemodialysis was not available.

The sociodemographic characteristics of patients included in the study are presented in Table 1. There was no statistically significant difference in these characteristics among the study population.

Table 1 Sociodemographic characteristics of the cases group and control patients

	Case (*n* = 81)	Control (*n* = 81)	*p*-value
Age	56 ± 17.1	53 ± 16.3	0.325
Sex			
Male	36 (44.5)	47 (58.0)	0.083
Female	45 (55.5)	34 (42.0)	
Race			
White	49 (60.5)	55 (68.0)	0.325
Nonwhite	32 (39.5)	26 (32.0)	
Educational level			
No education	21 (26.0)	14 (17.0)	0.198
Elementary	28 (34.5)	22 (27.0)	
High School	22 (27.0)	28 (35.0)	
Higher education	10 (12.5)	17 (21.0)	

Values are expressed as mean ± SD or *n* (%).

For clinical data related to dialysis treatment, the following variables were statistically significant ($p \leq 0.05$) in the initial analyses and were preselected for logistic regression: associated diseases (hypertension), previous treatment (history of peritoneal dialysis), current type of venous access, duration of current venous access, use of previous venous access, previous type and duration of tunneled hemodialysis CVC, previous use of antimicrobials, and previous hospitalization. Duration of previous venous access had a p-value of ≤0.05; however, it was not included in regression analysis because of its low frequency (Table 2).

Table 3 shows the results of logistic regression analysis. In univariate analysis, variables significantly associated with the occurrence of BSI were: hypertension, history of peritoneal dialysis, type and duration of current venous access, use of a tunneled hemodialysis CVC as previous venous access, previous use of antimicrobials, and previous hospitalization (whether there had been a previous hospitalization or not).

With multiple logistic regression analysis, current access (CVC) and previous hospitalization were independent risk factors for the occurrence of BSI. Patients who had a CVC showed an 11.2-fold (CI 95%: 5.17–24.29) greater chance of developing BSI compared with patients who had an AVF. Previous hospitalization increased the chance of developing a BSI 6.6-fold (CI 95%: 1.9–23.09).

The most prevalent microorganisms isolated in blood cultures taken from the case group were Gram-positive bacteria (72.8%), followed by Gram-negative bacteria (25.9%), and fungi (1.2%). Among the Gram-positive microorganisms, *S. aureus* was isolated in 32.1% of cases, and of these, 38.5% showed resistance to *methicillin*.

Table 2 Clinical variables of interest of the case group and control patients

	Case ($n=81$)	Control ($n=81$)	p-value
Comorbidities			
Hypertension	71(87.6)	59 (72.8)	0.018
Cardiovascular diseases	17 (20.9)	12 (14.8)	0.306
Diabetes mellitus	26 (32.0)	26(32.0)	1.000
Others*	27 (33.3)	22 (27.2)	0.421
Body mass index, Kg/m^2	24 ± 4.3	24 ± 3.9	0.945
Previous treatments	56 (69.1)	47 (58.0)	0.141
Type of previous treatments			
Conservative	36 (64.3)	30 (37.0)	0.337
Peritoneal dialysis	19 (33.9)	9 (11.1)	0.038
Hemodialysis	17 (30.4)	9 (11.1)	0.087
Transplant	15 (26.8)	8 (9,9)	0.115
Duration of hemodialysis treatment, months	29 ± 39.2	36 ± 42.1	0.276
Type of current venous access			
AVF**	25 (30.9)	64 (79.0)	<0.001
Tunneled hemodialysis CVC***	52 (64.2)	13 (16.0)	
Non-tunneled hemodialysis CVC	4 (4.9)	1 (1.2)	
PTFE Graft****	0 (-)	3 (3.7)	
Location of current venous access			
Upper arm	24 (29.6)	67 (82.7)	
Jugular vein	50 (61.7)	13 (16.0)	
Subclavian vein	7 (8.6)	0 (-)	
Femoral vein	0 (-)	1 (1.2)	
Duration of current venous access			
0–30	17 (21,0)	3 (3.7)	<0.001
30–180 days	27 (33.3)	8 (9.9)	
>180 days	37 (45.7)	70 (86.4)	
Previous venous access (6 months)	26 (32.1)	11 (13.6)	0.005
Number of previous accesses	1.2 ± 0.41	1.3 ± 0.46	0.744
Type of previous venous access			
AVF	7 (8.6)	3 (3.7)	0.192
Tunneled hemodialysis CVC	14 (17.3)	5 (6.2)	0.028
Non-tunneled hemodialysis CVC	5 (6.2)	6 (7.4)	0.755
PTEF Graft	5 (6.2)	1 (1.2)	0.210
Location of tunneled hemodialysis CVC			
Jugular vein	13 (16.0)	3 (3.7)	
Subclavian vein	0 (-)	1 (1.2)	
Location of non-tunneled hemodialysis CVC			
Jugular vein	4 (4.9)	6 (7.4)	
Subclavian vein	1 (1.2)	0	

Table 2 Clinical variables of interest of the case group and control patients *(Continued)*

	Duration of previous venous access			
	AVF			
	0–30	0	1 (1.2)	
	30–180 days	4 (4.9)	0 (-)	
	>180 days	3 (3.7)	2 (2.5)	
	Tunneled hemodialysis CVC			
	0–30	4 (4.9)	0 (-)	0.034
	30–180 days	6 (7.4)	5 (6.2)	
	>180 days	4 (4.9)	0 (-)	
	Non-tunneled hemodialysis CVC			
	0–30	1 (1.2)	6 (7.4)	
	30–180 days	3 (3.7)	0	
	>180 days	1 (1.2)	0	
	PTFE Graft**			
	0–30	0 (-)	0 (-)	
	30–180 days	1 (1.2)	0 (-)	
	>180 days	4 (4.9)	1 (1.2)	
Transfusions		11 (13.6)	7 (8.6)	0.317
Number of transfusions		1.9 ± 2.7	1 (-)	0.246
Hospitalizations due to infection		21 (25.9)		
Length of hospital stay		16.9 ± 16.4		
Previous use of antimicrobials		28 (34.6)	14 (17.3)	0.012
Previous hospitalizations		19 (23.5)	4 (4.9)	<0.001
Number of previous hospitalizations		1.5 ± 1.2	1(-)	0.259

Values are expressed as mean ± SD or *n* (%). *hypothyroidism, hyperthyroidism, neoplasm and *systemic lupus erythematosus*; **AVF: arteriovenous fistula; ***CVC: central venous catheter; ****PTFE, polytetrafluoroethylene.

Table 3 Univariate and multivariate logistic regression analyses

	Simple logistic regression		Multiple logistic regression	
	OR (IC 95%)	***p*-value**	**OR (IC 95%)**	***p*-value**
Diagnosis of hypertension	2.65 (1.16–6.03)	0.021		
Previous treatment (peritoneal dialysis)	2.45 (1.03–5.81)	0.042		
Type of current venous access				
CVC* vs. AVF**	10.72 (5.09–22.57)	<0.001	11.2 (5.17–24.29)	<0.001
Duration of current venous access				
0–30 vs. > 180 days	10.72 (2.95–38.96)	<0.001		
30–180 days vs. > 180 days	6.39 (2.64–15.45)	<0.001		
Use of previous venous access	3.01 (1.37–6.62)	0.006		
Tunneled CVC (previous access)	3.18 (1.09–9.28)	0.035		
Prior antimicrobial use	2.53 (1.21–5.28)	0.013		
Previous hospitalizations	5.90 (1.91–18.24)	0.002	6.63 (1.9–23.09)	0.003

*CVC: central venous catheter; **AVF: arteriovenous fistula.

The second most frequent Gram-positive organism was *S. epidermidis* (13.6%), with 100% resistance to *methicillin*. Of the Gram-negative microorganisms isolated, 13.6% were of the enterobacteriaceae family and 12.3% were non-fermenters. For Gram-negative microorganisms, 33.3% were multi-resistant (Table 4).

MRSA was isolated in 10 patients. Two of these patients had previous exposure to vancomycin and had a minimum inhibitory concentration to vancomycin of ≤0.05 μg/mL and 1.0 μg/mL.

With regard to progression for cases and controls, there were no significant differences in variables. Death occurred only in the cases group, retention in treatment was higher in controls, and shift to peritoneal dialysis showed a higher frequency in the cases group. Fifteen patients (46.7%) died from BSI, two (13.3%) from cardiovascular disease, and six (40%) from other causes, such as neoplasms, infections at other sites, and noninfectious complications at the vascular access. The median time to death after BSI was 4.6 ± 5.5 days (Table 5). Among the patients that died due to other causes, the death occurred from 45 to 672 days after the BSI.

Discussion

For patients undergoing renal replacement therapy, infection is the leading cause of morbidity and the second leading cause of mortality [1]. In Brazil, it is estimated that 97,586 patients currently receive chronic dialysis treatment [26]. According to North American data, the rates of BSI among hemodialysis patients range between 0.5 and 27.1 per 100 patients/month depending on the type of venous access used [2]. Results of a Brazilian study reported that rates varied between 0.55 and 7.32 per 1000 venous accesses/day [27].

Table 4 Microorganisms isolated in the cases group, and profiles of resistance

	MR	S	Total
Gram-positives	28 (47.5)	31 (52.5)	59 (72.8)
Staphylococcus aureus	10 (38.5)	16 (61.5)	26 (32.1)
Staphylococcus epidermidis	11 (100.0)	0 (-)	11 (13.6)
Staphylococcus coagulase negative non *S. epidermidis*	4 (57.1)	3 (42.9)	7 (8.6)
Enterococcus faecalis	1 (33.3)	2 (66.7)	3 (3.7)
Other Gram-positives*	3 (33.3)	9 (66.7)	12 (14.8)
Gram-negatives	7 (33.3)	14 (66.7)	21 (25.9)
Enterobacteriaceae**	4 (36.4)	7 (63.6)	11 (13.6)
Non-fermenters***	3 (30.0)	7 (70.0)	10 (12.3)
Fungi	0 (-)	1 (100.0)	1 (1.2)
Candida albicans	0 (-)	1 (100.0)	1 (1.2)
Total of microorganisms			81

Values are expressed as mean ± SD or *n* (%). MR: multi-resistant. S: sensitive. **Streptococcus acidominimus, Streptococcus agalactiae, Streptococcus anginosus, Streptococcus bovis, Streptococcus pyogenes, Staphylococcus simulans, Staphylococcus capitis, Staphylococcus haemolyticus, Staphylococcus lugdunensis*; **Enterobacteriaceae: *Enterobacter spp, Enterobacter aerogenes, Enterobacter cloacae, Escherichia coli, Klebsiella pneumoniae, Serratia marcescens, Proteus mirabilis*; ***Non-fermenters: *Acinetobacter baumannii, Pseudomonas aeruginosa, Stenotrophomonas maltophilia.*

Table 5 Progression of the patients, cause of death and time of death post-BSI

	Cases (*n* = 81)	Controls (*n* = 81)	*p*-value
Progression of the patients			
Death	15 (18.5)	0 (-)	<0.001
Transfer of care	9 (11.1)	5 (6.2)	0.263
Duration of treatment	41 (50.6)	70 (86.4)	<0.001
Peritoneal dialysis	9 (11.1)	1 (1.2)	0.009
Transplant	7 (8.6)	5 (6.2)	0.549
Cause of death in the cases			
BSI	7 (46.7)		
Cardiovascular diseases	2 (13.3)		
Other*	6 (40.0)		
Total	15		
Time of death post-BSI			
	4.6 ± 5.5		

Values are expressed as mean ± SD or *n* (%). *neoplasms, infections at other sites, cardiovascular diseases, and noninfectious complications in the vascular access.

In the present study, risk factors for BSI were evaluated in patients on hemodialysis at a hemodialysis service in São Paulo, Brazil. The study was a case–control design, which can analyze risk factors related to a determined condition. Patients presenting with BSI during the study period were included as cases, and controls were those patients who did not develop the studied event (pairing criteria: age, previous time on hemodialysis, and diagnosis of diabetes mellitus).

Use of a CVC compared with use of an AVF, and previous hospitalization were independent risk factors for the occurrence of BSI among patients on hemodialysis treatment. Use of a CVC was associated with an increased risk of developing BSI (OR: 11.2; CI 95%: 5.17–24.29; p < 0.001) compared with the use of an AVF. This finding aligns with previous trials of antimicrobial locks, which reported a higher occurrence of BSI among hemodialysis patients with CVC (3-4 cases per 1000 catheter-days) [28]. In a longitudinal cohort study, Xui *et al.* found that the rates of BSI in patients using CVC were three times higher than in patients using AVF (p < 0.001) [8]. A case–control study conducted at a university hospital in Greece demonstrated, through multivariate logistic regression, that patients using CVC had a higher risk of BSI compared with patients using AVF (OR: 2.93; p = 0.047) [10].

In the current study, only five patients (four cases and one control) used a non-tunneled hemodialysis CVC. In these patients, three had started hemodialysis within 60 days and were awaiting the manufacture of an AVF, and the other two had been undergoing treatment for a longer period of time and had spent longer with a non-tunneled hemodialysis CVC because of difficulties in the insertion of a tunneled hemodialysis CVC or the manufacture of an AVF.

Previous hospitalization increased the risk of BSI 5.33-fold (p = 0.003). There are few reports in the literature on the association between BSI and previous hospitalizations in patients undergoing hemodialysis treatment. Nguyen *et al.* in a study performed between 2005 and 2011, evaluated BSI from MRSA in patients on dialysis treatment, and found that 70% of patients who developed BSI were hospitalized at least once in the year prior to the infection [6]. In a study by Barbosa *et al.* the researchers reported that, in 320 chronic renal patients, previous hospitalization was an important risk factor for colonization of multi-resistant microorganisms (e.g., VRE) [29]. And Aktas *et al.* in a study of 70 patients on dialysis treatment, reported a higher colonization for MRSA in patients who had been hospitalized within the previous 6 months compared with those who had not [30].

In univariate logistic regression analysis, systemic arterial hypertension, peritoneal dialysis as a prior treatment, duration of venous access, presence of previous venous access, use of tunneled hemodialysis CVC as a previous access, and previous antimicrobials were associated with a higher occurrence of BSI. No data was found in the literature on the possible relationship between systemic arterial hypertension and previous peritoneal dialysis with the occurrence of BSI in this population.

For examination of time of duration of current venous access as a risk factor, BSI was found to be associated with access that had been gained within 30 days. Duration of current venous access was analyzed using three categories (0–30 days, 30–180 days, and >180 days). BSI was higher in those who had had the CVC inserted within 30 days, which underscores the need for greater care during the CVC insertion procedure. Napalkov *et al.* in a study that evaluated infectious and noninfectious complications in CVC, reported that the majority of BSI occurred within the first 90 days, with an incidence rate/1000 catheter-days of 5.1 (CI 95%: 3.7–4.3) [31]. There was also a higher risk of infection for catheters inserted within the 6 months following infection, reinforcing the need for care during this period.

The use of previous venous access and, primarily, previous access of tunneled hemodialysis CVC, was associated with a higher occurrence of BSI. As mentioned above, studies have reported that CVC use is associated with a higher incidence of BSI compared with the use of an AVF [8-10]. References to previous venous access as a risk factor for BSI were not found in the literature.

Previous use of antimicrobials was associated with a higher occurrence of BSI (OR: 2.53; p = 0.013). As with other variables, data were collected on the use of antimicrobials within 6 months before the event. We found no specific studies that related prior antimicrobial exposure to BSI in patients undergoing hemodialysis treatment. However, Lim *et al.* in a case–control study conducted with patients seen in the emergency department of a tertiary hospital in Australia, showed through multivariate analysis that prior antimicrobial use increased the risk of developing BSI by multi-resistant microorganisms (OR: 5.49; p < 0.001) [32]. According to the Centers for Disease Control and Prevention, the rational use of antimicrobials is an important measure for controlling the spread of multi-resistant microorganisms [23].

Gram-positive microorganisms were the most prevalent (72.8%) found in the current study. Among them, *S. aureus* was the most frequently isolated (32.1%), with about 38.5% resistant to oxacillin. Other studies have also reported a high prevalence of Gram-positive microorganisms in patients undergoing hemodialysis treatment, primarily *S. aureus* [7,10,11]. Despite the high prevalence of Gram-positive microorganisms observed in the current study, Gram-negative microorganisms accounted for 25.9% of isolates in blood cultures. In a university hospital in Spain, microorganisms isolated in blood cultures from patients with kidney disease were: Gram-negative bacteria, 52.3%; Gram-positive bacteria, 46.5%; and fungi, 1.2%. *Escherichia coli* was the most frequent microorganism (27%) [33].

With regard to resistance profiles, microorganisms such as MRSA and VRE have been isolated in surveillance cultures collected from patients on dialysis treatment [29,34,35]. Aktas *et al.* used molecular typing to show a high similarity between MRSA strains isolated from surveillance cultures and clinical cultures collected from patients on dialysis treatment [30]. And a study conducted at long-term care facilities in Hong Kong reported a significant dissemination of MRSA, reinforcing the need to adopt measures to reduce the transmission of this microorganism [36].

The independent risk factors for BSI identified in the current study were use of a CVC compared with use of an AVF, and previous hospitalization. Although previous studies have indicated a relationship between the presence of CVC and BSI, our study expands the characteristics of this group, highlighting the importance of care during the initial period and the period of up to 6 months of catheter duration. Furthermore, the study highlights the importance of previous hospitalization as a risk factor for BSI. To the best of the authors' knowledge, this factor has not been reported in previous studies and requires further research.

This study had some limitations inherent in the retrospective character of the data collection. However, patient records at the study institution were completed with significant caution, given the characteristics of a service dedicated to the treatment of chronic renal patients, and followed the high standards of the organization. Additionally, as there are standardized protocols for performing blood cultures for these patients, it is unlikely that events were underdiagnosed in the study period.

Preventative measures against BSI related to CVC should be strengthened and effectively applied to hemodialysis treatment units, as well as reducing the use of this device whenever possible, prioritizing the use of AVF. Considering that previous hospitalization was an independent risk factor for BSI, patients who developed BSI after hospitalization are probably infected by microorganisms during this period. Standard precautions should be enforced to prevent microorganism dissemination during hospitalization.

A reduction in the number of infections in this population may contribute to a decrease in hospital admissions, since infections are a leading cause of hospitalization in patients on hemodialysis treatment.

Conclusions

The risk factors for BSI in chronic renal disease patients receiving hemodialysis were previous hospitalization and use of a CVC. The most prevalent microorganisms were Gram-positive bacteria, of which 47.5% were multi-resistant. The results of this study suggest the need to intensify measures to prevent and control BSI in hemodialysis patients, among which are specific measures for insertion and maintenance of the CVC, and the judicious use of this device. Efforts should be made to reduce exposure of these patients to hospitalization to minimize the risk of BSI. Future research could evaluate the impact of surveillance cultures to prevent microorganism dissemination in this population.

Consent

Written informed consent was obtained from the patient for the publication of this report and any accompanying images.

Competing interests

The authors declare that they have no competing interests.

Authors' contributions

DF: principal researcher and participated in all steps of the study: development of the project, data collection, revision of the database, data analysis, and drafting and revising the manuscript. MFPO: development of the project, data analysis and article revision. MT: development of the project, data analysis and article revision. VP: development of the project, data analysis, and article revision. SRM: data collection and revision of the database. CG: revision of the database and article revision. AB: data analysis and article revision. RS: manuscript structure and article revision. DB: coordinated and conceived the study, participated in project design, supervision of data collection, data analysis, drafting and revision of the article. All authors read and approved the final version of the manuscript.

Authors' information

DF: Nurse, MSc and PhD; MFPO: Nurse, MSc and PhD; MT: Nurse, MSc, PhD and post- doctoral student (EPE/UNIFESP); VP: Physician, MSc and doctoral student (EPM/UNIFESP); SRM: Nurse, MSc and doctoral student (EPE/UNIFESP); CG: Nurse, PhD and post-doctoral student (EPE/UNIFESP); AB: Nurse, MSc, PhD and Adjunct Professor (EPE/UNIFESP); RS: Physician, MD, PhD and Associate Professor (EPM/UNIFESP); and, DB: Nurse, PhD, MSc and Associate Professor (EPE/UNIFESP).

Acknowledgements

We wish to acknowledge the Fundação de Amparo à Pesquisa do Estado de São Paulo FAPESP and Conselho Nacional de Desenvolvimento Científico e Tecnológico CNPq for the financial support for this study.

Author details

[1]School of Nursing, Paulista School of Nursing, Universidade Federal de São Paulo (Federal University of São Paulo – EPE/UNIFESP), R. Napoleão de Barros 754, São Paulo 04024-002, Brazil. [2]Infection Control Unit, Children's Institute and Institute for the Treatment of Childhood Cancer, School of Medicine, Universidade de São Paulo (University of São Paulo – ITACI/FMUSP), Av. Dr. Enéas Carvalho de Aguiar 647, São Paulo 05403-000, Brazil. [3]Division of Infectious Diseases, Escola Paulista de Medicina, Universidade Federal de São Paulo (Paulista School of Medicine, Federal University of São Paulo – EPM/ UNIFESP), R. Napoleão de Barros, 715, 7° andar, São Paulo 04024-002, Brazil. [4]Division of Dialysis, Hospital do Rim e Hipertensão, Fundação Oswaldo Ramos, (Kidney and Hypertension Hospital, Foundation Oswaldo Ramos - HRIM/FOR), R. Pedro de Toledo 282, São Paulo 04039-030, Brazil. [5]Division of Nephrology, Paulista School of Medicine, Universidade Federal de São Paulo (Federal University of São Paulo – EPM/UNIFESP), R. Botucatu 740, São Paulo 04023-900, Brazil.

References

1. United States Renal Data System. U.S. Renal Data System: USRDS 2013 Annual Data Report: Atlas of Chronic Kidney Disease and End-Stage Renal Disease in the United States, National Institutes of Health, National Institute of Diabetes and Digestive and Kidney Diseases. Bethesda, MD; 2013. [http://www.usrds.org/atlas.aspx]
2. Klevens RM, Edwards JR, Andrus ML, Peterson KD, Dudeck MA, Horan TC, et al. Dialysis Surveillance Report: National Healthcare Safety Network (NHSN)-data summary for 2006. Semin Dial. 2008;21 Suppl 1:24–8.
3. Centers for Diseases Control and Prevention. Vital signs: central line–associated blood stream infections— United States, 2001, 2008, and 2009. MMWR. 2011;60:243–8.
4. Patel PR, Yi SH, Booth S, Bren V, Downham G, Hess S, et al. Bloodstream infection rates in outpatient hemodialysis facilities participating in a collaborative prevention effort: a quality improvement report. Am J Kidney Dis. 2013;62 Suppl 2:322–30.
5. National action plan to reduce healthcare-associated infections [http:// www.hhs.gov/ash/initiatives/hai/actionplan/index.html]
6. Nguyen DB, Lessa FC, Belflower R, Mu Y, Wise M, Nadle J, et al. Invasive methicillin-resistant *Staphylococcus aureus* infections among patients on chronic dialysis in the United States, 2005-2011. Clin Infect Dis. 2013;57 Suppl 10:1393–400.
7. Gauna TT, Oshiro E, Luzio YC, Paniago AM, Pontes ER, Chang MR. Bloodstream infection in patients with end-stage renal disease in a teaching hospital in central-western Brazil. Rev Soc Bras Med Trop. 2013;46 Suppl 4:426–32.
8. Xue H, Ix JH, Wang W, Brunelli SM, Lazarus M, Hakim R, et al. Hemodialysis access usage patterns in the incident dialysis year and associated catheter-related complications. Am J Kidney Dis. 2013;61 Suppl 1:123–30.
9. Patel PR, Kallen AJ, Arduino MJ. Epidemiology, surveillance, and prevention of bloodstream infections in hemodialysis patients. Am J Kidney Dis. 2010;56 Suppl 3:566–77.
10. Fysaraki M, Samonis G, Valachis A, Daphnis E, Karageorgopoulos DE, Falagas ME, et al. Incidence, clinical, microbiological features and outcome of bloodstream infections in patients undergoing hemodialysis. Int J Med Sci. 2013;10 Suppl 12:1632–8.
11. Esmanhoto CG, Taminato M, Fram DS, Belasco AGS, Barbosa DA. Microorganisms isolated from patients on hemodialysis by central venous

catheter and related clinical evolution. Acta Paul Enferm. 2013;26 Suppl 5:413–20.
12. Fram D, Taminato M, Ponzio V, Manfredi SR, Grothe C, Batista RE, et al. Risk factors for morbidity and mortality of bloodstream infection in patients undergoing hemodialysis: a nested case-control study. BMC Res Notes. 2014;7(Supp1):882.
13. Fram DS, Taminato M, Ferreira D, Neves L, Belasco AGS, Barbosa DA. Prevention of Catheter-Related Bloodstream Infections in Patients on Hemodialysis. Acta Paul Enferm. 2009;22:564–8.
14. Pugh-Clarke K, Donlon S, McCann M. CE: continuing education article. Prevention of infection in patients with chronic kidney disease part 1: application of infection control principles to the renal care environment. J Ren Care. 2010;36 Suppl 4:191–8.
15. Centers for Disease Control and Prevention. Infection control requirements for dialysis facilities and clarification regarding guidance on parenteral medication vials. MMWR. 2008;57 Suppl 32:875–6.
16. Centers for Disease Control and Prevention. Recommendations for preventing transmission of infections among chronic hemodialysis patients. MMWR. 2001;50:1–43.
17. Centers for Disease Control and Prevention. Dialysis Event Surveillance Manual. Atlanta; 2013. [http://www.cdc.gov/nhsn/PDFs/pscManual/Dialysis-Manual.pdf]
18. Horan TC, Andrus M, Dudeck MA. CDC/NHSN surveillance definition of health care-associated infection and criteria for specific types of infections in the acute care setting. Am J Infect Control. 2008;36 Suppl 5:309–32.
19. Clinical and Laboratory Standards Institute. Performance Standards for Antimicrobial Susceptibility Testing; 23st Informational Supplement. CLSI document M100-S23. Wayne, PA: Clinical and Laboratory Standards Institute; 2013.
20. de Onis M, Habicht JP. Anthropometric reference data for international use: recommendations from a World Health Organization Expert Committee. Am J Clin Nutr. 1996;64(4):650–8.
21. Conterno LO, Wey SB, Castelo A. Risk factors for mortality in *Staphylococcus aureus* bacteremia. Infect Control Hosp Epidemiol. 1998;19 Suppl 1:32–7.
22. Lee CH, Chien CC, Liu JW. Timing of initiating glycopeptide therapy for methicillin-Resistant Staphylococcus aureus bacteremia: the impact on clinical outcome. Sci World J. 2013;2013:457435.
23. Center for disease control and prevention. Antibiotic resistance threats in the United States. Atlanta; 2013. [http://www.cdc.gov/drugresistance/threat-report-2013/pdf/ar-threats-2013-508.pdf]
24. Kallen AJ. Identifying and classifying bloodstream infections among hemodialysis patients. Semin Dial. 2013;26 Suppl 4:407–15.
25. Center for disease control and prevention: Guideline for Isolation Precautions. Preventing Transmission of Infectious Agents in Healthcare Settings. Atlanta; 2007. [http://www.cdc.gov/hicpac/pdf/isolation/Isolation2007.pdf]
26. Sociedade Brasileria de Nefrologia. Censo de Diálise. São Paulo; 2012. [http://www.censo-sbn.org.br/inicio]
27. de Albuquerque SE, Cavalcante RD, Ponce D, Fortaleza CM. Epidemiology of healthcare-associated infections among patients from a hemodialysis unit in southeastern Brazil. Braz J Infect Dis. 2014;18 Suppl 3:327–30.
28. James MT, Conley J, Tonelli M, Manns BJ, MacRae J, Hemmelgarn BR, et al. Meta-analysis: antibiotics for prophylaxis against hemodialysis catheter-related infections. Ann Intern Med. 2008;148 Suppl 8:596–605.
29. Barbosa D, Lima L, Silbert S, Sader H, Cendoroglo M, Draibe S, et al. Evaluation of the prevalence and risk factors for colonization by vancomycin-resistant *Enterococcus* among patients on dialysis. Am J Kidney Dis. 2004;44 Suppl 2:337–43.
30. Aktaş E, Pazarli O, Külah C, Cömert F, Külah E, Sümbüloğlu V. Determination of *Staphylococcus aureus* carriage in hemodialysis and peritoneal dialysis patients and evaluation of the clonal relationship between carriage and clinical isolates. Am J Infect Control. 2011;39 Suppl 5:421–5.
31. Napalkov P, Felici DM, Chu LK, Jacobs JR, Begelman SM. Incidence of catheter-related complications in patients with central venous or hemodialysis catheters: a health care claims database analysis. BMC Cardiovasc Disord. 2013;13:86.
32. Lim CJ, Cheng AC, Kong DC, Peleg AY. Community-onset bloodstream infection with multidrug-resistant organisms: a matched case-control study. BMC Infect Dis. 2014;14 Suppl 1:126.
33. Rojas L, Muñoz P, Kestler M, Arroyo D, Guembe M, Rodríguez-Créixems M, et al. Bloodstream infections in patients with kidney disease: risk factors for poor outcome and mortality. J Hosp Infect. 2013;85 Suppl 3:196–205.
34. Fram D, Castrucci FM, Taminato M, Godoy-Martinez P, Freitas MC, Belasco A, et al. Cross-transmission of vancomycin-resistant *Enterococcus* in patients undergoing dialysis and kidney transplant. Braz J Med Biol Res. 2010;43 Suppl 1:115–9.
35. Gómez-González MC, Campos R, Pascua J, Marigliano N, Lancho JM, Teno P. Colonization management of methicillin resistant *Staphylococcus aureus* in patients and health professional in the haemodialysis unit in a situation of high risk of endemic disease: looking for zero nasal carriers? Enferm Infecc Microbiol Clin. 2012;30 Suppl 3:124–30.
36. Cheng VC, Tai JW, Wong ZS, Chen JH, Pan KB, Hai Y, et al. Transmission of methicillin-resistant *Staphylococcus aureus* in the long term care facilities in Hong Kong. BMC Infect Dis. 2013;13:205.

7

Infectious tenosynovitis with bloodstream infection caused by *Erysipelothrix rhusiopathiae*, a case report on an occupational pathogen

Kristine Hofseth[1], Håvard Dalen[2,3,4], Leif Kibsgaard[1], Solrun Nebb[5], Angela Kümmel[5] and Arne Mehl[2,6*]

Abstract

Background: *Erysipelothrix rhusiopathiae* is an established animal pathogen, which may cause infections in humans. It is a gram-positive rod and found in the tonsils or the digestive tracts of animals. The bacterium is occupationally related, as usually only people with frequent animal contacts are infected. We report a case of a patient who was admitted with an infectious tenosynovitis with bloodstream infection due to *E. rhusiopathiae*, and to our knowledge, this is the first report of a tenosynovitis with systemic manifestation associated with this bacterium.

Case presentation: A 52-year old Norwegian man, who worked with transportation of swine cadavers, was admitted to the local hospital with sepsis and unknown focus of infection. A few days earlier he had an injury to the skin of one of his fingers that later proved to be infected with *E. rhusiopathiae*. There were no other causes for his symptoms than the infectious tenosynovitis with systemic manifestation. The infection resolved on treatment with antibiotics and surgery. A transoesophageal echocardiogram was performed to exclude endocarditis, which may be associated with this pathogen.

Conclusions: This case report highlights the importance of clinicians being aware of this bacterium, and we describe risk factors for infection, differences in the clinical manifestations of the disease, challenges with diagnosing the bacterium and adverse effects of immunosuppressive drugs. Recommended treatment is appropriate antibiotic therapy and adequate debridement and surgical drainage of the tendon sheath.

Keywords: *Erysipelothrix rhusiopathiae*, Infectious tenosynovitis, Sepsis, Bloodstream infection, Endocarditis, Surgical treatment, TNF-α inhibitor, Case report

Background

Erysipelothrix rhusiopathiae is described as a non-motile, non-sporulating, non-acid-fast, slender gram-positive rod with capsule, which is easily decolourised. The rod is recovered from the tonsils or the digestive tracts of different animals [1]. Swine is believed to be the major reservoir of *E. rhusiopathiae*, but rodents and birds are also frequently infected. The bacterium also grow and persist in mucoid exterior slime in fish [2]. Humans can be infected from contact with these animals, their secretions, wastes or products, or contaminated organic matter [1].

E. rhusiopathiae causes mainly three types of infections in humans. Firstly, a mild cutaneous infection (erysipeloid), described as a local cellulitis, usually on the hands or fingers. The disease is self-limiting within 3–4 weeks without therapy, but if not treated with antibiotics there is a risk of relapse. Secondly, it may cause a diffuse cutaneous infection where the patient experiences that the local lesions spread to other locations of the body and bullous lesions may coexist with systemic symptoms such as fever, malaise, headache, joint- and muscle pain. Some patients also experience polyarthritis. Lastly, *E. rhusiopathiae* may cause septicaemia and endocarditis [1, 2].

* Correspondence: Arne.Mehl@helse-nordtrondelag.no
[2]Department of Medicine, Levanger Hospital, Nord-Trøndelag Hospital Trust, Levanger, Norway
[6]Mid-Norway Sepsis Research Group, Norwegian University of Science and Technology, Trondheim, Norway
Full list of author information is available at the end of the article

Penicillin G is the drug of choice to treat infections caused by this bacterium [2].

Infectious tenosynovitis refers to the infection of a tendon and its synovial sheath. In the setting of tenosynovitis, the space between the inner visceral layer adherent to the tendon and an outer parietal layer may be filled with inflammatory or purulent fluid. Bacteria can enter the tendon sheath by direct inoculation via trauma or spread from infected adjacent soft tissues. It may also spread hematogenously. The most common pathogens are skin flora (i.e., gram-positive cocci such as *Staphylococcus aureus* and streptococci) [3, 4]. Recommended treatment for this type of infection is appropriate antibiotic therapy, adequate debridement and surgical drainage, a period of immobilisation and elevation of the extremity, and early mobilisation. Appropriate tetanus prophylaxis is necessary [4].

Hereby, we describe the successful management of a patient who was admitted with an infectious tenosynovitis with bloodstream infection due to *E. rhusiopathiae.* Only once in published literature there has been described tenosynovitis caused by this bacterium, as a local infection [5]. To our knowledge, this case report shed new light on the pathogenesis of this disease being the first known report of a tenosynovitis with systemic manifestation associated with this bacterium.

Case presentation

Admission

A 52-year-old man was admitted to the local hospital because of acute fever and poor general condition. By admittance he was septic with unknown focus of infection. He worked in the transportation business and mainly by transportation of cadavers, most often swine cadavers. He rarely used protective gloves. He had known ankylosing spondylitis since years and was treated with adalimumab injections every 14 days and ibuprofen. He had earlier experienced a reaction to penicillin with symptoms of urticaria. Five days before admission he got a cut on the volar side of the proximal inter phalangeal joint of the fourth finger on the left hand, but he could not remember how he got it. Two days later he had increasing pain in his finger and it swelled, but no pus was seen from the wound. The last 24 h before admission, he experienced fever with chills, increasing pain in the finger, nausea, diarrhoea and fatigue.

On physical examination at admission, his body temperature (after taking antipyretics) was 38.4°C, pulse rate was 93 beats per minute, respiratory rate was 20 per minute, and blood pressure was 147/92 mmHg. By auscultation the lung sounds were normal and there was no cardiac murmur. The abdomen was soft and free from pain by palpation. Examination of the fourth finger on the left hand showed a small, dry wound from the cut, some tenderness along the course of the flexor sheath, slightly flexed finger at rest, erythema and enlargement compared to the other digits.

Laboratory and imaging examinations showed white blood cells (WBC) 18.3×10^9/L, neutrophil granulocytes 16.4×10^9/L, haemoglobin 13.7 g/L, platelets 300×10^9/L, C-reactive protein (CRP) 15 mg/L, lactate dehydrogenase 287 U/L. Blood cultures (three bottles from one venipuncture) were sampled. The chest X-ray was normal and he had a normal urine dipstick test. In conclusion the patient fulfilled 4/4 systemic inflammatory response syndrome (SIRS) criteria and the most plausible explanation was sepsis due to a bacterial tenosynovitis in the fourth finger of the left hand. Based on this the patient was rapidly brought to the operating room.

Therapeutic intervention

In local anaesthetic ulnar and median nerve block an incision was made to reach the common synovial sheath 2–3 cm proximally to the basis of the fourth finger. Immediately accumulated fluid emptied the synovial sheath and a bacterial sample was collected. In accordance with Norwegian sepsis guidelines in patients allergic to penicillin, the patient was then given clindamycin and gentamicin intravenously. Furthermore, two incisions on the volar side of the proximal and distal interphalangeal joints through the synovial sheath were made and a drain tube was inserted into the sheath from the palm of the hand to the distal interphalangeal joint. The drain tube was connected to Ringer's acetate that flushed the tendon sheath until the next day.

Recovery and discharge

The day after the patient was feeling much better. He had no fever and did not appear septic. Laboratory examinations showed: WBC 19.7×10^9/L; CRP 73 mg/L. Three out of three blood cultures bottles were positive with gram-positive rods, and gram-positive cocci in clusters, probably staphylococci, were found in the sample from the synovial sheath. The patient was referred for transthoracic echocardiography to exclude endocarditis and the echocardiogram showed morphologically normal valves and chambers with no signs of vegetations. After 4 days of intravenous treatment with clindamycin 600 mg × 3/day and gentamicin 320 mg × 1/day, the patient was discharged in well-being. CRP had fallen to 11 mg/L and WBC to 9.3×10^9/L. He continued with clindamycin orally 300 mg × 3/day for 1 week. He was recommended to avoid the upcoming injection of adalimumab at discharge.

Five days after discharge, a transoesophageal echocardiogram was performed with no signs of valvular or endocardial manifestation of the disease. He was recommended to see his general practitioner for a clinical follow-up and removal of the stitches 1 week after discharge. At an outpatient control after three months and when we contacted him ten months after discharge, the patient reported no relapse of the infection and no persistent sequela.

Verifying the rod

A blood culture set including two aerobic bottles and one anaerobic bottle was sampled immediately at admission. Within the first 24 h of incubation in 35°C, all three bottles turned positive. The gram stain showed gram-positive rods (Fig. 1). Due to characteristic V-formation when visualised in the microscope, they could easily be mistaken for *Corynebacterium sp.* Because of this we did an initial susceptibility test, directly from positive bottles, based on antibiotics used on *Corynebacterium sp.* according to Nordic Committee on Antimicrobial Susceptibility Testing (NordicAST) guidelines with disc diffusion method [6]. The isolate was susceptible to penicillin, clindamycin, ciprofloxacin, linezolid and doxycycline and was resistant to gentamicin and rifampicin.

After six to eight hours there were signs of growth on agar plates, but not enough for further examination. After 24 h of incubation, there was growth on both aerobic and anaerobic agar plates. Identification of the isolate was achieved by automatically testing with BD Phoenix 100. It was identified as *E. rhusiopathiae* with 99% confidence value. Confirmation of the result by the Maldi-tof system was done at the regional university reference laboratory. Due to the patient's history, the isolation of this bacterium was expected.

A second susceptibility test was done from cultured bottles to determine the minimum inhibitory concentration value of the antibiotics (MIC), using NordicAST guidelines on non-species related breakpoints. MIC-testing showed the isolate was susceptible to penicillins, cephalosporins, ciprofloxacin, clindamycin, erythromycin and imipenem. The isolate was resistant to gentamicin, trimethoprim-sulfa and vancomycin.

During surgery two samples from the synovial sheath were collected and these were also cultured. One sample was sterile, *Staphylococcus aureus* alone was found in the other. The isolate was, among others, susceptible to clindamycin and gentamicin. This bacterium was not detected in the blood cultures.

Discussion

We have described a rare invasive *E. rhusiopathiae* infection and several lessons can be learned from this case.

Swine are the most important animal reservoir of *E. rhusiopathiae*, which is shed by infected animals in faeces, urine, saliva and nasal secretions [1]. Our patient worked with transportation of swine cadavers, and thus, he had an occupational risk for such infections. We know that 20–40% of healthy swine harbour this pathogen in their lymphoid tissue of the alimentary tract, particularly in the tonsils [1]. Infections caused by *E. rhusiopathiae* are strongly related to the occupation of the patient and almost 90% of patients with endocarditis due to this pathogen have an occupational risk of infection [7].

Most often infection with *E. rhusiopathiae* is initiated either by an injury to the skin with infective material or by contamination of a previous injury. There have also

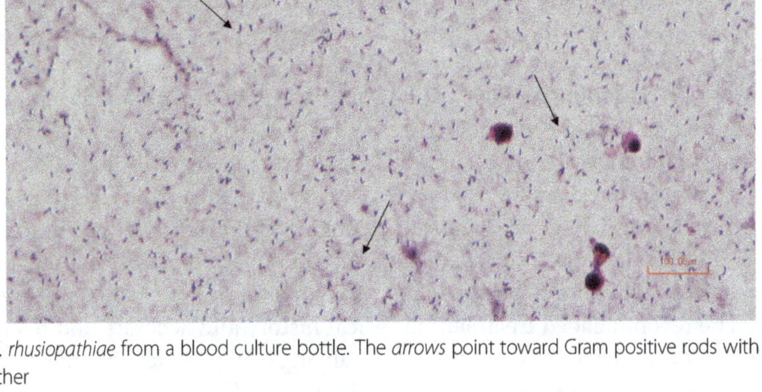

Fig. 1 Gram stain smear of *E. rhusiopathiae* from a blood culture bottle. The *arrows* point toward Gram positive rods with V-formation, a characteristic way the bacteria group together

been a few documented cases of penetration through the skin by this bacterium [1]. Our patient rarely used protective gloves, and he had a cut in one of his fingers a few days before admission. We believe that contamination of this injury was the cause of the infection. Due to changes in technology in the animal industry, it has been suggested that the frequency of human infection by this pathogen is decreasing [2]. However, in some environments, exposure to *E. rhusiopathiae* is maintained, and the threat of infections is present. Preventive initiatives include good hygiene with frequent hand washing, use of protective gloves and cleansing of wounds. Removal or regular disinfection of contaminated sources is important to limit the spread of the bacterium as well [1].

Our patient was diagnosed with ankylosing spondylitis since years and was treated with adalimumab, a tumour necrosis factor-alpha (TNF-α) inhibitor. TNF-α is an important component of the immune response to a variety of infections. Thus, the use of such medication has been associated with an increased risk of serious infections [8], including infective tenosynovitis [4]. As the American College of Rheumatology recommends not to administer TNF-α inhibitors to patients with active bacterial infections [9], our patient was instructed not to take the subsequent dose of adalimumab. Depression of the immune system predisposes to the development of systemic infections with among other *E. rhusiopathiae*, and thus, the risk of systemic infections, as endocarditis, is also increased [7].

Reports show that systemic infection with *E. rhusiopathiae* occur in less than 1% of cases, but in 90% of these there is an association with endocarditis [1, 7]. The first case of endocarditis with *E. rhusiopathiae* was reported in 1912, but since then no more than 80 cases of endocarditis caused by *E. rhusiopathiae* have been reported [7]. This cause of endocarditis is therefore extremely rare [7, 10]. However, endocarditis caused by *E. rhusiopathiae* has a high case fatality rate of approximately 40% [10, 11]. Due to these reasons the echocardiographic examinations included a transoesophageal approach as this is more sensitive to reveal endocardial manifestations, and an echocardiographic examination was repeated after 6 days. *E. rhusiopathiae* is reported to be susceptible to penicillin, cephalosporin, imipenem, clindamycin, and fluoroquinolones, but it is often nonsusceptible to macrolides and chloramphenicol, and resistant to sulphonamides, vancomycin and aminoglycosides [10]. The first-line empiric therapy for a presumed endocarditis in patients allergic to penicillin include vancomycin and aminoglycosides, which have no effect against *E. rhusiopathiae* [2, 7]. It is therefore important to reveal the correct diagnosis to avoid delayed administration of appropriate drugs. The recommended treatment in patients with endocarditis due to this bacterium is penicillin G given intravenously for a total duration of 4–6 weeks [2]. Alternatively, patients with an *E. rhusiopathiae* infection and coexisting allergy to penicillin can be treated with cephalosporin or fluoroquinolone [2, 12].

Due to sepsis and presumed allergy to penicillin, the patient was treated with an aminoglycoside, to which the bacterium was resistant, and clindamycin. Clindamycin may be bactericide in high concentrations [12]. Our patient responded well to the treatment and did not fill the SIRS-criteria the day after surgery. Thus, we decided to continue with clindamycin orally after discharge for one week. The patient received antibiotic therapy for 12 days in total. The optimal duration of antibiotic therapy for *E. rhusiopathiae* bloodstream infection is unknown and has not been evaluated in clinical trials. Thus, the duration of antibiotic therapy in patients with bacteremia, but without endocarditis, must be based on the clinical response to the treatment provided and the patient's underlying health condition.

The diagnosis of *E. rhusiopathiae* can be challenging. In this case the blood cultures revealed *E. rhusiopathiae*, but in the sample from the tendon sheath only *S. aureus* was found. This may be caused by the slow growth of the bacterium and the small sizes of its colonies. *E. rhusiopathiae* can be overgrown with secondary pathogens such as *S. aureus* and *S. pyogenes*. We believe that this is what happened with the cultured samples from the tendon sheath. The diagnosis of this pathogen can therefore be challenging if the bacteriologists are not aware of the clinical suspicion of potential contamination from animal contact [1]. Thus, infections with *E. rhusiopathiae* may be under-diagnosed.

According to our recommendations, two blood culture sets from two separate venipunctures should be drawn. In this case, probably because of time constraints, only one blood culture set including two aerobic bottles and one anaerobic bottle was sampled. We have still judged this case to be a real bloodstream infection, as it is unlikely that *E. rhusiopathiae* should occur as a skin contaminant at the venipuncture site.

Conclusion

This case report shed new light on the pathogenesis of infections with *E. rhusiopathiae* being the first known report of a tenosynovitis with bloodstream infection associated with this pathogen. Recommended treatment for this type of infection is appropriate antibiotic therapy and adequate debridement and surgical drainage. Due to the slow growth of the bacterium, the small sizes of its colonies, and the risk that it can be overgrown with secondary pathogens, the diagnosis of this pathogen is challenging if bacteriologists are not aware of the clinical suspicion of potential contamination from animal contact. This shows the importance of both comprehensive medical history and accurate and detailed information accompanying samples to the microbiology laboratory. Even though *E. rhusiopathiae* is a rare cause of endocarditis or other systemic infections, endocarditis is associated with high case fatality rate. *E. rhusiopathiae* is reported to be resistant to vancomycin and aminoglycosides, which represent the first-line empiric therapy for a presumed endocarditis in patients allergic to penicillin. This highlights the importance of revealing the correct diagnosis to avoid delayed administration of appropriate drugs.

Abbreviations

CRP: C-reactive protein; MIC: Minimum inhibitory concentration; NordicAST: Nordic committee on antimicrobial susceptibility testing; TNF-α inhibitors: Tumour necrosis factor-alpha inhibitors; WBC: White blood cell

Acknowledgements

Not applicable.

Funding

This work was not financially supported.

Authors' contributions

KH, LK and HD were responsible for the patient's management during hospitalization and follow-up after discharge. AM, SN and AK participated in the diagnostics and treatment of the disease. KH and SN prepared the manuscript. HD, AK and AM have reviewed and given significant contribution to the final version. All authors read and approved the final version of the manuscript.

Competing interests

The authors declare that they have no competing interests.

Consent for publication

The patient has provided his written informed consent for publication of this case report.

Author details

[1]Department of Orthopedic Surgery, Levanger Hospital, Nord-Trøndelag Hospital Trust, Levanger, Norway. [2]Department of Medicine, Levanger Hospital, Nord-Trøndelag Hospital Trust, Levanger, Norway. [3]Cardiac Exercise Research Group, Department of Circulation and Medical Imaging, Norwegian University of Science and Technology (NTNU), Trondheim, Norway. [4]Department of Cardiology, St. Olavs University Hospital, Trondheim, Norway. [5]Department of Laboratory Medicine, Levanger Hospital, Nord-Trøndelag Hospital Trust, Levanger, Norway. [6]Mid-Norway Sepsis Research Group, Norwegian University of Science and Technology, Trondheim, Norway.

References

1. Brooke CJ, Riley TV. Erysipelothrix rhusiopathiae: bacteriology, epidemiology and clinical manifestations of an occupational pathogen. J Med Microbiol. 1999;48(9):789–99.
2. Reboli AC, Farrar WE. Erysipelothrix rhusiopathiae: an occupational pathogen. Clin Microbiol Rev. 1989;2(4):354–9.
3. Small LN, Ross JJ. Suppurative tenosynovitis and septic bursitis. Infect Dis Clin N Am. 2005;19(4):991–1005.
4. Tsai E, Failla JM. Hand infections in the trauma patient. Hand Clin. 1999; 15(2):373–86.
5. Tolis K, Spyridonos S, Tsiplakou S, Fandridis E. Tenosynovitis of a digit due to Erysipelothrix rhusiopathiae: case report and review of the literature. New Microbes New Infect. 2015;8:128–30.
6. Nordic Committee on Antimicrobial Susceptibility Testing. Breakpoint tables for interpretation of MICs and zone diameters. Version 6.0, 2016. [http://www.nordicast.org/brytpunktstabeller]. Accessed 15 May 2016.
7. Tomaszuk-Kazberuk A, Kaminska M, Sobkowicz B, Hirnle T, Prokop J, Lewczuk A, Sawicki R, Musial W. Infective endocarditis caused by Erysipelothrix rhusiopathiae involving three native valves. Kardiol Pol. 2011;69(8):827–9.
8. Koo S, Marty FM, Baden LR. Infectious complications associated with immunomodulating biologic agents. Infect Dis Clin N Am. 2010;24(2):285–306.
9. Saag KG, Teng GG, Patkar NM, Anuntiyo J, Finney C, Curtis JR, Paulus HE, Mudano A, Pisu M, Elkins-Melton M, et al. American College of Rheumatology 2008 recommendations for the use of nonbiologic and biologic disease-modifying antirheumatic drugs in rheumatoid arthritis. Arthritis Rheum. 2008;59(6):762–84.
10. Hua P, Liu J, Tao J, Liu J, Yang Y, Yang S. Erysipelothrix rhusiopathiae-induced aortic valve endocarditis: case report and literature review. Int J Clin Exp Med. 2015;8(1):730–6.
11. Hill EE, Herijgers P, Claus P, Vanderschueren S, Herregods MC, Peetermans WE. Infective endocarditis: changing epidemiology and predictors of 6-month mortality: a prospective cohort study. Eur Heart J. 2007;28(2):196–203.
12. Venditti M, Gelfusa V, Tarasi A, Brandimarte C, Serra P. Antimicrobial susceptibilities of Erysipelothrix rhusiopathiae. Antimicrob Agents Chemother. 1990;34(10):2038–40.

8

Neonatal bloodstream infections in a Ghanaian Tertiary Hospital: Are the current antibiotic recommendations adequate?

Appiah-Korang Labi[1], Noah Obeng-Nkrumah[2*], Stephanie Bjerrum[3], Christabel Enweronu-Laryea[4] and Mercy Jemima Newman[5]

Abstract

Background: Diagnosis of bloodstream infections (BSI) in neonates is usually difficult due to minimal symptoms at presentation; thus early empirical therapy guided by local antibiotic susceptibility profile is necessary to improve therapeutic outcomes.

Methods: A review of neonatal blood cultures submitted to the microbiology department of the Korle-Bu Teaching Hospital was conducted from January 2010 through December 2013. We assessed the prevalence of bacteria and fungi involved in BSI and the susceptibility coverage of recommended empiric antibiotics by Ghana Standard Treatment guidelines and the WHO recommendations for managing neonatal sepsis. The national and WHO treatment guidelines recommend either ampicillin plus gentamicin or ampicillin plus cefotaxime for empiric treatment of neonatal BSI. The WHO recommendations also include cloxacillin plus gentamicin. We described the resistance profile over a 28-day neonatal period using multivariable logistic regression analysis with linear or restricted cubic splines.

Results: A total of 8,025 neonatal blood culture reports were reviewed over the four-year period. Total blood culture positivity was 21.9 %. Gram positive organisms accounted for most positive cultures, with coagulase negative staphylococci (CoNS) being the most frequently isolated pathogen in early onset infections (EOS) (59.1 %) and late onset infections (LOS) (52.8 %). Susceptibility coverage of early onset bacterial isolates were 20.7 % to ampicillin plus cefotaxime, 32.2 % to the combination of ampicillin and gentamicin, and 71.7 % to cloxacillin plus gentamicin. For LOS, coverage was 24.6 % to ampicillin plus cefotaxime, 36.2 % to the combination ampicillin and gentamicin and 63.6 % to cloxacillin plus gentamicin. Cloxacillin plus gentamicin remained the most active regimen for EOS and LOS after exclusion of BSI caused by CoNS. For this regimen, the adjusted odds of resistance decreased between 12-34 % per day from birth to day 3 followed by the slowest rate of resistance increase, compared to the other antibiotic regimen, thereafter until day 28. The trend in resistance remained generally unchanged after excluding data from CoNS. Multidrug resistant isolates were significantly (p-value <0.001) higher in LOS (62.4 %, $n = 555/886$) than in EOS (37.3 %, $n = 331/886$).

Conclusions: There is low antibiotic susceptibility coverage for organisms causing neonatal bloodstream infections in Korle-Bu Teaching Hospital when the current national and WHO recommended empiric antibiotics were assessed. A continuous surveillance of neonatal BSI is required to guide hospital and national antibiotic treatment guidelines for neonatal sepsis.

Keywords: Neonates, Bloodstream, Infections, Ghana, Antibiotics, Resistance

* Correspondence: successfulnoahforchrist@yahoo.com
[2]Microbiology Department, School of Biomedical and Allied Health Sciences, College of Health Sciences, University of Ghana, P.O. Box 4326, Accra, Republic of Ghana
Full list of author information is available at the end of the article

Background

The neonatal age represents a critical period in the life of an infant. The immature state of their immune system predisposes them to infections [1]. Of these, bloodstream infections (BSI) are the most important because of their association with increased cost, morbidity and mortality [1–3]. In Africa, neonatal bloodstream infection rates are estimated to be 20 per 1000 live births'; mainly ascribed to poor intra-partum and postnatal practices [4, 5]. Neonatal bloodstream infections may be of early or late onset. Early onset neonatal BSI (i.e. infections occurring within first 48 h of life) [3] is mostly due to vertical transmission from maternal flora during the perinatal period [6]. Group B Streptococcus is the typical organism isolated during this period in developed countries although other bacteria do play a role [3]. Late onset neonatal BSI (infections occurring past 48 h after birth) [3] are caused by organisms from the hospital or home environment [4, 6]. Commonly associated pathogens are *Staphylococcus* species and Gram negative bacteria mainly *Enterobacteriaceae* [1–3].

In neonates early signs and symptoms of BSI are minimal, making it difficult to diagnose [1, 3]. This means empirical antibiotic management of suspected BSI must be started immediately to reduce associated morbidity and mortality. The antibiotic of choice must cover commonly isolated organisms, and must take into account their known local antibiotic susceptibility patterns. However in developing countries, antimicrobial therapy is usually based on international recommendations without adaptation to local susceptibility patterns; although it has been shown that evidence based treatment improves treatment outcomes [7]. Rising incidence of multi-drug resistant bacteria worldwide [8], and the variability of antibiotic susceptibility patterns by location, means that local antibiotic susceptibility profiles are invaluable to effective empiric antibiotic therapy.

Very few published data on neonatal bloodstream infections exist in Ghana and the West African subregion. A study conducted among neonates in a major teaching Hospital in Ghana, described decreasing susceptibility of Gram negative organisms to aminoglycosides and cephalosporins [5]. The evolving nature of antibiotic resistance means that there is the need to regularly update antibiotic susceptibility data to guide empiric therapy. The aim of this study was to describe bacterial and fungal isolates from neonatal blood cultures processed at the Microbiology Department of the Korle-Bu Teaching Hospital (KBTH) over a four year period (2010–2013); with emphasis on antibiotic susceptibility patterns, multi-drug resistant isolates and coverage of antibiotics suggested by the current national standard treatment guidelines [9] and the World Health Organisation (WHO) [10] for treating neonatal sepsis. This information may contribute to improved management of neonatal sepsis and the development of local policies based on local epidemiological information.

Methods

Study design and setting

We conducted a retrospective review of neonatal blood cultures over a 4-year period from January 2010 through December 2013. Given that the current definition of neonatal BSI incorporate time thresholds that delimit infections between 0 and 28 days after birth, only blood cultures with information on age of patients at time of sampling were considered for review and analyses. Blood culture reports of newborn infants were collated from the bacteriology unit of the Microbiology Department of KBTH, which processes over 40,000 clinical cultures annually. We included blood culture results of neonates primarily receiving healthcare at the KBTH ($n = 7{,}594$) or secondarily referred to the laboratory from other health facilities for microbiological investigations ($n =$ 431). Blood cultures from KBTH were from the Babies Unit and neonatal intensive care units of the Department of Child Health. The Department of Child Health has a 55-bed neonatal intensive care unit; and a 40-bed Babies Unit for neonatal cases referred to KBTH [11]. The hospital annually records about 11,000 live births; and provides referral healthcare services to an estimated population of 24 million Ghanaians [11].

Laboratory procedures

Over the period under review the laboratory performed 8,025 neonatal blood cultures. For neonatal patients, the guideline is to inject between 1-3 mL of blood directly into Paediatric Bactec® culture vials (Becton Dickinson, USA). These are then submitted for laboratory diagnosis. Cultures are processed with the BACTEC 9240 blood culture system (Becton Dickinson, NJ, USA) according to manufacturer's instructions. Subcultures are typically made on to blood, chocolate, MacConkey and Saboraund agars; and incubated aerobically at 37 °C for 20 h. Identification of bacterial isolates was performed by Gram-stain microscopy and with routine biochemical methods. Bacteria speciation was done with the BBL Crystal identification system (Becton Dickinson, NJ, USA). Antibiotic susceptibility testing was performed using the Kirby Bauer Disc diffusion method in accordance to Clinical and Laboratory Standards Institute guidelines. Positive blood cultures for yeast and non-yeast fungi were identified on the basis of macromorphology (including estimation of radial growth on selected media) and microscopic examinations of sexual reproduction, conidiogenesis, and hyphal branching. Routinely at the laboratory, positive blood cultures are evaluated to determine whether they represent true bacteraemia, fungaemia, or contamination - they are each reviewed by the Clinical

Microbiologist for decisions on the significance of the organism and the appropriate antibiotic susceptibility data to report. The Clinical Microbiologists have access to patients' clinical information.

Review and analysis

Study data were collected by physician-assisted review of laboratory records. Information extracted included gender, age and year of infection, the isolated organism and antibiotic susceptibility data. For purposes of this study, positive blood cultures were those with bacteria or fungi (i) recovered and for which antibiotic susceptibility tests were performed (if isolates were bacteria); and (ii) identified as the first isolate per patients within the study period. If more than one organism was isolated from a single culture this was classified as a poly-microbial infection. Certain organisms, including *Micrococcus species*, *Bacillus species*, and diptheroids were classified as contaminants. Coagulase negative *Staphylococci* (CoNS) because of their possible role as pathogens in this age group were included in the overall data for analysis except where specified in the laboratory records as contaminants with no antimicrobial susceptibility data. Neonatal BSI was defined by at least one set of positive blood culture for bacteria or fungi in an infant 28 days old or younger. Bloodstream infections were sub-classified into early onset (EOS) if it occurred <48 h and late onset (LOS) if it occurred 2–28 days after birth. Positive cultures were further categorized into Gram-positive bacteria, Gram-negative organisms, and fungi.

Antimicrobial susceptibility

Empirical choice of antibiotics at the KBTH is varied and may involve ampicillin, cloxacillin, gentamicin, amikacin, or ceftotaxime in various combinations. However the national and WHO treatment guidelines recommend either ampicillin plus gentamicin or ampicillin plus cefotaxime for empiric treatment of neonatal BSI [9]. The WHO recommendations also include cloxacillin plus gentamicin [10]. Susceptibility of bacterial isolates to the recommended regimen was evaluated based on reported antibiogram. Isolates were described as susceptible to the combination regimens if they were reported susceptible in vitro to either one or both of the antibiotics recommended. Susceptibility profiles of isolates to different treatment regimens were repeated after excluding BSI with CoNS. We assessed the occurrence of multidrug resistant bacteria between early and late onset infections, focusing on six epidemiological bacterial pathogens: vancomycin resistant *Enterococcocus* species (VRE) [based on in vitro susceptibility to vancomycin disk (30ug)], methicillin resistant *Staphylococcus aureus* (MRSA) [based on in vitro susceptibility to cefoxitin disk (30ug)], penicillin resistant streptococci (PRS) [based on in vitro susceptibility to ampicillin disk (10ug)], cephalosporin resistant enterobacteria (Ceph-R Ent) [based on in vitro susceptibility to cefotaxime disk (30ug)], multi-drug resistant *Pseudomonas* species (MDR Ps.) and multi-drug resistant *Acinetobacter* species (MDR Act). Multidrug resistant (MDR) phenotype was defined according to the international standard definitions for acquired resistance, and relative to the panel of antibiotics tested for each isolate, as in vitro non-susceptibility to ≥1 agent in ≥3 antimicrobial categories: penicillins, cephalosporins, beta-lactamase inhibitor combinations, fluoroquinolones, aminoglycosides, chloramphenicol, folate pathway inhibitors, tetracyclines, macrolides and glycopeptides [12].

Statistics

Study data was captured into Microsoft Excel, and exported into Statistical Package for Social Sciences (SPSS, Version 20.0) for editing and statistical analyses. Where appropriate, data were compared between four consecutive study periods (2010 through 2013) so that trends could be ascertained. Comparisons between categorical data were conducted with Fisher's exact test or Chi-square with Marascuilo's post hoc tests for multiple comparisons. Changes in incidence over time were analyzed by Chi-square test for trend. Continuous data were compared using students' t-test with analyses of variance (ANOVA) for multiple comparisons. A multivariable logistic regression with linear or restricted cubic splines was used to model the association between the proportion of resistant bacteria causing BSI and the age of neonates at the time of blood culture sampling. The number and placement of spline knots was based on a previously published method by Blackburn et al., 2014 [13], using '*mkspline* functions' created in Stata version 12 (StataCorp., USA). Each linear spline incorporated one, two, three or four knots. Restricted cubic splines included four knots. Logistic regression models with the best fit were chosen based on the Akaike's Information Criterion (AIC). Models with least AIC values were preferred. Organisms, year of infections and patients' gender were included in the models as cross-factor random effects, continuous and binary variables, respectively. The likelihood ratio test was used to determine the statistical significance for outcomes in the regression models. Point estimates of statistical significance were indicated with 2-tailed p-values <0.05. Logistic regression analysis were repeated after excluding BSI with CoNS.

Results

From January 2010 through December 2013, we reviewed 8025 blood culture reports of neonates. Contaminants accounted for 3.6 % ($n = 294$); and these were more prevalent (p-value = 0.001) in newborns <48 h old (17.2 %;

n = 151/875) than in neonates 2–28 days old (12.1 %; *n* = 143/1182). Blood culture positivity was 21.9 % (*n* = 1763/8025), and remained significantly higher among neonates receiving care at KBTH (22.5 %, *n* = 1712/7594) compared to those referred to the laboratory from elsewhere (11.8 %, *n* = 51/431). In the proceeding analysis however, we have disregarded comparing results between the two sources of blood cultures due to few true positive cultures from the latter.

Isolates from neonatal BSI

Ranked distributions for reported organisms are presented in Table 1 for EOS and LOS. The data show a predominance (*p*-value <0.001) of LOS (13.0 %, *n* = 1039/8025) over EOS (9.0 %, *n* = 724/8025). Gram-positive organisms accounted for the majority of BSI and were significantly (*p*-value =0.001) more prevalent in EOS (84.2 %, *n* = 610/724) compared to LOS (78.1 %, *n* = 811/1039). Coagulase negative *Staphylococci* were the most frequent organism (EOS: 59.1 % > LOS: 52.8 %; *p*-value = 0.005), followed by *Staphylococcus aureus* (EOS: 10.5 % < LOS: 15.3 %; *p*-value = 0.003) and *Streptococcus* species (EOS: 8.1 % > LOS: 5.6 %; *p*-value = 0.003). For EOS *Citrobacter* (3.2 %, *n* = 23/724) and *Enterobacter* (2.6 %, *n* = 19/724) species were the most frequently reported Gram negative bacteria. *Citrobacter* species accounted for the majority of Gram negative bacteria reported in LOS (4.3 %, *n* = 44/1039). There was a trend towards increased incidence of CoNS in EOS, from 55.3 % in 2010 to 65.4 % in 2013 (Chi- square for trend analysis, *p*-value <0.001). In LOS, we observed a rise in *Candida* species from 0 in 2010 to 0.4 % (*n* = 1/261) in 2011, 0.6 % (*n* = 2/352) in 2012 and 3.3 % (*n* = 5/151) in 2013 (Chi- square for trend, *p*-value <0.001).

Antibiotic susceptibility

Table 2 compares in vitro susceptibility of bacterial isolates to empiric antimicrobials used for treatment of neonatal sepsis. In EOS, the susceptibility of all isolates was 20.7 % to ampicillin plus cefotaxime, 32.2 % to the combination of ampicillin and gentamicin and 71.6 % to cloxacillin plus gentamicin (Chi-square for trend, *p*-value <0.001). In Table 3 the antimicrobial profiles for all bacteria isolated from LOS showed that susceptibility was 24.6 % to ampicillin plus cefotaxime, 36.2 % to the combination ampicillin and gentamicin and 63.6 % to cloxacillin plus gentamicin (Chi-square for trend, *p*-value <0.001). For each treatment regimen, there was no significant difference in proportion of susceptible isolates between EOS and LOS. Overall, the combination of cloxacillin and gentamicin remained the most active regimen for EOS and LOS even after exclusion of BSI by CoNS. In EOS, when the analysis excluded data on CoNS, the susceptibility coverage of cloxacillin/gentamicin decreased by 7.7 % but this did not achieve statistical significance (*p*-value = 0.081). In LOS (Table 3), susceptibility to cloxacillin plus gentamicin significantly (*p*-value = 0.011) reduced from 63.6 % (*n* = 570/896) to 55.8 % (*n* = 204/365) after the exclusion of CoNS.

Changes in antibiotic susceptibility over 4-year study period

Resistance of blood culture isolates to ampicillin/gentamicin and to cloxacillin/gentamicin remained relatively unchanged from 2010 through 2013 (Fig. 1). In contrast, we identified significant increase in resistance to ampicillin/cefotaxime during the same study period. The yearly trend in resistance to each regimen remained unchanged after excluding data on CoNS.

Changes in antibiotic susceptibility over 28-day neonatal period

The relationship between resistance to each empiric antibiotic combinations and neonates' age was best described by linear spline functions incorporating one or four age breakpoints (knots) (Additional file 1: Table S1). After adjusting for gender, year of infection and bacterial isolates, the odds ratios from multivariable logistic regression showed evidence of association between resistance and age for each antibiotic regimen (*p*-value <0.008 for all antibiotic combinations) (Additional file 1: Table S2). The adjusted odds ratios (AOR) can be interpreted as resistance decreasing at varying rates between 12–26 % per day from birth (day 0) to day 7 for cloxacillin/gentamicin and ampicillin/cefotaxime, and to day 9 for ampicillin/gentamicin — followed by increasing resistance levels thereafter until day 28 (Fig. 2). Ampicillin/gentamicin recorded the slowest rate in decline of antibiotic resistance. The odds of resistance fell by 22 % between birth and day 3 followed by a similar decrease of 22 % per day from days 6–9. The rate of increase in resistance was slowest for cloxacillin/gentamicin — the rate increases each day by 24 % from days 7 through 14 and by 61 % thereafter until 28 days (Fig. 2). The trends in resistance over 28-day period remained generally unchanged after excluding data from CoNS, although increase in adjusted odds of resistance occurred within fewer days after birth (Additional file 1: Table S2). Resistance decreased between 29-49 % per day from birth to day 3 for all antibiotic combinations. The decrease in resistance was greatest for cloxacillin/gentamicin. For this regimen, the odds of resistance fell by 38 % from birth to day 1, with a further 11 % decrease in day 2 followed by increasing resistance thereafter until day 28 (Fig. 2)

Multidrug resistance

Figure 3 compares the occurrence of epidemiologically important bacterial phenotypes across EOS and LOS. No carbapenem resistant *Enterobacteriaceae* was isolated.

Table 1 Bacteria and fungi isolates from blood cultures of neonates <48 h and 2–28 days old

Organism	Total		EOS Number of isolates (%)				X^2 trend p-value	LOS Number of isolates (%)				X^2 trend p-value
	EOS	LOS	2010	2011	2012	2013		2010	2011	2012	2013	
Gram negatives	109 (14.9) [a]	220 (21.7) [b]	33 (14.0)	16 (11.1)	45 (17.2)	15 (17.8)	0.219	63 (22.9)	41 (15.7)	80 (22.7)	36 (20.5)	0.541
Enterobacteriacea	79 (10.9)	160 (15.3)	28 (11.9)	8 (5.5)	35 (13.4)	8 (9.5)	0.879	45 (16.4)	28 (10.7)	61 (17.3)	26 (17.9)	0.444
Escherichia coli	11 (1.5)	14 (1.3)	2 (0.9)	1 (0.7)	6 (2.2)	2 (2.4)	0.183	5 (1.8)	5 (1.9)	10 (2.8)	4 (2.6)	0.450
Klebsiella species	10 (1.4)	21 (2.0)	3 (1.2)	1 (0.7)	5 (1.9)	1 (1.2)	0.801	5 (1.8)	1 (0.4)	11 (3.1)	4 (2.6)	0.210
Kluyvera species	7 (0.9)	6 (0.6)	5 (2.1)	0	1 (0.4)	1 (1.2)	0.109	1 (0.3)	1 (0.4)	1 (0.2)	3 (2.0)	0.187
Citrobacter species	23 (3.2)	44 (4.3)	7 (2.9)	3 (2.1)	11 (4.2)	2 (2.4)	0.785	16 (5.8)	10 (3.8)	12 (3.4)	6 (4.0)	0.199
Enterobacter species	19 (2.6)	40 (3.9)	6 (2.5)	2 (1.4)	10 (3.8)	1 (1.2)	0.927	14 (5.1)	4 (1.5)	19 (5.4)	3 (2.0)	0.520
Proteus species	5 (0.7)	7 (0.6)	3 (1.2)	1 (0.7)	1 (0.4)	0	0.097	0	2 (0.6)	3 (0.9)	2 (1.3)	0.144
Salmonella species	3 (0.4)	10 (0.9)	1 (0.4)	0	1 (0.4)	1 (1.2)	0.698	3 (1.1)	3 (1.1)	3 (0.9)	1 (0.7)	0.506
Serratia species	1 (0.4)	8 (0.7)	1 (0.4)	0	0	0	0.089	1 (0.3)	2 (0.8)	2 (0.6)	3 (2.0)	0.216
Acinetobacter species	16 (2.2)	43 (4.1)	3 (1.2)	4 (2.7)	4 (1.5)	5 (5.9)	0.131	15 (5.4)	7 (2.6)	13 (3.7)	8 (5.3)	0.740
Pseudomonas species	11 (1.5)	16 (1.5)	2 (0.8)	2 (1.3)	5 (1.9)	2 (2.4)	0.300	3 (1.1)	6 (2.3)	5 (1.4)	2 (1.3)	0.934
Others	3 (0.4)	1 (0.09)	0	2 (1.3)	1 (0.4)	0	0.865	0	0	1	0	0.895
Gram positives	610 (84.2) [b]	811 (78.0) [a]	200 (85.1)	127 (88.2)	214 (81.9)	69 (82.1)	0.241	212 (77.1)	219 (83.9)	270 (76.7)	114 (75.5)	0.386
Enterococcus species	43 (5.9)	36 (3.4)	32 (13.7)	3 (2.1)	6 (2.3)	2 (2.4)	<0.001	23 (8.4)	5 (1.9)	6 (1.7)	2 (1.3)	<0.001
Micrococcus species	1 (0.4)	5 (0.4)	1 (0.4)	0	0	0	0.089	0	1 (0.4)	2 (0.6)	2 (1.3)	0.108
Staphylococcus aureus	76 (10.5)	159 (15.3)	24 (10.2)	20 (13.9)	24 (9.2)	8 (9.5)	0.570	43 (15.6)	51 (19.5)	46 (13)	19 (12.6)	0.142
CoNS	431 (59.5)	549 (52.8)	130 (55.3)	94 (65.2)	152 (58.2)	55 (65.4)	<0.001	133 (48.4)	150 (57.5)	195 (55.3)	71 (47.0)	0.844
Streptococcus species	59 (8.1)	58 (5.6)	13 (55.3)	10	32 (12.3)	4 (4.8)	0.162	13 (4.7)	12 (4.6)	21 (6.0)	4 (2.6)	0.698
Streptococcus pneumoniae	3 (0.4)	9 (0.9)	2 (0.8)	0	1 (0.4)	0	0.199	2 (0.6)	1 (0.4)	3 (0.9)	3 (2.0)	0.988
Streptococcus pyogenes	3 (0.4)	9 (0.9)	2 (0.8)	0	1 (0.4)	0	0.199	2 (0.6)	1 (0.4)	3 (0.9)	3 (2.0)	0.295
Streptococcus agalactiae	5 (0.7)	7 (0.6)	2 (0.8)	1 (0.7)	1 (0.4)	1 (1.2)	0.715	1 (0.3)	2 (0.8)	3 (0.9)	1 (1.3)	0.726
Viridans Streptococci	22 (3.0)	16 (1.5)	2 (0.8)	5 (3.5)	13 (4.9)	2 (2.4)	0.073	2 (0.6)	3 (1.1)	7 (1.9)	4 (2.6)	0.102
Other Streptococci	26 (3.6)	17 (1.6)	5 (2.1)	4 (2.8)	16 (6.1)	1 (1.2)	0.288	6 (2.0)	4 (1.5)	5 (1.4)	2 (1.3)	0.378
Streptomyces species	0	4 (0.3)	0	0	0	0	-	0	1 (0.4)	0	3 (2.0)	0.049
Fungi	5 (0.7) [a]	8 (0.7) [a]	5 (2.1)	1 (0.7)	2 (0.8)	0	0.053	0	1 (0.4)	2 (0.6)	6 (3.9)	<0.001
Aspergillus species	2 (0.2)	0	1 (0.4)	0	1 (0.4)	0	0.480	0	0	0	0	-
Candida albicans	3 (0.4)	8 (0.7)	1 (0.4)	1 (0.06)	1 (0.4)	0	0.467	0	1 (0.4)	2 (0.6)	5 (3.3)	<0.001
Total	724 (41.1)	1039 (58.9)	235	144	261	84		275	261	352	151	

*Differing superscripts across columns indicate significant difference at p-value <0.05; EOS, early onset infections; LOS, late onset infections; CoNS, coagulase negative staphylococci. Other Gram negatives included *Neisseria* species, *Stenophromonas* species and *Moraxella* species; Other Streptococci included *S. mitis, S. salivarius, S. oralis, S sanguinis group, S bovis, S milleri, S. anginosus, S. constellatus and S. intermedius*

Table 2 Susceptibility (of bacteria from blood cultures taken from neonates less than 48 h old) to antimicrobials used for empiric treatment of neonatal BSI

Organisms	Susceptibility							Regimen coverage
		Ampicillin + Gentamicin (A)		Ampicillin + Cefotaxime (B)		Cloxacillin + Gentamicin (C)		
	Number of isolates	Number Tested (%)	Number susceptible (%)	Number Tested (%)	Number susceptible (%)	Number Tested (%)	Number susceptible (%)	
Gram negatives	109	101 (92.6)	38 (37.6)^a	68 (62.4)	32 (47.1)^a	75 (68.8)	52 (69.3)^b	C > B = A; $p = 0.001$
Enterobacteriacea	79	74 (93.7)	24 (32.4)	55 (69.6)	27 (49.1)	53 (67.1)	37 (69.8)	
Acinetobacter species	16	16 (100)	10 (62.5)	13 (81.2)	5 (38.4)	13 (81.2)	8 (61.5)	
Pseudomonas species	11	11 (100)	4 (36.4)	-	-	9 (81.8)	7 (77.7)	
Others	3							
Gram positives	610	511 (83.8)	159 (31.1)^b	356 (58.4)	56 (15.7)^a	211 (34.6)	153 (72.5)^b	C > A > B; $p = 0.001$
Enterococcus species	43	37 (86.1)	8 (21.6)	37 (86.1)	7 (18.9)	-	-	
Staphylococcus aureus	76	67 (88.2)	34 (50.7)	59 (77.6)	5 (8.5)	69 (90.7)	46 (66.7)	
CoNS	431	376 (87.2)	107 (28.5)	226 (52.4)	26 (11.5)	111 (25.7)	93 (83.7)	C > A > B; $p = 0.001$
Streptococcus species	59	31 (52.5)	10 (32.3)	34 (57.6)	18 (30.5)	31 (52.5)	14 (45.2)	
Others	1							
Total	719	612 (85.1)	$_a$197 (32.2)^b	424 (58.9)	$_a$ 88 (20.7) ^{a}	286 (40.0)	$_a$205 (71.7)^c	C > A > B; $p = 0.001$
Total excluding CoNS	288	236 (81.9)	$_a$90 (38.1)^a	198 (68.8)	$_b$ 62 (31.3)^a	175 (60.7)	$_a$112 (64.0)^b	C > B = A; $p = 0.001$
Polymicrobial infections	20	19 (95.0)	4 (21)^a	18 (90.0)	2 (11.1)^a	20 (100.0)	5 (25.0)^a	C = B = A; $p = 0.540$
2 organisms	17	16 (94.1)	1 (6.3)	15 (88.2)	1 (6.7)	17 (100)	4 (23.5)	
3 organisms	3	3 (100)	3 (100)	3 (100)	1 (33.3)	3 (100)	1 (33.3)	

Based on in-vitro susceptibility. Data on isolates with insufficient numbers ($n \leq 5$) not shown. For polymicrobial infections, all isolates were susceptible to at least one of the treatment antibiotics

A, Ampicillin plus Gentamicin; B, Ampicillin plus cefotaxime; C, Cloxacillin plus gentamicin; CoNS, Coagulase negative *Staphylococcus* species. Other Gram-negatives included *Neisseria* species ($n = 1$), *Stenophromonas* species ($n = 1$) and *Moraxella* species ($n = 1$). Other Gram-positives included *Micrococcus* species

Differing superscripts across row denotes differences in the proportion of susceptible isolates to antimicrobial regimen. Differences in proportions computed by Chi square with Marascuilo's Post Hoc Multiple proportion comparisons at p-value <0.05. Differing subscripts within a column denotes differences in the proportion of susceptible isolates to antimicrobial regimen

Table 3 Susceptibility (of bacteria from blood cultures taken from neonates between 2 to 28 days) to antimicrobials used for empiric treatment of neonatal septicaemia

Organisms	Number of isolates	Susceptibility						
		Ampicillin + Gentamicin (A)		Ampicillin + Cefotaxime (B)		Cloxacillin + Gentamicin (C)		Regimen coverage
		Number Tested (%)	Number susceptible (%)	Number Tested (%)	Number susceptible (%)	Number Tested (%)	Number susceptible (%)	
Gram negatives	220	200 (90.9)	72 (36.0)^{a}	188 (85.4)	92 (48.9)^{a}	173 (0.78)	102 (46.3)^{b}	C > B = A; $p = 0.001$
Enterobacteriacea	160	145 (90.6)	44 (30.3)	149 (93.1)	75 (50.3)	131 (81.8)	78 (59.5)	
Acinetobacter species	43	40 (93.0)	22 (55.0)	39 (90.7)	17 (43.6)	31 (72.1)	17 (54.8)	
Pseudomonas species	16	15 (93.7)	6 (40.0)	-	-	11 (68.7)	7 (63.6)	
Others	1							
Gram positives	811	762 (93.9)	276 (36.3)^{b}	770 (94.9)	144 (18.7)^{a}	723 (89.1)	468 (64.7)^{c}	C > B < A; $p = 0.001$
Enterococcus species	36	29 (80.5)	8 (27.5)	34 (94.4)	9 (26.4)	-	-	
Staphylococcus aureus	159	143 (89.9)	64 (44.7)	151 (94.9)	22 (14.6)	142 (89.3)	82 (57.7)	
CoNS	549	539 (98.2)	183 (34.0)^{b}	540 (98.3)	97 (17.9)^{a}	531 (96.7)	366 (68.9)^{c}	C > B < A; $p = 0.001$
Streptococcus species	58	51 (97.9)	21 (41.0)	45 (77.5)	16 (35.5)	50 (86.2)	20 (40.0)	
Others	9							
Total	1031	962 (93.3)	$_{a}$348 (36.2)^{b}	958 (92.9)	$_{a}$236 (24.6)^{a}	896 (86.9)	$_{a}$570 (63.6)^{c}	C > B < A; $p = 0.001$
Total excluding CoNS	482	423 (87.8)	$_{a}$165 (39.0)^{b}	418 (86.7)	$_{b}$139 (33.2)^{a}	365 (75.7)	$_{b}$204 (55.8)^{c}	C > B < A; $p = 0.001$
Polymicrobial infections	25	16 (64.0)	3 (18.7)	14 (56.0)	3 (21.4)	16 (64.0)	6 (37.7)	C = B = A; $p = 0.431$
2 organisms	22	14 (63.6)	2 (14.2)	12 (54.5)	2 (16.7)	15 (68.2)	5 (33.3)	
3 organisms	3	2 (66.7)	1 (50.0)	2 (66.7)	1 (50.0)	1 (33.3)	1 (100.0)	

Based on in-vitro susceptibility. Data on isolates with insufficient numbers (n ≤ 5) not shown. For polymicrobial infections, all isolates were susceptible to at least one of the treatment antibiotics
A, Ampicillin plus Gentamicin; B, Ampicillin plus cefotaxime; C, Cloxacillin plus gentamicin; CoNS, Coagulase negative *Staphylococcus* species. Other Gram-negatives included *Neisseria* species (n = 1), *Stenophromonas* species (n = 1) and *Moraxella* species (n = 1). Other Gram-positives included *Micrococcus* species (n = 5), and *Sterptomyces* species (n = 4)
Differing superscripts across row denotes differences in the proportion of susceptible isolates to antimicrobial regimen. Differences in proportions computed by Chi square with Marascuilo's Post Hoc Multiple proportion comparisons at p-value <0.05. Differing subscripts within a column denotes differences in the proportion of susceptible isolates to antimicrobial regimen

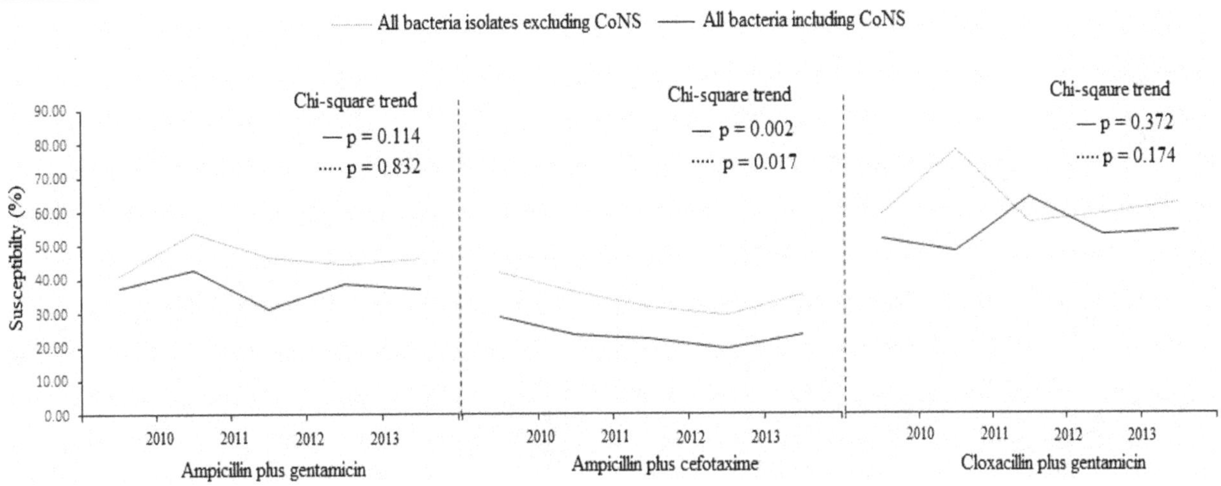

Fig. 1 Antibiotic resistance across study years. *CoNS, coagulase negative staphylococci; %, percentage.* Resistance of blood culture isolates (with or without CoNS) to ampicillin/cefotaxime significantly increased over study period. Resistance to ampicillin/gentamicin and cloxacillin/gentamicin remained relatively unchanged from 2010 through 2013

The incidence of Ceph-R Ent. and MDR Act. were significantly higher among LOS than in EOS. Meanwhile, VRE, MRSA, PRS and MDR Ps. were equally prevalent in LOS and EOS. Overall 53 % ($n = 917/1763$) of the total isolates exhibited MDR, accounting for about 50 % ($n = 886/1763$) of total bloodstream infections. Gram negative bacteria had more MDRs (71.7 %; $n = 236/329$) than GPB (47.9 %; $n = 681/1421$) (p-value =0.001). The MDRs were less prevalent (p-value <0.001) in EOS (37.3 %, $n = 331/886$) compared to LOS (62.4 %, $n = 555/886$). The yearly incidence of all MDRs remained relatively stable from 2010 through 2014 for EOS (Chi-square for trend, p-value = 0.284) and LOS (Chi-square for linear trend, p-value = 0.531).

Discussion

The rise in antibiotic resistance worldwide means that empirical therapy guided by local susceptibility is critical for improved therapeutic outcomes. In this study about a quarter of all neonatal blood cultures in our institution over a four year period were positive. We found a high prevalence of Gram-positive organisms which contrasts with previous findings in our hospital [5] and elsewhere [14, 15] where Gram-negative bacteria were the predominant organisms isolated. Coagulase negative *Staphylococcus* was the predominant organism identified in our study. The role played by CoNS in neonatal bloodstream infections is however not clear, as isolation from a single blood culture may represent true bacteraemia or contamination [16, 17]. Coagulase negative *Staphylococcus* have been found to play a significant role in bloodstream infections in neonates with low birth weight and gestational age [16–18] as well as in those with intravascular catheters insitu. In this study however, we were unable to ascertain the percentage of neonates with low birth weight; although anecdotally there is very low use of central catheters among neonates at the KBTH. Others have also suggested that a majority of blood cultures in neonates are performed in the first few days of life because of perceived risk factors of sepsis and not for clinical features of sepsis; and this may account for high rates of contamination with CoNS [19]. Thus it is possible that the high rate of isolation of CoNS from our study may point to high contamination rates from skin flora due to poor skin disinfection techniques. Despite this, other studies have reported high prevalence of CoNS among neonatal blood cultures [1, 2, 20].

Members of the *Enterobacteriaceae* were the commonest Gram negative organisms, with *Citrobacter* species, *Enterobacter* species and *Klebsiella* species accounting for the majority of organisms. This is in accordance with findings from other developing countries [1, 2, 14, 15, 21] as well as previous reports among neonates in KBTH [5]. The major role played by *Enterobacteriaceae* in neonatal sepsis may reflect a high rate of healthcare associated infections among our neonatal population, with these infections likely to have been transmitted from the environment by healthcare personnel and parents [4].

This study confirmed findings of low prevalence of *Streptococcus agalactaie* as a cause of EOS [5] This is contrary to findings in developed countries where EOS is mostly associated with *Streptococcus agalactiae* [3, 6]. However, similar findings of low prevalence have been made in other developing countries [2, 14, 15, 20, 21]. The prevalence of *Streptococcus agalactiae* in this study was low (0.68 %), despite a previous study showing *Streptococcus agalactiae* colonization rate of 19 % among pregnant women [22]. This finding may point to a minimal role

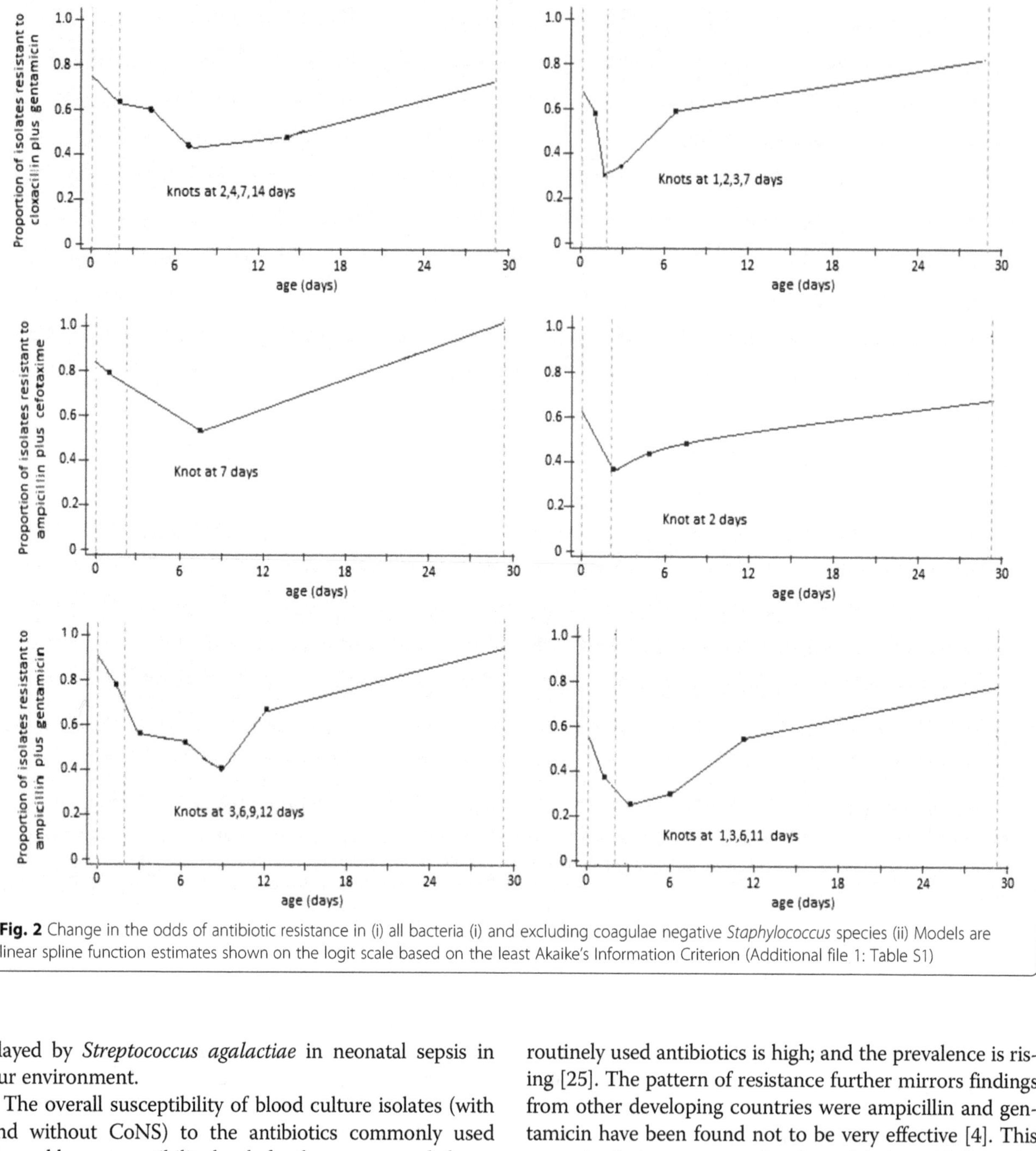

Fig. 2 Change in the odds of antibiotic resistance in (i) all bacteria (i) and excluding coagulae negative *Staphylococcus* species (ii) Models are linear spline function estimates shown on the logit scale based on the least Akaike's Information Criterion (Additional file 1: Table S1)

played by *Streptococcus agalactiae* in neonatal sepsis in our environment.

The overall susceptibility of blood culture isolates (with and without CoNS) to the antibiotics commonly used showed low susceptibility levels for the recommended regimens of ampicillin/gentamicin and ampicillin/cefotaxime [9, 10]. Cloxacillin/gentamicin had improved coverage over the national treatment guidelines, and remained the most active antibiotic combination despite a moderate coverage of <65.6 % for all bacterial isolates (with or without CoNS). This observation is in agreement with previous studies in Ghana and at Korle-Bu teaching Hospital, that found high resistance to ampicillin, gentamicin and cefotaxime among Gram negative isolates [23–25]. It is also the experience in KBTH that resistance to many routinely used antibiotics is high; and the prevalence is rising [25]. The pattern of resistance further mirrors findings from other developing countries were ampicillin and gentamicin have been found not to be very effective [4]. This suggests that current national antibiotic guidelines for neonatal sepsis may not be appropriate for management of neonatal infections in our study setting. Our results identified a pattern of resistance across neonatal age for all antibiotic combinations. When data excluded CoNS, we observed a decline in resistance for bacteria causing BSI in neonates aged <3 days for each of the antibiotic combinations. The rate in decrease of resistance was highest for cloxacillin/gentamicin. When data included CoNS, our results identified an age (9 days) beyond which antibiotic resistance appear to increase. This rate

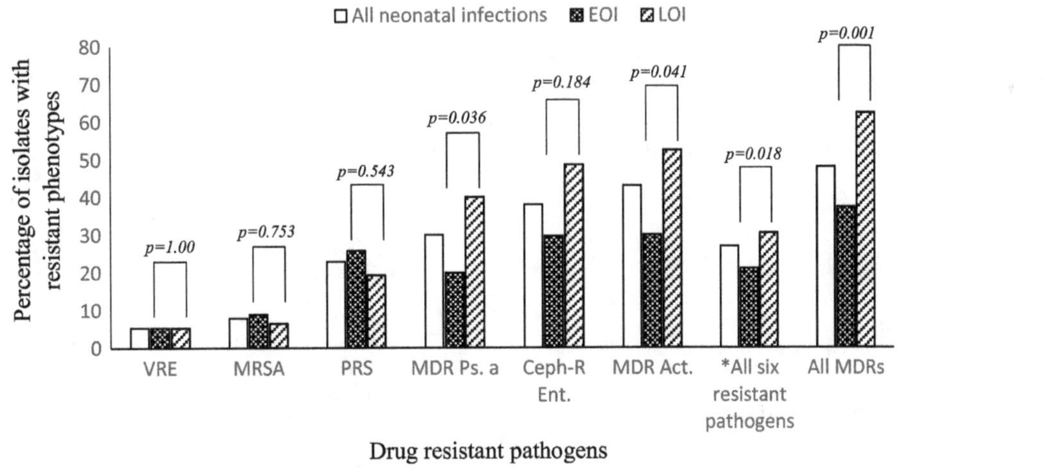

Fig. 3 Antimicrobial resistance phenotypes in early and late onset neonatal bloodstream infections. VRE, vancomycin resistant *Enterococci*; MRSA, methicillin resistant *Staphylococcus aureus*; PRS, penicillin resistant Streptococci; Cef-R Ent, cephalosporin resistant *Enterobacteriaceae*; MDR Ps, multidrug resistant *Pseudomonas aeruginosa*; MDR Act, multidrug resistant Acinetobacter species; * All six resistant pathogens is the pooled resistance for all six selected antibiotic drug resistance phenotypes

of increase in resistance was slowest for cloxacillin/gentamicin. Early onset resistance may point to the role played by resistant organisms of maternal origin, whilst increasing resistance over time may be indicative of increased role played by healthcare related infections which is associated with increased chances of antibiotic resistance [3]. This observation is reflected in our finding that GNB (which were more often MDRs; and are frequently associated with hospital flora) were dominant in LOS.

Also the study showed high levels of cefotaxime resistant *Enterobacteriaceae* which is a possible marker for extended spectrum beta lactamase (ESBL) production. However, data on ESBLs were not available for the study isolates. There was also high level of multi-drug resistant *Acinetobacter* species, but low levels of VRE and MRSA, and absence of carbapenem resistant *Enterobacteriaceae.* The KBTH has a higher prevalence (>40 %) of infections caused by ESBL-producers [25, 26] compared to MRSA (<10 %) [27]. High rates of ESBL-producers have been reported in community-acquired and neonatal bloodstream infections elsewhere in Ghana [28]. It is also anecdotal experience that CRE are encountered more often than VRE, but there are no published reports to document this evidence. This study shows that continuous surveillance of bloodstream infections among the neonatal populations in Ghana is needed to inform management strategies and policy which will contribute to the reduction of neonatal mortality from sepsis. The study had some limitations. Our study was retrospective thus affected by missing data including diagnosis of patients at time of sampling. Also, it was not possible to compare in vitro susceptibility testing of recommended antibiotic combinations with in vivo clinical efficacy.

Conclusion

From our study we observed a blood culture positivity rate of 21.9 % among neonates with most infections being of late onset. Coagulase negative *Staphylococcus* species were the commonly isolated organism in both early and late onset bacteraemia although their exact pathogenic role could not be determined. Whilst members of the *Enterobacteriaceae* (*Citrobacter* species, *Enterobacter* species, *Klebsiella* species) represented the commonest Gram negative organisms isolated. There was very high resistance to ampicillin/gentamicin and ampicillin/cefotaxime combinations among the isolated organism whilst relatively high susceptibility was observed to cloxacillin/gentamicin combination. Continuous surveillance of neonatal bloodstream infections is required to guide hospital and national antibiotic treatment guidelines to improve morbidity and mortality associated with neonatal bloodstream infections.

Abbreviations

µg: Microgram; AKL: Appiah-Korang Labi; ANOVA: Analysis of variance; BSI: Blood stream infections; CEL: Christabel Enweronu-Laryea; Ceph-R Ent: Cephalosporin resistant enterobacteria; CI: Confidence interval; CLSI: Clinical and Laboratory Standards Institute; GNB: Gram-negative bacteria; GPB: Gram-positive bacteria; KBTH: Korle-Bu Teaching Hospital; MDR Act: Multi-drug resistant *Acinetobacter* species; MDR Ps: Multi-drug resistant *Pseudomonas* species; MDR: Multidrug resistance; MDR: Multidrug resistant; MJN: Mercy Jemima Newman; MRSA: Methicillin resistant *Staphylococcus aureus*; NON: Noah Obeng-Nkrumah; PRS: Penicillin resistant streptococci; SB: Stephanie Bjerrum; SPSS: Statistical Package for Social Sciences; VRE: *Enterococcocus* species; VRE: *Enterococcocus* species

Acknowledgements

We thank the staff of the Microbiology Department of the Korle-Bu Teaching Hospital for their support.

Funding

The study received no specific gran.

Authors' contribution

LAK conceived the study; participated in its design, coordination, and collation of laboratory data; and helped to draft the manuscript. NON participated in the study design, coordination and collation of laboratory data; performed the statistical analysis; and helped to draft the manuscript. SB participated in drafting the manuscript. MJN, CEL participated in the study design and drafting of the manuscript. All authors read and approved the final manuscript.

Competing interests

The authors declare they have no competing interests.

Consent for publication

All authors have read the manuscript and provided consent for publication.

Ethics approval and consent to participate

The Department of Microbiology of KBTH routinely de-identifies patients from their laboratory records. The study authors were thus not privy to patients' laboratory data prior to anonymization. On receipt of de-identified laboratory data, we further anonymized all records to ensure complete obscurity from laboratory archives. We also allotted arbitrary numbers to all isolates assigned to the study. We did not review patients' clinical notes for further information. However given the anonymized data, as well as the retrospective nature of the study, we could not obtain patients' consent for use of the laboratory records. Ethical approval for isolates and laboratory data was not required as the study was regarded as part of routine surveillance measures for infection control.

Author details

[1]Department of Microbiology, Korle-Bu Teaching Hospital, P.O. Box 77, Accra, Republic of Ghana. [2]Microbiology Department, School of Biomedical and Allied Health Sciences, College of Health Sciences, University of Ghana, P.O. Box 4326, Accra, Republic of Ghana. [3]Department of Infectious Diseases, Institute of Clinical Research, Odense University Hospital, Sdr. Boulevard 29, Odense C, 5000 Odense, Denmark. [4]Department of Child Health, School of Medicine and Dentistry, College of Health Sciences, University of Ghana, P.O. Box 4326, Accra, Republic of Ghana. [5]Department of Medical Microbiology, School of Biomedical and Allied Health Sciences, University of Ghana, P.O. Box 147, Accra, Republic of Ghana.

References

1. Ballot DE, Nana T, Sriruttan C, Cooper PA. Bacterial bloodstream infections in neonates in a developing country. ISRN Pediatr. 2012;2012:508–12.
2. Morkel G, Bekker A, Marais BJ, Kirsten G, van Wyk J, Dramowski A. Bloodstream infections and antimicrobial resistance patterns in a South African neonatal intensive care unit. Paediatr Int Child Health. 2014;34:108–14.
3. Muller-Pebody B, Johnson AP, Heath PT, Gilbert RE, Henderson KL, Sharland M, iCAP Group (Improving Antibiotic Prescribing in Primary Care). Empirical treatment of neonatal sepsis: are the current guidelines adequate? Arch Dis Child - Fetal Neonatal Ed. 2011;96:F4–8.
4. Zaidi AKM, Huskins WC, Thaver D, Bhutta ZA, Abbas Z, Goldmann DA. Hospital-acquired neonatal infections in developing countries. Lancet. 2005;365:1175–88.
5. Enweronu-Laryea CC, Newman MJ. Changing pattern of bacterial isolates and antimicrobial susceptibility in neonatal infections in Korle-Bu Teaching hospital, Ghana. East Afr Med J. 2007;84:164–7.
6. Dagnew AF, Cunnington MC, Dube Q, Edwards MS, French N, Heyderman RS, Madhi SA, Slobod K, Clemens SAC. Variation in Reported Neonatal Group B Streptococcal Disease Incidence in Developing Countries. Clin Infect Dis. 2012;55:91–102.
7. Penno EC, Baird SJ, Crump JA. Cost-effectiveness of surveillance for bloodstream infections for sepsis management in low-resource settings. Am J Trop Med Hyg. 2015;93:850–60.
8. WHO: ANTIMICROBIAL RESISTANCE Global Report on Surveillance. Geneva: World Health Organisation; 2014.
9. Ministry of Health: Ghana Standard Treatment Guidelines. Sixth edit.; 2010.
10. Countdown Coverage Writing Group: Countdown to 2015 for Maternal, Newborn, and Child Survival: The 2008 Report on Tracking Coverage of Interventions. Volume 371; 2008
11. KBTH. Korle Bu Teaching Hospital, 2012 Annual Report. Accra, Ghana: Korle-Bu Teaching Hospital; 2013.
12. Magiorakos A, Srinivasan A, Carey RB, Carmeli Y, Falagas ME, Giske CG, Harbarth S, Hindler JF. bacteria : an international expert proposal for interim standard definitions for acquired resistance. Clin Microbiol Infect. 2012;18:268–81.
13. Blackburn RM, Verlander NQ, Heath PT, Muller-Pebody B. The changing antibiotic susceptibility of bloodstream infections in the first month of life: informing antibiotic policies for early- and late-onset neonatal sepsis. Epidemiol Infect. 2014;142:803–11.
14. West BA, Peterside O. Sensitivity pattern among bacterial isolates in neonatal septicaemia in port Harcourt. Ann Clin Microbiol Antimicrob. 2012;11:7–13.
15. Mhada TV, Fredrick F, Matee MI, Massawe A. Neonatal sepsis at Muhimbili National Hospital, Dar es Salaam, Tanzania; aetiology, antimicrobial sensitivity pattern and clinical outcome. BMC Public Health. 2012;12:904–7.
16. Healy CM, Baker CJ, Palazzi DL, Campbell JR, Edwards MS. Distinguishing true coagulase-negative Staphylococcus infections from contaminants in the neonatal intensive care unit. J Perinatol. 2013;33:52–8.
17. Jean-Baptiste N, Benjamin DK, Cohen-Wolkowiez M, Fowler VG, Laughon M, Clark RH, Smith PB. Coagulase-negative Staphylococcal Infections in the Neonatal Intensive Care Unit. Infect Control Hosp Epidemiol. 2011;32:679–86.
18. Isaacs D. A ten year, multicentre study of coagulase negative staphylococcal infections in Australasian neonatal units. Arch Dis Child Fetal Neonatal Ed. 2003;88:F89–93.
19. Blackburn RM, Muller-Pebody B, Planche T, Johnson A, Hopkins S, Sharland M, Kennea N, Heath PT. Neonatal sepsis–many blood samples, few positive cultures: implications for improving antibiotic prescribing. Arch Dis Child Fetal Neonatal Ed. 2012;97:F487–8.
20. Kohli-Kochhar R, Omuse G, Revathi G. A ten-year review of neonatal bloodstream infections in a tertiary private hospital in Kenya. J Infect Dev Ctries. 2011;5:218–25.
21. Kruse AY, Thieu Chuong DH, Phuong CN, Duc T, Graff Stensballe L, Prag J, Kurtzhals J, Greisen G, Pedersen FK. Neonatal bloodstream infections in a pediatric hospital in Vietnam: A cohort study. J Trop Pediatr. 2013;59:483–8.
22. Enweronu-Laryea CC, Damale NR, Newman MJ. Prevalence of group B streptococcus in pregnant women attending a tertiary hospital in Ghana in 2001. Parity. 2011;4:272–6.
23. Newman MJ, Frimpong E, Donkor ES, Opintan JA, Asamoah-Adu A. Resistance to antimicrobial drugs in Ghana. Infect Drug Resist. 2011;4:215–20.
24. Ayisi LA, Adu-Sarkodie Y. Extended-Spectrum-Beta-Lactamase (ESBL) production among Escherichia coli and Klebsiella species in Kumasi, Ghana. J Nat Sci Res. 2015;5:81–6.
25. Obeng-Nkrumah N, Twum-Danso K, Krogfelt KA, Newman MJ. High levels of extended-spectrum beta-lactamases in a major teaching hospital in Ghana: the need for regular monitoring and evaluation of antibiotic resistance. Am J Trop Med Hyg. 2013;89:960–4.
26. Oduro-Mensah D, Obeng-Nkrumah N, Bonney EY, Oduro-Mensah E, Twum-Danso K, Osei YD, Sackey ST. Genetic characterization of TEM-type ESBL-associated antibacterial resistance in Enterobacteriaceae in a tertiary hospital in Ghana. Ann Clin Microbiol Antimicrob. 2016;15:29–36.
27. Egyir B, Guardabassi L, Monecke S, Addo KK, Newman MJ, Larsen AR. Methicillin-resistant Staphylococcus aureus strains from Ghana include USA300. J Glob Antimicrob Resist. 2015;3:26–30.
28. Eibach D, Campos CB, Krumkamp R, Al-Emran HM, Dekker D, Gyau K, Kreuels B, Adu-sarkodie Y, Aepfelbacher M, Park SE, Panzner U, Marks F, May J. Extended spectrum beta-lactamase producing Enterobacteriaceae causing bloodstream infections in rural Ghana, 2007–2012. Int J Med Microbiol. 2016;306:249–54.

9

Trends in antimicrobial resistance and empiric antibiotic therapy of bloodstream infections at a general hospital in Mid-Norway

Arne Mehl[1,2,3*], Bjørn Olav Åsvold[3,4,5], Angela Kümmel[6], Stian Lydersen[7], Julie Paulsen[1,3,8], Ingvild Haugan[9], Erik Solligård[3,10,11], Jan Kristian Damås[3,8,12], Stig Harthug[13,14] and Tom-Harald Edna[2,15]

Abstract

Background: The occurrence of bloodstream infection (BSI) and antimicrobial resistance have been increasing in many countries. We studied trends in antimicrobial resistance and empiric antibiotic therapy at a medium-sized general hospital in Mid-Norway.

Methods: Between 2002 and 2013, 1995 prospectively recorded episodes of BSI in 1719 patients aged 16–99 years were included. We analyzed the antimicrobial non-susceptibility according to place of acquisition, site of infection, microbe group, and time period.

Results: There were 934 community-acquired (CA), 787 health care-associated (HCA) and 274 hospital-acquired (HA) BSIs. The urinary tract was the most common site of infection. *Escherichia coli* was the most frequently isolated infective agent in all three places of acquisition. Second in frequency was *Streptococcus pneumoniae* in CA and *Staphylococcus aureus* in both HCA and HA. Of the BSI microbes, 3.5% were non-susceptible to the antimicrobial regimen recommended by the National Professional Guidelines for Use of Antibiotics in Hospitals, consisting of penicillin, gentamicin, and metronidazole (PGM). In contrast, 17.8% of the BSI microbes were non-susceptible to cefotaxime and 27.8% were non-susceptible to ceftazidime.
Antimicrobial non-susceptibility differed by place of acquisition. For the PGM regimen, the proportions of non-susceptibility were 1.4% in CA, 4.8% in HCA, and 6.9% in HA-BSI ($p < 0.001$), and increasing proportions of non-susceptibility over time were observed in HA-BSI, 2.2% in 2002–2005, 6.2% in 2006–2009, and 11.7% in 2010–2013 ($p = 0.026$), mainly caused by inherently resistant microbes. We also observed increasing numbers of bacteria with acquired resistance, particularly *E. coli* producing ESBL or possessing gentamicin resistance, and these occurred predominantly in CA- and HCA-BSI.

Conclusions: Generally, antimicrobial resistance was a far smaller problem in our BSI cohort than is reported from countries outside Scandinavia. In our cohort, appropriate empiric antibiotic therapy could be achieved to a larger extent by replacing second- and third-generation cephalosporins with penicillin-gentamicin or piperacillin-tazobactam.

Keywords: Antibiotic therapy, Antimicrobial resistance, Bacteremia, Bacteraemia, Bloodstream infection, Empiric antibiotic treatment, Non-susceptibility, Sepsis

* Correspondence: arne.mehl@hnt.no
[1]Department of Medicine, Levanger Hospital, Nord-Trøndelag Hospital Trust, Post box 333, Levanger N-7601, Norway
[2]Unit for Applied Clinical Research, Department of Cancer Research and Molecular Medicine, NTNU, Norwegian University of Science and Technology, Trondheim, Norway
Full list of author information is available at the end of the article

Background

Bloodstream infection (BSI) contributes substantially to morbidity and mortality worldwide [1]. In Europe, the annual number of BSI episodes and deaths associated with BSI has been estimated to 1.2 million and 157,000, respectively [1]. Early diagnosis and early appropriate treatment is crucial. In severe sepsis, the case fatality increases for each hour the antibiotic treatment is delayed [2, 3]. Therefore, empirical antibiotic treatment has to be initiated before the results of blood cultures are available. However, as infections with resistant microbes is an escalating problem worldwide [4–6], it is increasingly challenging to maintain appropriate antibiotic regimens for initial empiric therapy. Resistant pathogenic bacteria are found less frequently in Norway and other Nordic countries, compared to the rest of Europe and other world regions [7, 8]. This probably reflects a relatively restrictive use of antimicrobial agents. In Norway, a regimen containing penicillin and gentamicin (PG), plus metronidazole (PGM) if an anaerobic infection is suspected, has been recommended for more than thirty years in sepsis with unknown focus and etiology [9–11]. In recent years, however, increasing numbers of infections with methicillin-resistant *Staphylococcus aureus* (MRSA), extended-spectrum beta-lactamase producing *Enterobacteriaceae* (ESBL-E), and vancomycin resistant enterococci have been detected [8]. Selection of inherently resistant microbes due to antibiotic use is also a challenge. Updated knowledge about the distribution of microbes in serious infections and their resistance against antimicrobial agents is needed to ensure appropriate empiric antimicrobial treatment regimens. It is also important to identify subgroups in which tailored regimens are required. Important differences in antibiotic resistance have been found with regard to place of acquisition [12, 13], and therefore, resistance statistics should specify results for community acquired (CA), health care-associated (HCA), and hospital acquired (HA) infections.

We conducted a prospective study to assess the occurrence and distribution of BSI microbes and their non-susceptibility to some common antibiotic regimens for initial empiric antimicrobial treatment of sepsis of unknown etiology. Particularly, we assessed microbes and antimicrobial resistance by place of acquisition (CA, HCA and HA-BSIs) and with regard to time trends over a 12-year period. We also studied the antibiotic regimens that were used for initial empiric treatment during the same time period and the degree to which they were appropriate.

Methods

Levanger Hospital serves a population of about 90,000 as an emergency facility in a defined geographical area of Mid-Norway. Since 1994, all positive blood cultures at the hospital have been prospectively recorded for surveillance purposes, and clinical information has been recorded, in the following way: whenever a positive blood culture was reported, a physician at the clinical ward filled out a registration form. A team of three research nurses, two subordinate doctors, and the main investigator reviewed all patients' records to verify the data and record additional variables. The present study includes BSIs that occurred between January 1, 2002 and December 31, 2013 in patients who were ≥16 years of age, and it is part of the Mid-Norway Sepsis Study.

The microbiology laboratory at Levanger Hospital is ISO 15189 accredited and participates in the national quality assurance schemes (ring tests). Blood cultures were performed in BACTEC 9240 Vacutainer Culture Bottles (Becton Dickinson Diagnostic Instrument Systems, Sparks, MD) [14], which in 2010 was replaced by BACTEC FX. No obvious changes in blood culture techniques or indications for drawing blood cultures have been done during the study period, but an increased focus on early detection of sepsis may have influenced the rate of blood culture sampling. Over the study period, the number of blood culture sets per 1000 hospital bed-days increased from 25.0 in 2002 to 59.5 in 2013.

Isolates were identified using standard methods [15]. Antimicrobial susceptibility testing was performed by the disc diffusion method (Neo-Sensitabs, Rosco Diagnostica, Taastrup, Denmark). For measurement of MIC, E-test (AB Biodisk, Solna, Sweden) was used. The results of antibacterial susceptibility testing were interpreted according to the Norwegian Working Group on Antibiotics (NWGA). For the antibiotics included in this study, the Norwegian breakpoints correspond to EUCAST (European Committee on Antimicrobial Susceptibility Testing) breakpoints [8, 16]. In this study, microbes intermediately susceptible to antibiotics were classified as non-susceptible [17–19], as only susceptible microbes can be regarded as being able to be managed by means of the respective antibiotic regimens. Microbes not tested in the laboratory because of known inherent non-susceptibility (e.g. enterococci are inherently resistant to cephalosporins) were classified as non-susceptible (see Additional file 1: Appendix 1 On inherent (natural) resistance in microbes).

An episode of BSI was defined by growth of one or more microbes from blood culture combined with clinical evidence of systemic infection. A new BSI episode with the same microbe in the same patient was recorded if an interval of at least 30 days had passed without signs of infection since an earlier episode [20]. If more than one organism was isolated from one or more blood cultures within a 72-h period, the BSI episode was classified as polymicrobial. One positive blood culture for organisms usually regarded as etiological agents was the requirement for inclusion. For coagulase-negative staphylococci or other possible skin contaminants, at least two identical isolates from separate venipunctures were required. Among alpha-hemolytic streptococci, *S. pneumoniae* and streptococci belonging to the *S. milleri* group were not considered as skin contaminants. Other alpha-hemolytic streptococci were included if they were found in two or more blood cultures from different venipuncture sites.

The place of acquisition was classified as hospital-acquired (HA), health care-associated (HCA) or community acquired (CA) [12, 21]. HA-BSI was diagnosed if the infection was detected >48 h after admission [22]. Patients who during the 30 days prior to hospital admission had (1) been hospitalized two or more days or (2) had received intravenous therapy or wound care at home or (3) hemodialysis or chemotherapy at hospital visits or (4) were nursing home residents, were categorized as having HCA-BSI. CA-BSI was diagnosed if the infection was detected <48 h after admission and none of the criteria for HCA-BSI were fulfilled.

A urinary focus was assigned when there was growth of the same microbe (s) from urine as well as from blood culture along with clinical signs/symptoms or risk factor for urinary infection, and no other source of infection was identified. A presumed pulmonary focus was diagnosed with clinical signs of lower respiratory infection accompanied by positive radiological findings. Focus in the biliary tract was ascertained based on clinical, biochemical and radiological findings. Signs of infection along with focal growth of the same microbe as in blood culture were

Table 1 Bloodstream infection (BSI) episodes in three time periods

	Total	2002–2005	2006–2009	2010–2013
All BSIs	1995 (100,0)	582 (100.0)	638 (100.0)	775 (100.0)
Place of acquisition				
Community acquired	934 (46.8)	317 (54.5)	280 (43.9)	337 (43.5)
Health care-associated	787 (39.4)	175 (30.1)	277 (43.4)	335 (43.2)
Hospital acquired	274 (13.7)	90 (15.5)	81 (12.7)	103 (13.3)
Microbial agent(s)				
Escherichia coli	686 (34.4)	186 (32.0)	231 (36.2)	269 (34.7)
Streptococcus pneumoniae	225 (11.3)	80 (13.8)	80 (12.5)	65 (8.4)
Staphylococcus aureus	218 (10.9)	72 (12.4)	55 (8.6)	91 (11.7)
Klebsiella spp.	135 (6.8)	22 (3.8)	44 (6.9)	69 (8.9)
Beta-hemolytic streptococci	104 (5.2)	33 (5.7)	35 (5.5)	36 (4.6)
Enterococcus spp.	89 (4.5)	28 (4.8)	26 (4.1)	35 (4.5)
Other mixed bacterial infections	68 (3.4)	21 (3.6)	19 (3.0)	28 (3.6)
Pseudomonas spp.	58 (2.9)	20 (3.4)	21 (3.3)	17 (2.2)
Viridans group streptococci	57 (2.9)	15 (2.6)	19 (3.0)	23 (3.0)
Coagulase-negative staphylococci	54 (2.7)	23 (4.0)	11 (1.7)	20 (2.6)
Proteus spp.	48 (2.4)	17 (2.9)	15 (2.3)	16 (2.1)
Anaerobic Gram-negative bacteria	45 (2.3)	14 (2.4)	16 (2.5)	15 (1.9)
Mixed Gram-negative aerobic or anaerobic bacteria	42 (2.1)	13 (2.2)	11 (1.7)	18 (2.3)
Enterobacter spp.	37 (1.9)	8 (1.4)	14 (2.2)	15 (1.9)
Other *Enterobacteriaceae*	37 (1.9)	7 (1.2)	12 (1.9)	18 (2.3)
Other aerobic Gram-negative bacteria	19 (1.0)	5 (0.9)	4 (0.6)	10 (1.3)
Haemophilus influenzae	17 (0.9)	6 (1.0)	8 (1.3)	3 (0.4)
Candida spp.	14 (0.7)	1 (0.2)	4 (0.6)	9 (1.3)
Anaerobic Gram-positive bacteria	11 (0.6)	3 (0.5)	4 (0.6)	4 (0.5)
Mixed gram-positive aerobic or anaerobic bacteria	11 (0.6)	1 (0.2)	4 (0.6)	6 (0.8)
Neisseria meningitidis	9 (0.5)	4 (0.7)	2 (0.3)	3 (0.4)
Listeria monocytogenes	8 (0.4)	2 (0.3)	2 (0.3)	4 (0.5)
Mixed bacterial and fungal infections	3 (0.2)	1 (0.2)	1 (0.2)	1 (0.1)

The table shows number (percent) of BSIs overall, by place of acquisition, and by microbial agent(s)

taken as a confirmation of infection in abdomen, skin, soft tissue or other sites. An unknown focus of infection was assigned when none of the criteria for ascertaining a focus were met.

Appropriate empiric antibiotic therapy (AEAT) was defined as correctly dosed intravenous antibiotic therapy with a regimen that was active in vitro against the microbe(s) isolated from blood culture (s). We assessed AEAT within 6 h and within 24 h of the time that the blood culture specimen was obtained.

Statistical analyses

Proportions of non-susceptibility across place of acquisition categories and time periods were assessed by a two-sided chi-square test. Trends in proportions were analyzed using Cochran-Armitage test. Two-sided p-values <0.05 were considered significant. Confidence intervals were calculated using Wilson's approximation to the binominal distribution [23]. The analyses were performed using SPSS 22, STATA 13, and StatXact 9.

Results

During the 12-year study period, a total of 1995 episodes of BSI occurred among 1719 individuals. CA-BSI episodes amounted to 46.8% of the total, HCA- and HA-BSI contributed 39.4% and 13.7%, respectively (Table 1). *Escherichia coli* was the predominating microbe (34.4%), followed by *Streptococcus pneumoniae* (11.3%) and *Staphylococcus aureus* (10.9%). The distribution of microbes by place of acquisition is shown in Fig. 1 and Additional file 1: Table S1. The distribution of microbes by infection site is shown in Additional file 1: Table S2. Totally, the number of BSIs increased across the three 4-year periods 2002–2005, 2006–2009, and 2010–2013 (Table 1). Most microbes contributed essentially similar proportions of the BSIs in each of the three time periods. However, the proportions of BSI from *Klebsiella* spp. (3.8% vs. 8.9%) and *Candida* spp. (0.3% vs. 1.3%) increased from the first to the third period. Conversely, the proportion of BSI from *Streptococcus pneumoniae* decreased from 13.8 to 8.4%.

In vitro susceptibility to antibiotics

Overall, 6.1% of the microbes were non-susceptible to a regimen consisting of penicillin and gentamicin (PG), and 3.5% were non-susceptible to a triple agent regimen including penicillin, gentamicin, and metronidazole (PGM) (Table 2). The proportions not susceptible to imipenem, piperacillin-tazobactam (PIP/TAZ), and cefotaxime, were 4.5%, 7.6%, and 17.8%, respectively. A broad-spectrum combination containing PIP/TAZ, gentamicin, and metronidazole had the lowest degree of non-susceptibility (2.6%), whereas ceftazidime had the highest (27.8%) (Table 2).

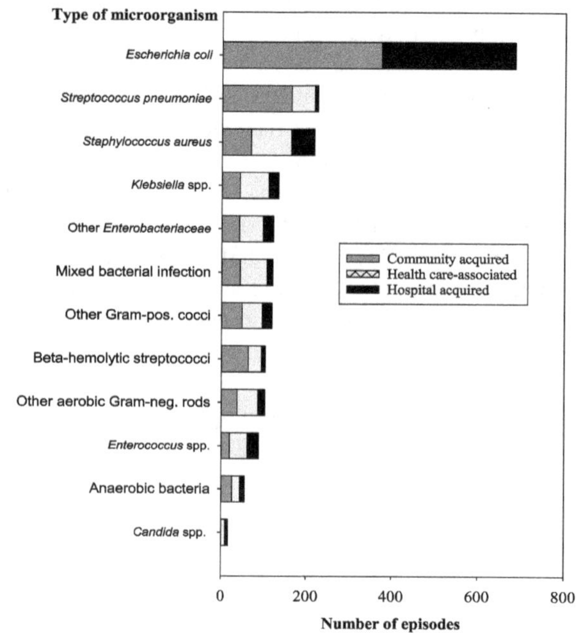

Fig. 1 Distribution of microbes from 1995 bloodstream infection episodes by place of acquisition. (Additional file 1: Table S1 shows microbial agents by place of acquisition in more detail)

The non-susceptibility to PGM was higher in HA-BSI (6.9%) and HCA-BSI (4.8%) than in CA-BSI (1.4%) ($p < 0.001$). Similar differences across place of acquisition were seen for imipenem, PIP/TAZ, and cefotaxime (Fig. 2, Table 2, Additional file 1: Table S3). The proportions of microbes non-susceptible to PGM increased through the three time periods in HA-BSI (2.2%, 6.2%, and 11.7%; $p = 0.026$), but we observed no significant time trends in antibiotic susceptibility for other antibiotic regimens (Table 2). Proportions of non-susceptibility by microbe are shown in Table 3. Non-susceptibility by site of infection is shown in Additional file 1: Table S4.

Among seventy BSI episodes with microbes non-susceptible to PGM (Fig. 3; Additional file 1: Table S5), *Candida* spp. accounted for 17 episodes, *E. coli* 16, and *Enterococcus faecium* and *Staphylococcus epidermidis* for 9 episodes each. The great majority of episodes with *Candida* spp., *Enterococcus faecium* or *Staphylococcus epidermidis* occurred in HCA or HA-BSI, and the highest numbers were recorded in the third time period. Regarding *E. coli* not susceptible to PGM (which means not susceptible to gentamicin), seven episodes occurred in CA, eight in HCA, and one in HA-BSI. The number of *E. coli* isolates non-susceptible to gentamicin was one (0.5%) in 2002–2005, six (2.6%) in 2006–2009, and nine (3.3%) in 2010–2013 (Additional file 1: Table S6).

The proportions of *E. coli* producing extended-spectrum beta-lactamase (ESBL) were 0% in 2002–05,

Table 2 The proportion (%) of bloodstream infection (BSI) episodes with microbe(s) non-susceptible to some common antibiotic regimens

	Total	2002–2005[a]	2006–2009	2010–2013	p for trend
Penicillin-gentamicin					
Total	6.1	4.4	6.1	7.5	0.011
Community acquired	4.3	2.2	5.7	5.0	0.22
Health care-associated	6.7	7.4	5.8	7.2	0.16
Hospital acquired	10.2	4.4	8.6	16.5	0.023
p for trend	0.006	0.058	0.46	0.003	
Penicillin-gentamicin-metronidazole					
Total	3.5	1.9	3.0	5.2	<0.001
Community acquired	1.4	0.3	1.8	2.1	0.28
Health care-associated	4.8	4.6	3.2	6.3	0.045
Hospital acquired	6.9	2.2	6.2	11.7	0.026
p for trend	<0.001	0.007	0.15	0.001	
Piperacillin/tazobactam					
Total ($n = 1413$)	7.6		7.4	7.7	0.25
Community acquired ($n = 617$)	3.6		2.9	4.2	0.27
Health care-associated ($n = 612$)	8.8		9.4	8.4	0.31
Hospital acquired ($n = 184$)	8.8		9.4	17.0	0.31
p for trend	<0.001		<0.001	<0.001	
Piperacillin/tazobactam-gentamicin					
Total ($n = 1413$)	3.0		2.4	3.6	0.21
Community acquired ($n = 617$)	1.0		0.7	1.2	0.69
Health care-associated ($n = 612$)	3.3		3.2	3.3	0.98
Hospital acquired ($n = 184$)	9.2		4.9	12.6	0.12
p for trend	<0.001		0.037	<0.001	
Piperacillin/tazobactam-gentamicin-metronidazole					
Total ($n = 1413$)	2.6		1.7	3.4	0.065
Community acquired ($n = 617$)	0.5		0.0	0.9	0.26
Health care-associated ($n = 612$)	2.9		2.5	3.3	0.64
Hospital acquired ($n = 184$)	8.7		4.9	11.7	0.12
p for trend	<0.001		0.004	<0.001	
Imipenem					
Community acquired	1.1	1.6	0.7	0.9	0.59
Health care-associated	6.5	9.1	5.8	5.7	0.39
Hospital acquired	10.6	11.1	7.4	12.6	0.14
p for trend	<0.001	<0.001	0.001	<0.001	

Table 2 The proportion (%) of bloodstream infection (BSI) episodes with microbe(s) non-susceptible to some common antibiotic regimens *(Continued)*

Cefotaxime					
Total	17.8	17.5	18.7	17.3	0.68
Community acquired	10.8	11.0	11.4	10.1	0.69
Health care-associated	21.3	25.1	22.7	18.2	0.18
Hospital acquired	31.4	25.6	29.6	37.9	0.31
p for trend	<0.001	<0.001	<0.001	<0.001	
Ceftazidime					
Total	27.8	29.0	24.8	29.4	0.25
Community acquired	18.5	20.2	15.4	19.6	0.42
Health care-associated	31.3	36.0	28.2	31.3	0.37
Hospital acquired	49.6	46.7	45.7	55.3	0.46
p for trend	<0.001	<0.001	<0.001	<0.001	

[a]Piperacillin/tazobactam was not adopted in the first time period
The BSIs are stratified by place of acquisition and by time period (the total number in each cell is shown under the heading Place of acquisition in Table 1)

2.0% in 2006–09, and 1.7% in 2010–13 (Additional file 1: Table S7). Only one episode of methicillin-resistant *Staphylococcus aureus* (MRSA) was found, and only in two (0.9%) of 225 BSIs with *Streptococcus pneumoniae*, the microbe was non-susceptible to penicillin (Additional file 1: Table S3).

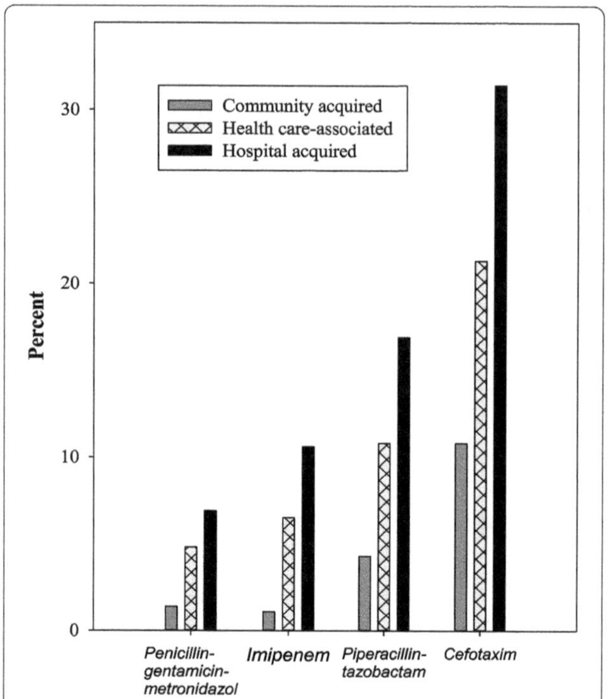

Fig. 2 Proportion of bloodstream infection microbes non-susceptible to four antibiotic regimens by place of acquisition

Initial empiric antibiotic therapy

The use of second- and third generation cephalosporins as initial empiric therapy decreased through the study periods. Cefuroxime was used as monotherapy or in combination in 19.6% and 5.3% of the BSI episodes in the first and in the third time period, respectively. The corresponding proportions for cefotaxime were 18.1% and 15.7% (Table 4). In contrast, the use of ampicillin or penicillin plus gentamicin increased from 14.1% to 19.9%. PIP/TAZ was not used in the first period, but was the second most used empiric therapy in the third period (17.3%). The proportions of patients who received appropriate empiric antibiotic therapy (AEAT) within 6 h and within 24 h were larger in the third period than in the first and second periods (Table 5). The proportions of patients who received AEAT within 6 h in the third period were 67.1% in CA, 67.2% in HCA, and 59.0% in HA-BSI. The corresponding proportions who received AEAT within 24 h were 88.4%, 84.4%, and 83.1%, respectively.

Discussion

In this prospective study of 1995 consecutive BSIs at a medium-sized Norwegian hospital between 2002 and 2013, antimicrobial resistance was a far smaller problem than reported in most studies [7, 17, 24, 25]. Except for third-generation cephalosporins, antimicrobial resistance to regimens recommended for sepsis of unknown etiology was low. In less than 4% of BSI episodes, microbes were non-susceptible to PGM, consistent with previous findings at our hospital [26] and in other Norwegian studies [10, 27]. However, the proportion of antibiotic non-susceptibility was higher in HA and HCA than in CA-BSI. For PGM, an increase in non-susceptibility

Table 3 Proportions (%) of different microbes or microbe groups non-susceptible to some commonly recommended antibiotics and antibiotic regimens

Microbe/microbe group	Antibiotics and antibiotic combinations (2002–2013)							P/T alone or in combinations (2006–2013)			
	PG	PGM	Imi-penem	Cefo-taxime	Cefta-zidime	Cipro-floxa-cin	Total N	P/T	P/T-G	P/T-G-M	Total N
Streptococcus pneumoniae§	0.9	0.9	0.0	0.4	0.4	NRT	226	0.7	0.7	0.7	146
Beta-hemolytic streptococci	0.0	0.0	0.0	0.0	100.0	NRT	104	0.0	0.0	0.0	71
Viridans streptococci	0.0	0.0	0.0	3.5	8.8	NRT	57	0.0	0.0	0.0	42
Staphylococcus aureus#	0.5	0.5	0.0	0.0	100.0 (IR)	NRT	218	0.0	0.0	0.0	146
Coagulase-negative staphylococci	13.0	13.0	38.9	38.9	100.0 (IR)	NRT	54	41.9	19.4	19.4	31
Enterococcus spp.	9.0	9.0	11.2	100.0 (IR)	100.0 (IR)	NRT	89	11.5	9.8	9.8	61
Listeria monocytogenes	0.0	0.0	0.0	100.0 (IR)	100.0 (IR)	NRT	8	0.0	0.0	0.0	6
Escherichia coli	1.9	1.9	0.1	1.9	1.9	3.3	686	6.0	0.8	0.8	500
Klebsiella spp. or *Proteus* spp.	0.0	0.0	5.5	2.2	2.2	4.7	182	7.0	0.0	0.0	143
Other enterobacteria	1.4	1.4	9.5	20.3	21.6	2.9	74	16.9	100.0	100.0	59
Pseudomonas spp.	1.7	1.7	6.9	100.0 (IR)	3.4	8.2	58	5.3	2.6	2.6	38
Other aerobic Gram-negatives	8.9	8.9	8.9	31.1	28.9	6.7	45	23.3	0.0	0.0	30
Anaerobic bacteria	66.1	3.6	0.0	96.4	96.4	NRT	56	5.1	7.7	0.0	39
Mixed bacterial infection	24.8	11.6	13.2	48.8	50.4	NRT	121	11.6	8.1	4.7	86
Candida spp. single or in mixed infection	100.0 (IR)	100.0 (IR)	100.0 (IR)	100.0 (IR)	100.0 (IR)	100.0 (IR)	17	100.0 (IR)	100.0 (IR)	100.0 (IR)	15
Total	6.1	3.5	4.5	17.8	27.8	NRT	1995	7.6	3.0	2.6	1413

§two isolates of penicillin-non-susceptible pneumococci were detected
#one single isolate of methicillin-resistant *Staphylococcus aureus* (MRSA) and one single isolate of gentamicin-resistant *S. aureus* were detected
IR, inherently resistant (see Additional file 1: Appendix 1 On inherent (natural) resistance in microbes); NRT, not routinely tested; PG, penicillin-gentamicin; PGM, penicillin-gentamicin-metronidazole; P/T, piperacillin-tazobactam; P/T-G, piperacillin-tazobactam plus gentamicin; P/T-G-M, piperacillin-tazobactam plus gentamicin plus metronidazole
Piperacillin-tazobactam (P/T) was adopted in 2006

through the study period was observed in HA-BSI, mainly caused by inherently resistant microbes. A slightly increasing number of bacteria with acquired resistance was also detected, particularly *E. coli* producing ESBL or possessing gentamicin resistance. In our cohort, appropriate empiric antibiotic therapy could be achieved to a larger extent by replacing cephalosporins with PG or PIP/TAZ.

Strengths of this study include the prospective registration of BSIs within a well-defined area, and the handling of blood cultures at one microbiology laboratory. We present susceptibility data by microbe, by place of acquisition, and by site of infection. Most authors have presented susceptibility data only by microbe, which is generally unknown at the time the physician has to decide on the initial antimicrobial therapy. We included microbes with known inherent resistance in the presentation in order to give guidance for empirical treatment before the microbial etiology is known. Our use of one single institution as the study site limits the generalizability of our results, but regarding antibiotic resistance patterns as basis for treatment guidelines, our results may be relevant for other general hospitals in Scandinavia.

The low proportions of non-susceptibility in our BSI microbes are likely explained by a relatively strict use of antibiotics in Norway [8, 28, 29]. All antibiotics used in humans are prescribed by physicians, and penicillins and aminoglycosides are the preferred drugs in severe bacterial infections. The increasing non-susceptibility in BSI microbes by place of acquisition and, for HA-BSI, by time period, was mainly due to a shift towards microbes with natural (inherent) resistance, particularly *Candida* spp., *Enterococcus faecium*, and *Staphylococcus epidermidis*. We attribute this shift to the increasing use of chemotherapy and other immunosuppressive treatments (Additional file 1, Table S9), which results in more prevalent infections and antibiotic treatments, giving rise to selection of

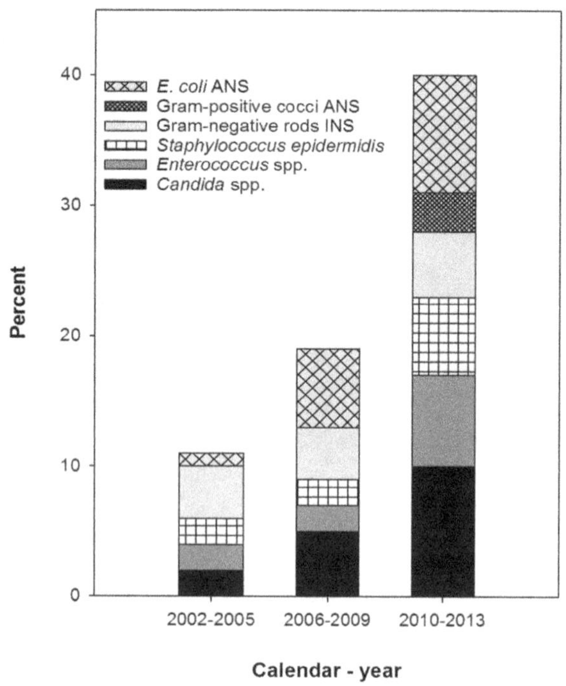

Fig. 3 Microbes non-susceptible to penicillin-gentamicin-metronidazole (PGM) through three time periods. (Additional file 1: Table S5 shows the PGM non-susceptible microbes in detail) ANS, acquired non-susceptibility; INS, inherent non-susceptibilty

resistant microbes. A higher proportion of non-susceptible microbes in HA and HCA than in CA-BSI is well known from other studies [12, 13], but this cautionary knowledge does not seem to have been sufficiently heeded by clinicians and guideline makers. The national Norwegian surveillance data on the distribution of different microbes isolated from blood cultures show no time trend towards increasing occurrence of natural resistant microbes from 2004 to 2014

Table 4 The most commonly used initial empiric antibiotic regimens (percent) through three time periods

Initial antibiotic regimen	2002–2005 ($n = 582$)	2006–2009 ($n = 638$)	2010–2013 ($n = 775$)
Cefotaxime	18.1	18.2	15.7
Penicillin/ampicillin-gentamicin	14.1	14.6	19.9
Penicillin	14.1	14.3	8.1
Piperacillin-tazobactam	0	8.6	17.3
Cefuroxime-metronidazole	9.8	8.1	4.1
Cefotaxime-metronidazole	3.6	5.6	5.5
Mecillinam	5.0	4.7	4.9
Cefuroxime	9.8	3.4	1.2
Penicillin-gentamicin-metronidazole	5.9	3.4	1.7

A complete table showing initial treatment in 1995 bloodstream infection episodes is found in Additional file 1: Table S8

Table 5 Appropriate empiric antibiotic therapy (AEAT) through three time periods by place of acquisition

	2002–2005 ($n = 582$)	2006–2009 ($n = 638$)	2010–2013 ($n = 775$)
AEAT within 6 h			
Community acquired BSI	61.7	63.4	67.1
Health care-associated BSI	64.0	53.6	67.2
Hospital acquired BSI	43.9	46.4	59.0
AEAT within 24 h			
Community acquired BSI	84.2	89.4	88.4
Health care-associated BSI	76.7	81.3	84.4
Hospital acquired BSI	72.2	73.9	83.1

Percent of patients with bloodstream infection (BSI) receiving AEAT within 6 h and within 24 h

[8, 30], but do not distinguish between CA, HCA, and HA infection. The European Antimicrobial Resistance Surveillance Network (EARS-Net) reported increasing occurrence of *Enterococcus faecium* from 2002 to 2008 [7], but *Candida* spp. and *S. epidermidis* are not included in the EARS-Net surveillance.

Acquired resistance was uncommon in our BSI cohort, but an increasing proportion of *E. coli* was non-susceptible to gentamicin, and they occurred in CA as well as in HCA-BSIs. Nationwide, a worrying increase in resistance to gentamicin has emerged from 2003 to 2014 (0.6% to 7.7%) [8]. The EARS-Net has reported 5.2% and 9.9% aminoglycoside resistance in *E. coli* in 2002 and 2013, respectively [7, 24], but the proportion of aminoglycoside resistance was much higher in the south-eastern region (32.1% in Bulgaria in 2013). The proportion of *E. coli* producing ESBL has increased from 2008 to 2014 (1.5% to 5.8%) according to the national data [8], and according to EARS-Net data, the proportion of ESBL-producing *E. coli* in Europe increased from 2.0% in 2002 [24] to 12.6% in 2013 (39.6% in Bulgaria) [7].

One single isolate of MRSA and two pneumococci intermediately susceptible to penicillin were found in our cohort. Nationwide, the proportion of MRSA in blood cultures has been low in the corresponding time period (0.3% and 0.8% in 2002 and 2014, respectively). The low occurrence of MRSA in the Nordic countries and in the Netherlands clearly distinguishes from the other European countries, where MRSA accounted for >25% of the *S. aureus* BSIs in 2007 [25] but had decreased to 18% in 2013 [7]. The nationwide proportion of invasive pneumococci non-susceptible to penicillin was 0.9% in 2002 and 5.5% in 2014 [8, 30]. In Europe, the proportion of penicillin-non-susceptible isolates in 2013 ranged from 1.1% (the Netherlands) to 40.0% (Cyprus) [7]. Comparisons of trends in acquired non-susceptibility in the current study and in surveillance data from Norway and other European countries are shown in Table 6.

Empirical antibiotic treatment regimens have to be continuously evaluated in accordance with national and local microbe resistance patterns. The initial empiric treatment for sepsis of unknown origin recommended by the National Professional Guidelines for Use of Antibiotics in Hospitals in Norway consists of penicillin and gentamicin, plus metronidazole (PGM) if an anaerobic infection is suspected [11]. PGM was not effective in vitro against 3.5% of the microbes isolated from blood cultures in the present study. In patients with HA-BSI, however, the proportion of microbes not susceptible to PGM was 11.7% in the third time period. In defined subgroups we have to be aware of PGM resistant microbes and include vancomycin (e.g., suspected central venous catheter infection) or an antifungal drug (if suspected candida infection, e.g., long lasting broad-spectrum antibiotic therapy, long time stay in a ICU, particularly after gastrointestinal surgery), in our recommendations. Use of carbapenems in empiric therapy should be restricted to patients infected with bacteria resistant (known or suspected) to PIP/TAZ and in whom aminoglycoside therapy is contraindicated.

Enterococci are inherently resistant to cephalosporins and staphylococci are not susceptible to ceftazidime. In our BSI cohort, staphylococci and enterococci contributed to 30% of HA-BSI episodes. Noteworthy, the percentages of microbes non-susceptible to cefotaxime and ceftazidime in HA-BSI in the third period were as high as 37.9 and 55.3%, respectively. Therefore, none of these appears suitable for use as monotherapy in sepsis of unknown microbial origin. The emergence of ESBL in Gram-negative bacteria has made it even more risky to choose a third-generation cephalosporin as monotherapy for severe infections with unknown etiology.

Even though the National Professional Guidelines [11] recommend PG (or PGM) as the regimen of first choice in sepsis of unknown etiology, the PG (or PGM) combination was given in no more than 20% of the episodes in our BSI cohort, yet the proportion was increasing with time. There are mainly two reasons for prescribing antibiotic treatment that does not include an aminoglycoside: (1) Aminoglycosides are potentially nephrotoxic and ototoxic. Therefore, there is a tendency to avoid them even in cases where they should not be contraindicated. (2) Use of an aminoglycoside requires measurement of aminoglycoside serum concentrations, which is resource consuming, and knowledge and experience is needed for assessment of the results. In a busy day, it is much simpler to administer a beta-lactam-antibiotic, where dosing is simple and the risk of toxicity is negligible.

In Norway, we lack national data for antibacterial treatment given in cases of bloodstream infection or sepsis.

Table 6 Comparisons of trends in acquired non-susceptibility in *Escherichia coli*, *Staphylococcus aureus*, and *Streptococcus pneumoniae*

Microbe	Type of non-susceptibility	Surveillance Area	Trends in proportions of non-susceptibility (Time period)	
E. coli	Gentamicin non-susceptibility	Levanger Hospital	0.5% (2002–05)	3.3% (2010–13)
		Iceland	2.9% (2010)	4.1% (2013)
		Norway	0.6% (2003)	7.7% (2014)
		EU/EEA	5.2% (2002)	9.9% (2013)
		Bulgaria	15.8% (2003)	32.1% (2013)
E. coli	Resistance to 3rd generation cephalosporins	Levanger Hospital	0 (2002–05)	1.7% (2010–13)
		Norway	1.5% (2008)	5.8% (2014)
		EU/EEA	2.0% (2002)	12.6% (2013)
		Bulgaria	24.8% (2010)	39.6% (2013)
S. aureus	MRSA	Levanger Hospital	0 (2002–05)	1.0% (2010–13)
		Norway	0.3% (2002)	0.8% (2014)
		EU/EEA	25.6% (2007)	18.0% (2013)
		Malta	52.0% (2007)	51.8% (2013)
		Romania	39.1% (2010)	64.5% (2013)
S. pneumoniae	PNSP	Levanger Hospital	0 (2002–05)	3.0% (2010–13)
		Netherlands	2.0% (2010)	1.1% (2013)
		Norway	0.9% (2002)	5.5% (2014)
		Cyprus	41.7% (2010)	40.0% (2013)

MRSA, meticillin-resistant *Staphylococcus aureus*; PNSP, penicillin non-susceptible pneumococci
Proportions of non-susceptibility from the current study (Levanger Hospital) are compared with data from Norway (the national surveillance system [8, 30], the European Union/the European Economic Area (EU/EEA), and with countries which have extraordinary low or high proportions of non-susceptibility [7, 24, 25]

Regarding antibiotic use in Norwegian hospitals, the national surveillance data [8] show that the proportion of aminoglycoside use was less than 5% in 2015 (3.3 out of 73 DDD/100 bed-days), indicating that avoiding aminoglycosides in favor of beta-lactam antibiotics is a common mode of acting countrywide.

The drawback of avoiding aminoglycosides is increased risk of antimicrobial resistance, as particularly cephalosporins are far more resistance driving than aminoglycosides. Therefore, a further shift in favor of aminoglycosides is desirable. As the use of aminoglycosides in our hospital and nationwide is still relatively low, overuse of aminoglycosides is unlikely to explain the observed increase in non-susceptibility to gentamicin in *E. coli*.

During the three time periods, we observed that the use of second- and third- generation cephalosporins decreased, whereas ampicillin or penicillin plus gentamicin were more frequently given. PIP/TAZ was introduced at our hospital in 2006, and the use of it has been increasing, particularly in the third period. Nationwide, the use of aminoglycosides and particularly piperacillin/tazobactam has increased during the last ten years, whereas the use of second-generation cephalosporins has decreased. The use of third-generation cephalosporins and fluoroquinolones peaked in 2011–2012 and have since then declined [8]. These changes are in accordance with the national [11] and local antibiotic policy, in order to achieve regimens that are less resistance driving and also cover the BSI microbes to a larger extent.

Conclusions

Antimicrobial resistance was a far smaller problem in our BSI cohort than is reported from countries outside Scandinavia. The antibiotic regimen recommended by Norwegian Health Authorities [11], consisting of penicillin and gentamicin, and with metronidazole added when an anaerobic infection is suspected, is so far effective in vitro against a great majority of microbes isolated from BSI patients in this region. In our cohort, appropriate empiric antibiotic therapy was achieved to a larger extent by replacing second- and third-generation cephalosporins with penicillins and gentamicin. We must, however, be aware of an increasing occurrence of inherently resistant microbes, particularly in HA infection. There are also indications of increasing numbers of bacteria with acquired resistance, particularly *E. coli* producing ESBL and/or possessing gentamicin resistance, and these occurred predominantly in CA and HCA infections.

Additional file

Additional file 1: Table S1. Number (percent) of bloodstream infection episodes stratified by microbe(s)/microbe group and by place of acquisition. **Table S2.** Number (percent) of bloodstream infection episodes stratified by microbe(s)/microbe group and by infection focus. **Table S3.** Proportions of bloodstream infection episodes with microbe(s) non-susceptible to four commonly used antibiotic regimens by place of acquisition. **Table S4.** Percent of bloodstream infection episodes with microbe(s) non-susceptible to commonly recommended sepsis regimens by site of infection. **Table S5.** Number of microbes not susceptible to penicillin-gentamicin-metronidazole by place of acquisition through three time periods. **Table S6.** Number of BSIs with *Escherichia coli* susceptible, intermediately susceptible or resistant to gentamicin through three time periods. **Table S7.** Number of BSIs with *Escherichia coli* non-susceptible to cefotaxime through three time periods. **Table S8.** Antimicrobial agents (single or in combinations) given as initial treatment in 1995 episodes of bloodstream infection. **Table S9.** Use of antibacterial agents and antineoplastic agents, measured in DDD/100 bed-days, at Levanger Hospital 2006 to 2013. **Appendix 1 On inherent (natural) resistance in microbes.** Rules for assessment of non-susceptibility in microbes not tested against antimicrobial agents in the laboratory. (DOCX 78 kb)

Abbreviations

AEAT: Appropriate empiric antibiotic therapy; BSI: Bloodstream infection; CA: Community acquired; EARS-Net: The European Antimicrobial Resistance Surveillance Network; ESBL: Extended-spectrum beta-lactamase; ESBL-E: Extended-spectrum beta-lactamase producing *Enterobacteriaceae*; EUCAST: European Committee on Antimicrobial Susceptibility Testing; HA: Hospital acquired; HCA: Health care-associated; NWGA: Norwegian Working Group on Antibiotics; PG: Penicillin plus gentamicin; PGM: Penicillin, gentamicin, and metronidazole; PIP/TAZ: Piperacillin-tazobactam

Acknowledgments

We would like to thank our research nurses for diligent and accurate work in the data collection process. We would also like to thank the staff at the Microbiology Laboratory, Levanger Hospital, for consecutively including cases and sending registration forms to physicians treating the patients at the wards.

Funding

This work is supported by the Unit for Applied Clinical Research, Norwegian University of Science and Technology; the Liaison Committee between the Central Norway Regional Health Authority (RHA) and the Norwegian University of Science and Technology (NTNU); St Olav's University Hospital; the Norwegian Surveillance Programme for Antimicrobial Resistance; and by Nord-Trøndelag Hospital Trust's Fund for Research and Improvement.

Authors' contributions

AM conceived the study and participated in design, data collection, statistical analysis, interpretation of the data, and drafting of the manuscript. BOÅ participated in design, statistical analysis, data interpretation, and drafting of the manuscript. AK participated in design, data interpretation, and drafting of the manuscript. SL participated in design, statistical analysis, data interpretation, and drafting of the manuscript. JP participated in design, data collection and drafting of the manuscript. ES contributed to design, interpretation of the data, and drafting of the manuscript. JKD participated in study design, data interpretation and drafting of the manuscript. SH participated in design, data interpretation, and drafting of the manuscript. THE participated in design, data collection, statistical analysis, and drafting of the manuscript. All the authors read and approved the final manuscript.

Competing interests

The authors declare that they have no competing interests.

Consent for publication

Not applicable

Author details
[1]Department of Medicine, Levanger Hospital, Nord-Trøndelag Hospital Trust, Post box 333, Levanger N-7601, Norway. [2]Unit for Applied Clinical Research, Department of Cancer Research and Molecular Medicine, NTNU, Norwegian University of Science and Technology, Trondheim, Norway. [3]Mid-Norway Sepsis Research Group, Faculty of Medicine, NTNU, Norwegian University of Science and Technology, Trondheim, Norway. [4]Department of Public Health, NTNU, Norwegian University of Science and Technology, Trondheim, Norway. [5]Department of Endocrinology, St Olavs Hospital, Trondheim University Hospital, Trondheim, Norway. [6]Department of Laboratory Medicine, Levanger Hospital, Nord-Trøndelag Hospital Trust, Levanger, Norway. [7]Regional Centre for Child and Youth Mental Health and Child Welfare – Central Norway, NTNU, Norwegian University of Science and Technology, Trondheim, Norway. [8]Centre of Molecular Inflammation Research, Department of Cancer Research and Molecular Medicine, NTNU, Norwegian University of Science and Technology, Trondheim, Norway. [9]Department of Medical Microbiology, St Olavs Hospital, Trondheim University Hospital, Trondheim, Norway. [10]Clinic of Anesthesia and Intensive Care, St Olavs Hospital, Trondheim University Hospital, Trondheim, Norway. [11]Department of Circulation and Medical Imaging, NTNU, Norwegian University of Science and Technology, Trondheim, Norway. [12]Department of Infectious Diseases, St Olav's Hospital, Trondheim University Hospital, Trondheim, Norway. [13]Department of Research and Development, Haukeland University Hospital, Bergen, Norway. [14]Department of Clinical Science, University of Bergen, Bergen, Norway. [15]Department of Surgery, Levanger Hospital, Nord-Trøndelag Hospital Trust, Levanger, Norway.

References

1. Goto M, Al-Hasan MN. Overall burden of bloodstream infection and nosocomial bloodstream infection in North America and Europe. Clin Microbiol Infect. 2013;19(6):501–9.
2. Ferrer R, Martin-Loeches I, Phillips G, Osborn TM, Townsend S, Dellinger RP, Artigas A, Schorr C, Levy MM. Empiric antibiotic treatment reduces mortality in severe sepsis and septic shock from the first hour: results from a guideline-based performance improvement program. Crit Care Med. 2014;42(8):1749–55.
3. Kumar A, Roberts D, Wood KE, Light B, Parrillo JE, Sharma S, Suppes R, Feinstein D, Zanotti S, Taiberg L, et al. Duration of hypotension before initiation of effective antimicrobial therapy is the critical determinant of survival in human septic shock. Crit Care Med. 2006;34(6):1589–96.
4. Nathan C, Cars O. Antibiotic resistance-problems, progress, and prospects. N Engl J Med. 2014;371(19):1761–3.
5. World Health Organization: Antimicrobial resistance: Global report on surveillance. Geneva; 2014. http://www.who.int/drugresistance/documents/surveillancereport/en.
6. Levy SB, Marshall B. Antibacterial resistance worldwide: causes, challenges and responses. Nat Med. 2004;10(12 Suppl):S122–9.
7. EARS-Net. European Centre for Disease Prevention and Control: Antimicrobial resistance surveillance in Europe 2013. In: Annual Report of the European Antimicrobial Resistance Surveillance Network (EARS-Net). Stockholm: ECDC; 2014.
8. NORM/NORM-VET. Usage of Antimicrobial Agents and Occurrence of Antimicrobial Resistance in Norway 2015. Oslo: Tromsø; 2016. ISSN:1502–2307 (print)/1890-9965(electronic).
9. Solberg CO. Treatment of sepsis. Tidsskr Nor Laegeforen. 1978;98:1764–6.
10. Vorland LH, Lingaas E, Ragnhildstveit E. The resistance of microorganisms in bacteremia. Tidsskr Nor Laegeforen. 1988;108(2):130–1.
11. The Norwegian Directorate of Health: National Professional Guidelines for Use of Antibiotics in Hospitals. https://helsedirektoratet.no/retningslinjer/antibiotikabruk-i-sykehus. Accessed 15 July 2014.
12. Siegman-Igra Y, Fourer B, Orni-Wasserlauf R, Golan Y, Noy A, Schwartz D, Giladi M. Reappraisal of community-acquired bacteremia: a proposal of a new classification for the spectrum of acquisition of bacteremia. Clin Infect Dis. 2002;34(11):1431–9.
13. Cardoso T, Almeida M, Carratala J, Aragao I, Costa-Pereira A, Sarmento AE, Azevedo L. Microbiology of healthcare-associated infections and the definition accuracy to predict infection by potentially drug resistant pathogens: a systematic review. BMC Infect Dis. 2015;15:565.
14. Nolte FS, Williams JM, Jerris RC, Morello JA, Leitch CD, Matushek S, Schwabe LD, Dorigan F, Kocka FE. Multicenter clinical evaluation of a continuous monitoring blood culture system using fluorescent-sensor technology (BACTEC 9240). J Clin Microbiol. 1993;31(3):552–7.
15. Murray PR, Baron EJ, Jorgensen JH, Pfaller MA, Yolken RH. Manual of Clinical Microbiology. 8th ed. Washington: American Society for Microbiology; 2003.
16. EUCAST: European Committee on Antimicrobial Susceptibility Testing: Clinical breakpoints. https://eucast.org. Accessed 15 Jan 2012.
17. Reacher MH, Shah A, Livermore DM, Wale MC, Graham C, Johnson AP, Heine H, Monnickendam MA, Barker KF, James D, et al. Bacteraemia and antibiotic resistance of its pathogens reported in England and Wales between 1990 and 1998: trend analysis. BMJ. 2000;320(7229):213–6.
18. Hernandez C, Cobos-Trigueros N, Feher C, Morata L, De La Calle C, Marco F, Almela M, Soriano A, Mensa J, Del Rio A, et al. Community-onset bacteraemia of unknown origin: clinical characteristics, epidemiology and outcome. Eur J Clin Microbiol Infect Dis. 2014;33(11):1973–80.
19. Livermore DM, Hope R, Brick G, Lillie M, Reynolds R, Surveillance BWPoR. Non-susceptibility trends among Enterobacteriaceae from bacteraemias in the UK and Ireland, 2001–06. J Antimicrob Chemother. 2008;62(2):ii41–54.
20. Haug JB, Harthug S, Kalager T, Digranes A, Solberg CO. Bloodstream infections at a Norwegian university hospital, 1974–1979 and 1988–1989: changing etiology, clinical features, and outcome. Clin Infect Dis. 1994;19(2):246–56.
21. Friedman ND, Kaye KS, Stout JE, McGarry SA, Trivette SL, Briggs JP, Lamm W, Clark C, MacFarquhar J, Walton AL, et al. Health care-associated bloodstream infections in adults: a reason to change the accepted definition of community-acquired infections. Ann Intern Med. 2002;137(10):791–7.
22. Weinstein MP, Reller LB, Murphy JR, Lichtenstein KA. The clinical significance of - positive blood cultures: a comprehensive analysis of 500 episodes of bacteremia and fungemia in adults. I. Laboratory and epidemiologic observations. Rev Infect Dis. 1983;5:35–53.
23. Lydersen S, Fagerland MW, Laake P. Categorical data and contingency tables. In: Veierød S, Lydersen S, Laake P, editors. Medical statistics in clinical and methodological research. Oslo: Gyldendal akademisk; 2012. p. 48–89.
24. De Kraker ME, Jarlier V, Monen JC, Heuer OE, van de Sande N, Grundmann H. The changing epidemiology of bacteraemias in Europe: trends from the European Antimicrobial Resistance Surveillance System. Clin Microbiol Infect. 2013;19(9):860–8.
25. De Kraker ME, Davey PG, Grundmann H, group Bs. Mortality and hospital stay associated with resistant Staphylococcus aureus and Escherichia coli bacteremia: estimating the burden of antibiotic resistance in Europe. PLoS Med. 2011;8(10):e1001104.
26. Hallan S, Naustdal T. Bacteremia at a medium-sized Norwegian hospital. Tidsskr Nor Laegeforen. 1994;114(18):2102–6.
27. Leegaard TM, Bevanger L, Jureen R, Lier T, Melby KK, Caugant DA, Oddvar Froholm L, Hoiby EA. Antibiotic sensitivity still prevails in Norwegian blood culture isolates. Int J Antimicrob Agents. 2001;18(2):99–106.
28. Berild D, Haug JB. Rational use of antibiotics in hospitals. Tidsskr Nor Laegeforen. 2008;128(20):2335–9.
29. Haug JB, Berild D, Walberg M, Reikvam A. Increased antibiotic use in Norwegian hospitals despite a low antibiotic resistance rate. J Antimicrob Chemother. 2011;66(11):2643–6.
30. NORM/NORM-VET. Usage of Antimicrobial Agents and Occurrence of Antimicrobial Resistance in Norway 2006. Oslo: Tromsø; 2007. ISSN:1502–2307 (print)/1890-9965(electronic).

10

A prospective multicenter evaluation of direct molecular detection of blood stream infection from a clinical perspective

A. E. Nieman[1,9], P. H. M. Savelkoul[1,2], A. Beishuizen[3,4], B. Henrich[5], B. Lamik[5], C. R. MacKenzie[5], D. Kindgen-Milles[6], A. Helmers[7], C. Diaz[7], S. G. Sakka[8] and R. P. Schade[1*]

Abstract

Background: Rapid diagnosis and appropriate antimicrobial therapy are of major importance to decrease morbidity and mortality in patients with blood stream infections (BSI). Blood culture, the current gold standard for detecting bacteria in blood, requires at least 24–48 hours and has limited sensitivity if obtained during antibiotic treatment of the patient. The aim of this prospective multicenter study was to clinically evaluate the application of a commercial universal 16S/18S rDNA PCR, SepsiTest™ (PCR-ST), directly on whole blood.

Methods: In total 236 samples from 166 patients with suspected sepsis were included in the study. PCR-ST results were compared to blood culture, the current gold standard for detecting BSI. Because blood cultures can give false-negative results, we performed an additional analysis to interpret the likelihood of bloodstream infection by using an evaluation based on clinical diagnosis, other diagnostic tests and laboratory parameters.

Results: Clinical interpretation of results defined the detected organism to be contaminants in 22 of 43 positive blood cultures (51.2 %) and 21 of 47 positive PCR-ST results (44.7 %). Excluding these contaminants resulted in an overall sensitivity and specificity of the PCR-ST of 66.7 and 94.4 % respectively. Of the 36 clinically relevant samples, 11 BSI were detected with both techniques, 15 BSI were detected with PCR-ST only and 10 with blood culture only. Therefore, in this study, SepsiTest™ detected an additional 71 % BSI compared to blood culture alone.

Conclusions: More clinically relevant BSI were diagnosed by molecular detection, which might influence patient treatment. An improved SepsiTest™ assay suited for routine use can have additional value to blood culture in diagnosing bacteremia in septic patients.

Keywords: SepsiTest™, PCR, Blood stream infection, Sepsis, Bacteremia, Molecular, 16S

Background

Blood stream infection is a serious clinical condition with high morbidity and mortality rates. Sepsis, severe sepsis and septic shock are associated with high mortality, ranging from 20 to 60 % depending on severity and underlying disease [1–4]. Sepsis is defined as a systemic inflammatory response syndrome (SIRS) in addition to documented or presumed infection. Severe sepsis is sepsis associated with organ dysfunction, hypoperfusion, or hypotension. Septic shock is the persistence of hypotension and perfusion abnormalities despite adequate resuscitation therapy [5]. Bacteremia, the presence of bacteria within the bloodstream, which leads to SIRS or sepsis, is associated with high morbidity and mortality. Rapid diagnosis of BSI and early initiation of appropriate antimicrobial treatment significantly decreases morbidity and mortality. Appropriate therapy in septic patients within the first hour of documented hypotension was associated with a survival rate of 80 %, with an average decrease of 7,6 % in survival every hour, up to 6 h, that antibiotics were delayed [6]. Empiric antimicrobial therapy is correct in approximately 85–90 % of blood stream infections [7–10]. As soon as

* Correspondence: r.schade@vumc.nl
[1]Department of Medical Microbiology and Infection control, VU University Medical Center, Amsterdam, The Netherlands

microbiological results are available, inappropriate antibiotics can be adjusted.

Currently, automated blood culture systems are the standard technique to diagnose BSI, however, blood cultures have several disadvantages. First, the minimum time to detection and identification of the causative organism is 24–48 h. Secondly, the sensitivity is approximately 70 % for critically ill patients and even lower for fastidious microorganisms [11]. Thirdly, prior administration of antibiotics significantly reduces the sensitivity of blood culture, sometimes even up to 100 % [12–15].

These disadvantages can potentially be overcome by molecular techniques performed directly on blood without culture. Polymerase chain reaction (PCR) targeting microbial DNA performed directly on blood is a rapid technique with a processing time of only a few hours. PCR detection of bacterial or fungal DNA is not dependent on the presence of replicating organisms and can be detected from intact dead or living bacteria. The major technological drawback to apply PCR assays for diagnosing blood stream infection is inhibition of the PCR amplification by relatively large amounts of proteins and human DNA in whole blood samples that currently limits the sample volume to approximately 200 µl of whole blood [14]. Human DNA in leukocytes and proteins, like immunoglobulin G, heme in erythrocytes and lactoferrin in leukocytes all interfere with the process by binding DNA polymerase or binding the nucleic acids [16–21]. However, optimization of DNA isolation and new methods that selectively purify microbial DNA to circumvent inhibition by human DNA have been developed. In this way higher volumes of blood can be processed which theoretically reduces sampling error and increases sensitivity. SepsiTest™ is not the only technique in this field, several other commercial tests have been developed that use PCR or time-of flight mass spectrometry for fast identification of pathogens, i.e. SeptiFast, MALDI-TOF on blood culture and more recently PCR ESI/MS (IRIDICA). The SeptiFast assay is a multiplex PCR performed directly on whole blood. Sensitivity compared to blood culture was 12–67 % depending on the microorganism, with a specificity of 81–98 % [22, 23] and the clinical sensitivity of the SeptiFast assay, excluding contaminants, was 62–70 % [24]. A recent randomized trial showed a significant reduction in the time required from sampling to providing pathogen identification to the clinician, with a mean duration of 15.9 h for PCR compared to 38.1 h for blood culture [25]. A drawback of this technique is the limited number of bacterial and fungal pathogens, 25 in total, in this multiplex PCR, and the low sensitivity. The next technique, MALDI-TOF in combination with the commercial Sepsityper kit allows identification on positive blood cultures with a reliable detection of 76 % of Gram-positive microorganisms and 90 % of Gram-negative microorganisms [26]. Of course the major drawback of this method is the necessity to culture first, which takes approximately 1–2 days and delays the time-to-result compared to direct tests on blood. More recently IRIDICA has been developed, a technique that combines multiplex PCR directly on whole blood with electrospray ionization mass spectrometry (PCR ESI/MS). Sensitivity and specificity compared to blood culture were 83 and 78–94 % and sensitivity and specificity of the test compared with the clinical infection criterion were 91 and 87 % [27, 28]. This seems a promising technique, however publications so far are limited.

We here present a prospective multicenter study that investigates the SepsiTest™ assay (Molzym, Bremen, Germany) in 1 ml of whole blood from patients on intensive care units with clinically suspected sepsis. The SepsiTest™ assay selectively degrades human DNA, before isolation of the microbial DNA. SepsiTest™ can provide a positive or negative result within 4 h and needs additional sequencing to identify the microorganism, which takes another 2–3 h if sequencing is available in the laboratory. Clinical relevance and routine applicability of this approach was evaluated by comparing the PCR results to blood culture, C-reactive protein, other microbiological investigations and patient data. This study shows that molecular detection of BSI has a potential benefit for patients suffering from sepsis however, several improvements of the technique are still required.

Methods

This study was conducted as a multicenter trial with patients suspected of sepsis. From each patient routine blood cultures and EDTA blood for PCR with the SepsiTest™ assay were taken. The study was performed in three participating centers: Medical Center Cologne-Merheim, University Witten/Herdecke in Cologne, Germany; Heinrich Heine University Hospital in Düsseldorf, Germany and VU University Medical Center in Amsterdam, The Netherlands. The study was approved by the Institutional Ethical Board of each center. Blood sampling was incorporated in routine patient care, without additional written informed consent. Blood samples for PCR-ST were collected; DNA extraction, PCR and sequencing were performed retrospectively. As this was an observational study, results of PCR-ST were not shared with the clinicians. Treatment of the patient was based on cultures and clinical signs and symptoms.

Patient selection

In total 166 patients were included in the three centers. The collection period was 5 months for each center, in the time period from November 2010 to September 2012. Inclusion criteria were patients ≥18 years old, admitted to the intensive care unit with systemic inflammatory response syndrome (SIRS) or suspected sepsis. If the treating physician had a clinical suspicion of SIRS or sepsis, blood was taken for culture and PCR-ST.

Sample and data collection

Samples for blood culture and PCR-ST were collected from the same blood vessel puncture according to the hospital's standardized aseptic procedures. For blood culture 10 ml of blood was drawn into an aerobic and anaerobic blood culture bottle each, and inoculated in BACTEC™ FX (Beckton Dickinson) or BacT/ALERT® (bioMérieux) depending on the participating center. Blood cultures were incubated for a maximum of 5 days. For PCR-ST, an additional volume of 4 ml of EDTA blood was collected. Identification of the organism in positive blood culture was performed with conventional methods as customary in each laboratory. All laboratories were certified according to the national quality standard for clinical microbiological laboratories.

Other samples were taken according to the suspected cause of infection, e.g. sputum, wound swabs, pus or urine. C-reactive protein and leucocyte count were recorded on the day of blood sample collection. Primary and secondary diagnosis, antibiotics used in the past 48 h and hospital inpatient mortality were registered.

DNA isolation with SepsiTest™

Fresh EDTA blood was divided into two aliquots of 1 ml and processed according to the SepsiTest™ manufacturer's manual. In short, a chaotropic buffer was first added to the blood samples that selectively lysed the blood cells. Then, the released nucleic acids were degraded by adding MolDNase. After enrichment by centrifugation, the sediment was treated with BugLysis and ß-mercaptoethanol to lyse cell walls of potentially present bacteria and yeasts. Proteinase K and a final chaotropic buffer was added for extra cell lysis and denaturation of proteins. The pathogen DNA was isolated by a bind-wash-elute procedure and eluated in a final volume of 100 μl. All materials used during these steps were sterile and nucleic acid-free to avoid laboratory and handling contamination. Sterile and nucleic acid free buffers and tubes were provided in the SepsiTest™ kit. Sterile pipette tips were used. Handling of samples was performed in a laminar flow cabinet that was disinfected and treated with UV light after each use.

PCR and amplicon detection

The protocol for PCR-ST was performed according to the manufacturer's manual. Mastermixes for universal PCR, internal control, and negative and positive controls were available in the kit. Five μl of eluate (~50 μl EDTA blood) of each duplicate sample were tested, with internal inhibition tested separately. All PCR-STs were performed on Piko Thermal Cyclers (Finnzymes). Amplicons were detected with electrophoresis on 2 % agarose gel. A sample was considered positive if at least one of the duplicates was positive with a blank negative control.

Sequencing

Positive amplicons were purified with QIAquick PCR Purification Kit (Qiagen) and sent to GATC Biotech (Germany) for sequencing with primers provided in the kit. Acquired sequences were identified with SepsiTest™ BLAST, or with NCBI BLAST when results were not available in SepsiTest™ BLAST. The organism was identified at a genus level if the sequence homology was ≥97 and <99 % and at a species level if ≥99 % according to the manufacturer's manual. For samples with weak bands on agarose gel and insufficient quality of sequencing results, the PCR, amplicon detection and sequencing were repeated. If sequencing results still had insufficient quality, the sample was considered negative.

Definitions

Positive samples were divided into 4 categories: true, probable, possible and questionable bacteremia. Identical bacteria detected both in blood culture and PCR-ST was considered as true bacteremia. For discordant results an interpretation of the likelihood of bacteremia was made according to the following definitions: bacteremia was considered probable if the pathogen was also cultured in other specimens of the same patient and consistent with the clinical diagnosis; possible if the pathogen was not confirmed in other cultures, but considered to be consistent with the clinical diagnosis. The result was interpreted as questionable bacteremia if the microorganism was not confirmed by other microbiological results and was not considered a likely cause of sepsis. In this case we defined the microorganism as a contaminant.

Results of other specimens, i.e. urine culture, wound swabs etc., were taken into account when sampled within 48 h before or after the positive blood culture or positive PCR-ST.

A polymicrobial result, i.e. a sample which yielded more than one microorganism in the same sample, was considered as true, probable or possible bacteremia, when one of the detected microorganisms met the definitions for true, probable or possible.

Statistical analysis

Sensitivity and specificity of PCR-ST by using blood culture as gold standard were calculated both on sample and patient level. Statistics were calculated based on paired samples, i.e. blood culture with corresponding PCR-ST sample. Subsequently, to investigate the potential additional value of PCR-ST in diagnosing BSI, the sensitivity and specificity of the PCR-ST were also calculated including clinical interpretation of results. Based on the above definitions, positive samples were divided into: true, probable, possible and questionable BSI. True, probable and possible BSI were regarded as positive, and questionable as negative for the calculation of an adjusted sensitivity and specificity.

Results

In this study, 166 patients were included with a total of 236 blood samples. The mean age of the patients was 65 years, with a range from 26 to 92 years. Sixty-three women were included (38 %). From all blood samples 43 of the 236 were positive by blood culture (18.2 %) and 47 were positive by PCR-ST (19.9 %). Samples matched in 72 % of cases. After excluding contaminants 91 % of the samples matched.

Sensitivity and specificity of the SepsiTest™ assay compared to blood culture was 25.6 and 82.9 % respectively, with negative and positive predictive values of 84.7 and 23.4 % (sample level, Table 1). When analyzed for the 166 patients, sensitivity and specificity were 28.9 and 79.7 %, with a negative and positive predictive value of 81.0 and 27.5 % (patient level).

The majority of detected microorganisms were staphylococci in both blood culture and PCR-ST (Table 2). Coagulase negative staphylococci (CoNS) were found in blood cultures in 30 of the 43 positive cultures (69.8 %). *Staphylococcus aureus* was found in 2 blood cultures. For PCR-ST, identification to species level was not always possible. CoNS were detected by PCR-ST in 13 of 47 positive samples (27.7 %) whereas *S. aureus* was detected in 6 cases (12.8 %). *Staphylococcus* spp. not further identified, were detected in an additional 9 samples (19.1 %). It was not possible to distinguish between coagulase negative staphylococci or *Staphylococcus aureus* for these 9 samples, due to insufficient quality of the sequencing fragment at the site of distinction. In total, 32 staphylococci (74.4 %) were detected with blood culture compared to 28 (59.6 %) with PCR-ST. Gram-negative rods were found in two samples with blood culture (4.7 %) and in six samples with PCR-ST (12.8 %). Candida was found in only one sample with each technique, however in different samples.

Table 1 Results of BC and PCR-ST without clinical interpretation

	BC positive	BC negative	Total
PCR-ST positive	11 + 3[a]	33	47
PCR-ST negative	29	160	189
Total	43	193	236

Abbreviations: *BC* blood culture, *PCR-ST* polymerase chain reaction with SepsiTest™
[a]Three samples were positive in both BC and PCR-ST, however the microorganisms detected were different. For calculating sensitivity and specificity of PCR-ST compared to BC only concordant results were included

Table 2 Microorganisms detected in sepsis patients with PCR-ST alone, blood culture alone or detected with both methods

True, probable and possible bacteremia			
	PCR-ST	BC	both
Monomicrobial			
Staphylococcus aureus	3	1	1
Coagulase negative *Staphylococci* (CoNS)	2	3	5[a]
Staphylococcus spp.	1	0	1
Enterococcus spp.	1	3	3[b]
Streptococcus pneumoniae	1	0	0
Escherichia coli	1	1	0
Klebsiella oxytoca	0	0	1
Candida albicans	1	1	0
Polymicrobial[c]	5	1	0
Questionable bacteremia			
	PCR-ST	BC	
Monomicrobial			
Coagulase negative *Staphylococci*	5	20	
Staphylococcus spp.	3	0	
Propionibacterium spp.	0	2	
Streptococcus spp.	4	0	
Enterococcus spp.	1	0	
Lactococcus lactis	1	0	
Rickettsia symbiont	1	0	
Corynebacterium spp.	1	0	
Polymicrobial[c]	5	0	
	PCR-ST	BC	both
Total	36	32	11

Abbreviations: *PCR-ST* polymerase chain reaction with SepsiTest™, *BC* blood culture, *spp.* species
[a]one sample contained CoNS in blood culture and CoNS + Corynebacterium in PCR-ST
[b]one sample contained *Enterococcus faecalis* in blood culture and *Enterococcus* + *Streptococcus* spp in PCR-ST
[c]for microorganisms detected in polymicrobial samples, see Table 3
In total 236 samples were analyzed of which 79 were positive in one or both methods. Results are presented by likelihood of bacteremia, true/probable/possible versus questionable bacteremia

Polymicrobial samples, i.e. samples with more than one microorganism, were detected in only one blood culture (2.3 %), but were common in the PCR-ST results (12 samples, 25.5 %) (Table 3). It is to be noted that 9 out of 12 polymicrobial PCR-ST results were found in one center (75 %).

Evaluation of PCR-ST results to blood culture as gold standard may result in lower sensitivity when clinically contaminated blood cultures are defined as positive. On the other hand, specificity may be hampered by false negative blood cultures due to antibiotic therapy or bacteria that are difficult to culture. Based on the combination of lab results and clinical interpretation of the

Table 3 Microorganisms detected in polymicrobial samples with PCR-ST and blood culture

True, probable and possible bacteremia		
	PCR-ST	BC
Polymicrobial		
Enterococcus spp, Coagulase negative *Staphylococci*	0	1
Staphylococcus aureus, Lactobacillus spp.	1	0
Escherichia coli, Streptococcus mitis group	1	0
Pseudomonas aeruginosa, Acinetobacter lwoffii, Staphylococcus warneri, Streptococcus equi	1	0
Escherichia coli, Edwardsiella ictaluri, Enterococcus faecium, Staphylococcus aureus	1	0
Streptococcus agalactiae, Enterococcus spp, *Propionibacterium* acnes, *Staphylococcus* spp.	1	0
Questionable bacteremia		
	PCR-ST	BC
Polymicrobial		
Lactobacillus spp., *Enterococcus mundtii*	1	0
Haemophilus parainfluenzae, Haemophilus ducreyi, Neisseria wadsworthii, Lactococcus lactis	1	0
Staphylocccus spp., *Streptococcus* spp	1	0
Lactobacillus spp., *Staphylocccus* spp., *Streptococcus* spp.	1	0
Abiotropha paraadiacens/Granulicatella adiacens, Staphylococcus spp., *Streptococcus* spp.	1	0
	PCR-ST	BC
Total	10[a]	1

Abbreviations: *PCR-ST* polymerase chain reaction with SepsiTest™, *BC* blood culture, *spp.* species
[a]Two additional polymicrobial PCR-ST results are listed in Table 2: these samples contained two microorganisms in the PCR-ST and one concordant microorganism in the corresponding BC
A polymicrobial sample, a sample that yielded more than one microorganism, was considered as true, probable or possible bacteremia, when one of the detected microorganisms met the definitions for true, probable or possible, regardless of the meaning of the other microorganisms

microorganism with respect to the patient's disease, 22 of 43 positive blood cultures of in total 236 samples were considered to be contaminants. This is 51,2 % of positive blood cultures and 9,3 % of all blood cultures. For PCR-ST 21 of 47 positive results were considered to be contaminants (44,7 %), i.e. 8,9 % of all samples. For example, a septic patient with the clinical signs of a thrombophlebitis of the lower arm and a *Staphylococcus aureus* detected in both blood culture and PCR-ST, was considered to have a true bacteremia. A patient with peritonitis and a negative blood culture, however *Enterococcus* spp. detected with PCR-ST that had also *Enterococcus faecium* in peritoneal cultures was considered to have probable bacteremia. On the other hand, a *Corynebacterium* detected with PCR-ST that was not detected in any other culture and is known to be a common contaminant, was considered as questionable bacteremia. After clinical interpretation of all positive results (Table 4), the adjusted sensitivity and specificity on sample level was 66.7 and 94.4 %. The negative and positive predictive value was 96.7 and 53.8 % respectively. In total 36 samples were considered clinically relevant as detected by PCR-ST, blood culture or both. Of these 36 samples, 11 microorganisms were detected by both methods, 15 were detected by PCR-ST only and 10 by blood culture only.

Of 28 patients with clinically relevant positive blood samples, 13 (47 %) had a respiratory or an intra-abdominal cause of sepsis (Table 5). From these patients 22/28 (78.6 %) had received antibiotics in the 48 h prior to testing. Of discordant results, i.e. a positive result in either blood culture or PCR-ST alone, 8 patients with previous antibiotics had a PCR-ST positive result only, compared to 6 patients with positive blood cultures only.

This study clearly indicates that clinical interpretation of PCR-ST results is important, as is true for blood culture. The additional value of PCR-ST in diagnosing BSI is substantial; an extra 15 bacteremias confirming the clinical perspective were detected compared to 21 with blood culture alone (71 %). These results may

Table 4 Results of BC and PCR-ST after excluding contaminants

	BC positive	BC negative	Total
PCR-ST positive	14[a]	12	26
PCR-ST negative	7	203	210
Total	21	215	236

Abbreviations: *BC* blood culture, *PCR-ST* polymerase chain reaction with SepsiTest™
[a]Three samples were positive in both BC and PCR-ST, however the microorganisms detected were different. Since both microorganisms were considered clinically relevant these samples were included as possible/probable blood stream infections in the adjusted sensitivity

Table 5 Focus of infection in patients with positive blood culture and/or PCR results considered true, probable or possible

Focus of infection	Number of patients
Intra-abdominal	8
Respiratory	5
Cardiac	3
Central nervous system	3
Skin	2
Postoperative fever	2
Trauma	2
Intravascular catheter	1
Multiorgan failure	1
Bone	1
Total	28

influence antimicrobial therapy in terms of type, dose and duration.

Discussion

A rapid diagnosis of BSI is of major importance for patient outcome. A direct PCR on whole blood, instead of blood culture, should theoretically reduce the time to diagnosis and implementation of adequate antimicrobial therapy.

In this multicenter study we have evaluated the performance of a universal PCR assay in patients suspected of sepsis. Sensitivity and specificity were based on comparing PCR-ST with blood culture, on both sample and patient level. To determine the actual clinical relevance of these PCR-ST results, all positive samples were also analyzed after a clinical interpretation of the microorganism detected in respect to other diagnostic tests, and the patient's disease. Despite the fact that the total numbers of relevant microorganisms were small, with 21 relevant blood cultures and 26 relevant PCR-ST results in a total of 236 samples, the performance of the SepsiTest™ within a clinical context was verified.

Sensitivity of PCR-ST compared to blood culture, without clinical interpretation of results, was only 33 % with a specificity of 83 % (sample level). A previous study showed similar specificity (85.8 %), but much higher sensitivity (87 %) of the SepsiTest™ assay compared to blood culture [29]. The same test and a comparable patient population were evaluated but we found a higher number of blood cultures with coagulase negative staphylococci that were considered to be a contamination (47 % of positive BC). In routine application, clinical interpretation of results is crucial for clinical use of both blood culture as well as PCR-ST. In 9 of 47 positive PCR-ST results *Staphylococcus* spp. were found. Due to insufficient quality of the sequencing fragment at the site of distinction it was not possible to differentiate between *Staphylococcus aureus* and coagulase negative staphylococci. This is a shortcoming of the test, since coagulase negative staphylococci are often contaminants while *Staphylococcus aureus* is a clinically relevant pathogen. More than 40 % of positive results in both blood culture and PCR-ST were considered contaminants, based on clinical diagnosis, laboratory parameters and other microbiological tests performed in the same individual. In the majority of these results coagulase negative staphylococci were found in blood culture and staphylococci and streptococci were found in PCR-ST. A recent study of 1334 patients with positive blood cultures also showed significant numbers of contaminants. In this study 55,8 % of blood cultures were considered bacterial contamination, compared to 44,2 % true blood stream infections [15]. After clinical interpretation of results, the adjusted sensitivity and specificity were 66.7 and 94.4 % respectively. For clinical interpretation we made some assumptions as described in the methods. Questionable bacteremia as defined in this study may actually be true bacteremia and possible bacteremia may be actually contaminants. This is a drawback of the calculated adjusted sensitivity and specificity. However, in daily practice it is very common to make a clinical evaluation of the microorganism found in the blood culture, especially for coagulase negative staphylococci and certain streptococci. For PCR-ST a clinical interpretation is also important. Interpretation errors may limit these calculations.

In studies evaluating PCR directly on whole blood, other than SepsiTest™, low sensitivities were also found compared to blood culture results. For the SeptiFast assay, Josefson and Grif showed a sensitivity on sample level of 12–67 and 63 % respectively [22, 23]. Clinical sensitivity, after excluding contaminants, was 62–70 % (Bravo et al.) [24]. In these studies a multiplex PCR with a select number of microorganisms was used to detect bacteremia. Bacteria that were not included in the multiplex PCR were logically not detectable with this approach. However, this explained only in part the low sensitivity since the majority of microorganisms missed were included in the PCR panel but were only detected by blood culture [22–24, 30].

An explanation for the low sensitivity in most studies as well as in our study is possibly the large difference in input volume used in blood culture compared to PCR. For one blood culture bottle, 8–10 ml of blood was used. For PCR, an amount equal to 50 μl of whole blood was tested. This means that the amount of blood tested in one blood culture bottle is around 200 times more than in one PCR reaction. The chance of sampling error in PCR is therefore much higher, especially when low amounts of bacteria are present in the blood of the patient. This can be improved by using 50 μl of eluate and

10 μl of DNA in the PCR although the amount of blood tested in a blood culture bottle will still be 50 times more. If higher input volumes for PCR can be used, sensitivity of PCR on blood will increase [16–21].

Specificity was more in line with blood culture, however it is debatable whether blood culture is a reliable gold standard. In our samples we found many staphylococci and considered more than 50 % of positive blood cultures (mostly CoNS) clinically irrelevant. On the other hand, blood cultures may be false negative. The sensitivity of blood culture increases if more blood cultures are obtained, from approximately 65–73 % for 1 set of blood culture bottles (20 ml), 80–90 % for two sets and 95–99 % for 3 sets of blood cultures. As a consequence one negative blood culture cannot exclude BSI [31, 32]. Therefore, the presence of microorganisms detected by PCR may reflect actual disease. Moreover, the microorganisms can truly be temporarily present in blood, as is known for short bacteremias after dental procedures [33–35] and surgical procedures [36, 37]. Mostly, these bacteremias do not cause a systemic inflammatory response syndrome and therefore no BSI. These are true bacteremias, but not clinically relevant. Of course, in a universal PCR technique the chance of contamination of the sample in the laboratory is also substantial. Clean handling of samples throughout the entire procedure from withdrawal to PCR is of utmost importance. Obviously, for both PCR-ST and blood culture, the detected microorganisms need to be evaluated in the clinical context to decide whether the result is more likely to be clinically relevant or contamination.

Theoretically, the advantage of blood culture is that one viable bacterium is sufficient for a positive result. High volumes of blood can be tested at once, and the possibility of testing antibiotic susceptibility makes blood culture a valuable technique. PCR on the other hand is useful for microorganisms that are difficult or impossible to culture, after the initiation of antibiotic therapy and can be performed directly on whole blood, thus eliminating the incubation time, which is important for early adequate antimicrobial therapy.

The SepsiTest™ assay is a complex method with many buffers, enzymes and reagents to be added and several centrifugation steps before the eluate is obtained. Hands-on-time and the possibility of laboratory contamination can be reduced by automation of this procedure and replacing gel electrophoresis by melting curve analysis to detect positive samples. The SepsiTest™ assay is now designed as a positive or negative result with subsequent sequencing to identify the bacteria. DNA extraction and PCR-ST can be performed within 4 h and produces a negative or positive result. Only a positive result needs to be sequenced for identification of the microorganism. This adds 2 to 3 h to the time-to-results, provided that sequencing is available in the laboratory. In our study, sequencing was outsourced which increased the turnaround time. In routine practice however this could be performed within 6–7 h until complete identification. The test can be used without sequencing, with only a positive or negative result. However, owing to the substantial chance of contamination, a clinical interpretation of results is necessary and therefore the identification of the microorganism. With the current setup of this method, the theoretical advantage of a fast PCR directly on whole blood is reduced by the complex handling procedure and the need for sequencing to identify the microorganism.

Conclusions

This study in 166 patients with sepsis indicates that direct molecular detection of bacteria is of added value to blood culture in detecting blood stream infections. An additional 71 % of BSI were detected by the SepsiTest™ assay (PCR-ST) compared to blood culture alone. Furthermore, after antibiotic therapy, slightly more BSI were detected by PCR-ST than by blood culture. Overall, PCR-ST results may influence the administration of adequate antimicrobial therapy and diminish patient's morbidity and mortality. Although the SepsiTest™ PCR directly on blood is a promising technique, the input volume of blood should be increased to lower sampling error, and a faster procedure to identify the microorganism is of importance. The current universal microbial PCR is not a substitute for blood culture but may be of additional clinical value in diagnosing BSI. In general, from a clinical perspective a rapid molecular whole blood test is of added value for patient treatment.

Abbreviations

BC, blood culture; BSI, blood stream infection (s); CoNS, coagulase negative staphylococci; ESI/MS, electrospray ionization mass spectrometry; MALDI-TOF, matrix assisted laser desorption/ionization time-of-flight (mass spectrometry); PCR, polymerase chain reaction; PCR-ST, universal PCR with SepsiTest™; SIRS, systemic inflammatory response syndrome

Acknowledgments

This work was performed in collaboration with the ESCMID Study Group on Molecular Diagnostics (ESGMD), Basel, Switzerland. The SepsiTest™ kits were supplied by the manufacturer, Molzym (Bremen, Germany).

Funding

There was no funding for this study.

Authors' contributions

AN performed laboratory tests in Amsterdam, analyzed the data and drafted the manuscript. PS participated in the design and coordination of the study in Amsterdam and supervised drafting the manuscript. AB participated in coordination of the study at the intensive care unit in Amsterdam. BH participated in the design and coordination of the study in the laboratory in Düsseldorf. BL performed the laboratory tests. CM participated in the design and coordination of the study in the laboratory in Düsseldorf. DK coordination and supervision of the clinical aspect of the study on the intensive care unit in Düsseldorf. AH participated in the coordination of the study in the laboratory in Cologne and performed laboratory tests. CD participated in the coordination of the study in the laboratory in Cologne and performed laboratory tests. SS participated in the design and coordination of the study at the intensive care unit in Cologne and analyzed the data. RS participated in the design and coordination of the study in Amsterdam and supervised drafting the manuscript. All authors read and approved the manuscript.

Competing interests

The authors declare that they have no conflict of interest.

Author details

[1]Department of Medical Microbiology and Infection control, VU University Medical Center, Amsterdam, The Netherlands. [2]Department of Medical Microbiology, Maastricht University Medical Center, Maastricht, The Netherlands. [3]Department of Intensive Care Medicine, VU University Medical Center, Amsterdam, The Netherlands. [4]Department of Intensive Care, Medisch Spectrum Twente, Enschede, The Netherlands. [5]Institute of Medical Microbiology and Hospital Hygiene, University Clinic of Heinrich-Heine University Düsseldorf, Düsseldorf, Germany. [6]Department of Anesthesiology, University Clinic of Heinrich-Heine University Düsseldorf, Düsseldorf, Germany. [7]Department of Microbiology, Merheim Zentrallabor, MVZ synlab Leverkusen GmbH, Leverkusen, Germany. [8]Department of Anesthesiology and Intensive Care Medicine, Medical Center Cologne-Merheim, University Witten/Herdecke, Cologne, Germany. [9]Laboratory for Medical Microbiology, Immunology and Infection Control, Elisabeth-TweeSteden Hospital, Tilburg, The Netherlands.

References

1. Machado FR, Mazza BF. Improving mortality in sepsis: analysis of clinical trials. Shock. 2010;34 Suppl 1:54–8.
2. Mann E a, Baun MM, Meininger JC, Wade CE. Comparison of mortality associated with sepsis in the burn, trauma, and general intensive care unit patient: a systematic review of the literature. Shock. 2012;37:4–16.
3. Martin GS, Mannino DM, Eaton S, Moss M. The epidemiology of sepsis in the united states from 1979 through 2000. N Engl J Med. 2003;348:1546–54.
4. Angus DC, Linde-Zwirble WT, Lidicker J, Clermont G, Carcillo J, Pinsky MR. Epidemiology of severe sepsis in the united states: analysis of incidence, outcome, and associated costs of care. Crit Care Med. 2001;29:1303–10.
5. Bone RC, Balk RA, Cerra FB, Dellinger RP, Fein AM, Knaus WA, et al. Definitions for sepsis and organ failure and guidelines for the use of innovative therapies in sepsis. Crit Care Med. 1992;20:864–74.
6. Kumar A, Roberts D, Wood KE, Light B, Parrillo JE, Sharma S, et al. Duration of hypotension before initiation of effective antimicrobial therapy is the critical determinant of survival in human septic shock. Crit Care Med. 2006;34:1589–96.
7. Flaherty SK, Weber RL, Chase M, Dugas AF, Graver AM, Salciccioli JD, Cocchi MN, Donnino MW: Septic Shock and Adequacy of Early Empiric Antibiotics in the Emergency Department. J Emerg Med. 2014;47:601-7.
8. Macarthur RD, Miller M, Albertson T, Panacek E, Johnson D, Teoh L, et al. Adequacy of early empiric antibiotic treatment and survival in severe sepsis: experience from the MONARCS trial. Clin Infect Dis. 2004;38:284–8.
9. Miano TA, Powell E, Schweickert WD, Morgan S, Binkley S, Sarani B. Effect of an antibiotic algorithm on the adequacy of empiric antibiotic therapy given by a medical emergency team. J Crit Care. 2012;27:45–50.
10. Sligl WI, Dragan T, Smith SW: Nosocomial Gram-Negative Bacteremia in Intensive Care: Epidemiology, Antimicrobial Susceptibilities and Outcomes. Int J Infect Dis. 2015;37:129-34.
11. Beutz M, Sherman G, Mayfield J, Fraser VJ, Kollef MH. Clinical utility of blood cultures drawn from central vein catheters and peripheral venipuncture in critically ill medical patients. Chest. 2003;123:854–61.
12. Glerant JC, Hellmuth D, Schmit JL, Ducroix JP, Jounieaux V. Utility of blood cultures in community-acquired pneumonia requiring hospitalization: influence of antibiotic treatment before admission. Respir Med. 1999;93:208–12.
13. McKenzie R, Reimer LG. Effect of antimicrobials on blood cultures in endocarditis. Diagn Microbiol Infect Dis. 1987;8:165–72.
14. Peters RPH, Van Agtmael M a, Gierveld S, Danner S a, Groeneveld a BJ, Vandenbroucke-Grauls CMJE, et al. Quantitative detection of staphylococcus aureus and enterococcus faecalis DNA in blood to diagnose bacteremia in patients in the intensive care unit. J Clin Microbiol. 2007;45:3641–6.
15. Ruiz-Giardín JM, Martin-Díaz RM, Jaqueti-Aroca J, Garcia-Arata I, San Martín-López JV, Sáiz-Sánchez Buitrago M. Diagnosis of bacteraemia and growth times. Int J Infect Dis. 2015;41:6–10.
16. Al-Soud WA, Rådström P. Purification and characterization of PCR-inhibitory components in blood cells. J Clin Microbiol. 2001;39:485–93.
17. Hansen WLJ, Bruggeman CA, Wolffs PFG. Evaluation of new preanalysis sample treatment tools and DNA isolation protocols to improve bacterial pathogen detection in whole blood. J Clin Microbiol. 2009;47:2629–31.
18. Hedman J, Rådström P: Overcoming Inhibition in Real-Time Diagnostic PCR. In *PCR Detection of Microbial Pathogens: Second Edition, Methods in Molecular Biology. Volume 943*; 2013:17–49.
19. Morata P, Queipo-Ortuño MI, de Dios Colmenero J. Strategy for optimizing DNA amplification in a peripheral blood PCR assay used for diagnosis of human brucellosis. J Clin Microbiol. 1998;36:2443–6.
20. Smith K, Diggle M a, Clarke SC. Comparison of commercial DNA extraction kits for extraction of bacterial genomic DNA from whole-blood samples. J Clin Microbiol. 2003;41:2440–3.
21. Wilson IG. Inhibition and facilitation of nucleic acid amplification. Appl Environ Microbiol. 1997;63:3741–51.
22. Grif K, Fille M, Würzner R, Weiss G, Lorenz I, Gruber G, et al. Rapid detection of bloodstream pathogens by real-time PCR in patients with sepsis. Wien Klin Wochenschr. 2012;124:266–70.
23. Josefson P, Strålin K, Ohlin a, Ennefors T, Dragsten B, Andersson L, et al. Evaluation of a commercial multiplex PCR test (SeptiFast) in the etiological diagnosis of community-onset bloodstream infections. Eur J Clin Microbiol Infect Dis. 2011;30:1127–34.
24. Bravo D, Blanquer J, Tormo M, Aguilar G, Borrás R, Solano C, et al. Diagnostic accuracy and potential clinical value of the LightCycler SeptiFast assay in the management of bloodstream infections occurring in neutropenic and critically ill patients. Int J Infect Dis. 2011;15:326–31.
25. Tafelski S, Nachtigall I, Adam T, Bereswill S, Faust J, Tamarkin A, et al. Randomized controlled clinical trial evaluating multiplex polymerase chain reaction for pathogen identification and therapy adaptation in critical care patients with pulmonary or abdominal sepsis. J Int Med Res. 2015;43:364–77.
26. Morgenthaler NG, Kostrzewa M. Rapid identification of pathogens in positive blood culture of patients with sepsis: review and meta-analysis of the performance of the sepsityper Kit. Int J Microbiol. 2015;2015:1–10.
27. Bacconi A, Richmond GS, Baroldi M a, Laffler TG, Blyn LB, Carolan HE, et al. Improved sensitivity for molecular detection of bacterial and Candida infections in blood. J Clin Microbiol. 2014;52:3164–74.
28. Jordana-Lluch E, Giménez M, Quesada MD, Rivaya B, Marcó C, Domínguez MJ, et al. Evaluation of the broad-range PCR/ESI-MS technology in blood specimens for the molecular diagnosis of bloodstream infections. PLoS One. 2015;10, e0140865.
29. Wellinghausen N, Kochem A-J, Disqué C, Mühl H, Gebert S, Winter J, et al. Diagnosis of bacteremia in whole-blood samples by use of a commercial universal 16S rRNA gene-based PCR and sequence analysis. J Clin Microbiol. 2009;47:2759–65.
30. Pasqualini L, Mencacci A, Leli C, Montagna P, Cardaccia A, Cenci E, et al. Diagnostic performance of a multiple real-time PCR assay in patients with suspected sepsis hospitalized in an internal medicine ward. J Clin Microbiol. 2012;50:1285–8.
31. Cockerill FR, Wilson JW, Vetter EA, Goodman KM, Torgerson CA, Harmsen WS, et al. Optimal testing parameters for blood cultures. Clin Infect Dis. 2004;38:1724–30.
32. Lee A, Mirrett S, Reller LB, Weinstein MP: Detection of Bloodstream Infections in Adults: How Many Blood Cultures Are Needed? J Clin Microbiol. 2007;45:3546–8.
33. Cobe HM. Transitory bacteremia. Oral Surg Oral Med Oral Pathol. 1954;7:609–15.
34. Tomás I, Diz P, Tobías A, Scully C, Donos N. Periodontal health status and bacteraemia from daily oral activities: systematic review/meta-analysis. J Clin Periodontol. 2012;39:213–28.

35. Forner L, Larsen T, Kilian M, Holmstrup P. Incidence of bacteremia after chewing, tooth brushing and scaling in individuals with periodontal inflammation. J Clin Periodontol. 2006;33:401–7.
36. Wilson W, Taubert K a, Gewitz M, Lockhart PB, Baddour LM, Levison M, et al. Prevention of infective endocarditis: guidelines from the American heart association: a guideline from the American heart association rheumatic fever, endocarditis, and Kawasaki disease committee, council on cardiovascular disease in the young, and the Co. Circulation. 2007;116: 1736–54.
37. Dajani AS, Taubert KA, Wilson W, Bolger AF, Bayer A, Ferrieri P, et al. Prevention of bacterial endocarditis: recommendations by the American heart association. Clin Infect Dis. 1997;25:1448–58.

11

Genetic relatedness and risk factor analysis of ampicillin-resistant and high-level gentamicin-resistant enterococci causing bloodstream infections in Tanzanian children

Håvard Aamodt[1,2], Stein Christian Mohn[2], Samuel Maselle[3], Karim P Manji[4], Rob Willems[5], Roland Jureen[6], Nina Langeland[1,2] and Bjørn Blomberg[1,2*]

Abstract

Background: While enterococci resistant to multiple antimicrobials are spreading in hospitals worldwide, causing urinary tract, wound and bloodstream infections, there is little published data on these infections from Africa.

Methods: We assessed the prevalence, susceptibility patterns, clinical outcome and genetic relatedness of enterococcal isolates causing bloodstream infections in children in a tertiary hospital in Tanzania, as part of a prospective cohort study of bloodstream infections among 1828 febrile children admitted consecutively from August 2001 to August 2002.

Results: Enterococcal bacteraemia was identified in 2.1% (39/1828) of admissions, and in 15.3% (39/255) of cases of culture-confirmed bloodstream infections. The case-fatality rate in children with *Enterococcus faecalis* septicaemia (28.6%, 4/14) was not significantly different from those with *Enterococcus faecium* septicaemia (6.7%, 1/15, $p = 0.12$). *E. faecium* isolates commonly had combined ampicillin-resistance and high-level gentamicin resistance (HLGR), (9/17), while *E. faecalis* frequently displayed HLGR (6/15), but were ampicillin susceptible. None of the tested enterococcal isolates displayed vancomycin resistance by Etest or PCR for *vanA* and *vanB* genes. Multi-locus sequence-typing (MLST) showed that the majority of *E. faecium* (7/12) belonged to the hospital associated Bayesian Analysis of Population Structure (BAPS) group 3–3. Pulsed-field gel electrophoresis (PFGE) indicated close genetic relationship particularly among *E. faecium* isolates, but also among *E. faecalis* isolates. There was also correlation between BAPS group and PFGE results. Risk factors for enterococcal bloodstream infection in univariate analysis were hospital-acquired infection and clinical diagnosis of sepsis with unknown focus. In multivariate analysis, neonates in general were relatively protected from enterococcal infection, while both prematurity and clinical sepsis were risk factors. Malnutrition was a risk factor for enterococcal bloodstream infection among HIV negative children.

Conclusion: This is the first study to describe bloodstream infections caused by ampicillin-resistant HLGR *E. faecium* and HLGR *E. faecalis* in Tanzania. The isolates of *E. faecium* and *E. faecalis*, respectively, showed high degrees of relatedness by genotyping using PFGE. The commonly used treatment regimens at the hospital are insufficient for infections caused by these microbes. The study results call for increased access to microbiological diagnostics to guide rational antibiotic use in Tanzania.

Keywords: *Enterococcus*, *Enterococcus faecalis*, *Enterococcus faecium*, Microbial drug resistance, Sepsis, Bacteremia, Pulsed-field gel electrophoresis, Multilocus sequence typing, Tanzania, Africa

* Correspondence: bjorn.blomberg@k2.uib.no
[1]Department of Clinical Science, University of Bergen, Bergen, Norway
[2]Center for Tropical Infectious Diseases, Department of Medicine, Haukeland University Hospital, Bergen, Norway
Full list of author information is available at the end of the article

Background

Enterococci are normal inhabitants of human and animal intestine [1-3]. They were previously considered innocent commensal organisms as compared to more virulent organisms, such as *Streptococcus pyogenes* and *Staphylococcus aureus.* In recent years enterococci, first *Enterococcus faecalis* [4] and more recently *Enterococcus faecium* [5,6], have emerged as major pathogens causing nosocomial infections, particularly urinary tract, wound and bloodstream infections. Enterococci tend to cause infections in immunocompromised hosts and seriously ill patients and patients with indwelling devices, such as catheters [7]. There is evidence that enterococci are a significant cause of bacteraemia in people with HIV infection [8]. Enterococci are intrinsically resistant to cephalosporins [9-11] and have reduced susceptibility to aminoglycosides [12]. Enterococci also have great ability to acquire antimicrobial resistance through mutations and exchange of genetic material [3]. High consumption of cephalosporins tends to select for enterococci and favour their spread in hospital settings [13-15]. Resistance to anti-enterococcal first-line drugs such as ampicillin and the combination ampicillin/gentamicin, commonly used empirically for sepsis, is increasing rapidly [16,17]. Vancomycin-resistant enterococci (VRE) have spread globally [16] and have become a very important cause of nosocomial infections. Treatment of VRE infections is hampered by the fact that many isolates are resistant to multiple other agents as well [18,19]. Typing of *E. faecium* strains by multi-locus sequence typing (MLST) has identified hospital-adapted subpopulations, initially coined clonal complex 17 (CC17), as being associated with serious infections and nosocomial outbreaks worldwide [16,20-22]. Further analysis on the population genetics of *E. faecium* indicated the existence of three hospital lineages (17, 18, and 78), that group in two Bayesian Analysis of Population Structure (BAPS) groups, BAPS 2–1 (lineage 78) and BAPS 3–3 (lineage 17 and 18) [23]. Recent whole genome-based phylogeny suggests that these hospital-lineages are all part of a single clade, called A1 [24].

Little is known about the role of enterococci in bloodstream infections in East Africa, their resistance patterns, and whether certain clonal complexes are associated with more disease in this setting. However, carriage of high-level gentamicin-resistant (HLGR) enterococci has been described in Zimbabwe [25] and South Africa [26]. Outbreaks of infections caused by VRE have been reported from South Africa [27] and VRE are often found in milk, beef, and chicken in Botswana [28].

The purpose of this study was to assess the prevalence, resistance patterns, and genetic relatedness of enterococcal isolates causing bloodstream infections in children at Muhimbili National Hospital, Dar es Salaam, Tanzania, and risk factors for such infections.

Methods

The study took place from August 2001 to August 2002 at the Paediatric Department at Muhimbili National Hospital, a tertiary referral hospital in Dar es Salaam, Tanzania. A cohort of 1828 consecutive admissions of a total of 1787 children presenting with clinical features of systemic infection were included in the study as described elsewhere [29]. The inclusion criteria were fever, hypothermia and other signs and symptoms described in the World Health Organization's program for Integrated Management of Childhood Illness (IMCI) [30], including general danger signs such as convulsions, lethargy, inability to drink or breastfeed, vomiting, and other signs of infection, such as neck stiffness, bulging fontanelles, cough, tachypnoea, difficulty breathing, chest in-drawings, nasal flaring, grunting, diarrhoea, dehydration, ear or eye discharge, lymphadenopathy, and, in neonates, signs of infection in the skin and umbilicus. The attending clinician recorded patient data using a standardized case report form. Medical records and departmental registries for admissions, discharges and deaths were reviewed with the purpose of quality-assuring the data.

The protocol was approved by The Research and Publications Committee of Muhimbili University College of Health Sciences and by the National AIDS Control Programme. Since the study subjects were young children aged 0–7 years, the parents or other accompanying, responsible family members were asked for written consent on behalf of the patient. Written informed consent was obtained before including the patient in the study and before taking blood tests. In some circumstances, in the case of critically ill patients, blood specimens were taken based on verbal consent, since these investigations are strongly recommended as routine investigations for severely ill febrile children, and since it would be inappropriate to delay management of such patients due to paperwork. The responsible family member was then approached in retrospect for written consent to use these specimens. The Tanzanian national language, Kiswahili, was used for obtaining consent.

Blood specimens were examined for growth of bacteria, mycobacteria and fungi by the use of BACTEC™ MYCO/F Lytic culture vials. Isolates were identified by standard microbiological methods as described in Mackie & McCartney Practical Medical Microbiology [31]. *E. faecalis* and *E. faecium* species identification was confirmed by polymerase chain reaction (PCR) of the *ddl* gene [32]. Susceptibility was tested by the disk diffusion method according to the guidelines of the National Committee for Clinical Laboratory Standards (NCCLS, now CLSI - Clinical and Laboratory Standards Institute) [33] for doxycycline and chloramphenicol. Testing for minimum inhibitory concentration (MIC) was performed by Etest (BioMerieux, Craponne, France, previously AB Biodisk, Solna, Sweden) for ampicillin, high-level gentamicin-resistance, vancomycin, linezolid, and quinupristin-dalfopristin. Resistance to ampicillin was defined as MIC ≥ 16 (mcg/ml) and high-level gentamicin-resistance as MIC > 500 (mcg/ml) as assessed by Etest. PCR for *vanA* and *vanB* genes was performed to detect vancomycin resistance.

Genetic relatedness of the isolates was assessed by pulsed field gel electrophoresis (PFGE). This was performed on SmaI (Promega Corp, Madison, WI) digested genomic DNA as previously described [34] and modified by Dahl et al. [35]. The PFGE patterns were analysed with Bionumerics, version 3.0 (Applied Maths, Kortrijk, Belgium). The Dice coefficient of similarity was calculated, and unweighted pair group method with arithmetic averages (UPMGA) was used for cluster analysis. Twelve *E. faecium* isolates were also investigated by MLST. MLST was carried out with a standard set of primers that amplify the 7 genes included in the *E. faecium* MLST scheme [36]. Information on these loci, the latest set of primers, amplification conditions, and details of all isolates are available on the MLST Web site (http://pubmlst.org/efaecium/).

Community-acquired (CA) infection was defined as bloodstream infection (BSI) with growth of pathogenic bacteria in a blood-culture obtained within the first 48 hours after admission [37]. A neonate who was born in hospital within the last 10 days was considered as having hospital-acquired (HA) infection. HIV testing was performed by ELISA as previously described and confirmed by PCR for children <18 months [29]. For the univariate analysis, Chi-square test and student *t*-test was used to compare proportions and means, respectively. Multivariate analysis was performed by stepwise backwards logistic regression with threshold $p = 0.2$ for removal from the model and $p = 0.05$ for inclusion. Risk factors were removed one-by-one starting with the least significant factor until remaining with only factors significant to the level of $p < 0.2$. Since only about half (n = 942) of the study participants consented to be HIV tested, and the many missing values would affect the logistic regression model, we present two different models; one where HIV status is removed from the model (n = 1603), and one where HIV status is locked in the model (n = 842). Statistical analysis was performed in Stata 13 (Stata Corp, College Station, Texas, US).

Results

Thirty-nine of 1828 cases (2.1%) had growth of enterococcal isolates in blood culture. The clinical presentation of patients with enterococcal bacteraemia was assessed as clinical sepsis without certain focus in 45% (n = 15), pneumonia in 21% (n = 7), urinary tract infection in 11% (n = 4), and non-specific infection without sepsis-symptoms in 21% (n = 7), while six patients could not be evaluated due to missing clinical information. Enterococcal isolates contributed to 15.3% (39/255) of the total number of identified episodes of bacteraemia in the study, 17 caused by *E. faecium*, 15 by *E. faecalis* and 7 by enterococcal isolates that were not available for speciation. Since some patients had more than one isolate of *E. faecium*, the total number of *E. faecium* isolates was 21. Twenty-three percent (9/39) of the patients had enterococci as part of a polymicrobial infection, involving other enterococcal isolates as well as 2 isolates of Candida species, 3 klebsiellae isolates and single isolates of *Salmonella enteritidis*, *Staphylococcus aureus* and *Streptococcus viridans*. The majority of *E. faecium* bacteraemia episodes (10/17) were hospital-acquired, i.e. obtained in blood-cultures taken ≥48 hours after admission, while the majority of *E. faecalis* bacteraemia episodes (10/15) were community-acquired.

The antimicrobial susceptibility of the isolates is shown in Table 1. Nine of 17 *E. faecium* isolates showed combined ampicillin-resistance and HLGR. Six of 15 *E. faecalis* isolates were HLGR, but none of these were resistant to ampicillin. All except one of the HLGR isolates were also resistant to chloramphenicol. The resistant strains were recovered from different wards, including the neonatal ward. All isolates were sensitive to vancomycin by disk-diffusion testing and Etest, and none of the 22 tested isolates were positive on PCR for *vanA* or *vanB* genes.

Twenty-one isolates of *E. faecium* and 15 isolates of *E. faecalis* were available for PFGE. The majority of the *E. faecium* and *E. faecalis* isolates were closely related as assessed visually from PFGE (Figure 1). From the figure 11/15 *E. faecalis* cluster at 72% similarity and 13/21 *E. faecium* at 80% similarity (Some duplicate strains are analysed in the dendrogram, resulting in totals of 12/16 similarly clustering *E. faecalis* and 17/25 similarly clustering *E. faecium* banding patterns). To assess whether the *E. faecium* isolates belonged to previously described, globally dispersed hospital subpopulations, MLST was performed on 12 *E. faecium* isolates and identified 7 different sequence types (STs) of which ST132 (5 isolates) and ST18 (2 isolates) were found in multiple isolate. These two STs, involving 7/12 isolates belong to lineage-18, which is contained in the global hospital-associated BAPS group 3–3. In the current study, persons with hospital-acquired infection accounted for 4 of 6 isolates in BAPS group 3–3. All 5 isolates of ST132 came from the same ward (neonatal ward). Isolates with ST125 and ST169, belonging to BAPS 3–1, and ST170 and ST171 belonging to BAPS 2–3 are also evolutionary related. Isolate 1064, ST178, belongs to BAPS 1, which is significantly associated with human commensal isolates in the community. Isolates with STs belonging to BAPS 3–3 were also related by PFGE. All isolates with STs belonging to BAPS 3–3 as well as isolate 2118 (ST125) belonging to BAPS 3–1 were ampicillin resistant, while the

Table 1 Antimicrobial susceptibility of enterococci causing bloodstream infection among febrile children admitted to Muhimbili National Hospital

Antibiotic	Susceptibility						
	E. faecium			*E. faecalis*			*Enterococci*
Antibiotic	CA	HA	All	CA	HA	All	All
Etest							
Ampicillin	25%	11%	19%	100%	100%	100%	53%
High-level Gentamicin	67%	33%	52%	56%	67%	60%	56%
Vancomycin*	100%	100%	100%	100%	100%	100%	100%
Linezolid	100%	100%	100%	100%	100%	100%	100%
Quinupristin-dalfopristin	100%	100%	100%	0%	17%	7%	61%
Disk-diffusion							
Chloramphenicol	50%	11%	32%	38%	33%	36%	33%
Doxycycline	9%	0%	5%	25%	0%	14%	9%

*Confirmed by negative PCR for *vanA* and *vanB* genes.
CA = community-acquired, HA = hospital-acquired.

other isolates were ampicillin susceptible. None of the isolates carried the esp gene.

Time in hospital from admission until blood cultures were obtained was not significantly longer among patients with BSI caused by *E. faecium* (median 3 days, range 0–10, p = 0.06) or *E. faecalis* (median 4 days, range 0–20, p = 0.56) compared to those with BSI caused by other microbes (median 2 days, range 0–34).

Table 2 shows univariate and multivariate analysis of risk factors for enterococcal BSI. HIV status was only known for 51.5% (n = 942) of patients, among which 18.7% (n = 176) were positive. As including HIV status in the multivariate analysis would eliminate close to half of the observations, we present two different multivariate models; one without HIV status (n = 1603 evaluable patients) and one with HIV status locked in the model (n = 842). Apart from factors shown in the table, all recorded clinical diagnoses and symptoms were assessed as risk factors.

Hospital-acquired infection (i.e. positive blood-culture drawn >48 hours after admission) was a risk factor for enterococcal BSI compared to community-acquired clinical infections (i.e. positive blood-culture drawn <48 hours after admission) in univariate analysis (Odds ratio (OR): 1.9, 95% confidence interval (95% CI): 1.01-3.61, p = 0.046), but did not remain a significant risk factor in multivariate analysis (OR: 2.0, 95% CI: 0.96-4.00, p = 0.066) (Table 2). There was no difference in proportions of hospital-acquired infection between enterococcal BSI compared to patients with other culture-proven BSI (44%, 17/39 vs 51%, 111/216, p = 0.37). Community-acquired and hospital-acquired *E. faecium* isolates did not have different rates of ampicillin-resistance (75% 9/12 vs 89%, 8/9, p = 0.42) or high-level gentamicin resistance (38%, 8/21 vs 53%, 8/15, p = 0.36).

A clinical diagnosis of sepsis with unspecified focus of infection was a borderline significant risk factor for enterococcal infection in univariate analysis (OR: 2.0, 95% CI: 1.00-4.00, p = 0.050) and a significant risk factor in multivariate analysis (OR: 2.9, 95% CI: 1.36-6.20, p = 0.006). In the multivariate analysis on the subset with known HIV status, sepsis remained a significant risk factor. Clinical diagnoses of urinary tract infection or pneumonia were not significant risk factors.

Prematurity was a significant risk factor for enterococcal bacteraemia in multivariate analysis (OR: 4.4, 95% CI: 1.06-18.1, p = 0.041), although this relationship was not significant in univariate analysis. Being a neonate appeared relatively protective in multivariate analysis (OR: 0.4, 95% CI: 0.14-0.98, p = 0.046), although again this was not significant in the univariate analysis. Within the cohort of neonates (children < 1 month of age), enterococcal BSI accounted for almost a quarter of BSI episodes in premature babies (23.1%, 3/13), and, despite the small numbers, the premature babies had a significantly increased risk of enterococcal BSI compared to babies born to term (5.8% vs 1.4%, OR 4.3, 95% CI: 1.03-17.55, p = 0.045). Prematurity remained a significant risk factor in the multivariate analysis on the subset of children with known HIV status.

The proportion of malnourished children was 21% in children with enterococcal BSI and 15% in controls, but this difference was not significant, neither in the univariate nor in the overall multivariate analysis. However, in the multivariate analysis on patients with known HIV status, malnutrition was indeed a significant risk factor for enterococcal BSI (OR 3.7, 95% CI 1.24-11.28, p = 0.019). The selection of children with known HIV status may have been skewed in the sense that malnourished and HIV positive patients may share clinical features, and thus more malnourished children may have been

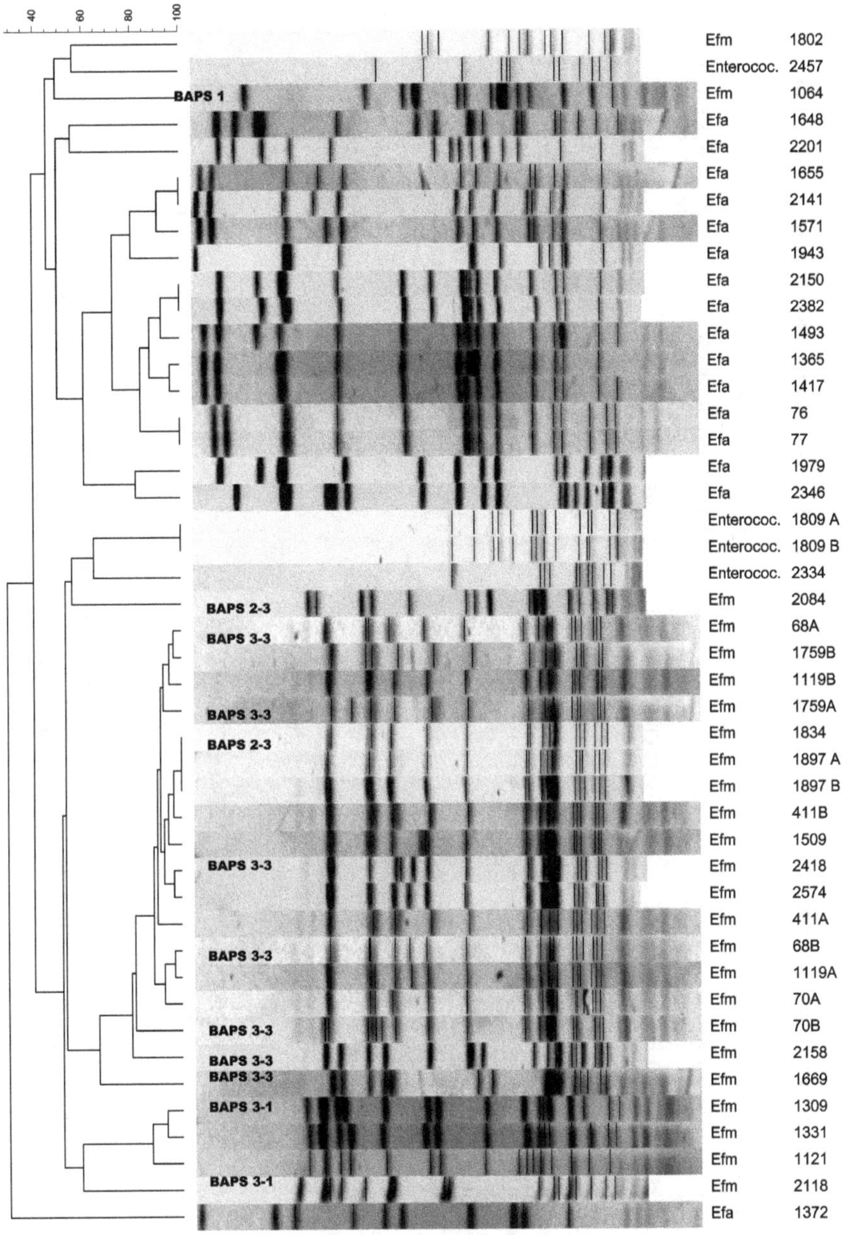

Figure 1 Genetic relatedness of enterococcal isolates causing bloodstream infections in Tanzanian children. The dendrogram shows genetic relatedness based on pulsed-field gel electrophoresis analysis on SmaI digested genomic DNA. Genetic relatedness was also assessed by multi-locus sequence typing and corresponding Bayesian Analysis of Population Structure (BAPS) groups are indicated in the dendrogram.

tested for HIV on clinical suspicion. Indeed, within the cohort of HIV negative children, malnourishment was a statistically significant risk factor for enterococcal BSI (6.6% (5/76) vs 2,3% (14/606), OR: 3.0, 95% CI: 1.04-8.51, p = 0.042), while there was no such association in HIV positive children (1.7% (1/60) vs 2.0% (2/100), OR: 0.83, 95% CI: 0.07-9.36, p = 0.881).

Altogether, HIV status was known for 51.5% (942/1828) of the total number of admission during the study (corresponding to 51.0% of patients (911/1787), and for 59% (23/39) of those with enterococcal BSI. There was no significant difference in HIV positivity rate between patients with enterococcal BSI (13.0%, 3/23) and all other patients with known HIV status (18.8%, 173/919, p = 0.486), and neither compared to those with BSI of other aetiologies (22.0%, 28/127, p = 0.33). Neither cephalosporin use, nor other antibiotic use prior to obtaining blood-culture, were significant risk factors for enterococcal

Table 2 Univariate and multivariate† analysis of risk factors for enterococcal bloodstream infection among febrile children admitted to Muhimbili National Hospital (n = 1828)*

	Univariate anlysis			Multivariate analyses†	
				All patients with clinical information (n = 1603)	All patients with known HIV status (n = 842)
Variable	Enterococci	Others	OR (95% CI) P	OR (95% CI) P	OR (95% CI) P
Neonate	28.2% (11/39)	29.3 (524/1789)	0.9 (0.47-1.92) 0.883	0.4 (0.14-0.98) 0.046	‡g
Prematurity	9.1 (3/33)	3.2 (51/1570)	3.0 (0.88 - 10.08) 0.079	4.4 (1.06-18.1) 0.041	4.7 (1.19-18.8) 0.019
Male sex	61.5 (24/39)	55.4 (992/1789)	1.3 (0.67 - 2.47) 0.450	‡e	2.9 (1.03-7.91) 0.043
Hospital acquired infection#	48.7 (19/39)	33.2 (594/1789)	1.9 (1.01 - 3.61) 0.046	2.0 (0.96– 4.00) 0.066	1.8 (0.73-4.29) 0.209
Antibiotic use before blood culture	66.7 (26/39)	57.0 (1020/1789)	1.5 (0.77 – 2.95) 0.231	‡c	‡b
Cephalosporin use before blood culture	5.1 (2/39)	4.0% (71/1789)	1.3 (0.31 – 5.53) 0.715	‡a	‡c
Diagnoses					
Malnutrition	21.2 (7/33)	15.4 (241/1570)	1.5 (0.64 - 3.46) 0.360	‡f	3.7 (1.24-11.28) 0.019
HIV infection	13.0 (3/23)	18.8 (173/919)	0.6 (0.19 – 2.20) 0.486	§	0.5 (0.14-2.04) 0.363§
Urinary tract infection	12.1% (4/33)	11.4% (179/1570)	1.1 (0.37- 3.08) 0.898	‡b	‡a
Pneumonia	21.2% (7/33)	20.1% (315/1570)	1.1 (0.46- 2.49) 0.871	‡d	‡e
Sepsis with unknown focus	45.5% (15/33)	29.4% (462/1570)	2.0 (1.00- 4.00) 0.050	2.9 (1.36-6.20) 0.006	2.6 (1.06-6.55) 0.037
Congenital heart disease	6.1% (2/33)	2.3% (36/1570)	2.7 (0.63- 11.93) 0.177	‡g	‡d
Acute watery diarrhoea	9.1 (3/33)	21.8 (343/1570)	0.4 (0.11 - 1.18) 0.091	0.3 (0.09-1.07) 0.065	‡f

OR = Odds ratio, 95% CI = 95% confidence interval, *There are varying numbers of patients evaluated for each risk factor because, among the 1828 study persons, we only have information on HIV status for n = 942 and sufficient clinical information for n = 1603. #Hospital acquired = blood culture taken >48 hours after admission †Multivariate analysis was performed by stepwise backwards logistic regression with threshold p = 0.2 for removal from the model and p = 0.05 for inclusion, ‡Risk factors were removed in a stepwise fashion in the sequence of ascending letters from "a" to "g", §HIV was removed from the first logistic regression because the many missing values would affect the model, HIV was locked in the second model although number of observations were reduced.

BSI. Male sex was associated with enterococcal BSI in the multivariate analysis of the subset with known HIV status, but not in univariate or overall multivariate analysis (Table 2).

Clinical outcome was known for 89.3% (1632/1828) of the admissions. Among those with known outcome, the case-fatality rate in children with *E. faecalis* septicaemia (28.6%, 4/14) was not significantly higher than for those with *E. faecium* septicaemia (6.7%, 1/15, $p = 0.12$). Children with enterococcal BSI received inappropriate chemotherapy due to antimicrobial resistance in 44.1% (15/39) of the cases, but this was not significantly different from BSI due to other agents (41.6%, 77/185, $p = 0.8$). The case fatality rate was 20% (3/15) for enterococcal BSI treated with inappropriate antibiotics, and 10% (2/19) for those treated with appropriate antibiotics, however, the numbers were small and the difference was not statistically significant ($p = 0.439$). Among patients with *E. faecalis* bacteraemia, two had concomitant malaria parasitaemia detected on microscopy, both of whom died. Among patients with *E. faecium* bacteraemia, one had concomitant growth of *S. aureus,* two had *Candida* species in blood culture, and two had concomitant malaria parasitaemia, none of whom died.

Discussion

Recent studies from Tanzania have described enterococci in urinary tract infections [38,39], but, to our knowledge, there are no published clinical studies on enterococcal bloodstream infections from this country. Although the data from the current study were collected some years ago, the study provides insight in prevalence, resistance patterns, and risk factors of enterococcal bloodstream infections in Tanzania, confirming similar trends as seen in Europe and the USA, and sets a benchmark for future studies. Surprisingly, we do not find that prior use of cephalosporins or other antibiotic use is a risk factor for enterococcal BSI in this study. This may be due to small numbers.

Enterococci are a prevalent aetiology for bloodstream infections in Tanzania, comprising 15.3% of the total number of identified episodes of bacteraemia in the current study. Information on antimicrobial use was available for 85.2% (1557/1828) of admissions and at least two-thirds (67.2%, 1046/1557) received antibiotics before blood-culture was taken. This may have selected more resistant clones in our study. All ampicillin-resistant HLGR *E. faecium* isolates were susceptible to vancomycin, linezolid and quinupristin/dalfopristin. All HLGR *E. faecalis* isolates were sensitive to vancomycin, linezolid and ampicillin.

As expected, the majority of *E. faecium* isolates were hospital-acquired, and hospital-acquired infection was a significant risk factor for enterococcal infections in univariate analysis. In accordance with other studies, most isolates associated with hospital-acquired infections clustered in BAPS group 3–3 based on MLST. The patient with ST178/ BAPS 1, a BAPS group significantly associated with human commensals in the community, had a clinical diagnosis of tuberculosis/pneumonia and anaemia.

A clinical diagnosis of sepsis, but not pneumonia and urinary tract infection, was a significant risk factor for enterococcal BSI. While neonates in general were not particularly at risk, premature babies had significantly increased risk of enterococcal BSI. Malnutrition was a significant risk factor for enterococcal BSI in sub-analysis of children with known HIV status (multivariate analysis), particularly among those with known negative HIV test (univariate analysis).

Among the 14 patients with *E. faecium* recovered from blood culture (and known outcome) only one died, this was a two months old boy with suspected meningitis who was admitted with fever, convulsions and neck stiffness. The isolate was resistant to ampicillin and chloramphenicol, and high-level gentamicin-resistant. The patient received antimicrobial treatment with penicillin and chloramphenicol, to which the enterococcal isolate was resistant. Chloramphenicol is largely abandoned in developed countries due to the risk of aplastic anaemia, although it has been used to treat VRE. Chloramphenicol is still widely used in Africa for the treatment of a number of bacterial infections including meningitis and typhoid fever. It was, however, uncertain whether the *E. faecium* isolate was the cause of the meningitis, which was thought to be the main diagnosis.

Among the patients with *E. faecalis* bacteraemia, four died. Two of those who died had concomitant malaria parasitaemia on microscopy, one of which received quinine (for the other therapy was unknown). Two of them had HLGR, including one of the patients with malaria parasitaemia. The given antimicrobial therapy was known for three of the patients, one of which received inappropriate antibiotic treatment (chloramphenicol), and two of which received at least one appropriate antibiotic (ampicillin) and one inappropriate (gentamicin) for HLGR.

Conclusions

Consistent with global trends showing increasing importance of *E. faecium* as a cause of human infections relative to *E. faecalis* [22,40], our study found that more than half of the enterococcal bloodstream infections were caused by *E. faecium* in this hospital. This first clinical study of enterococcal bloodstream infections from Tanzania has identified septicaemia caused by ampicillin-resistant and HLGR enterococci as common nosocomial infections with a considerable case-fatality rate. Premature babies and malnourished children, and those with a clinical diagnosis of sepsis with unknown focus appeared at particular risk. These infections constitute a therapeutic problem as the commonly used treatment regimens at the hospital (ampicillin and gentamicin or penicillin and chloramphenicol) are insufficient for infections caused by ampicillin-resistant HLGR enterococci. Vancomycin is the empirical drug of choice for proven *E. faecium* bloodstream infections. However, in a resource-constrained setting such as Tanzania, limited access to microbiological laboratories and expensive second-line antimicrobials may render such recommendations futile. Furthermore, escalating empirical use of broad-spectrum antibiotics may be ecologically detrimental in a setting where microbiological laboratory services are scarce and patients rarely get a bacteriologically confirmed diagnosis. In this context, it is crucial to counteract further emergent antibiotic resistance by infection control measures and prudent antibiotic use based on best available data from surveillance activities, sentinel surveys, and, whenever possible, microbiological diagnosis for the individual patient.

Abbreviations

95% CI: 95% confidence interval; AIDS: Acquired immune deficiency syndrome; BAPS: Bayesian Analysis of Population Structure; BSI: Bloodstream infection; CA: Community-acquired; CC17: Clonal complex 17; CLSI: Clinical and Laboratory Standards Institute; ELISA: Enzyme-linked immunosorbent assay; HA: Hospital-acquired; HIV: Human immunodeficiency virus; HLGR: High-level gentamicin-resistance; IMCI: Integrated management of childhood illnesses; MIC: Minimum inhibitory concentration; MLST: Multi-locus sequence-typing; NCCLS: National Committee for Clinical Laboratory Standards; OR: Odds ratio; PCR: Polymerase chain reaction; PFGE: Pulsed-field gel electrophoresis; ST: Sequence type; UPMGA: Unweighted pair group method with arithmetic averages; VRE: Vancomycin-resistant enterococci.

Competing interests

The authors declare that they have no competing interests.

Authors' contributions

BB, NL, KPM and SYM conceived and designed the study. BB, KPM and SYM supervised the data collection. BB, SCM, RJ and RW performed phenotypic and molecular microbiological analysis. RW performed multi-locus sequence-typing. HA and BB analysed the data. All authors contributed to the interpretation of the data and writing of the manuscript. All authors read and approved the final manuscript.

Acknowledgements

The study received funding from grant 100675 from the Norwegian Research Council and from the Norwegian Council for Higher Education's Programme for Development Research and Education under project number 44003 PRO 42.2.91. We are grateful to Dr Kristine Mørch, Head of the National Centre for Infectious Tropical Diseases, for support during data-analysis and writing of the manuscript. We would like to thank all doctors, nurses, laboratory technicians and other staff at Muhimbili National Hospital who contributed to the study.

Author details

[1]Department of Clinical Science, University of Bergen, Bergen, Norway. [2]Center for Tropical Infectious Diseases, Department of Medicine, Haukeland University Hospital, Bergen, Norway. [3]Department of Microbiology and Immunology, Muhimbili University of Health and Allied Sciences, Dar es Salaam, Tanzania. [4]Department of Pediatrics and Child Health, Muhimbili University of Health and Allied Sciences, Dar es Salaam, Tanzania. [5]Department of Medical Microbiology, University Medical Center Utrecht, Utrecht, Netherlands. [6]National University Health System, Singapore City, Singapore.

References

1. Sghir A, Gramet G, Suau A, Rochet V, Pochart P, Dore J. Quantification of bacterial groups within human fecal flora by oligonucleotide probe hybridization. Appl Environ Microbiol. 2000;66(5):2263–6.
2. Damborg P, Top J, Hendrickx AP, Dawson S, Willems RJ, Guardabassi L. Dogs are a reservoir of ampicillin-resistant Enterococcus faecium lineages associated with human infections. Appl Environ Microbiol. 2009;75(8):2360–5.
3. Witte W, Wirth R, Klare I. Enterococci. Chemotherapy. 1999;45(2):135–45.
4. Low DE, Keller N, Barth A, Jones RN. Clinical prevalence, antimicrobial susceptibility, and geographic resistance patterns of enterococci: results from the SENTRY Antimicrobial Surveillance Program, 1997–1999. Clin Infect Dis. 2001;32 Suppl 2:S133–45.
5. Treitman AN, Yarnold PR, Warren J, Noskin GA. Emerging incidence of Enterococcus faecium among hospital isolates (1993 to 2002). J Clin Microbiol. 2005;43(1):462–3.
6. Bonten MJ, Willems RJ. [Vancomycin-resistant enterococcus–chronicle of a foretold problem]. Nederlands Tijdschrift Voor Geneeskunde. 2012;156(38):A5233.
7. Oppenheim BA. The changing pattern of infection in neutropenic patients. J Antimicrob Chemother. 1998;41 Suppl D:7–11.
8. Pedro-Botet ML, Modol JM, Valles X, Romeu J, Sopena N, Gimenez M, et al. Changes in bloodstream infections in HIV-positive patients in a university hospital in Spain (1995–1997). Int J Infect Dis. 2002;6(1):17–22.
9. Kristich CJ, Little JL, Hall CL, Hoff JS. Reciprocal regulation of cephalosporin resistance in Enterococcus faecalis. mBio. 2011;2(6):e00199–00111.
10. Kristich CJ, Little JL. Mutations in the beta subunit of RNA polymerase alter intrinsic cephalosporin resistance in Enterococci. Antimicrob Agents Chemother. 2012;56(4):2022–7.
11. Georgopapadakou NH, Liu FY. Binding of beta-lactam antibiotics to penicillin-binding proteins of Staphylococcus aureus and Streptococcus faecalis: relation to antibacterial activity. Antimicrob Agents Chemother. 1980;18(5):834–6.
12. Moellering Jr RC, Weinberg AN. Studies on antibiotic syngerism against enterococci. II. Effect of various antibiotics on the uptake of 14 C-labeled streptomycin by enterococci. J Clin Invest. 1971;50(12):2580–4.
13. Paterson DL. "Collateral damage" from cephalosporin or quinolone antibiotic therapy. Clin Infect Dis. 2004;38 Suppl 4:S341–5.
14. Pallares R, Pujol M, Pena C, Ariza J, Martin R, Gudiol F. Cephalosporins as risk factor for nosocomial Enterococcus faecalis bacteremia. A matched case–control study. Arch Intern Med. 1993;153(13):1581–6.
15. Dahms RA, Johnson EM, Statz CL, Lee JT, Dunn DL, Beilman GJ. Third-generation cephalosporins and vancomycin as risk factors for postoperative vancomycin-resistant enterococcus infection. Arch Surg. 1998;133(12):1343–6.
16. Willems RJ, Top J, van Santen M, Robinson DA, Coque TM, Baquero F, et al. Global spread of vancomycin-resistant Enterococcus faecium from distinct nosocomial genetic complex. Emerg Infect Dis. 2005;11(6):821–8.
17. Cattoir V, Leclercq R. Twenty-five years of shared life with vancomycin-resistant enterococci: is it time to divorce? J Antimicrob Chemother. 2013;68(4):731–42.
18. Huycke MM, Sahm DF, Gilmore MS. Multiple-drug resistant enterococci: the nature of the problem and an agenda for the future. Emerg Infect Dis. 1998;4(2):239–49.
19. McCracken M, Wong A, Mitchell R, Gravel D, Conly J, Embil J, et al. Molecular epidemiology of vancomycin-resistant enterococcal bacteraemia: results from the Canadian Nosocomial Infection Surveillance Program, 1999–2009. J Antimicrob Chemother. 2013;68(7):1505–9.
20. Hsieh YC, Lee WS, Ou TY, Hsueh PR. Clonal spread of CC17 vancomycin-resistant Enterococcus faecium with multilocus sequence type 78 (ST78) and a novel ST444 in Taiwan. Eur J Clin Microbiol Infect Dis. 2010;29(1):25–30.
21. Laverde Gomez JA, van Schaik W, Freitas AR, Coque TM, Weaver KE, Francia MV, et al. A multiresistance megaplasmid pLG1 bearing a hylEfm genomic island in hospital Enterococcus faecium isolates. Int J Med Microbiol. 2011;301(2):165–75.
22. Top J, Willems R, Blok H, de Regt M, Jalink K, Troelstra A, et al. Ecological replacement of Enterococcus faecalis by multiresistant clonal complex 17 Enterococcus faecium. Clin Microbiol Infect. 2007;13(3):316–9.
23. Willems RJ, Top J, van Schaik W, Leavis H, Bonten M, Siren J, et al. Restricted gene flow among hospital subpopulations of Enterococcus faecium. mBio. 2012;3(4):e00151–00112.
24. Lebreton F, van Schaik W, McGuire AM, Godfrey P, Griggs A, Mazumdar V, et al. Emergence of epidemic multidrug-resistant Enterococcus faecium from animal and commensal strains. mBio. 2013;4(4):e00534–13.

25. Patterson JE, Barry M, Gallant J, Mangine LS, Farrel P, Latif A. Epidemiology of high-level gentamicin resistant enterococcal isolates from Zimbabwe. Am J Trop Med Hyg. 1990;43(4):397–9.
26. Keddy KH, Klugman KP, Liebowitz LD. Incidence of high-level gentamicin resistance in enterococci at Johannesburg Hospital. S Afr Med J. 1996;86(10):1273–6.
27. McCarthy KM, Van Nierop W, Duse A, Von Gottberg A, Kassel M, Perovic O, et al. Control of an outbreak of vancomycin-resistant Enterococcus faecium in an oncology ward in South Africa: effective use of limited resources. J Hosp Infect. 2000;44(4):294–300.
28. Chingwaru W, Mpuchane SF, Gashe BA. Enterococcus faecalis and Enterococcus faecium isolates from milk, beef, and chicken and their antibiotic resistance. J Food Prot. 2003;66(6):931–6.
29. Blomberg B, Manji KP, Urassa WK, Tamim BS, Mwakagile DS, Jureen R, et al. Antimicrobial resistance predicts death in Tanzanian children with bloodstream infections: a prospective cohort study. BMC Infect Dis. 2007;7:43.
30. IMCI Integrated Management of Childhood Illness. Model Chapter for Textbooks. Document no. WHO/FCH/CAH/01.01. Accessible from http://whqlibdoc.who.int/hq/2001/WHO_FCH_CAH_01.01.pdf. Geneva: World Health Organization; 2001.
31. Collee JG, Marmion BP, Irvine R, Fraser AG, Simmons A. Mackie & McCartney Practical Medical Microbiology. 14th ed. New York: Churchill Livingstone; 1996.
32. Angeletti S, Lorino G, Gherardi G, Battistoni F, De Cesaris M, Dicuonzo G. Routine molecular identification of enterococci by gene-specific PCR and 16S ribosomal DNA sequencing. J Clin Microbiol. 2001;39(2):794–7.
33. NCCLS. Performance standards for antimicrobial disk susceptibility tests. Approved standard M2-M7. Wayne, Pa, USA 1997 (7th edition).
34. Murray BE, Singh KV, Heath JD, Sharma BR, Weinstock GM. Comparison of genomic DNAs of different enterococcal isolates using restriction endonucleases with infrequent recognition sites. J Clin Microbiol. 1990;28(9):2059–63.
35. Dahl KH, Simonsen GS, Olsvik O, Sundsfjord A. Heterogeneity in the vanB gene cluster of genomically diverse clinical strains of vancomycin-resistant enterococci. Antimicrob Agents Chemother. 1999;43(5):1105–10.
36. Homan WL, Tribe D, Poznanski S, Li M, Hogg G, Spalburg E, et al. Multilocus sequence typing scheme for Enterococcus faecium. J Clin Microbiol. 2002;40(6):1963–71.
37. Siegman-Igra Y, Fourer B, Orni-Wasserlauf R, Golan Y, Noy A, Schwartz D, et al. Reappraisal of community-acquired bacteremia: a proposal of a new classification for the spectrum of acquisition of bacteremia. Clin Infect Dis. 2002;34(11):1431–9.
38. Masinde A, Gumodoka B, Kilonzo A, Mshana SE. Prevalence of urinary tract infection among pregnant women at Bugando Medical Centre, Mwanza, Tanzania. Tanzan J Health Res. 2009;11(3):154–9.
39. Moyo SJ, Aboud S, Kasubi M, Maselle SY. Bacterial isolates and drug susceptibility patterns of urinary tract infection among pregnant women at Muhimbili National Hospital in Tanzania. Tanzan J Health Res. 2010;12(4):236–40.
40. Iwen PC, Kelly DM, Linder J, Hinrichs SH, Dominguez EA, Rupp ME, et al. Change in prevalence and antibiotic resistance of Enterococcus species isolated from blood cultures over an 8-year period. Antimicrob Agents Chemother. 1997;41(2):494–5.

12

Incidence of and factors associated with catheter-related bloodstream infection in patients with advanced solid tumors on home parenteral nutrition managed using a standardized catheter care protocol

Pankaj G. Vashi, Natasha Virginkar, Brenten Popiel, Persis Edwin and Digant Gupta*

Abstract

Background: Catheter-related bloodstream infections (CRBSIs) are associated with high morbidity and mortality as well as increased medical costs. Cancer patients, who are often immunocompromised, are susceptible to CRBSI while receiving home parenteral nutrition (HPN). We evaluated the incidence of and factors associated with CRBSIs in cancer patients undergoing HPN managed using a standardized catheter care protocol.

Methods: This is a retrospective cohort study of 335 cancer patients receiving HPN between January 2012 and July 2015. The primary outcome of interest was the incidence of CRBSI expressed as events per 1000 HPN days. HPN days were calculated from the start date with the home infusion provider until the discontinuation of HPN, or the removal of the venous access device (VAD), or the death of the patient. The VADs used were either peripherally inserted central catheters (PICCs) or a subcutaneous implanted port or tunneled central catheters (TCCs). Univariate Poisson regression analyses were used to determine the variables associated with CRBSIs.

Results: Of 335 patients, 193 were females and 142 were males. The most common cancer types were colorectal, pancreatic, ovarian and stomach. A total of 408 VADs in 335 patients were studied, covering a total of 29,403 HPN days. Of 408 VADs, 206 (50.5%) were ports, 191 (46.8%) were PICCs, and 7 (2.7%) were TCCs. The median duration of HPN was 54 days. A total of 16 CRBSI episodes were recorded (8 in ports, 7 in PICCs and 1 in TCCs). The median duration from the start of HPN to the development of CRBSI episodes was 43.5 days. The overall incidence of CRBSI per 1000 HPN days was 0.54 (95% confidence interval: 0.32–0.86). Upon univariate analysis, no variables were found to be statistically significantly associated with CRBSI incidence.

Conclusions: We found a low rate of CRBSI following a standardized catheter maintenance protocol in a high-risk oncology population undergoing HPN.

Keywords: Bloodstream infections, Cancer, Home parenteral nutrition, Standardized protocol

* Correspondence: gupta_digant@yahoo.com
Cancer Treatment Centers of America® (CTCA) at Midwestern Regional Medical Center, 2520 Elisha Ave, Zion, Illinois 60099, USA

Background

Cancer patients often require central venous access for continuous infusion of chemotherapeutic agents, hydration, and parenteral nutrition (PN) [1]. Other indications for the placement of these catheters in patients with cancer include poor peripheral access, frequent need to administer blood products or antibiotics or to draw blood, a prolonged treatment course and use of vesicant drugs [2].

Earlier, long-term venous access devices (VADs) were described by Broviac et al. and then by Hickman et al. [3, 4]. Central venous devices are either simple catheters, such as tunneled Hickman catheters, or catheters linked to a subcutaneous port. Both types of VADs, simple or port catheter, are placed percutaneously via a subclavian route or a jugular route under sonographic guidance [5]. Implanted subcutaneous ports or tunneled catheters are placed in the operating room or a designated minor procedure room in order to adhere to an aseptic environment and strict sterile technique. Intraoperative fluoroscopy is often used to guide the catheter into the correct position. Peripherally inserted central catheters (PICCs), on the other hand, are usually placed ultrasound guided in the intervention radiology department using sterile precautions.

Although the use of long-term VADs has enhanced the lives of oncology patients, it has added a new set of challenges [6]. While totally implantable access ports have the advantages of not requiring an external dressing, allowing more patient activity and requiring only monthly maintenance flushing [7, 8], these devices still have a reported complication rate of 11% to 25% [7, 9, 10]. Complications of catheterization include those associated with VAD insertion such as pneumothorax and arterial and nerve injuries as well as those associated with long-term VAD use such as thrombosis and catheter-related bloodstream infection (CRBSI) [11–14]. Other complications include embolization of a ruptured distal part of the catheter, migration of the tip of the catheter, fibrin-sheath obstruction of the catheter, embolization of a guidewire during placement of the central venous device and leakages [5, 15].

Cancer patients, who are often immunocompromised, are more susceptible to CRBSI while receiving total parenteral nutrition [16]. The major causes of CRBSI are migration of the skin organisms at the insertion site into the catheter tract and contamination of the catheter hub [17]. This incidence of CRBSI ranges from 0.05 to 6.8 infections per 1000 catheter days [17, 18]. Success rates of 60% to 91% have been reported using antimicrobial therapy to treat CRBSIs, although often the device has to be removed [19]. The organisms most commonly cultured are gram-positive (70%; Coagulase negative Staphylococci, *Staphylococcus aureus* and Enterococci], gram-negative (15%; *Escherichia coli*), fungal (8%; Candida), and anaerobic bacteria (7%) [20].

Few observational studies (with none conducted in the US) have quantified the incidence of CRBSI in patients with solid tumors receiving active oncologic treatment while undergoing home parenteral nutrition (HPN) [18, 21–25]. The aims of the present study were to evaluate the following in a case series of patients with advanced solid tumors treated at a tertiary care cancer center in the US: 1) The incidence of CRBSI while receiving HPN using a standardized catheter care protocol; 2) Factors associated with CRBSI development.

Methods

Study design and patient population

This is a retrospective cohort study of a consecutive case series of patients with solid tumors receiving HPN between January 2012 and July 2015 while being treated at Cancer Treatment Centers of America® (CTCA) at Midwestern Regional Medical Center. We included a consecutive case series of patients to avoid non-response and minimize the probability of selection bias. The criteria for receiving HPN were based on the American Society for Parenteral and Enteral Nutrition (ASPEN) guidelines [26] and included the following: (1) Patients receiving active anticancer treatment who are malnourished and who are anticipated to be unable to ingest and/or absorb adequate nutrients for a prolonged period of time; (2) Eastern Cooperative Oncology Group (ECOG) performance status score of <= 2 (minimum score of 0 indicates a normal person with no limitations, whereas a maximum score of 5 indicates a dead person); (3) Evaluation and approval by a multi-disciplinary nutrition and metabolic support team (NMST) comprised of a physician, dietitian, nurse, pharmacist and care manager.

The present study was conducted according to the guidelines laid down in the Declaration of Helsinki and was approved by the Institutional Review Board (IRB) at CTCA Midwestern Regional Medical Center. The need for informed consent was waived by the IRB because there was no direct patient contact in this study. This study involved collection of existing data from patient records in such a manner that subjects cannot be identified, directly or through identifiers linked to the subjects. Patient records/information was anonymized and de-identified prior to analysis.

Venous access devices

The VADs used in our patients were either PICCs, or a subcutaneous implanted port or tunneled central catheters (TCCs). The choice of the type of VAD used in each patient was primarily based on the provider's preference. The ports were inserted by a surgical oncologist. All ports were inserted in the upper chest through a subclavian vein approach. The placement was confirmed by an X-ray before using the port. The PICC lines were inserted under ultrasound guidance into the brachial or basilic veins by a trained nurse or an interventional radiologist. The TCCs were inserted by a surgeon. All VADs were inserted with maximal barrier precautions and skin antisepsis with 2% chlorhexidine swabs as part of a prepackaged kit. The barrier precautions used for VADs depended upon the type of access. All the ports were inserted in the sterile operation room by the surgeon. After washing the hands with soap and water with scrubbing, the surgeon wore a sterile gown and gloves for the procedure like any major surgery. The PICC and TCC lines were inserted in the designated interventional radiology room by the interventional radiologist who also followed the same routine as the surgeons for sterile barrier. Sterile solution (2% chlorhexidine) was used for all the patients as a barrier with sterile draping covering up the insertion site. The appropriate central position of the tip of the catheter was consistently verified, either by fluoroscopy during the procedure or by chest X-ray after the procedure.

Standardized VAD care protocol

All patients received HPN from a single home infusion company. Patients were managed by 12 different branches of the same home infusion company across the country. Patients received detailed pre-discharge teaching by a team of hospital and home infusion nurses, registered dietitians, and a dedicated case manager prior to going home with PN. Every patient was evaluated for the presence of a suitable environment at home for HPN which included clean running water, designated area in the refrigerator to store the PN bags, access of communication (cell phone or a land line), clean designated area for preparation of the PN bag, and good family support system that understands the steps for sterile infusion and basic monitoring devices like a weighing machine, thermometer to check temperature and blood sugar monitoring device in selected patients. Every patient had to have a responsible caregiver at home which was defined as someone who understood step-by-step PN preparation process, troubleshooting and identifying any potential complications.

Written as well as visual instructions on step-by-step process of caring for the VAD were given to the patient and the caregiver before their transition to HPN. A home health nurse for each patient was arranged by the same infusion company. Patients in the study were managed using a specific catheter care protocol that included: a strict aseptic flushing and dressing change procedure; weekly sterile dressing changes with use of Chloraprep®; and the application of MicroClave® connectors and SwabCaps® on all lumens that were not in use. A weekly assessment was performed that provided details about the patients' clinical status, compliance with catheter care and HPN, and catheter status. Complete blood count and serum chemistry were conducted weekly and critical values were reported to the metabolic support team immediately. Printed materials and custom multimedia videos were used to reinforce infusion technique and patient/caregiver compliance with catheter maintenance protocol. A member of the NMST was available to answer any questions regarding these videos.

CRBSI diagnosis and management

The diagnosis and management of CRBSI were conducted according to the clinical practice guidelines provided by the Infectious Diseases Society of America (IDSA) [27]. Any patient who developed unexplained high grade fever (101 degrees F or higher) was evaluated for CRBSI by performing blood cultures. The blood cultures (both peripheral and central) were performed in the local emergency room. In the case of a positive blood culture, antibiotics were selected according to the sensitivity of the responsible microorganism(s). Antibiotic administration and catheter removal were conducted according to the IDSA guidelines [27].

Statistical analysis

The *primary outcome* of interest was the incidence of CRBSI. Incidence rates of CRBSI were expressed as events per 1000 HPN days. This is the ratio of the number of VAD-related episodes of infection to the total number of HPN days during the study period multiplied by 1000. Follow-up continued until either the VAD was removed or HPN stopped. Loss to follow-up was considered when contact with the patient was lost while still receiving HPN. HPN days were calculated from the start date with the home infusion provider until the discontinuation of HPN, or the removal of the VAD, or the death of the patient. The *primary independent variable* of interest was the type of VAD. The following variables were evaluated as potential *covariates* or *confounders* because of their potential to be associated with the key outcome of interest (incidence of CRBSI): age, gender, tumor type, Subjective Global Assessment (SGA), ECOG performance status, stage at diagnosis, body mass index (BMI) and serum albumin. The SGA is a clinical technique that combines data from subjective and objective aspects of medical history (weight change, dietary intake change, gastrointestinal symptoms, and changes in functional capacity) and physical examination (loss of subcutaneous fat, muscle wasting, ankle or sacral edema, and ascites). After evaluation, patients were categorized into 3 distinct classes of nutritional status; well nourished (SGA-A), moderately malnourished (SGA-B) and severely malnourished (SGA-C) as described by Detsky et al. [28]. The distribution of these potential confounders across the different types of VADs was examined using the computation of standardized mean differences in accordance with the guidance provided by Austin 2011 [29]. A standard difference of less than 0.2 was taken to indicate a negligible difference in the mean or prevalence of a covariate between VAD types. The duration of VADs was compared across the different types of VADs using the non-parametric Kruskal-Wallis test with pair-wise comparisons. CRBSI incidence rates across the VAD types were compared using the Fisher and Mid-P exact tests adjusted for HPN-days (using the number of HPN days as the denominator).

Univariate Poisson regression was used to determine which variables were associated with CRBSIs. Since the amount of exposure to the risk of developing CRBSI was different across patients, the "natural log of HPN days" was added as an "offset" variable in all Poisson regression analyses. The Pearson dispersion statistic was used to evaluate the presence of overdispersion in the models. Values of Pearson dispersion statistic greater than 1 were taken to indicate overdispersion. In such a scenario, scaling of standard errors and robust (or sandwich) variance estimators were employed, to adjust for overdispersion in the models. When using scaling or robust variance estimators, the parameter estimates are the same as in the previous model fit, but the standard errors are increased, resulting in more conservative statistical tests. Scaling or applying a robust variance estimate allows the fit of the model to better reflect the true underlying distribution. The effect of individual variables on the incidence of CRBSI was expressed as incidence rate ratios (IRRs) calculated by exponentiating the estimated parameters of the Poisson models. The corresponding 95% confidence intervals (CIs) and p-values were also reported.

No formal sample size calculations were conducted for this analysis. All data were analyzed using IBM SPSS version 23.0 (IBM, Armonk, NY, USA). All analyses were two-tailed, and a difference was considered to be statistically significant if the p value was <= 0.05.

Results

Patient characteristics

The final study sample consisted of 335 consecutive patients of which 193 were females (57.6%) and 142 were males (42.4%) with an overall mean age of 53.7 years. All eligible patients during the study period were included with no exclusions at any stage. There were no losses to follow-up and all patients were included in the final analysis. The most common cancer types were colorectal, pancreatic, ovarian, and stomach. The majority of our patient population was moderately to severely malnourished (81.5%) at baseline and had received chemotherapy or radiotherapy during HPN (73.1%). The median duration of HPN was 54 days. Tables 1 and 2 describe the baseline characteristics of our patient cohort in greater detail.

The primary indications for using HPN in these patients were poor oral intake in spite of aggressive nutrition counseling by a dietitian, failure of oral supplementations and appetite stimulants (n = 123; 36.7%), weight loss/malnutrition (n = 84; 25.1%), bowel obstruction (n = 42; 12.5%) and post cytoreductive surgery and hyperthermic intraperitoneal chemotherapy (n = 33; 9.9%). All patients were followed up until either the VAD was removed or HPN stopped. HPN was discontinued in most patients on recovery of oral nutrition (n = 120; 35.8%), worsening of clinical state (n = 85; 25.4%), death (n = 77; 23%) and transfer to other facility (n = 33; 9.9%); the reasons for HPN discontinuation were not statistically significantly different across the 3 VAD types.

Table 1 Baseline patient characteristics (Categorical Variables); N = 335

Characteristic	Categories	Number (Percent)
Gender	Male	142 (42.4)
Cancer site	Colorectal	71 (21.2)
	Pancreas	59 (17.6)
	Ovary	35 (10.4)
	Stomach	29 (8.7)
	Cervix	17 (5.1)
	Esophagus	16 (4.8)
	Lung	15 (4.5)
	Others	93 (27.8)
Cancer stage at diagnosis	Stage 0	1 (0.3)
	Stage I	26 (7.8)
	Stage II	53 (15.8)
	Stage III	98 (29.3)
	Stage IV	157 (46.9)
Chemotherapy during HPN	Yes	208 (62.1)
Radiotherapy during HPN	Yes	73 (21.8)
SGA at HPN Start	Well-nourished	62 (18.5)
	Moderately Malnourished	175 (52.2)
	Severely Malnourished	98 (29.3)
ECOG performance status	0	11 (3.3)
	1	86 (25.7)
	2	132 (39.4)
	3	101 (30.1)
	4–5	5 (1.5)

ECOG Eastern Cooperative Oncology Group, *HPN* home parenteral nutrition, *SGA* Subjective Global Assessment

Table 2 Baseline patient characteristics (Continuous Variables); $N = 335$

Characteristic	Mean (SD)	Median	Range
Age (years) at start of HPN	53.7 (9.3)	55.2	22.8–84.5
Weight (kg) at start of HPN	69.2 (18.2)	67.7	31–145.4
BMI (kg/m^2) at start of HPN	24.2 (6.2)	23.1	12.2–57.1
Albumin (g/dl) at start of HPN	2.7 (0.64)	2.7	0.9–5.9
HPN Duration (days)	87.7 (108.4)	54	0–972

BMI body mass index, *g/dl* grams per deciliter, *HPN* home parenteral nutrition, *kg* kilograms, *kg/m^2* kilograms per meter squared, *SD* standard deviation

VADs

All the VADs placed in this study were used for HPN. In those patients who were receiving HPN and chemotherapy, the VAD was used for both but never at the same time. Among the 335 unique patients described above, the study included 408 VADs covering a total of 29,403 HPN days (median 46 days). Of the 408 VADs, 206 (50.5%) were ports, 191 (46.8%) were PICCs, and 11 (2.7%) were TCCs. Ports and PICCs were the only two VADs offered at our institution. The 11 TCCs were placed at a different institution before those patients visited us. Table 3 displays the characteristics of VADs in greater detail (this table is based on the total number of VADs and not the total number of unique patients). The median duration of HPN for ports was significantly greater than the median HPN duration for PICCs (53 days versus 41 days; $p = 0.02$). Table 4 displays the standardized mean differences in the distribution of baseline characteristics across the 3 VAD types. A standardized mean difference of greater than equal to 0.20 in a particular baseline characteristic was considered to indicate an imbalance between the 2 VAD groups. As can be seen from Table 4, the Port and PICC groups were different from each other with regard to BMI; the PICC and TCC groups were different from each other with regard to age, gender, cancer stage and ECOG performance status; the Port and TCC groups were different from each other with regard to age, BMI, gender, cancer stage and ECOG performance status.

CRBSIs

Incidence

Of 335 patients, 15 (4.5%) patients experienced CRBSI. One patient experienced 2 episodes of CRBSI. As a result, for a total of 408 VADs, the number of CRBSI cases was 16 (3.9%). Table 3 displays the overall incidence of CRBSI as well as incidence stratified by the 3 VAD types. The overall incidence of CRBSI per 1000 HPN days was 0.54 (95% CI: 0.32 to 0.86). Of the 16 CRBSI cases, 8 occurred in ports, 7 in PICCs and 1 in TCCs. There were no statistically significant differences in the incidence rates of CRBSI across the 3 types of VADs. The median

Table 3 Characteristics of and Infections Associated with VADs; $N = 408$

	Port	PICC	TCC	Total
Characteristics				
Number (%) of VADs	206 (50.5)	191 (46.8)	11 (2.7)	408 (100)
Median HPN Days#	53	41	88	46
Total HPN Days	16,929	11,401	1073	29,403
Mean Age (years)	53.6	53.9	58.6	53.8
Mean BMI (kg/m^2)	23.5	25.1	25.3	24.3
Mean Serum Albumin (g/dl)	2.8	2.8	2.9	2.8
Gender, % Male	43.7	43.5	54.5	43.9
Cancer Stage at Diagnosis, % Stage IV	51.5	43.5	27.3	47.1
SGA at HPN Start, % well-nourished	23.3	19.9	18.2	21.6
ECOG Performance Status, % 0–2	67	71.7	81.8	69.6
Infection				
Number of CRBSI	8	7	1	16
Number of CRBSI/1000 HPN Days (95% CI)*	0.47 (0.20–0.93)	0.61 (0.25–1.3)	0.93 (0.02–5.2)	0.54 (0.32–0.86)
Days to CRBSI, Median (Range)	83.5 (13–420)	30 (0–95)	187 (187–187)	43.5 (0–420)

CI confidence interval, *CRBSI* catheter-related bloodstream infection, *ECOG* Eastern Cooperative Oncology Group, *HPN* home parenteral nutrition, *PICC* peripherally inserted central catheter, *SGA* Subjective Global Assessment, *TCC* tunneled central catheter, *VAD* venous access device

#Port versus PICC $p = 0.02$
Port versus TCC $p = 0.99$
PICC versus TCC $p = 0.34$
*Port versus PICC $p = 0.61$
Port versus TCC $p = 0.52$
PICC versus TCC $p = 0.65$

Table 4 Standardized Mean Differences in Baseline Characteristics across VADs; $N = 408$

Characteristics	Port vs. PICC	PICC vs. TCC	Port vs. TCC
Mean Age (years)	0.03	0.52*	0.58*
Mean BMI (kg/m^2)	0.27*	0.04	0.35*
Mean Serum Albumin (g/dl)	0.00	0.16	0.16
Gender, % Male	0.00	0.22*	0.22*
Cancer Stage at Diagnosis, % Stage IV	0.16	0.34*	0.51*
SGA at HPN Start, % well-nourished	0.08	0.04	0.13
ECOG Performance Status, % 0–2	0.10	0.24*	0.34*

BMI body mass index, *ECOG* Eastern Cooperative Oncology Group, *g/dl* grams per deciliter, *HPN* home parenteral nutrition, *kg/m2* kilograms per meter squared, *PICC* peripherally inserted central catheter, *SGA* Subjective Global Assessment, *TCC* tunneled central catheter, *VAD* venous access device
*Values >0.20

duration from the start of HPN to the development of CRBSI episodes was 43.5 days.

The majority of cases with CRBSIs were either moderately malnourished ($n = 6$) or severely malnourished ($n = 6$) at the start of HPN therapy. Eight cases occurred in males and 8 in females. Ten (62.5%) cases occurred in patients with stage 4 disease. Fourteen (87.5%) cases received chemotherapy during HPN while only 3 (18.8%) received radiotherapy. In 15 out of 16 cases of CRBSI, the VAD was removed because of infection. Similarly, in 15 out of 16 cases, patients were hospitalized because of infection. The case in whom the VAD was not removed was not the one who was not hospitalized. With respect to microbiology, CRBSIs were caused by *Staphylococcus epidermidis* (6 cases), candida (3 cases), Coagulase-negative Staphylococci (3 cases), Methicillin-resistant *Staphylococcus aureus* (1 case), *Klebsiella pneumoniae* (1 case), *Escherichia coli* (1 case) and Enterococcus faecium (1 case).

Factors associated with CRBSI

Table 5 displays the results of univariate Poisson regression analyses evaluating the factors associated with CRBSI. No variables were found to be statistically significantly associated with CRBSI incidence. Type of VAD had no effect on the incidence of CRBSI. Severely malnourished patients and those with metastatic disease had almost twice the risk of CRBSI compared to well-nourished and non-metastatic patients respectively; however the results did not attain statistical significance. Similarly, serum albumin <3.5 g/dl was associated with almost thrice the risk of CRBSI compared to serum albumin > = 3.5 g/dl, however, the finding was not statistically significant. No multivariate Poisson regression analyses were conducted.

Table 5 Univariate Poisson Regression Analysis of the Factors Associated with CRBSI; $N = 408$

Variables	Univariate model IRR (95% CI)
Type of VAD	
Port (reference)	
PICC	1.3 (0.36–4.7)
TCC	1.9 (0.14–27.2)
Gender	
Female (reference)	
Male	1.1 (0.33–3.9)
SGA at HPN Start	
Well-nourished (reference)	
Moderately malnourished	0.94 (0.22–4.1)
Severely malnourished	2.3 (0.53–10.1)
ECOG performance status	
0–2 (reference)	
3–5	1.04 (0.25–4.3)
Stage at diagnosis	
Non-metastatic (reference)	
Metastatic	2.0 (0.59–6.7)
Age at HPN Start (years)	0.99 (0.93–1.1)
BMI at HPN Start (kg/m^2)	1.005 (0.9–1.1)
Albumin at HPN start (g/dl)	
> =3.5 g/dl (reference)	
< 3.5 g/dl	2.7 (0.47–15.5)

BMI body mass index, *CI* confidence interval, *CRBSI* catheter-related bloodstream infection, *ECOG* Eastern Cooperative Oncology Group, *g/dl* grams per deciliter, *HPN* home parenteral nutrition, *IRR* incidence rate ratio, *kg/m^2* kilograms per meter squared, *PICC* peripherally inserted central catheter, *SGA* Subjective Global Assessment, *TCC* tunneled central catheter, *VAD* venous access device

Discussion

Little US comparative data exists on the incidence of CRBSIs in HPN patients with a cancer diagnosis who are actively undergoing oncologic treatments. In this study, we evaluated the incidence of CRBSI and the factors associated with it in cancer patients undergoing HPN at a tertiary care cancer center in the US.

We found an overall CRBSI incidence of 0.54 per 1000 HPN days following a standardized catheter care protocol. Several studies have evaluated the incidence of CRBSI in cancer patients receiving HPN. A prospective study by Cotogni et al. evaluated 269 PICCs in 250 cancer patients for a total of 55,293 catheter days, and found a CRBSI rate of 0.05 per 1000 catheter days. Seventy-one percent patients received chemotherapy during the study period [18]. Another prospective study by the same research group, found a CRBSI rate of 0.35 per 1000 catheter days and 0.60 per 1000 HPN days [23]. Other studies have reported CRBSI rates ranging from 0.41 to 1.7 per 1000 catheter days [21, 22, 24, 25, 30]. We did not find any significant difference in the incidence of CRBSI across the three types of VAD, though it is to be noted that of a total of 408 VADs in this study, only 11 (2.7%) were TCCs. This finding could also possibly suggest that the incidence of CRBSI in patients receiving HPN might not be a function of the type of VAD, but rather the catheter care protocols used in these patients. Clearly, this finding needs to be investigated further in future studies.

The majority of previous studies were conducted in Europe with one originating in Japan and none in the US. Only two studies, both by Cotogni et al. [18, 23], were conducted exclusively in cancer patients, while all other studies used a heterogeneous patient population with cancer patients being a subset of the entire study sample. Combining patients with different disease types can lead to erroneous conclusions regarding the incidence rate of CRBSI in a specific population of interest. Our study is different from the above studies in 2 important ways. Our study is the first observational study based out of the US using a large sample of cancer patients. We focused exclusively on cancer patients, 73% of whom were undergoing active oncologic treatments. This patient population is at a high-risk of experiencing CRBSI and has not been adequately investigated in the literature. Having said that, our study is very comparable to that by Cotogni et al. [23] in terms of the patient population investigated and the overall incidence rate of CRBSI reported (0.54 per 1000 HPN days in our study versus 0.60 per 1000 HPN days in the Cotogni study).

Unfortunately, HPN in the US is provided by multiple companies with variable level of expertise and experience. While ASPEN has come up with HPN guidelines, they are not mandated by any private or government insurance agencies. Once the insurer has approved HPN, any provider can deliver the services. This explains why there is a lack of good US-based studies reporting the incidence of CRBSI in HPN patients.

We also evaluated several factors for their association with the incidence of CRBSI. The factors investigated were type of VAD, age, gender, SGA, ECOG performance status, stage at diagnosis, BMI and serum albumin. Upon univariate analysis, no factors were found to be statistically significantly associated with the incidence of CRBSI.

Several risk factors for CRBSI have been reported in the literature. These factors either relate to the patient (type of underlying disease), or the type of VAD (catheter caliber, number of lumens), or the PN therapy (number of HPN days per week), or education (good training given to the patient and caregiver) or follow-up (involvement of a home care nurse) [17]. However, no studies in the literature have investigated the association between baseline nutritional parameters and the risk of CRBSI. Serum albumin is a commonly used parameter to assess nutritional status in cancer and has been described as an independent prognosticator of survival in lung, pancreatic, gastric, colorectal, and breast cancers [31]. In the hospital setting, higher levels of serum albumin have also been found to be correlated with lower in-hospital mortality, lower length of stay (LOS), higher quality of life, and lower rates of nosocomial infection [32, 33]. Although our study did not find a statistically significant association between serum albumin and the incidence of CRBSI, future studies should attempt to further explore this finding using larger sample sizes.

CRBSI is one of the most frequently occurring, extremely costly to treat and potentially life-threatening complications associated with the use of VADs. The risk of CRBSI is even higher in oncology patients who are actively receiving oncologic therapies due to their immunocompromised status. As a result, developing strategies that would prevent or minimize the incidence of CRBSIs has been a continual challenge for healthcare providers. Working in collaboration with a home infusion company that can help implement standardized catheter care protocol can potentially reduce the CRBSI incidence in such patients. These data can serve as a benchmark for potential use by other hospitals in preventing CRBSIs in these patients.

There are some limitations of this study which require careful acknowledgment. This was a retrospective observational study using data not primarily collected for research purposes. As a result, we did not have data available on all potential confounding variables (such as patient and caregiver training, involvement of a home care nurse, assessment of adherence to the catheter care protocol, patient educational status, patient smoking status, steroid use during treatment, liver function tests, and white blood cell counts) that could have impacted the incidence rate of CRBSI. Moreover, all VADs in our study were not specifically placed for the purpose of HPN. In some patients, VADs were initially placed for the purpose of delivering chemotherapy. However, we did not have data on the duration (or number of days) of VAD which can also potentially affect the occurrence of CRBSI. Our study population consisted of heterogeneous non-hospitalized patients with solid tumors from a single institution. As a result, the findings might not be generalizable to all cancer patients, especially those with hematological malignancies and those receiving HPN in a hospital setting. Finally, the humanistic and economic aspects related to the use of VADs were not investigated.

There are some strengths and unique features of our study. By using a consecutive case series of all eligible patients seen at our institution during a fixed time period, we minimized the possibility of selection bias in our study. Most of our patients were receiving active anticancer treatments while undergoing HPN. All VADs were inserted using the same evidence-based protocol and all patients received the same standardized catheter care protocol at home. Our study had a long follow-up period and no patients were lost to follow-up. To the best of our knowledge, this is the first and the largest US-based study reporting the incidence of and factors associated with CRBSI in a consecutive case series of non-hospitalized cancer patients undergoing HPN.

Conclusions

We found a low incidence rate of CRBSI following a standardized catheter maintenance protocol in a high-risk oncology population undergoing HPN.

Abbreviations

BMI: Body mass index; CI: Confidence interval; CRBSI: Catheter-related bloodstream infection; ECOG: Eastern Cooperative Oncology Group; g/dl: grams per deciliter; HPN: Home parenteral nutrition; IDSA: Infectious Diseases Society of America; IRB: Institutional Review Board; IRR: Incidence rate ratio; kg/m^2: kilograms per meter squared; PICC: Peripherally inserted central catheter; SD: Standard deviation; SGA: Subjective Global Assessment; TCC: Tunneled central catheter; VAD: Venous access device

Acknowledgements

The authors thank Diane Ottersen, chief of Cancer Registry, for providing us with reliable and updated demographic data. The authors also thank Melinda Parker and Melissa Leone from CORAM home infusion company for their assistance with the development and implementation of standardized catheter care protocols.

Funding

This study was funded by Cancer Treatment Centers of America®.

Authors' contributions

PGV participated in concept, design, data interpretation, writing and general oversight of the study. NV, BP and PE participated in data collection, data interpretation and writing. DG participated in data analysis, data interpretation and writing. All authors read and approved the final manuscript.

Competing interests

The authors declare that they have no competing interests.

Consent for publication

Not applicable.

References

1. Hoffer EK, Borsa J, Santulli P, Bloch R, Fontaine AB. Prospective randomized comparison of valved versus nonvalved peripherally inserted central vein catheters. AJR Am J Roentgenol. 1999;173:1393–8.
2. Shapiro CL. Central venous access catheters. Surg Oncol Clin N Am. 1995;4:443–51.
3. Broviac JW, Cole JJ, Scribner BH. A silicone rubber atrial catheter for prolonged parenteral alimentation. Surg Gynecol Obstet. 1973;136:602–6.
4. Hickman RO, Buckner CD, Clift RA, Sanders JE, Stewart P, Thomas ED. A modified right atrial catheter for access to the venous system in marrow transplant recipients. Surg Gynecol Obstet. 1979;148:871–5.
5. Bessoud B, de Baere T, Kuoch V, Desruennes E, Cosset MF, Lassau N, et al. Experience at a single institution with endovascular treatment of mechanical complications caused by implanted central venous access devices in pediatric and adult patients. AJR Am J Roentgenol. 2003;180:527–32.
6. Rauthe G, Altmann C. Complications in connection with venous port systems: prevention and therapy. Eur J Surg Oncol. 1998;24:192–9.
7. Eastridge BJ, Lefor AT. Complications of indwelling venous access devices in cancer patients. J Clin Oncol. 1995;13:233–8.
8. Moureau N, Poole S, Murdock MA, Gray SM, Semba CP. Central venous catheters in home infusion care: outcomes analysis in 50,470 patients. J Vasc Interv Radiol. 2002;13:1009–16.
9. Grannan KJ, Taylor PH. Early and late complications of totally implantable venous access devices. J Surg Oncol. 1990;44:52–4.
10. Hartkamp A, van Boxtel AJ, Zonnenberg BA, Witteveen PO. Totally implantable venous access devices: evaluation of complications and a prospective comparative study of two different port systems. Neth J Med. 2000;57:215–23.
11. Abdullah BJ, Mohammad N, Sangkar JV, Abd Aziz YF, Gan GG, Goh KY, et al. Incidence of upper limb venous thrombosis associated with peripherally inserted central catheters (PICC). Br J Radiol. 2005;78:596–600.
12. Anderson AJ, Krasnow SH, Boyer MW, Cutler DJ, Jones BD, Citron ML, et al. Thrombosis: the major Hickman catheter complication in patients with solid tumor. Chest. 1989;95:71–5.
13. Bern MM, Lokich JJ, Wallach SR, Bothe A Jr, Benotti PN, Arkin CF, et al. Very low doses of warfarin can prevent thrombosis in central venous catheters. A randomized prospective trial. Ann Intern Med. 1990;112:423–8.
14. Lokich JJ, Becker B. Subclavian vein thrombosis in patients treated with infusion chemotherapy for advanced malignancy. Cancer. 1983;52:1586–9.
15. Lam AW, Chen YM, Yang KY, Tsai CM, Perng RP. Disconnection of a venous Port-A-Cath followed by embolization after saline flush: rare case report. Jpn J Clin Oncol. 1999;29:643–5.
16. Hanna HA, Raad II, Hackett B, Wallace SK, Price KJ, Coyle DE, et al. Antibiotic-impregnated catheters associated with significant decrease in nosocomial and multidrug-resistant bacteremias in critically ill patients. Chest. 2003;124:1030–8.
17. Dreesen M, Foulon V, Spriet I, Goossens GA, Hiele M, De PL, et al. Epidemiology of catheter-related infections in adult patients receiving home parenteral nutrition: a systematic review. Clin Nutr. 2013;32:16–26.
18. Cotogni P, Barbero C, Garrino C, Degiorgis C, Mussa B, De FA, et al. Peripherally inserted central catheters in non-hospitalized cancer patients: 5-year results of a prospective study. Support Care Cancer. 2015;23:403–9.
19. Bagnall-Reeb H. Evidence for the use of the antibiotic lock technique. J Infus Nurs. 2004;27:118–22.
20. O'Grady NP, Alexander M, Dellinger EP, Gerberding JL, Heard SO, Maki DG, et al. Guidelines for the prevention of intravascular catheter-related infections. The Hospital Infection Control Practices Advisory Committee, Center for Disease Control and Prevention, U.S. Pediatrics. 2002;110:e51.
21. Christensen LD, Rasmussen HH, Vinter-Jensen L. Peripherally inserted central catheter for use in home parenteral nutrition: a 4-year follow-up study. JPEN J Parenter Enteral Nutr. 2014;38:1003–6.
22. Botella-Carretero JI, Carrero C, Guerra E, Valbuena B, Arrieta F, Calanas A, et al. Role of peripherally inserted central catheters in home parenteral nutrition: a 5-year prospective study. JPEN J Parenter Enteral Nutr. 2013;37:544–9.
23. Cotogni P, Pittiruti M, Barbero C, Monge T, Palmo A, Boggio BD. Catheter-related complications in cancer patients on home parenteral nutrition: a prospective study of over 51,000 catheter days. JPEN J Parenter Enteral Nutr. 2013;37:375–83.
24. Crispin A, Thul P, Arnold D, Schild S, Weimann A. Central venous catheter complications during home parenteral nutrition: a prospective pilot study of 481 patients with more than 30,000 catheter days. Onkologie. 2008;31:605–9.
25. Bozzetti F, Mariani L, Bertinet DB, Chiavenna G, Crose N, De Cicco M, et al. Central venous catheter complications in 447 patients on home parenteral nutrition: an analysis of over 100.000 catheter days. Clin Nutr. 2002;21:475–85.
26. August DA, Huhmann MB. A.S.P.E.N. clinical guidelines: nutrition support therapy during adult anticancer treatment and in hematopoietic cell transplantation. JPEN J Parenter Enteral Nutr. 2009;33:472–500.

27. Mermel LA, Allon M, Bouza E, Craven DE, Flynn P, O'Grady NP, et al. Clinical practice guidelines for the diagnosis and management of intravascular catheter-related infection: 2009 update by the Infectious Diseases Society of America. Clin Infect Dis. 2009;49:1–45.
28. Detsky AS, McLaughlin JR, Baker JP, Johnston N, Whittaker S, Mendelson RA, et al. What is subjective global assessment of nutritional status? JPEN J Parenter Enteral Nutr. 1987;11:8–13.
29. Austin PC. An introduction to propensity score methods for reducing the effects of confounding in observational studies. Multivariate Behav Res. 2011;46:399–424.
30. Shirotani N, Iino T, Numata K, Kameoka S. Complications of central venous catheters in patients on home parenteral nutrition: an analysis of 68 patients over 16 years. Surg Today. 2006;36:420–4.
31. Gupta D, Lis CG. Pretreatment serum albumin as a predictor of cancer survival: a systematic review of the epidemiological literature. Nutr J. 2010;9:69. doi:10.1186/1475-2891-9-69.
32. Gupta D, Vashi PG, Lammersfeld CA, Braun DP. Role of nutritional status in predicting the length of stay in cancer: a systematic review of the epidemiological literature. Ann Nutr Metab. 2011;59:96–106.
33. Lis CG, Gupta D, Lammersfeld CA, Markman M, Vashi PG. Role of nutritional status in predicting quality of life outcomes in cancer–a systematic review of the epidemiological literature. Nutr J. 2012;11:27. doi:10.1186/1475-2891-11-27.

13

Factors related to outcome of bloodstream infections due to *Candida parapsilosis* complex

Francesco Barchiesi[1*], Elena Orsetti[1], Patrizia Osimani[3], Carlo Catassi[2], Fabio Santelli[4] and Esther Manso[5]

Abstract

Background: Although *Candida albicans* is the most common cause of fungal blood stream infections (BSIs), infections due to *Candida* species other than *C. albicans* are rising. *Candida parapsilosis* complex has emerged as an important fungal pathogen and became one of the main causes of fungemia in specific geographical areas. We analyzed the factors related to outcome of candidemia due to *C. parapsilosis* in a single tertiary referral hospital over a five-year period.

Methods: A retrospective observational study of all cases of candidemia was carried out at a 980-bedded University Hospital in Italy. Data regarding demographic characteristics and clinical risk factors were collected from the patient's medical records. Antifungal susceptibility testing was performed and MIC results were interpreted according to CLSI species-specific clinical breakpoints.

Results: Of 270 patients diagnosed with *Candida* BSIs during the study period, 63 (23 %) were infected with isolates of *C. parapsilosis* complex which represented the second most frequently isolated yeast after *C. albicans*. The overall incidence rate was 0.4 episodes/1000 hospital admissions. All the strains were in vitro susceptible to all antifungal agents. The overall crude mortality at 30 days was 27 % (17/63), which was significantly lower than that reported for *C. albicans* BSIs (42 % [61/146], $p = 0.042$). Being hospitalized in ICU resulted independently associated with a significant higher risk of mortality (HR 4.625 [CI95% 1.015–21.080], $p = 0.048$). Conversely, early CVC removal was confirmed to be significantly associated with a lower risk of mortality (HR 0.299 [CI95% 0.102–0.874], $p = 0.027$). Finally, the type of primary antifungal therapy did not influence the outcome of infection.

Conclusions: Candidemia due to *C. parapsilosis* complex, the second most commonly causative agent of yeast BSIs in our center, is characterized by a non-negligible mortality at 30 days. An early CVC removal is associated with a significant reduced mortality.

Keywords: *Candida paraspilosis* complex, Candidemia, Risk factors, Mortality, Antifungal agents

Background

Candida is an important cause of bloodstream infections (BSIs) and it is the main agent of invasive fungal infection in hospitalized patients [1, 2]. Although *Candida albicans* is the most common cause of invasive candidiasis, infections due to *Candida* species other than *C. albicans* are rising [3, 4]. In particular, *Candida parapsilosis* complex, which includes *C. parapsilosis* sensu strictu (the most frequent), *Candida orthopsilosis* and *Candida metapsilosis*, has emerged as an important fungal pathogen and became one of the main causes of fungemia in tertiary-care hospitals [5–9]. Although the mortality rate due to this species is generally lower than that reported for other *Candida* species, *C. parapsilosis* complex possesses several distinct features, such as its ability to develop biofilms on intravascular devices, high affinity for parenteral nutrition, and an intrinsic low susceptibility to echinocandins [10–12].

* Correspondence: f.barchiesi@univpm.it
[1]Clinica Malattie Infettive; Università Politecnica delle Marche, Azienda Ospedaliero-Universitaria, Ospedali Riuniti Umberto I°- G.M. Lancisi – G. Salesi, Ancona, Italy

Table 1 Comparison of epidemiological, clinical characteristics and outcome of patients with BSIs due to *Candida parapsilosis* and *Candida albicans*

Variables	Patients with BSIs due to:		
	C. parapsilosis ($n = 63$)	*C. albicans* ($n = 146$)	*P* value[a]
Age (years), median (IQR)[b]	67 (43–76)	51 (66–77)	0.133
Neonates (<3 months)	1 (2)	5 (3)	0.465
Elderly (>65 years)	32 (51)	72 (49)	0.844
Male sex, *n (%)*	35 (56)	91 (63)	0.358
Ward			
Internal Medicine, *n (%)*	25 (40)	52 (36)	0.448
Surgery, *n (%)*	17 (27)	32 (22)	
Intensive Care Unit, *n (%)*	21 (33)	62 (43)	
Comorbidities, *n (%)*	57 (90)	137 (94)	0.387
Chronic pulmonary diseases, *n (%)*[c]	9 (14)	11 (8)	0.127
Haematological malignancy, *n (%)*	1 (2)	8 (5)	0.203
Cardiovascular diseases, *n (%)*[d]	27 (43)	67 (46)	0.685
Neurological diseases, *n (%)*[e]	10 (16)	24 (16)	0.919
Gastrointestinal diseases, *n (%)*[f]	21 (33)	43 (29)	0.576
Diabetes mellitus, *n (%)*	8 (13)	28 (19)	0.254
Solid tumors, *n (%)*	15 (24)	43 (30)	0.403
Chronic renal failure, n (%)	7 (11)	12 (8)	0.504
Previous surgery (<30 days), *n (%)*	32 (51)	67 (46)	0.514
Gastrointestinal surgery, *n (%)*	8 (13)	19 (13)	0.950
Cardiovascular surgery, *n (%)*	13 (21)	28 (19)	0.807
Other surgery, *n (%)* [g]	12 (19)	24 (16)	0.646
Central venous catheter, *n (%)*	56 (89)	127 (87)	0.702
BSI CVC-related, *n (%)*	36 (64)	57 (45)	0.015
Other devices, *n (%)*[h]	57 (90)	129 (88)	0.653
Previous invasive procedures (<72 h), *n (%)*[i]	16 (25)	44 (30)	0.486
Parenteral nutrition, *n (%)*	43 (68)	105 (72)	0.592
Immunosuppressive therapy, *n (%)*[j]	18 (29)	56 (34)	0.174
Neutropenia, *n (%)*	4 (6)	7 (5)	0.644
Septic shock, *n (%)*	2 (3)	12 (8)	0.180
Prior antibiotic therapy, *n (%)*	58 (92)	139 (95)	0.370
Previous antifungal therapy (<30 days), *n (%)*	5 (8)	21 (14)	0.195
Concomitant bacteriemia, *n (%)*	15 (24)	40 (27)	0.588
Other coinfections, *n (%)*[k]	39 (62)	89 (61)	0.897
Appropriate antifungal therapy, *n (%)*[l]	38 (60)	92 (63)	0.712
Primary azole therapy	41 (65)	77 (53)	0.098
Primary echinocandin therapy	7 (11)	34 (23)	0.041
Primary polyene therapy	1 (2)	3 (2)	0.820
None	14 (22)	32 (22)	0.961

Table 1 Comparison of epidemiological, clinical characteristics and outcome of patients with BSIs due to *Candida parapsilosis* and *Candida albicans (Continued)*

Overall mortality, *n (%)*	17 (27)	61 (42)	0.042
Early mortality (days 1–7), *n (%)*	4 (6)	24 (17)	0.049
Late mortality (days 8–30), *n (%)*	13 (21)	37 (25)	0.464

[a]Comparisons between groups were performed using Wilcoxon rank sum test for quantitative variables and Chi-Square test (or Fisher Exact Test when expected frequencies were less than five) for qualitative variables
[b]IQR, Interquartile range
[c]Chronic pulmonary diseases include asthma, chronic bronchitis, emphysema and lung fibrosis
[d]Cardiovascular diseases include heart failure, ischemic heart disease, endocarditis and arrhythmia
[e]Neurological diseases include Parkinson's disease, Alzheimer's disease and paralysis
[f]Gastrointestinal diseases include Crohn's disease, ulcerative colitis, chronic pancreatitis and gallbladder stones
[g] Other surgery includes plastic surgery, thoracic surgery, orthopaedic surgery, urological surgery and neurosurgery
[h] Other devices include urinary catheter, surgical drainage, cutaneous gastrostomy and tracheostomy tube
[i]Previous invasive procedures include endoscopy and positioning of any device
[j]Immunosuppressive therapy include corticosteroids, calcineurin inhibitors and monoclonal antibodies
[k]Other coinfections include bacterial and/or fungal infections in sites other than blood
[l]Appropriate antifungal therapy was considered when the appropriate drug with adequate dosage was started ≤ 72 h from the first blood culture performed

The aim of this study was to analyze the factors related to outcome of candidemia due to *C. parapsilsosis* complex in a single institution over a five-year period.

Methods

Study population and data collection

A retrospective observational study of all cases of candidemia was carried out from January 1, 2010 to December 31, 2014 (5-year period) in a single 980-bedded referral University Hospital in Ancona, Italy. A case of *Candida* BSI was defined as a peripheral isolation of *Candida* species from blood culture in a patient with temporally related clinical signs and symptoms of infection. All *Candida* BSIs were identified through the microbiological laboratory database. Data regarding demographic characteristics and clinical risk factors were collected from the patient's medical records. Appropriate antifungal therapy was considered when an appropriate drug (based on subsequent in vitro susceptibility testing results) with adequate dosage was started within 72 h from the first blood culture performed. Adequate dosage of an antifungal agent was defined according to IDSA 2009 guidelines [13]. Early central venous catheter (CVC) removal was defined a removal of the line within 48 h from drawing blood culture. Mortality was calculated after 7 and 30 days from the occurrence of the episode of *Candida* BSI.

Candida species were isolated from blood samples using BacT/ALERT (bioMérieux) and identified with standard techniques. Each of the three species of *C. parapsilosis* sensu lato was identified using the MALDI-TOF Biotyper™ [14]. Antifungal susceptibility testing was performed using the SensitreYeastOne colorimetric plate (SYO) (Trek Diagnostic System) and MIC results were interpreted according to latest species-specific CBPs as established by the CLSI [15].

The present research has been performed in accordance with the ethical standards of the 1964 Declaration of Helsinki and its later amendements. The Institutional Review Board of the Azienda Ospedaliero-Universitaria Ospeadali Riuniti Umberto I°-Lancisi-Salesi granted retrospective access to the data without need for individual informed consent.

Statistical analysis

Quantitative data were shown as the median with interquartile ranges (Q1–Q3). Qualitative variables were expressed as absolute and relative frequencies. Categorical variables were compared using the $\chi 2$ test, whereas Mann–Whitney U test or Fisher exact test were applied for continuous variables. Variables with a $p \leq 0.05$ at the descriptive analysis were analyzed by Cox regression. All statistical analyses were performed using the statistical package SPSS for Windows v. 20 (SPSS Inc., Chicago, IL, USA). A P value of ≤0.05 was considered to represent statistical significance and all statistical tests were two-tailed.

Results

Of 270 patients diagnosed with *Candida* BSIs during the study period, 63 (23 %) were infected with isolates of *C. parapsilosis* complex (95 *C. parapsilosis* sensu lato, 3 *C. orthopsilsosis* and 2 % *C. metapsilosis*). This species represented the second most frequently isolated yeast after *C. albicans* (146 [54 %]). The remaining infections were due to *C. tropicalis* (23 [9]), *C. glabrata* (10 [4]) and other *Candida species* (10 [4 %]). Although C. *albicans* represented the most commonly isolated species, its percentage significantly decreased from 68 % to 48 % in the time period considered ($p = 0.040$). On the opposite, there was a significant increase of the percentage of *C. parapsilosis* isolation from 8 % (2010) to 30 % (2014) ($p = 0.036$). The overall incidence rate of BSIs due to *C. parapsilosis* was 0.4 episodes/1000 hospital admissions.

Demographics and clinical characteristics of 63 patients infected with isolates of *C. parapsilosis* complex were compared with those of 146 patients infected with

Table 2 Outcome of 63 patients with BSIs due to *Candida parapsilosis* complex considered in this study

Characteristics	30-day outcome		
	Survival ($n = 46$)	Death ($n = 17$)	*P* value[a]
Age (years), median (IQR)[b]	62 (31–75)	76 (63–78)	0.046
Male sex, *n (%)*	24 (52)	11 (65)	0.374
Ward			
Internal Medicine, *n (%)*	21 (46)	4 (24)	0.033
Surgery, *n (%)*	14 (30)	3 (18)	
Intensive Care Unit, *n (%)*	11 (24)	10 (59)	
Comorbidities, *n (%)*	40(87)	17(100)	0.117
Chronic pulmonary diseases, *n (%)*[c]	5(11)	4 (24)	0.235
Haematological malignancy, *n (%)*	1 (2)	0 (0)	0.540
Cardiovascular diseases, *n (%)*[d]	15 (33)	12(71)	0.006
Neurological diseases, *n (%)*[e]	9 (20)	1(6)	0.263
Gastrointestinal diseases, *n (%)*[f]	16 (35)	5 (29)	0.688
Diabetes mellitus, *n (%)*	4 (9)	4 (24)	0.195
Solid tumors, *n (%)*	9 (20)	6 (35)	0.193
Chronic renal failure, *n (%)*	5 (11)	2 (12)	1.000
Previous surgery (<30 days), *n (%)*	23(50)	9(53)	0.835
Gastrointestinal surgery, *n (%)*	5(11)	3(18)	0.671
Cardiovascular surgery, *n (%)*	7(15)	6(35)	0.080
Other surgery, *n (%)*[g]	11(24)	1 (6)	0.154
Central venous catheter, *n (%)*	41(89)	15 (88)	0.920
BSI CVC-related, *n (%)*	25 (61)	11 (73)	0.460
Early central venous catheter removal, *n (%)*[h]	41 (100)	11 (73)	<0.0001
Other devices, *n (%)*[i]	40 (87)	17(100)	0.178
Previous invasive procedures (<72 h), *n (%)*[j]	9 (20)	7 (41)	0.080
Parenteral nutrition, *n (%)*	29 (63)	14 (82)	0.143
Immunosuppressive therapy, *n (%)*[k]	13(28)	5(29)	0.920
Neutropenia, *n (%)*	3 (7)	1 (6)	1.000
Septic shock, *n (%)*	1(2)	1(6)	0.470
Prior antibiotic therapy, *n (%)*	42 (91)	16 (94)	0.713
Previous antifungal therapy, *n (%)*	4 (9)	1 (6)	0.713
Concomitant bacteriemia, *n (%)*	12(26)	3(18)	0.487
Other coinfections, *n (%)*[l]	28 (61)	11(65)	0.780

Table 2 Outcome of 63 patients with BSIs due to *Candida parapsilosis* complex considered in this study *(Continued)*

Appropriate antifungal therapy[m]	30 (65)	8 (47)	0.190
Primary azole therapy	32 (70)	9 (53)	0.219
Primary echinocandin therapy	5 (11)	2 (12)	1.000
Primary polyene therapy	1 (2)	0 (0)	1.000
None	8 (17)	6 (35)	0.129

[a]Comparisons between groups were performed using Wilcoxon rank sum test for quantitative variables and Chi-Square test (or Fisher Exact Test when expected frequencies were less than five) for qualitative variables
[b] IQR, Interquartile range
[c]Chronic pulmonary diseases include asthma, chronic bronchitis, emphysema and lung fibrosis
[d]Cardiovascular diseases include heart failure, ischemic heart disease, endocarditis and arrhythmia
[e]Neurological diseases include Parkinson's disease, Alzheimer's disease and paralysis
[f]Gastrointestinal diseases include Crohn's disease, ulcerative colitis, chronic pancreatitis and gallbladder stones
[g]Other surgery includes plastic surgery, thoracic surgery, orthopaedic surgery, urological surgery and neurosurgery
[h] Early CVC removal was considered occurring within 48 h from blood cultures drawing
[i] Other devices include urinary catheter, surgical drainage, cutaneous gastrostomy and tracheostomy tube
[j] Previous invasive procedures include endoscopy and positioning of any device
[k]Immunosuppressive therapy include corticosteroids, calcineurin inhibitors and monoclonal antibodies
[l] Other coinfections include bacterial and/or fungal infections in sites other than blood
[m]Appropriate antifungal therapy was considered when the appropriate drug with adequate dosage was started within 72 h the first blood culture performed

isolates of *C. albicans* and the results are shown in Table 1. Median patients age was 67 years. Male accounted for 56 % of the population. Twenty-five isolates were recovered from patients hospitalized in medical wards, 21 from patients hospitalized in ICUs and 17 from patients hospitalized in surgical wards. The majority of patients (90 %) suffered from multiple comorbidities (range 2 to 4) being the most common cardiovascular (43) and gastrointestinal (33 %) diseases. A total of 51 % of patients underwent a surgical intervention within 30 days from the onset of candidemia. In comparison with *C. albicans*, BSIs due to *C. parapsilosis* were significantly more often associated with the use of CVC ($p = 0.015$). The overall crude mortality at 30 days was higher in patients infected with *C. albicans* than *C. parapsilosis* (42 % *vs* 27 %, respectively, $p = 0.042$).

Factors related to outcome of 63 patients with BSIs due to *C. parapsilosis* are reported in Table 2. Older age ($p = 0.046$), being hospitalized in ICU or in medical wards rather than in surgical wards ($p = 0.033$), being recently diagnosed with a cardiovascular disease ($p = 0.006$), and the lack of an early CVC removal ($p = 0.003$) were all factors associated with a significant higher probability of death at the descriptive analysis. On multivariate analysis, being hospitalized in ICU resulted independently associated with a significant higher risk of mortality (HR 4.625 [CI95% 1.015–21.080], $p = 0.048$). Conversely, early CVC removal was confirmed to be significantly associated with a lower risk of mortality (HR 0.299 [CI95% 0.102–0.874], $p = 0.027$).

Table 3 shows the results of antifungal susceptibility testing to nine antifungal agents as routinely performed by the SYO method which was developed to provide an easy alternative to the CLSI procedure. With the exception of one isolate that showed to be susceptible dose dependent to fluconazole (MIC 4 μg/ml) and two isolates which were found to have non-wild type phenotype for flucytosine (MIC 1 μg/ml), all isolates showed to be fully susceptible to all antifungals according to the CLSI interpretation [15].

Table 3 In vitro susceptibilities of *Candida parapsilosis* complex isolates considered in this study

Antifungal agents	MIC range (μg/ml)	MIC_{50} (μg/ml)	MIC_{90} (μg/ml)	% of isolates in the indicated category according to CLSI[a]					
				S	SDD	I	R	WT	Non-WT
Amphotericin B	≤0.12–1	0.5	0.5	-	-	-	-	100	0
Flucytosine	≤0.06–1	≤0.06	0.25	-	-	-	-	97	3
Fluconazole	≤0.12–4	0.25	1	98.4	1.6	-	0	-	-
Itraconazole	≤0.015–0.25	0.06	0.12	-	-	-	-	100	0
Voriconazole	≤0.008–0.06	≤0.008	0.015	100	0	-	0	-	-
Posaconazole	≤0.008–0.12	0.03	0.06	-	-	-	-	100	-
Caspofungin	0.06–1	0.25	0.5	100	-	0	0	-	-
Anidulafungin	0.12–2	0.5	2	100	-	0	0	-	-
Micafungin	0.12–2	1	2	100	-	0	0	-	-

[a]Category was interpreted according to CLSI breakpoints as reported in ref. 15. S, susceptible; *SDD* susceptible dose dependent, *I* intermediate, *R* resistant, *WT* wild type

Discussion and conclusions

Although *C. albicans* remains the most common fungal isolate from blood, longitudinal studies showed a trend toward an increased prevalence of other *Candida* spp. with a larger proportion of *C. glabrata* in the United States and *C. parapsilosis* in some European (i.e.: Italy or Spain) and Latin American countries [3–9]. As far, few studies focused on the specific predictors influencing the outcome of BSIs due to *C. parapsilosis* [16–18].

First, we confirmed that the mortality due to this species is somewhat lower than that reported for *C. albicans*, having found a rate of 27 % at 30 days. This figure is consistent with literature data in which the 30-day mortality due to this species ranges from 23 % to 30 % [14, 19–21].

Second, hospitalization in ICU showed to be independently associated with higher risk of mortality. Our data are in agreement with a large study showing a mortality rate increasing from 29 % to 47 % in patients with BSIs due to *Candida* spp. hospitalized, respectively, in non-ICU and ICU wards [22]. ICU stay would represent a surrogate marker of illness severity thereby facilitating the poor outcome of this population group.

Third, we showed that early CVC removal is protective in BSIs due to *C. parapsilosis.* Although the impact of CVC management has been extensively investigated on the outcome of patients with candidemia, few studies have examined this issue across individual *Candida* species. Two recent studies showed that CVC removal exerted a protective effect on the outcome of candidemia due to *C. parapsilosis* [14, 20]. Since this species is characterized by a high propensity to develop biofilms on intravascular devices, their early removal play a fundamental role in determining the outcome of infection.

Fourth, we found that the outcome was not influenced by an appropriate antifungal therapy. Despite this finding is somewhat divergent from that reported by the current literature [23–25], there is a paucity of data considering the infection outcome of individual *Candida* species. In this regard, there are two important factors to consider. First, being *C. parapsilosis* less pathogenic than other *Candida* species (i.e.: *C. albicans* and *C. tropicalis*) [17], BSIs due to this entity could be more deeply affected by a correct general management (i.e.: prompt removal of any central line) rather than an early therapeutic intervention. Second, we defined appropriate antifungal therapy as the appropriate drug with adequate dosage started within 72 h from the first blood culture performed. Since *C. parapsilosis* has a time to positivity of blood cultures longer than those reported for *C. albicans* and *C. tropicalis* [26], preliminary blood culture showing the growth of yeast-like fungal pathogen could be delayed thereby determining an initial, although adequate, antifungal treatment after this time interval.

Interestingly, we found that primary antifungal treatment (i.e.: triazoles or echinocandins) did not influence the outcome of *C. parapsilosis* BSIs. Although, this *Candida* species possesses a natural low susceptibility profile to echinocandins [12] and there is still a debate on the use of these molecules in infections caused by this species, either randomized or not-randomized clinical trials have shown not significant differences in the success rates between arms [27–30]. Our data, although with a limited number of patients, corroborated these findings.

The present study have some limitations. First, being a single-center study, the number of patients considered is low. This feature has certainly weakened the statistical power of the study. Nevertheless, we have made all attempts to collect and analyze as many as clinical data as possible to reveal useful information for the management of patients infected with this *Candida* species. Second, being a retrospective study encompassing several departments and medical disciplines over a five years period, there was not a univocal management of each individual case. In this respect, serial follow-up blood cultures were not systematically performed and we were unable to include important parameters, other then 30-day mortality, such as the persistence of positive blood cultures after the initiation of antifungal therapy.

In conclusion, our study shows that candidemia due to *C. parapsilosis* complex, the second most commonly causative agent of yeast BSIs in our center, is characterized by a non-negligible mortality at 30 days. While an early CVC removal is associated with significant reduced mortality, the type of primary antifungal therapy does not influence the outcome. Further prospective studies including higher number of patients are needed to corroborate these findings.

Abbreviations

BSIs, bloodstream infections; CBP, clinical breakpoints; CLSI, Clinical and Laboratory Standards Institute; CVC, central venous catheter; HR, hazard ratio; ICUs, Intensive Care Units; IDSA, Infectious Disease Society of America; MALDI-TOF, Matrix Assisted Laser Desorption/Ionization Time of Flight Mass Spectrometry; MICs, minimum inhibitory concentrations; Q1-Q3, interquartile range; spp, species; h, hours.; SPSS, Statistical Package for the Social Sciences; SYO, SensitreYeastOne colorimetric plate

Authors' contributions

FB designed the study, analyzed data and wrote the article. EO, performed the acquisition of data, analyzed data and wrote the article. PO, CC, and FS, provided the clinical data. EM, provided the laboratory data. All authors drafted the article, revised it critically for important intellectual content, and approved the final article.

Competing of interests

The authors declare that they have no competing interests. The authors alone are responsible for the content and the writing of the paper.

Consent for publication
Not applicable.

Author details
[1]Clinica Malattie Infettive; Università Politecnica delle Marche, Azienda Ospedaliero-Universitaria, Ospedali Riuniti Umberto I°- G.M. Lancisi – G. Salesi, Ancona, Italy. [2]Clinica Pediatrica; Università Politecnica delle Marche, Azienda Ospedaliero-Universitaria, Ospedali Riuniti Umberto I°- G.M. Lancisi – G. Salesi, Ancona, Italy. [3]Pediatria, Azienda Ospedaliero-Universitaria, Ospedali Riuniti Umberto I°- G.M. Lancisi – G. Salesi, Ancona, Italy. [4]Anestesia e Rianimazione Pediatrica, Azienda Ospedaliero-Universitaria, Ospedali Riuniti Umberto I°- G.M. Lancisi – G. Salesi, Ancona, Italy. [5]Laboratorio di Microbiologia, Azienda Ospedaliero-Universitaria, Ospedali Riuniti Umberto I°- G.M. Lancisi – G. Salesi, Ancona, Italy.

References

1. Cornely OA, Bassetti M, Calandra T, et al. ESCMID guideline for the diagnosis and management of *Candida* diseases 2012: non-neutropenic adult patients. Clin Microbiol Infect. 2012;18:19–37.
2. Lionakis MS, Netea MG. *Candida* and host determinants of susceptibility to invasive candidiasis. PLoS Pathog. 2013;9:e1003079.
3. Nieto MC, Tellería O, Cisterna R. Sentinel surveillance of invasive candidiasis in Spain: epidemiology and antifungal susceptibility. Diagn Microbiol Infect Dis. 2015;81:34–40.
4. Bassetti M, Righi E, Costa A, et al. Epidemiological trends in nosocomial candidemia in intensive care. BMC Infect Dis. 2006;6:21.
5. Barchiesi F, Orsetti E, Gesuita R, Skrami E, Manso E, Candidemia Study Group. Epidemiology, clinical characteristics, and outcome of candidemia in a tertiary referral center in Italy from 2010 to 2014. Infection. 2016;44:205–13.
6. Tortorano A, Prigitano A, Lazzarini C, et al. A 1-year prospective survey of candidemia in Italy and changing epidemiology over one decade. Infection. 2013;41:655–62.
7. Montagna MT, Caggiano G, Lovero G, et al. Epidemiology of invasive fungal infections in the intensive care unit: results of a multicenter Italian survey (AURORA Project). Infection. 2013;41:645–53.
8. Trofa D, Gàcser A, Nosanchuk JD. *Candida parapsilosis*, an emerging fungal pathogen. Clin Microbiol Rev. 2008;21:606–25.
9. Nucci M, Queiroz-Telles F, Alvarado-Matute T, et al. Epidemiology of candidemia in Latin America: a laboratory-based survey. PLoS One. 2013;8:e59373.
10. Cantòn E, Pemàn J, Quindòs G, et al. Prospective multicenter study of the epidemiology, molecular identification, and antifungal susceptibility of *Candida parapsilosis*, *Candida orthopsilosis*, and *Candida metapsilosis* isolated from patients with candidemia. Antimicrob Agents Chemother. 2011;55: 5590–6.
11. Borghi E, Sciota R, Iatta R, et al. Characterization of *Candida parapsilosis* complex strains isolated from invasive fungal infections. Eur J Clin Microbiol Infect Dis. 2011;30:1437–4.
12. Pfaller MA, Diekema DJ, Andes D, et al. Clinical breakpoints for the echinocandins and *Candida* revisited: integration of molecular, clinical, and microbiological data to arrive at species-specific interpretive criteria. Drug Resist Updat. 2011;14:164–76.
13. Pappas PG, CA K m, Andes D, et al. Clinical practice guidelines for the management of candidiasis: 2009 update by the Infectious Diseases Society of America. Clin Infect Dis. 2009;48:503–35.
14. Chen CY, Sheng WH, Huang SY, et al. Clinical characteristics and treatment outcomes of patients with candidaemia due to *Candida parapsilosis* sensu lato species at a medical centre in Taiwan, 2000–12. J Antimicrob Chemother. 2015;70:1531–8.
15. Pfaller MA, Diekema DJ. Progress in antifungal susceptibility testing of *Candida* spp. by use of Clinical and Laboratory Standards Institute broth microdilution methods, 2010 to 2012. J Clin Microbiol. 2012;50:2846–56.
16. Andes DR, Safdar N, Baddley JW, et al. Impact of treatment strategy on outcomes in patients with candidemia and other forms of invasive candidiasis: a patient-level quantitative review of randomized trials. Clin Infect Dis. 2012;54:1110–22.
17. Girmenia C, Martino P, De Bernardis F, et al. Rising incidence of *Candida parapsilosis* fungemia in patients with hematologic malignancies: clinical aspects, predisposing factors, and differential pathogenicity of the causative strains. Clin Infect Dis. 1996;23:506–14.
18. Miranda LD, Rodrigues EC, Costa SF, et al. *Candida parapsilosis* candidaemia in a neonatal unit over 7 years: a case series study. BMJ Open. 2012;2:4. 10. 1136/bmjopen-2012-000992.
19. Almirante B, Rodríguez D, Cuenca-Estrella M, et al. Epidemiology, risk factors, and prognosis of *Candida parapsilosis* bloodstream infections: case-control population-based surveillance study of patients in Barcelona, Spain, from 2002 to 2003. J Clin Microbiol. 2006;44:1681–5.
20. Fernández-Ruiz M, Aguado JM, Almirante B, et al. Initial use of echinocandins does not negatively influence outcome in *Candida parapsilosis* bloodstream infection: a propensity score analysis. Clin Infect Dis. 2014;58:1413–21.
21. Fortún J, Martín-Dávila P, Gómez-García de la Pedrosa E, et al. Emerging trends in candidemia: a higher incidence but a similar outcome. J Infect. 2012;65:64–70.
22. Wisplinghoff H, Bischoff T, Tallent SM, et al. Nosocomial bloodstream infections in US hospitals: analysis of 24,179 cases from a prospective nationwide surveillance study. Clin Infect Dis. 2004;39:309–17.
23. Bassetti M, Molinari MP, Mussap M, Viscoli C, Righi E. Candidemia in internal medicine departements: the burden of a rising problem. Clin Microbiol Infect. 2013;19:e281–4.
24. Garey KW, Rege M, Pai MP, et al. Time to initiation of fluconazole therapy impacts mortality in patients with candidemia: a multi institutional study. Clin Infect Dis. 2006;43:25–31.
25. Morrell M, Fraser VJ, Kollef MH. Delaying the empiric treatment of *Candida* bloodstream infection until positive blood culture results are obtained: a potential risk factor for hospital mortality. Antimicrob Agents Chemother. 2005;49:3640–5.
26. Kim SH, Yoon YK, Kim MJ, Sohn JW. Clinical impact of time to positivity for Candida species on mortality in patients with candidaemia. J Antimicrob Chemother. 2013;68:2890–7.
27. Mora-Duarte J, Betts R, Rotstein C, et al. Comparison of caspofungin and amphotericin B for invasive candidiasis. N Engl J Med. 2002;347:2020–9.
28. Reboli AC, Rotstein C, Pappas PG, et al. Anidulafungin versus fluconazole for invasive candidiasis. N Engl J Med. 2007;356:2472–82.
29. Kuse ER, Chetchotisakd P, da Cunha CA, et al. Micafungin versus liposomal amphotericin B for candidaemia and invasive candidosis: a phase III randomised double-blind trial. Lancet. 2007;369:1519–27.
30. Pappas PG, Rotstein CM, Betts RF, et al. Micafungin versus caspofungin for treatment of candidemia and other forms of invasive candidiasis. Clin Infect Dis. 2007;45:883–93.

14

Characteristics of neonates with culture-proven bloodstream infection who have low levels of C-reactive protein (≦10 mg/L)

Mei-Yin Lai[1,3], Ming-Horng Tsai[2,3], Chiang-Wen Lee[4,5], Ming-Chou Chiang[1,3], Reyin Lien[1,3], Ren-Huei Fu[1,3], Hsuan-Rong Huang[1,3], Shih-Ming Chu[1,3,6*] and Jen-Fu Hsu[1,3,6*]

Abstract

Background: Elevated C-reactive protein (CRP) level is widely used in clinical practice as a marker to distinguish between neonates with or without sepsis. However, some neonates with bacteremia have a CRP level within the normal range and they are not well characterized.

Methods: All episodes of neonatal culture-proven bloodstream infections (BSIs) between July 2004 and June 2012 were enrolled. Patients characteristics were compared for three CRP groups (low, ≤ 10 mg/L; intermediate, 11–100 mg/L; and high, > 100 mg/L) using the Chi-square test and one-way ANOVA. The sepsis-attributable mortality rates were compared using logistic regression analyses.

Results: Of 986 episodes of neonatal BSI, 247 (25.1 %) had CRP ≤10 mg/L at the onset of clinical sepsis. In the low CRP group, patients had lower gestational age and birth weight, and an earlier occurrence of BSI. Patients with underlying gastrointestinal pathology, renal disorders, cholestasis, and pulmonary hypertension had a non-significant elevated CRP level at the onset of sepsis. In the blood culture of the low CRP group, coagulase-negative staphylococci (CoNS) were relatively more common (55.9 %, $p < 0.001$) than the other two groups, although one-fourth were infected with gram-negative bacilli (19.0 %), fungi (2.8 %), or polymicrobial pathogens (3.6 %). Of the BSIs with initial low CRP, 29.1 % were treated with inadequate antibiotics, 13.0 % progressed to septic shock, and 5.3 % had infectious complications. The sepsis-attributable mortality rate was lower in the low CRP group (4.9 %) than in the high CRP group (13.6 %).

Conclusions: A considerable proportion of neonatal BSIs had a normal or low initial CRP level (≤10 mg/L), which was more likely to occur in low birth weight or extremely preterm infants, those with earlier onset of sepsis, and those infected with CoNS. Plasma CRP level should not be used to rule out severe culture-proven sepsis or guide the empirical choice of antibiotics.

Background

The incidence of culture-proven bloodstream infection (BSI) in the neonatal intensive care unit (NICU) is around 37 episodes per 10,000 neonate-hospital days [1–4]. Neonatal BSI is associated with significant morbidity, worse long-term outcomes, and a reported mortality rate of 12–20 % [1, 5–8]. Early and appropriate antibiotic treatment is the cornerstone of treatment [9, 10], which highlights the importance of a high index of suspicion based on clinical and laboratory parameters long before the blood culture results are known. However, some neonatal BSIs may present with nonspecific symptoms and several laboratory predictors have been investigated for better identification of bacteremia in the NICU [11–15].

C-reactive protein (CRP) is an acute-phase protein of hepatic origin that increases following interleukin-6 secretion from macrophages and T-cells [16, 17]. The synthesis of CRP in response to inflammation starts very rapidly, and serum concentration rises to > 5 mg/L after 6 h and peaks at 48 h [18, 19]. The CRP reference values in neonates reported in the literature are 1.5–20 mg/L and have a wide range of sensitivities and specificities [19, 20]. Although some studies have demonstrated that

* Correspondence: kz6479@cgmh.org.tw; jeff0724@gmail.com
[1]Division of Pediatric Neonatology, Department of Pediatrics, Chang Gung Memorial Hospital, Taoyuan, Taiwan
Full list of author information is available at the end of the article

at least 2 CRP levels, both ≤ 10 mg/L and obtained 24 h apart, are needed to identify infants unlikely to be infected [19, 21], the high cut-off value associated with bacterial infection in neonates is still uncertain. Conversely, a small proportion of patients with bacteremia have CRP levels within the normal range [22, 23]. To date, this issue has not been well studied in the NICU. The present study was therefore conducted to characterize outcomes in neonates with culture-proven BSI and a CRP plasma level ≤ 10 mg/L.

Methods

We identified all episodes of culture-proven BSI in the NICU of Chang Gung Memorial Hospital (CGMH), a tertiary-level medical center in a university-affiliated teaching hospital in northern Taiwan, between 1 July 2004 and 30 June 2012. Only infants with late-onset sepsis, defined as clinical sepsis with a positive blood culture obtained after 3 days of life [1, 3, 24], were enrolled. The NICU has 3 units that include 49 beds equipped with mechanical ventilators and 28 beds in special-care nurseries. All babies under 34–35 weeks of completed gestation or birth weight < 2 kg or > 5 kg or those with any clinical signs of respiratory distress or cardiovascular, gastrointestinal, or neurological problems requiring surgical or intensive treatment were eligible for admission to our NICU. This study was approved by the institutional review board of Chang Gung Memorial Hospital, with a waiver of informed consent because all patient records/information was anonymized and de-identified prior to analysis.

Data retrieval and study database

Information for the NICU database was recorded by a full-time nurse specialist dedicated to following up neonates from birth (or admission if the neonate was transferred from another hospital) until discharge or death, and this nurse specialist has maintained the database every weekday for > 10 y. The NICU database contained information about basic demographic data, a summary of the patient's hospital course, discharge diagnosis, and complications during prematurity. Medical records were reviewed to characterize the detailed courses of every episode of BSI, including the clinical manifestations, laboratory results, progression of septic conditions, concurrent infectious focus, treatment, infectious complications, and outcomes. The severity of illness was evaluated at the most severe period during the course of BSI using the neonatal therapeutic intervention scoring system (NTISS) [25].

Definitions

An episode of BSI was defined according to the presence of clinical sepsis and identification of pathogens, which included any bacteria isolated from at least one blood culture and not pertaining to the saprophytic skin flora as significant. Growth of *Corynebacterium* spp., *Propionibacterium* spp., *Penicillium* spp., or *Diphtheroids* spp. in the blood cultures were considered contaminants and were excluded. The microbiology assay system in our hospital is a matrix-assisted laser desorption ionization time-of-flight (MALDI-TOF) system (Bruker's flagship FLEX series). For coagulase-negative staphylococci (CoNS) BSI, the diagnosis required clinical signs of sepsis, a blood culture positive for CoNS, and administration of intravenous antibacterial therapy for at least 5 days after the blood culture or until death [1, 2, 7].

An episode of clinical sepsis was defined if a patient had a positive blood culture treated with antibiotic therapy for 5 or more days or treated for a shorter period if the patient died, and the presence of at least two of the following clinical symptoms of sepsis: fever or hypothermia, hyper- or hypoglycemia, apnea or tachypnea, frequent desaturation with an increased requirement for ventilator support, bradycardia and/or cyanosis, feeding intolerance, abdominal distension, seizure, decreased activity, skin mottling and hypotension [1, 7, 9].

All co-morbidities of prematurity, including respiratory distress syndrome (RDS), intra-ventricular hemorrhage (IVH), broncho-pulmonary dysplasia (BPD), necrotizing enterocolitis (NEC), and peri-ventricular leukomalacia (PVL) were based on the latest updated diagnostic criteria [26]. Congenital anomalies included all neonates with either documented or undocumented syndrome, chromosome abnormalities, and genetic or metabolic disorders, but not simple cleft palate or polydactyly. Persistent bacteremia or fungemia was defined as three or more consecutive positive blood cultures, at least 48 h apart, during a single episode of sepsis [27]. All concurrent infectious foci, including NEC, ventilator associated pneumonia (VAP), catheter-related bloodstream infection (CRBSI), or meningitis were also recorded based on the strict diagnostic criteria of the Centers for Disease Control and Prevention and previous official publications [28, 29].

Infectious complications were defined as a new-onset infectious focus, empyema, abscess, venous thrombosis, or vegetation directly related to bacteremia or major organ dysfunction within 1 week after the onset of bacteremia. Empirical antibiotic therapy was considered inappropriate if the treatment regimen did not include at least 1 antibiotic active in vitro against the infecting microorganisms administered within 24 h of blood culture collection. For patients who died during hospitalization, the cause of death was recorded according to the clinician's assessment. Sepsis-attributable mortality was defined as neonates who expired within 3 days after the onset of sepsis and those who died of infectious complications or clinically progressive deterioration following the onset of BSI.

Data on CRP

The CRP plasma level was measured with an immunoturbidimetric instrument (Modular P, Roche, Germany). We excluded episodes of BSI for which CRP was not measured on the date of BSI onset. If more than 1 CRP measurement was done on the date of BSI, we used the measurement conducted closest to the time when blood culture samples were drawn. In the laboratory, a CRP level ≤ 5 mg/L was considered within the normal range. The low limit of detection of CRP in our hospital is > 0.5 mg/L, and there is no upper limit of CRP detection. All BSI episodes were divided into 3 CRP groups: low (CRP ≤ 10 mg/L), intermediate (CRP 11–100 mg/L), and high (CRP > 100 mg/L).

Statistical analysis

The patient characteristics by CRP group were computed in contingency tables. Differences in categorical and continuous variables were tested by the χ^2 test and one-way ANOVA, respectively. For continuous variables with large standard deviations, the nonparametric Kruskal–Wallis H test was applied. Trends in proportions of microorganisms in the 3 CRP groups were analyzed using the χ^2 test for trend. Statistical significance was set at $P < 0.05$.

The sepsis-attributable mortality rate by CRP group was examined using a logistic regression model. Univariate and multivariate analyses, including the covariables of sex, gestational age, underlying chronic co-morbidities, and bacterial subgroups, were performed. Because of the strong correlation between birth weight and gestational age, the risk factor of body weight at birth was excluded from the analysis. Estimates were expressed as odds ratios (ORs) with 95 % confidence intervals (CIs). All statistical analyses were performed using SPSS version 15.0 (SPSS, Chicago, IL, USA).

Results

During the study period, 1010 episodes of BSI (late-onset sepsis) in 793 neonates from the NICU were identified. Those with incomplete medical records ($n = 8$), no CRP measurement at BSI onset ($n = 12$), or transfer to another hospital ($n = 4$) were excluded, leaving a total of 986 BSI episodes in 772 neonates. Among these, 247 (25.1 %) had a plasma CRP level ≤ 10 mg/L, 563 (57.1 %) had a plasma CRP level of 11–100 mg/L, and 176 (17.8 %) had a plasma CRP level > 100 mg/L.

Patients in the low CRP group had a lower birth body weight and gestational age and an earlier onset of BSI than patients in the intermediate and high CRP groups (Table 1). There were no significant differences in the perinatal history and most underlying chronic co-morbidities among the 3 CRP groups. However, patients with gastrointestinal pathology, pulmonary hypertension, renal disorders, or cholestasis were more likely to have high CRP at BSI onset. When the clinical symptoms or signs were compared, significantly more patients in the high CRP group had apnea, bradycardia with or without cyanosis, feeding intolerance, hyper- or hypoglycemia, or septic shock compared to those in the low CRP group (Table 1). These clinical symptoms were not significantly different between the low and intermediate CRP groups.

Episodes of BSI in the high CRP group had a significantly higher rate of abnormal laboratory findings, including leucopenia, anemia, thrombocytopenia, and metabolic acidosis compared to those in the low CRP group. The severity of illness, judged by NTISS score, was also significantly higher in the high CRP group than in the low CRP group. These demographics, clinical features, and laboratory findings were not significantly different between neonatal BSIs in the low and intermediate CRP groups as determined by post hoc analyses (data not shown). However, neonatal BSIs in the low CRP groups occurred significantly earlier than in both the intermediate and high CRP groups. Episodes of BSI with concurrent meningitis, ventilator-associated pneumonia, and catheter-related BSI also had elevated CRP at the onset of clinical sepsis (Table 1).

Microbiology

In the low CRP group, gram-positive, gram-negative, fungal, and polymicrobial pathogens accounted for 74.5, 19.0, 2.8, and 3.6 % of infections, respectively. CoNS was significantly more common in the blood cultures of the low CRP group compared to the other groups. A lower proportion of most gram-negative bacteria occurred in the low CRP group (Table 2). However, for gram-positive bacteria, there were significantly fewer patients with Group B *Streptococcus* BSI and comparable numbers of *Staphylococcus aureus* BSI in the low CRP group.

Of the 247 patients with an initial plasma CRP level ≤ 10 mg/L, 178 had at least 1 more CRP measurement during the days following BSI onset. Among these, 82 (46.1 %) developed a CRP response > 10 mg/L (median [IQR]: 35.0 mg/L [22.8–52.5 mg/L]) at a median of 2.8 days (range 1–7 days) after antibiotic treatment. Of the 138 episodes of CoNS BSI with an initial CRP plasma level ≤ 10 mg/L, 58 (42.0 %) were treated with initial antibiotics that were inadequate and had repeated positive blood cultures. Among the 96 episodes of neonatal BSIs with repeated CRP data that still had a CRP level ≤ 10 mg/L, 31 (32.3 %) had CoNS in their blood cultures.

Table 1 Episodes of bloodstream infection stratified according to low (CRP 0–10 mg/L), intermediate (CRP 11–100 mg/L) and high (CRP > 100 mg/L) level

Characteristics	CRP 0–10 mg/L (*n* = 247)	CRP 11–100 mg/L (*n* = 563)	CRP > 100 mg/L (*n* = 176)	*p* value
Demographic characteristics				
Birth weight (g), mean ± SD	1310 ± 746	1507.9 ± 809	1725.2 ± 959	0.004
median (IQR)	1310 (920–1740)	1530 (885–1975)	1685 (923–2610)	
Gestational age (weeks), mean ± SD	30.2 ± 4.3	30.5 ± 4.6	31.4 ± 5.2	0.036
median (IQR)	30.0 (27.0–33.0)	30.0 (27.0–34.0)	30.0 (27.0–36.0)	
Male sex, n (%)	140 (56.7)	292 (51.9)	88 (50.0)	0.154
Onset of BSI (day), median (IQR)	23.0 (15.0–43.0)	30.0 (18.0–56.0)	32.5 (19.0–63.8)	<0.001
Perinatal history				
NSD/CS	112 (45.3)/135 (54.7)	220 (39.1)/343 (60.9)	81 (46.0)/95 (54.0)	0.901
Inborn/outborn	163 (66.0)/84 (34.0)	381 (67.7)/182 (32.3)	112 (63.6)/64 (36.4)	0.697
Low apgar score at 5 min (≦7)	111 (44.9)	255 (45.3)	70 (39.8)	0.344
Perinatal asphyxia	18 (7.3)	48 (8.5)	11 (6.3)	0.738
Underlying chronic conditions[a]				
Congenital anomalies	15 (6.1)	35 (6.2)	18 (10.2)	0.128
Neurological comorbidities	35 (14.2)	63 (11.2)	31 (17.6)	0.443
Complicated congenital heart disease (CHD)	8 (3.2)	23 (4.1)	4 (2.3)	0.696
Acyanotic CHD with heart failure	5 (2.0)	9 (1.6)	7 (4.0)	0.234
Bronchopulmonary dysplasia	66 (26.7)	188 (33.4)	60 (34.1)	0.087
Pulmonary hypertension	3 (1.2)	18 (3.2)	11 (6.3)	0.004
Gastrointestinal pathology	4 (1.6)	47 (8.3)	15 (8.5)	0.002
Renal	6 (2.4)	17 (3.0)	12 (6.8)	0.024
Cholestasis[b]	30 (12.1)	117 (20.8)	41 (23.3)	0.002
Clinical septic symptoms				
Fever (temperature > 38 °C)	99 (40.1)	228 (40.5)	84 (47.7)	0.135
Apnea ± bradycardia and/or cyanosis	158 (64.0)	385 (68.4)	139 (79.0)	0.001
Abdominal distension ± feeding intolerance	130 (52.6)	328 (58.3)	139 (79.0)	<0.001
Tachycardia	55 (22.3)	134 (23.8)	35 (19.9)	0.652
Hyper- or hypoglycemia	53 (21.5)	157 (27.9)	55 (31.3)	0.020
Septic shock	32 (13.0)	93 (16.5)	45 (25.6)	0.001
Disseminated intravascular Coagulopathy	12 (4.9)	45 (8.0)	30 (17.0)	<0.001
Laboratory parameter				
Leukopenia (WBC count < 4000/uL)	25 (10.1)	109 (19.4)	38 (21.6)	0.001
Leukocytosis (WBC count > 20,000/uL)	62 (25.1)	151 (26.8)	64 (36.4)	0.017
WBC shift to left (immature WBC ≥ 20 % total)	13 (5.3)	65 (11.5)	44 (25.0)	<0.001
Anemia (hemoglobin < 11.0 mg/dL)	79 (32.5)	217 (38.5)	98 (55.7)	<0.001
Thrombocytopenia (platelet < 80,000/uL)	41 (16.6)	197 (35.0)	110 (62.5)	<0.001
Metabolic acidosis	26 (10.7)	104 (18.5)	60 (34.1)	<0.001
Prolonged PT and/or aPTT	34 (14.0)	150 (26.6)	70 (39.8)	<0.001
NTISS score, mean ± SD	16.3 ± 4.2	16.9 ± 4.6	18.2 ± 5.1	<0.001
Sequences of BSI during hospitalization				0.014
First episode	204 (82.6)	412 (73.2)	128 (72.7)	
2nd episode	29 (11.7)	95 (16.9)	31 (17.6)	
>2nd episode	14 (5.7)	56 (9.9)	17 (9.7)	

Table 1 Episodes of bloodstream infection stratified according to low (CRP 0–10 mg/L), intermediate (CRP 11–100 mg/L) and high (CRP > 100 mg/L) level *(Continued)*

Concomitant infectious focus[c]				
Meningitis	12 (4.9)	20 (3.6)	23 (13.1)	0.001
Catheter-related bloodstream infection	12 (4.9)	30 (5.3)	20 (11.4)	0.012
Necrotizing enterocolitis (≥ stage II)[d]	4 (1.6)	10 (1.8)	7 (4.0)	0.126
Ventilator associated pneumonia	7 (2.8)	18 (3.2)	15 (8.5)	0.007
Others[e]	1 (0.4)	3 (0.5)	3 (1.7)	-

All data were expressed as number (percentage %), unless indicated otherwise
NTISS neonatal therapeutic intervention scoring system, *IQR* interquartile range, *SD* standard deviation, *BSI* bloodstream infection, *NSD* natural vaginal delivery, *C/S* cesarean section
[a]Indicating the presence of chronic conditions or comorbidities at onset of bloodstream infection, and some patients had > 1 underlying chronic conditions. Each patient with an underlying chronic condition is compared with those without that specific condition
[b]Indicating direct bilirubin ≥ 1.5 mg/dL or more than 50 % of the total bilirubin
[c]Indicating the diagnosis of a infectious focus was concurrent with onset of bacteremia
[d]Based on modified Bell's staging criteria
[e]Included osteomyelitis (2), septic arthritis (2), left thigh cellulitis (1), and urinary tract infection (2)

Treatments and outcomes

Neonates who experienced BSI episodes and had higher CRP levels had significantly more invasive intubation or high-frequency oscillatory ventilator use (Table 3). The rates of inadequate antibiotic treatment were comparable among the 3 CRP groups. The overall sepsis-attributable mortality rate was 7.4 % and occurred in 4.9, 6.6, and 13.6 % in the low, intermediate, and high CRP groups, respectively. Neonates in the high CRP group had a significantly higher sepsis-attributable mortality compared with those in the intermediate and low CRP groups ($P < 0.05$ by log-rank test) (Fig. 1).

There was no difference in the sepsis-attributable mortality rate between those with CRP ≤ 10 mg/L and those with CRP of 11–100 mg/L. The CRP level was a predictor of sepsis-attributable mortality (OR 3.09, 95 % CI 1.50–6.37) in the high CRP group compared to the low CRP group. The difference between these 2 groups remained unchanged even after adjustments for birth weight, sex, gestational age, bacterial subgroups, and several underlying chronic morbidities (data not shown).

Discussion

Approximately one-fourth of the cases of neonatal BSI—which is a surprisingly high proportion in the

Table 2 Pathogens causing neonatal bloodstream infections in the three CRP groups

Pathogens	CRP 0–10 mg/L (*n* = 247)	CRP 11–100 mg/L (*n* = 563)	CRP > 100 mg/L (*n* = 176)	*P* value
Gram-positive organisms	184 (74.5)	322 (57.2)	63 (35.8)	<0.001
Coagulase-negative staphylococci (CoNS)	138 (55.9)	227 (40.3)	24 (13.6)	<0.001
Staphylococcus aureus	34 (13.8)	62 (11.0)	23 (13.1)	0.715
Enterococcus spp.	8 (3.2)	18 (3.2)	1 (0.6)	0.130
Group-B streptococcus	3 (1.2)	13 (2.3)	15 (8.5)	<0.001
Others[a]	1 (0.4)	2 (0.4)	0 (0)	-
Gram-negative organisms	47 (19.0)	174 (30.9)	91 (51.7)	<0.001
E coli	12 (4.9)	41 (7.3)	23 (13.1)	0.003
Klebsiella spp.	18 (7.3)	66 (11.7)	32 (18.2)	0.001
Enterobacter spp.	4 (1.6)	26 (4.6)	11 (6.3)	0.015
Acinetobacter baumannii	6 (2.4)	23 (4.1)	12 (6.8)	0.028
Pseudomonas spp.	3 (1.2)	6 (1.1)	6 (3.4)	0.103
Serratia marscences	3 (1.2)	7 (1.2)	1 (0.6)	0.574
Others[b]	2 (0.8)	5 (0.9)	6 (3.4)	0.113
Fungemia	7 (2.8)	38 (6.7)	11 (6.3)	0.090
Polymicrobial bloodstream infection	9 (3.6)	29 (5.2)	11 (6.3)	0.214

[a]Including *Streptococcus pneumonia* (1), and non-enterococcal group D streptococcus (2)
[b]Including *Citrobacter freundii* (3), *Stenotrophomonas maltophilia* (3), *Hafnia alvei* (2), Neisseria Meningitidis (2), *Chryseobacterium meningoseptium* (1) *Flavobacterium* (1) and *Morganella morganii* (1)

Table 3 Treatment and outcomes of neonatal bloodstream infections among the three CRP groups

	CRP 0–10 mg/L (*n* = 247)	CRP 11–100 mg/L (*n* = 563)	CRP > 100 mg/L (*n* = 176)	*P* value
Treatment				
Invasive intubation	106 (42.9)	254 (45.1)	95 (54.0)	0.042
High frequency oscillatory ventilator	18 (7.3)	57 (10.1)	25 (14.2)	0.021
Inadequate antibiotic treatment with the first 24 h	72 (29.1)	150 (26.6)	42 (23.9)	0.463
Outcomes				
Infectious complications	13 (5.3)	49 (8.7)	42 (23.9)	<0.001
Sepsis attributable mortality	12 (4.9)	37 (6.6)	24 (13.6)	0.001

current cohort—had a CRP level of ≤ 10 mg/L at the onset of clinical sepsis. Low birth weight neonates, very low gestational age infants, and those in whom the occurrence of BSI episodes occurred earlier in life were more likely to have normal CRP at the onset of clinical sepsis. We found a high CRP level (>100 mg/L) was significantly associated with more severe clinical symptoms and worse outcomes. Although CoNS accounts for more than half of the episodes of BSI with normal CRP, in our cohort approximately one-fourth of those with normal CRP were infected with gram-negative bacteria, polymicrobial pathogens, or fungus. Furthermore, approximately 30 % of those with normal CRP were treated with inadequate initial antibiotics, and 13 % progressed to septic shock and 4.9 % had sepsis-attributable mortality.

It is reasonable to hypothesize that causative pathogens affect CRP level because some pathogens, especially gram-negative bacilli or *Pseudomonas* spp., tend to have a fulminant course [1, 7, 9], which can result in more severe tissue damage and inflammation. The findings here are consistent with a recent study conducted by Knudtzen et al., who found that CoNS BSI is more common in the low CRP group and that approximately 25–35 % of all CoNS BSI have normal CRP at the onset of clinical sepsis [22]. Because drawing 2 sets of blood culture at the same time is not routinely done and the second blood culture may become negative if vancomycin was

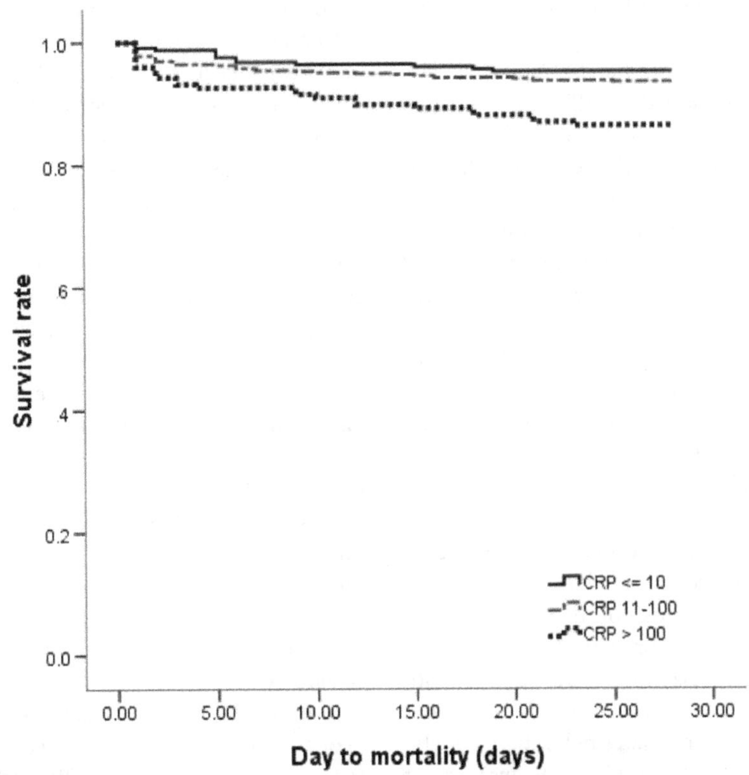

Fig. 1 Survival following positive blood culture from 986 episodes of neonatal culture-proven bloodstream infection. The Kaplan-Meier graph is stratified by three different CRP groups: low, ≤ 10 mg/L; intermediate, 11–100 mg/L; and high, > 100 mg/L

initially administrated, the lack of 2 positive blood cultures for documentation of CoNS BSI is a limitation of this study. Some possibly represent bacterial contaminations. To reduce the false positive cases of CoNS BSI, strict criteria for CoNS BSI have been applied, including requiring more than 2 septic symptoms or signs, as in previous studies [1, 2, 8]. Besides, more than three-fourths of the CoNS BSIs have elevated CRP or abnormal laboratory findings.

Because the initial symptoms of neonatal sepsis may be nonspecific and subtle and may become fulminant if appropriate antibiotics are not administered in time, the role of plasma CRP level in adequately predicting serious bacterial infection in neonates has recently become the topic of several studies [30–33]. Although we found that significantly more infectious complications and sepsis-attributable mortality occurred in the CRP group with > 100 mg/L, a possibly delayed elevation and inadequate sensitivity of CRP testing highlight the importance of investigating other predictors, including new laboratory markers [30–35] and clinical scores [36–38] and maintaining high alertness for the development of severe sepsis. Several studies report a sensitivity and specificity of 48–78 % and 71–88 %, respectively, for a single determination of CRP at 4–12 h after symptom onset [31–35]. Therefore, taken together, using the CRP level as a guide for empirical choice of antibiotics or to rule out serious infections or withhold antibiotic therapy is not recommended.

This study also investigated whether BSI episodes with initially low CRP levels developed a CRP response later. In contrast to a recent study in which 84 % of BSIs with initially normal CRP mounted a CRP response [22], the current study reveals that only 46 % have elevated subsequent CRP. This may be due to the high rate of initial effective antibiotic therapy and, possibly, the presence of CoNS as a low-level pathogenic bacterium that causes less tissue damage and inflammation. In a cohort of 60 neonates with early-onset sepsis, Ehl et al. [39] demonstrated that the CRP values decrease 16 h after successful antibiotic therapy. Some cases without CRP response in our cohort presented with a very fulminant course and hepatic failure, which was similar to a finding in a previous study [40].

The value of CRP as a predictive marker for bacterial infection in neonates has been studied with varying results [30–34, 38]. However, most of these studies focused on serious bacterial sepsis or critically ill neonates. This study aimed to characterize the NICU patients with normal or low CRP levels at the onset of sepsis and compared them with other neonates who had an elevated CRP level. We found the differences were most significant between neonatal BSIs in the low CRP group and those in the high CRP (>100 mg/L) group. The nonsignificant difference between the low CRP and the intermediate CRP groups by post hoc analyses (data not shown) implied that initial CRP level cannot be the sole predictor of final mortality. In this study, patients in the high CRP group treated with inappropriate antibiotics in the first 24 h were at especially higher risk of infectious complications and sepsis attributable mortality. However, those in the low CRP group had a relatively smooth clinical course even though they were initially treated with delayed effective antibiotics. Therefore, CRP still has a reference value as an indicator of severe infection.

We found that patients with lower gestational age or lower birth body weight tended to have a low CRP value at the onset of BSI. Because CRP is the end product of cytokine response after tissue injury, it is likely that extremely preterm or very low birth weight infants have less pronounced immunomodulatory or pre-inflammatory proteins after bacterial infection [41, 42]. Of interest, we found this cytokine response less severe in earlier life, but further investigation to validate these differences is required because the CRP level can also be affected by various factors, including pathogens, severity of illness, concomitant infectious focus, and some underlying chronic comorbidities.

There are some limitations in this study. Although a set of strict criteria was used to define true BSI, the lack of 2 positive blood cultures for CoNS as documentation of BSI is a weakness of this study. This was a retrospective, single-center cohort study, which inevitably restricts its generalizability compared to that of a prospective, multicenter study. The timing of blood sampling for culture and CRP also was not uniform because some septic work-up may be delayed because the initial septic symptoms were nonspecific and subtle. Furthermore, some CRP levels may have been falsely low because they were obtained too early before they started to rise around 4–6 h after sepsis onset. Lastly, a group with elevated CRP but without infection was not enrolled as controls. Thus, a prospective study is warranted to scientifically delineate the sensitivity and specificity of CRP as a predictive marker of neonatal sepsis.

Conclusion

Nearly one-forth of neonatal bloodstream infections had a normal or low initial CRP level (<=10 mg/L), which was more likely to occur in low birth weight or extremely preterm infants, those with earlier onset of sepsis, and those infected with coagulase-negative Staphylococcus. Although initial low CRP level was significantly with less severity of illness and better outcome, some critically ill neonates had CRP not significantly elevated at onset of sepsis. Therefore, plasma CRP level should not be used to rule out severe culture-proven sepsis or guide the empirical choice of antibiotics.

Abbreviations

BSI: Bloodstream infection; CDC: Center for disease control; BPD: Bronchopulmonary dysplasia; CI: Confidence interval; CRBSI: Catheter-related bloodstream infection; CoNS: Coagulase negative Staphylococcus; CRP: C-reactive protein; CVC: Central venous catheter; ESBL: Extended-spectrum β-lactamase; GBS: Group B streptococcus; IQR: Interquartile range; GPC: Gram-positive cocci; MALDI-TOF: Matrix-assisted laser desorption ionization time-of-flight; NEC: Necrotizing enterocolitis; NICU: Neonatal intensive care unit; NTISS: Neonatal therapeutic intervention scoring system; OR: Odds ratio; PVL: Periventricular leukomalacia; RDS: Respiratory distress syndrome; TPN: Total parenteral nutrition; VAP: Ventilator associated pneumonia (VAP).

Competing interests

The authors declare that they have no competing interests.

Authors' contributions

M-YL: Dr. Lai conceptualized and designed the study, drafted the initial manuscript, and approved the final manuscript as submitted. M-HT: Dr. Tsai took care of these patients, collected and verified the data and had been involved in drafting the manuscript. C-WL: Dr. Lee designed the data collection instruments, coordinated and supervised data collection, and had been involved in drafting the manuscript. M-CC: Dr. Chiang took care of these patients, helped data verification, and had been involved in drafting the manuscript. RL: Dr. Lien took care of these patients, approved the agreement of interstitial review board, and had been involved in drafting the manuscript. R-HF: Dr. Fu took care of these patients, helped data verification, and had been involved in drafting the manuscript. H-RH: Dr. Huang took care of these patients, carried out the initial analyses, and had been involved in drafting the manuscript. S-MC: Dr. Chu took care of these patients, collected and verified the data, critically reviewed the manuscript, revised the manuscript, and approved the final manuscript as submitted J-FH: Dr. Hsu critically reviewed the manuscript, revised the manuscript, and approved the final manuscript as submitted. All authors have read and approve of the final version of the manuscript.

Acknowledgements

All authors thank Mrs. Chiao-Ching Chiang for keeping the database of our NICU, and all nursing staff working in our NICUs for keeping extremely detailed patient records, which contributed greatly to the completion of this research. We want to thank Miss Chun-Chun Cheng and Mr. Yu-Jr Lin for statistical consultation, who was supported by grants from Biostatistical Center for Clinical Research, Chang Gung Memorial Hospital (CLRPG340599).

Author details

[1]Division of Pediatric Neonatology, Department of Pediatrics, Chang Gung Memorial Hospital, Taoyuan, Taiwan. [2]Division of Neonatology and Pediatric Hematology/Oncology, Department of Pediatrics, Chang Gung Memorial Hospital, Yunlin, Taiwan. [3]College of Medicine, Chang Gung University, Taoyuan, Taiwan. [4]Department of Nursing, Division of Basic Medical Sciences, and Chronic Diseases and Health Promotion Research Center, Chang Gung University of Science and Technology, Chia-Yi, Taiwan. [5]Research Center for Industry of Human Ecology, Chang Gung University of Science and Technology, Taoyuan, Taiwan. [6]Linkou Chang Gung Memorial Hospital, No. 5, Fu-Shin Rd., Kwei-Shan, Taoyuan, Taiwan.

References

1. Tsai MH, Hsu JF, Chu SM, Lien R, Huang HR, Chiang MC, et al. Incidence, clinical characteristics, and risk factors of adverse outcome in neonates with late-onset sepsis. Pediatr Infect Dis J. 2014;33:e7–13.
2. Makhoul IR, Sujov P, Smolkin T, Lusky A, Reichman B. Epidemiological, clinical, and microbiological characteristics of late-onset sepsis among very low birth weight infants in Israel: a national survey. Pediatrics. 2002;109:34–9.
3. Verstraete E, Boelens J, De Coen K, Claeys G, Vogelaers D, Vanhaesebrouck P, et al. Healthcare-associated bloodstream infections in a neonatal intensive care unit over a 20-year period (1992–2011): trends in incidence, pathogens, and mortality. Infect Control Hosp Epidemiol. 2014;35:511–8.
4. Stoll BJ, Hansen N, Fanaroff AA, Wright LL, Carlo WA, Ehrenkranz RA, et al. Late-onset sepsis in very low birth weight neonates: the experience of the NICHD Neonatal Research Network. Pediatrics. 2002;110:285–91.
5. Mitha A, Foix-L'Helias L, Arnaud C, Marret S, Vieux R, Aujard Y, et al. Neonatal infection and 5-year neurodevelopmental outcome of very preterm infants. Pediatrics. 2013;132:e372–80.
6. Stoll BJ, Hansen NI, Adams-Chapman I, Fanaroff AA, Hintz SR, Vohr B, et al. Neurodevelopmental and growth impairment among extremely low-birth-weight infants with neonatal infection. JAMA. 2004;292:2357–65.
7. Tsai MH, Chu SM, Lee CW, Hsu JF, Huang HR, Chiang MC, et al. Recurrent late-onset sepsis in the neonatal intensive care unit: incidence, clinical characteristics, and risk factors. Clin Microbiol Infect. 2014;20:O928–35.
8. Padula MA, Dewan ML, Shah SS, Padula AM, Srinivasan L, McGowan KL, et al. Risk factors associated with laboratory-confirmed bloodstream infections in a tertiary neonatal intensive care unit. Pediatr Infect Dis J. 2014;33:1027–32.
9. Tsai MH, Chu SM, Hsu JF, Lien R, Huang HR, Chiang MC, et al. Risk factors and outcomes for multidrug-resistant Gram-negative bacteremia in the NICU. Pediatrics. 2014;133:e322–9.
10. Tsai MH, Chu SM, Hsu JF, Lien R, Huang HR, Chiang MC, et al. Breakthrough bacteremia in the neonatal intensive care unit: incidence, risk factors, and attributable mortality. Am J Infect Control. 2015;43:20–5.
11. Escobar GJ, Puopolo KM, Wi S, Turk BJ, Kuzniewicz MW, Walsh EM, et al. Stratification of risk of early-onset sepsis in newborn ≧ 34 weeks' gestation. Pediatrics. 2014;133:30–6.
12. Schlapbach LJ, Graf R, Woerner A, Fontana M, Zimmermann-Baer U, Glauser D, et al. Pancreatic stone protein as a novel marker for neonatal sepsis. Intensive Care Med. 2013;39:754–63.
13. Mikhael M, Brown LS, Rosenfeld CR. Serial neutrophil values facilitate predicting the absence of neonatal early-onset sepsis. J Pediatr. 2014;164:522–8.
14. Olaciregui I, Hernandez U, Munoz JA, Emparanza JI, Landa JJ. Markers that predict serious bacterial infection in infants under 3 months of age presenting with fever of unknown origin. Arch Dis Child. 2009;94:501–5.
15. Verstraete EH, Blot K, Mahieu L, Vogelaers D, Blot S. Prediction models for neonatal health care-associated sepsis: a meta-analysis. Pediatrics. 2015;135:e1002–14.
16. Worthmann H, Tryc AB, Dirks M, Schuppner R, Brand K, Klawonn F, et al. Lipopolysaccharide binding protein, interleukin-10, interleukin-6 and C-reactive protein blood levels in acute ischemic stroke patients with post-stroke infection. J Neuroinflammation. 2015;12:13.
17. Cekic C, Arabul M, Alper E, Pakoz ZB, Saritas E, Yuksel, et al. Elevation of the relationship between serum ghrelin, C-reactive protein and interleukin-6 levels, and disease activity in inflammatory bowel diseases. Hepatogastroenterology. 2014;61:1196–200.
18. Povoa P. C-reactive protein: a valuable marker of sepsis. Intensive Care Med. 2002;28:235–43.
19. Hofer N, Zacharias E, Muller W, Resch B. An update on the use of C-reactive protein in early-onset neonatal sepsis: current insights and new tasks. Neonatology. 2012;102:25–36.
20. Chiesa C, Panero A, Osborn JF, Simonetti AF, Pacifico L. Diagnosis of neonatal sepsis: a clinical and laboratory challenge. Clin Chem. 2004;50:279–87.
21. Hengst JM. The role of C-reactive protein in the evaluation and management of infants with suspected sepsis. Adv Neonatal Care. 2003;3:3–13.
22. Knudtzen FC, Nielsen SL, Gradel KO, Lassen AT, Kolmos HJ, Lensen TG, et al. Characteristics of patients with community-acquired bacteremia who have low levels of C-reactive protein (<=20 mg/L). J Infect. 2014;68:149–55.
23. Benitz WE, Han MY, Madan A, Ramachandra P. Serial serum C-reactive protein levels in the diagnosis of neonatal infection. Pediatrics. 1998;102:E41.
24. Berardi A, Rossi C, Guidotti I, Vellani G, Lugli L, Bacchi Reggiani ML, et al. Factors associated with intrapartum transmission of group B streptococcus. Pediatr Infect Dis J. 2014;33:1211–5.
25. Gray JE, Richardson DK, McCormick MC, Workman-Daniels K, Goldmann DA. Neonatal therapeutic intervention scoring system: a therapy-based severity-of-illness index. Pediatrics. 1992;90:561–7.
26. Gleason CA, Devaskar SU. Avery's disease of the newborn. 9th ed. Philadelphia, PA: Elsevier Saunders; 2011.
27. Horan TC, Andrus M, Dudeck MA. CDC/NHSN surveillance definition of health care-associated infection and criteria for specific types of infections in the acute care setting. Am J Infect Control. 2008;36:309–32.

28. Apisarnthanarak A, Holzmann-Pazgal G, Hamvas A, Olsen MA, Fraser VJ. Ventilator-associated pneumonia in extremely preterm neonates in a neonatal intensive care unit: characteristics, risk factors and outcomes. Pediatrics. 2003;112:1283–9.
29. Tsai MH, Lien R, Wang JW, Huang HR, Chiang CC, Chu SM, et al. Complication rates with percutaneously central venous catheters inserted at femoral and non-femoral sites in very low birth weight infants. Pediatr Infect Dis J. 2009;28:966–70.
30. Keane M, Fallon R, Riordan A, Shaw B. Markedly raised levels of C-reactive protein are associated with culture proven sepsis or necrotizing enterocolitis in extremely preterm neonates. Acta Paediatr. 2015;104:e289–e293.
31. Enguix A, Rey C, Concha A, Medina A, Coto D, Dieguez MA. Comparison of procalcitonin with C-reactive protein and serum amyloid for the early diagnosis of bacterial sepsis in critically ill neonates and children. Intensive Care Med. 2001;27:211–5.
32. Stein M, Schachter-Davidov A, Babai I, Tasher D, Somekh E. The accuracy of C-reactive protein, procalcitonin, and s-TREM-1 in the prediction of serious bacterial infection in neonates. Clin Pediatr (Phila). 2015;54:439–44.
33. Andreola B, Bressan S, Callegaro S, Liverani A, Plebani M, Da Dalt L. Procalcitonin and C-reactive protein as diagnostic markers of severe bacterial infections in febrile infants and children in the emergency department. Pediatr Infect Dis J. 2007;26:672–7.
34. Chacha F, Mirambo MM, Mushi MF, Karange N, Zuechner A, Kidenya BR, et al. Utility of qualitative C-reactive protein assay and white blood cells counts in the diagnosis of neonatal septicaemia at Bugando Medical Centre, Tanzania. BMC Pediatr. 2014;14:248.
35. Laborada G, Rego M, Jain A, Guliano M, Stavola J, Ballabh P, et al. Diagnostic value of cytokines and C-reactive protein in the first 24 hours of neonatal sepsis. Am J Perinatol. 2003;20:491–501.
36. Hsu JF, Chu SM, Huang YC, Lien R, Huang HR, Lee CW, Chiang MC, Fu RH, Tsai MH. Predictors of clinical and microbiological treatment failure in neonatal bloodstream infections. Clin Microbiol Infect. 2015;21:482.e9–482.e17.
37. Mahieu LM, De Muynck AO, De Dooy JJ, Laroche SM, Van Acker KJ. Prediction of nosocomial sepsis in neonates by means of a computer-weighted bedside scoring system (NOSEP score). Crit Care Med. 2000;28:2026–33.
38. Luzzani A, Polati E, Dorizzi R, Rungatscher A, Pavan R, Merlini A. Comparison of procalcitonin and C-reactive protein as markers of sepsis. Crit Care Med. 2003;31:1737–41.
39. Ehl S, Gehring B, Pohlandt F. A detailed analysis of changes in serum C-reactive protein levels in neonates treated for bacterial infection. Eur J Pediatr. 1999;158:238–42.
40. Amon S, Litmanovitz I, Regev R, Lis M, Shainkin-Kestenbaum R, Dolfin T. The prognostic virtue of inflammatory markers during late-onset sepsis in preterm infants. J Perinat Med. 2004;32:176–80.
41. Skogstrand K, Hougaard DM, Schendel DE, Bent NP, Svaerke C, Thorsen P. Assocation of preterm birth with sustained postnatal inflammatory respones. Obstet Gynecol. 2008;111:1118–28.
42. Dembinski J, Behrendt D, Martini R, Heep A, Bartmann P. Modulation of pro- and anti-inflammatory cytokine production in very preterm infants. Cytokine. 2003;21:2006.

15

Central-line associated bloodstream infections in a tertiary care children's University hospital

Elisabetta Venturini[1†], Carlotta Montagnani[1†], Alessandra Benni[1], Sabrina Becciani[1], Klaus Peter Biermann[2], Salvatore De Masi[2], Elena Chiappini[1], Maurizio de Martino[1], Luisa Galli[1,2,3*] and on behalf of the CLABSI (central-line associated bloodstream infections) study group

Abstract

Background: The central-line associated bloodstream infections (CLABSI) are the most common healthcare-associated infections in childhood. Despite the international data available on healthcare-associated infections in selected groups of patients, there is a lack of large and good quality studies. The present survey is the first prospective study monitoring for 6 months the occurrence of central-line associated bloodstream infections in all departments of an Italian tertiary care children's university hospital.

Methods: The study involved all children aged less than 18 years admitted to Meyer Children's University Hospital, Florence, Italy who had a central line access between the October 15th, 2014 and the April 14th, 2015. CLABSI were defined according to the Center for Disease Control and Prevention criteria. CLABSI incidence rates with 95% confidence limits were calculated and stratified for the study variables. For each factor the relative risk and 95% confidence intervals were evaluated. Statistical analysis was performed using the statistical software SPSS for Windows, version 22.0 (SPSS Inc., Chicago, IL), $p < 0.05$ was considered statistically significant.

Results: CLABSI rate was 3.73/1000 (95% CI: 2.54–5.28) central line-days. A higher CLABSI incidence was seen with female gender ($p = 0.045$) and underlying medical conditions (excepting prematurity, surgical diseases and malignancy) ($p = 0.06$). In our study 5 infections, were caused by extended-spectrum β-lactamase producing organisms and in one case by carbapenem-resistant *Klebsiella pneumoniae*.

Conclusions: Our study confirms the spreading of multi-resistant pathogens as causes of healthcare associated infections in children. An increased incidence rate of CLABSI in our study was related to underlying medical conditions. Pediatric studies focusing on healthcare infections in this type of patients should be done in order to deepen our understanding on associated risk factors and possible intervention areas.

Keywords: CLABSI, Children, Central-line, Infection

Background

The central line associated bloodstream infections (CLABSI) are the most common healthcare-associated infections (HAIs) in childhood. The results of the *International Nosocomial Infection Control Consortium* surveillance study from January 2007 to December 2012 in pediatric intensive care units (PICU) in Latin America, Asia, Africa and Europe, showed CLABSI rate of 6.1/1000 (95% CI: 5.7–6.5) central line-days [1]. The 2014 report of the *European Centre for Disease Prevention and Control* (ECDC) estimated a mean device-adjusted rate in patients staying in an ICU for more than two days was 3.0 CLABSI episodes per 1000 central line-days (IQR: 0.5–4.1) [2]. A cohort study performed from 2007 to 2012 in 173 neonatal intensive care unit (NICU) and 64 PICU reporting data to the *Centers for Disease Control and Prevention's*

* Correspondence: luisa.galli@unifi.it
†Equal contributors
[1]Department of Health Sciences, University of Florence, Meyer Children's University Hospital, Florence, Italy
[2]Meyer Children's Hospital Healthcare Associated Infection Control Committee, Florence, Italy
Full list of author information is available at the end of the article

National Healthcare Safety Network in United States, showed a reduction of CLABSI rates from 4.9 to 1.5/1000 central line-days in NICU and from 4.7 to 1.0/1000 central line-days in PICU in 5 years time [3]. A trend of infection rate reduction was seen also in a prospective 2-year quality improvement British project conducted in 21 PICU with overall 34,635 central line-days analyzed [4].

Despite the international data available on HAIs in selected groups of patients, there is a lack of large and good quality studies. The best methodology to obtain reliable data would be a continuous prospective study. However, this type of study would require dedicated staff and enormous financial resources. Short prospective study or Point-prevalence survey are possible strategies. In the first case, data are collected about a certain period of time, giving a good estimate of the global burden and being cost-saving. The point-prevalence survey gives a punctiform picture (usually a day), allows collecting data in an easy and low-cost way but it is less accurate than the previous method. A Canadian point-prevalence survey was done on about 1353 pediatric patients with central-line access or with assisted-ventilation. Data were collected for 24 h in 30 hospitals. One hundred-eighteen patients (8.7%) had a HAI, of those 38 events (30.7%) were CLABSI [5]. A prospective study performed in 29 NICU in United States between October 2006 and December 2007 found that the risk of CLABSI is very low during the first week of catheterization and especially with lines inserted in the jugular vein, whereas it is increased in oncological and gastrointestinal patients and in case of prolonged catheterization [6]. Further recent studies estimated that CLABSI results in additional hospital costs on a per-case basis of 45,000 dollars [7–9]. The available studies are usually limited to selected groups of patients as oncological children or patients admitted to PICU. There are few prospective studies performed in a whole hospital in order to investigate the global incidence of HAIs. A Swiss study performed in a single institution between April 2008 and March 2009 on 152 patients showed an overall CLABSI incidence of 0.95/1000 central line-days. In this study, CLABSI incidence varied by type of catheter and by patient's age, with the highest risk in neonates with Silastic® percutaneous central line [10].

Available data regarding children's HAIs in Italy are limited to selected group of patients. A study done in Naples on 120 oncologic children found a positivity of blood cultures from central line in about one third (28.3%; 128/425 samples) of cases clinically suspected for infection [11]. There are two prospective studies performed in Turin: the first included 748 oncologic or immunologic patients within 7 years, registering 174 episodes of CLABSI [12], whereas the second enrolled 153 children with previous cardio-surgery, founding a CLABSI incidence of 11.7/1000 central line-days [13]. The only point-prevalence survey available in the Italian pediatric population was set in a large tertiary care children's hospital in Rome between 2007 and 2010. A two-weeks period monitoring was performed each year of the study, with 1506 patients included. Overall, 102 (6.8%) HAIs were identified, one third of which were CLABSI [14].

The present study is the first prospective study monitoring for 6 months the occurrence of CLABSI in all departments of a tertiary care children's University hospital.

Methods

Study setting

The Meyer Children's University Hospital is a 198-bed tertiary care university hospital in Florence, Italy. It is the Tuscany Region Pediatric Hospital, but one fourth of children come from other Italian Regions or from abroad. The hospital is structured for intensity of care, with two intensive care units (NICU and PICU), and Departments of oncology, surgery, neuroscience unit (including also neurosurgery patients) and a bone marrow transplant unit. Moreover, there are two medical wards for 14 pediatric medicine sub-specialties, and an unit for elective specialty admissions. The annual hospital inpatient admissions were 8898 in 2014, for overall 53,988 admission-days.

Study population

The study involved prospectively children aged less than 18 years admitted to Meyer Children's University Hospital who had a central line access inserted between the October 15th 2014 and April 14th 2015.

Data collection

During the study period the global number of children admitted to the hospital was monitored daily and the patients meeting the inclusion criteria were enrolled in the study. The data were collected daily by the trained healthcare staff involved in hospital infection control. Ethical approval was not required because the survey was carried out for surveillance purposes according to the criteria of hospital good clinical practice. The surveillance of CLABSI was performed in all the intensive care, medical, surgical and neonatal wards. The data were collected using a standardized format. The data were collected anonymously and entered in the study database, following the international guidelines for data protection.

For each child the following data were entered into the study database: demographic data, reason for admission, underlying illness, type of device, antibiotic treatment. Reasons to stop the follow-up were: hospital discharge, device removal or infection event related to the device.

Clinical, hematological and microbiological criteria for diagnosis were recorded in case of infection. The pathogen identified was also documented.

Case definitions

CLABSI were defined according to the Center for Disease, Control and Prevention (CDC) criteria [15]. CLABSI are defined as laboratory-confirmed bloodstream infection where central line or umbilical catheter was in place for >2 calendar days on the date of event and the line was in place on the date of event or the day before [15]. In order to capture data only about infections acquired during the hospitalization, the definition of CLABSI was considered valid only if the positive blood culture and clinical signs/ symptoms of infection occurred after at least 48 h from admission.

Statistical analysis

Median and interquartile range (IQR) was calculated for continuous measurement in the study groups (i.e., age). Categorical data were compared using the Chi-squared test (or Fisher's exact test, when expected cell sizes were smaller than five). CLABSI incidence rates with 95% confidence limits were calculated and stratified for the study variables. Specifically, the variables included in the analysis were: age, gender, underlying illness, type of device, treatment. For each factor the relative risk (RR) and 95% confidence intervals (95% CI) were evaluated. Statistical analysis was performed using the statistical software SPSS for Windows, version 22.0 (SPSS Inc., Chicago, IL), $p < 0.05$ was considered statistically significant.

Results

Overall, 388 children with central line access were enrolled during their hospital stay, resulting in 7783 catheter observation-days. The median age was 21 months (IQR: 3–105.5). The underlying conditions of the children enrolled in the study were: medical ($n = 135$, 34.8%), oncological ($n = 118$, 30.4%), surgical ($n = 116$, 29.9%) and prematurity ($n = 19$, 4.9%). Median catheter dwell time during hospital admission was 4 days (IQR: 2–9).

During the study period there were 29 episodes of CLABSI in 26 patients. In particular, two children had respectively 2 and 3 infections during the observation period. The characteristics of the children with CLABSI are reported in Table 1.

The global incidence of CLABSI was 3.73/1000 (95% CI: 2.54–5.28) central line-days.

The risk of infection in our study population was significantly correlated to female gender (RR = 2.17, 95% CI: 1.02–4.86, $p = 0.045$). Considering the catheter type, the incidence of CLABSI appeared higher for Broviac and short-term catheters, resulting almost double than Port-a-Cath and peripherally inserted central catheters (PICC). This difference could be explained because in our setting PICC are used mostly for antibiotic treatment compared to Broviac catheters which are mainly used for parenteral nutrition and in oncology patients.

Table 1 Characteristics of the 26 children with CLABSI during the study period

Age (months), median [IQR]	11.5 [4–37]
Gender, n (%)	
- Male	10 (38.5)
- Female	16 (61.5)
Underlying disease, n (%)	
- Medical	15 (57.7)
- Oncological	6 (23.1)
- Surgical	4 (15.4)
- Neonatological	1 (3.8)
Catheter type, n (%)[a]	
- Port-a-Cath	2 (6.9)
- PICC	3 (10.4)
- Short term	11 (37.9)
- Broviac	13 (44.8)
Catheter days, median [IQR]	13 [4–20]
Ward, n (%)[a]	
- ICU	9 (31)
- NICU	4 (13.8)
- Medical wards	9 (31)
- Oncology	4 (13.8)
- Neurology and Neurosurgery	1 (3.5)
- Surgery	2 (6.9)
Treatment, n (%)[a]	
- Yes	24 (82.8)
- No	2 (6.9)
- Unknown	3 (10.3)

IQR interquartile range, *PICC* peripherally inserted central catheters, *ICU* intensive care unit, *NICU* neonatal intensive care unit
[a]calculated on the total number of CLABSI event ($n = 29$)

The highest rate of CLABSI resulted in children with an underlying medical condition (i.e., respiratory, renal or cardiac diseases, neurological or metabolic conditions). In this group of patients, the number of infections were 16 for 2951 central line-days, with an incidence rate of 5.42/1000 catheter-days (IQR 3.10–8.80) and a RR of 2.01 (95% CI: 0.96–4.28), $p = 0.06$. The risk of CLABSI was significantly higher in patients within the respiratory sub-group compared to all the other conditions (RR = 4.38, 95% CI: 1.30–11.74, $p = 0.021$). Patients admitted to intensive care unit and to medical wards had a higher rate of infection (respectively 5.42 and 5.69/1000 catheter-days) compared with the other units; however, this result was not statistically significant. The incidence of CLABSI by population characteristics is reported in Table 2.

In more than half of the patients the pathogens identified were *Enterobacteriaceae* and *Candida spp.* The complete list of the microorganisms found is displayed in Fig. 1.

Discussion

The present study is designed to assess the incidence rate of CLABSI in a whole pediatric children tertiary care hospital in a 6-months prospective surveillance. In our study CLABSI rate is 3.73/1000 (95% CI: 2.54–5.28) central line-days. Comparing studies on CLABSI is challenging due to different study population and methodology used. Only another prospective study, conducted in a whole pediatric hospital, is available in literature [10]. This study included 152 patients for overall 14,752 catheter observation days, with a CLABSI rate of 0.95/1000 central line-days [10]. This lower CLABSI rate should be interpreted considering that, differently from our survey, Wagner and colleagues enrolled mainly neonatal, hematological/oncological and surgical patients. If we consider only these types of patients in our study, the CLABSI rate decreases to 2.69/1000 catheters-days (95% CI: 1.43–4.60). Moreover, the authors concluded that the heterogeneous case mix of the patients enrolled, including also out-patients settings, accounts for the low CLABSI rate found [10]. On the contrary, our study is conducted on inpatients only; therefore, the case mix index of our study population could be estimated on the basis of the average diagnosis-related group (DRG) weight, which was 1.48 in 2014.

Moreover, the present study can be compared with two previous one-month prospective surveys carried out in 2012 and in 2013 in our tertiary-care children's university hospital [16]. The data collected were respectively

Table 2 Distribution of CLABSI incidence by population characteristics

Population characteristics	Catheter days (n)	CLABSI (n)	Incidence of CLABSI (n/1000 catheter days)	95% CI
Age:				
- ≤ 1 year	3196	14	4.38	2.39, 7.35
- >1 year	4587	15	3.27	1.83, 5.39
Gender:				
- Male	4149	10	2.41	1.15, 4.43
- Female	3634	19	5.23	3.15, 8.16
Underlying disease:				
- Medical	2951	16	5.42	3.10, 8.80
- Oncological	2923	8	2.74	1.18, 5.39
- Surgical	1577	4	2.54	0.68, 6.49
- Neonatological	332	1	3.01	0.04, 16.76
Catheter type:				
- Port-a-Cath	775	2	2.58	0.29, 9.32
- PICC	1269	3	2.36	0.47, 6.90
- Short term catheter	2432	11	4.52	2.25, 8.09
- Broviac	2959	13	4.39	2.34, 7.51
- Umbilical vein catheter	105	0	–	–
- Unknown	243	0	–	–
Ward:				
- ICU	1660	9	5.42	2.47, 10.29
- NICU	1377	4	2.90	0.78, 7.44
- Medical ward	1581	9	5.69	2.60, 10.81
- Oncology and BMT	2015	4	1.98	0.53, 5.08
- Neurology and Neurosurgery	449	1	2.23	0.03, 12.39
- Surgery	587	2	3.41	0.38, 12.30
- Speciality ward	114	0	–	–

CI confidence interval, *CLABSI* central-line associated bloodstream infections, *PICC* peripherally inserted central catheter, *ICU* intensive care unit, *NICU* neonatal intensive care unit, *BMT* bone marrow transplant

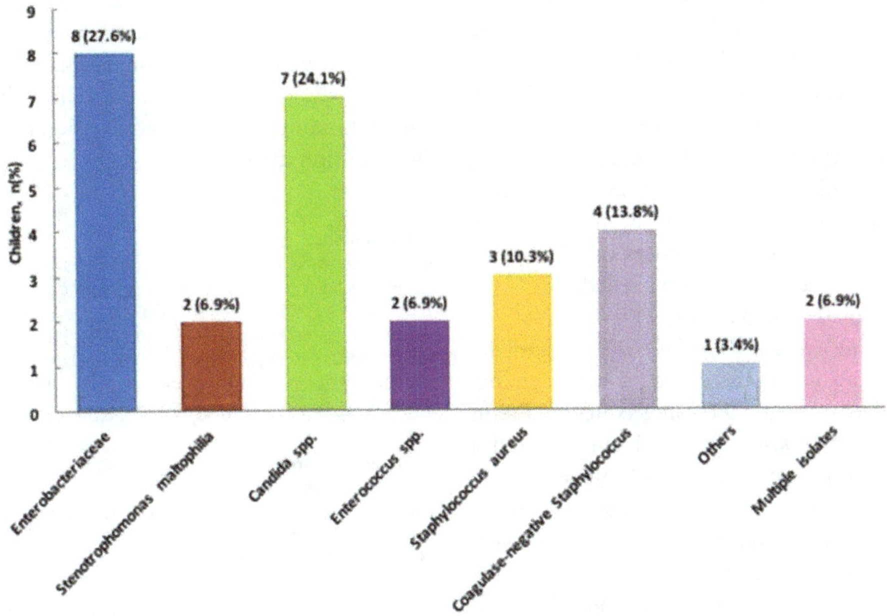

Fig. 1 Microorganisms identified in children with CLABSI. The complete list of the microorganisms found is displayed in the figure. The pathogens isolated in patients with CLABSI are mainly *Enterobacteriaceae* and *Candida spp*. Five infections, out of the 9 cases caused by *Enterobactriaceae* identified are due to extended-spectrum β-lactamase producing organisms (3 *Escherichia coli*, 2 *Klebsiella pneumoniae*) and in one case by carbapenem-resistant *Klebsiella pneumoniae*. Specifically, *Candida albicans* has been identified in 5 (71.4%) patients and *Candida parapsilosis* in other 2 (28.6%) children

on 97 children with CLABSI (935 central line-days) in 2012 and on 122 children (1123 central line-days) in 2013. CLABSI incidence rate found in the two reports was respectively 3.21/1000 catheter days (95% CI: 1.03–9.95) in 2012 and 1.78 (95% CI: 0.45–7.12) in 2013 [16]. CLABSI incidence rate find in the present study almost overlaps with the one found in 2012 survey, but it results higher than the 2013 ones. This fact is probably due to the increasing case mix of our hospital, objectively documented by hospital DRG, as explained above. However, an important limitation of the previous surveys performed in our hospital was the short length of the study, which explains the wide confidence intervals obtained and may justified this difference.

In 2012, our hospital participated to the point prevalence survey coordinated by the ECDC, resulting to have a prevalence of HAIs of 8% (LC 95% 3.9–14.1), 9.1% of those were CLABSI (prevalence 1.8%, 95% CI –0,7–4.2%) [17]. On the other hand, the rate of HAIs in our hospital in 2014 was retrospectively estimated on the basis of laboratory-derived microbiological isolates, resulting 5.6/1000 hospital stay-days (300 infections during 53,988 days of hospitalization, 95% CI 4.9–6.2). Specifically, the analysis of microbiological data showed 39 positive blood cultures in children with central line access, with a CLABSI incidence of 0.51/1.000 central line-days (7605 central line- day, estimated by the prospective study), lower than the incidence of 3.4/1.000 central line-days in 2013. However, the retrospective methodology might underestimate the incidence of CLABSI.

Interestingly, our study points the attention on underlying medical conditions as an important risk factor for developing CLABSI. In the available literature this type of patients was poorly studied, as the attention focused mainly on intensive care and oncological patients [1, 3, 4, 6, 11, 12]. However, in this wide group are included children with high risk of developing catheter related infections for different reasons. For example, in gastroenterological disorders (i.e., short bowel syndrome or inflammatory bowel disease), the parenteral nutrition was seen to be an adjunctive risk for infections [10, 18]. Unfortunately, this information has not been collected in our study. Moreover, in chronic disorders as renal diseases (chronic renal failure, dialysis patients), chronic respiratory conditions (bronchodysplasia, congenital tracheobronchial anomalies) and metabolic diseases the infection risk might be increased by possible immunosuppressive mechanisms in these chronic diseases. Moreover, patients with polymalformative syndromes might require multiple devices for enteral feeding and respiratory support. These conditions could increase the risk of bacteremia and catheter colonization. The risk of infection seems to be particularly higher in the sub-group of respiratory patients. This might be related to the complexity of these patients, who might require a superior intensity of care [19–21].

The risk of developing CLABSI in our study population is almost double in patient with Broviac and short term catheters compared to Port-a-Cath and PICC. Despite few pediatric studies available on CLABSI incidence in patients with PICC [19, 21], studies directly comparing differences by catheter type are limited [10, 22]. Moreover, comparison of unrelated studies is difficult because of heterogeneity in study populations and study methods [23]. Large pediatric prospective studies focuses on identifying the device with lower infections rate are needed.

The pathogens isolated in patients with CLABSI are mainly *Enterobacteriaceae* and *Candida spp. Enterobacteriaceae* spread is an emergent cause of severe infections. These pathogens are of increasing concern due to the rise of carbapenem resistance, which has created a generation of organism resistant to multiple antibiotic classes [24]. In Italy, gram negative resistance rate to third generation cephalosporins is between 30 and 56% [25], whereas the rate of carbapenem resistant Klebsiella is around 34% in invasive infections [26]. There is a lack of prevalence data in pediatric patients.

In our study 5 infections, out of the 9 cases identified are caused by extended-spectrum β-lactamase producing organisms (3 *Escherichia coli*, 2 *Klebsiella pneumoniae*) and in one case by carbapenem-resistant *Klebsiella pneumoniae.* In our surveillance no methicillin resistant *Staphylococcus aureus* nor vancomycin resistant *Enterococcus* infections were detected. The CLABSI caused by *Candida spp.* are beyond the neonatal period thanks to the spreading use of fluconazole prophylaxis. Specifically, *Candida albicans* has been identified in 5 (71.4%) patients and *Candida parapsilosis* in other 2 (28.6%) children.

Regarding CLABSI rate, our study is designed to assess the incidence rate during patients' hospital admission. Therefore, our results could not be extrapolated as an overall CLABSI incidence for each central line implanted, as this rate might differ if the follow-up was extended to the outpatient clinics and to the home-care. Moreover, our results might not necessarily reflect the HAIs incidence of other Italian hospitals because of different settings and case complexity. Monitoring HAIs is the best way to assess the risk factors for infection globally and specifically for each institution. Moreover, it helps in planning preventive interventions to reduce patient's morbidity and mortality, to save costs and to control resistant-microorganisms spread. Point prevalence surveys are cheaper and easier to conduct than long prospective studies, but might underestimate the real risk. Cost-effectiveness balance should be done to choose the best monitoring strategy for each setting.

Conclusions

Our study confirms the spreading of multi-resistant pathogens as causes of healthcare associated infections in children. An increased incidence rate of CLABSI in our study was related to underlying medical conditions. Pediatric studies focusing on healthcare infections in this type of patients should be done in order to deepen our understanding on associated risk factors and possible intervention areas.

Abbreviations

CDC: Center for disease, control and prevention; CI: Confidence interval; CLABSI: Central-line associated bloodstream infections; DRG: Diagnosis-related group; ECDC: European centre for disease prevention and control; HAIs: Healthcare-associated infections; IQR: Interquartile range; NICU: Neonatal intensive care unit; PICC: Peripherally inserted central catheters; PICU: Paediatric intensive care unit; RR: Relative risk

Acknowledgments

CLABSI study group. Alterini M[1], Anziati M[11], Baccini C[2], Bardelli T[3], Baroni M[4], Catarzi F[5], Ciriello E[1], Cozza S[5], Diani G[6], Ficozzi L[2], Francini S[7], Gervaso P[11], Guidozzi L[5], Ingargiola A[8], Lega L[8], Lenzi L[3], Lodi A[9], Loru S[1], Morganti M[6], Morrione T[8], Neri C[7], Paoli F[1], Pierucci E[6], Prato M[11], Putrino R[10], Sollai S[11], Tintori V[1], Tondo A[1], Trefoloni D[3]

1 Oncology Department, Meyer Children's University Hospital, Florence, Italy
2 Healthcare associated infections control committee, Meyer Children's University Hospital, Florence, Italy
3 Pediatric Medicine Department, Meyer Children's University Hospital, Florence, Italy
4 Accreditation and quality assurance, Meyer Children's University Hospital, Florence, Italy
5 Outpatients Department, Meyer Children's University Hospital, Florence, Italy
6 Pediatric Intensive Care Unit, Meyer Children's University Hospital, Florence, Italy
7 Neurology and Neurosurgery ward, Meyer Children's University Hospital, Florence, Italy
8 Neonatal Intensive Care Unit, Meyer Children's University Hospital, Florence, Italy
9 Surgery ward, Meyer Children's University Hospital, Florence, Italy
10 Week Hospital, Meyer Children's University Hospital, Florence, Italy
11 Infectious diseases Division, Pediatric Medicine Department, Meyer Children's University Hospital, Florence, Italy

Funding

Not applicable.

Authors' contributions

EV drafted the manuscript. SB and AB contributed in the acquisition of data, or analysis and interpretation of data. CM, EC, KPB and SDM participated in the design of the study and performed the statistical analysis. LG and MdM conceived of the study, and participated in its design and coordination and helped to draft the manuscript. All authors read and approved the final manuscript.

Competing interests

The authors declare that they have no competing interests.

Consent for publication

Not applicable.

Author details

[1]Department of Health Sciences, University of Florence, Meyer Children's University Hospital, Florence, Italy. [2]Meyer Children's Hospital Healthcare Associated Infection Control Committee, Florence, Italy. [3]Pediatric Infectious Diseases Division, Department of Pediatric Medicine, Meyer Children's University Hospital, viale Pieraccini 24, I-50139 Florence, Italy.

References

1. Rosenthal VD, Maki DG, Mehta Y, Leblebicioglu H, Memish ZA, Al-Mousa HH, et al. International Nosocomial Infection Control Consortium (INICC) report, data summary of 43 countries for 2007–2012, Device-associated module. Am J Infect Control. 2014;42:942–56.
2. European Centre for Disease Control and Prevention. Annual epidemiological report 2014-Antimicrobial resistance and healthcare-associated infections. 2014. http://ecdc.europa.eu/en/publications/surveillance_reports/annual_epidemiological_report/Pages/epi_index.aspx. Accessed 27 Jun 2016.
3. Patrick SW, Kawai AT, Kleinman K, Jin R, Vaz L, Gay C, et al. Health care-associated infections among critically ill children in the US, 2007–2012. Pediatrics. 2014;134:705–12.
4. Bion J, Richardson A, Hibbert P, Beer J, Abrusci T, McCutcheon M, et al. 'Matching Michigan': a 2-year stepped interventional programme to minimise central venous catheter-blood stream infections in intensive care units in England. BMJ Qual Saf. 2013;22:110–23.
5. Rutledge-Taylor K, Matlow A, Gravel D, Embree J, Le Saux N, Johnston L, et al. A point prevalence survey of health care-associated infections in Canadian pediatric inpatients. Am J Infect Control. 2012;40:491–6.
6. Niedner MF, Huskins WC, Colantuoni E, Muschelli J, Harris 2nd JM, Rice TB, et al. Epidemiology of central line-associated bloodstream infections in the pediatric intensive care unit. Infect Control Hosp Epidemiol. 2011;32:1200–8.
7. Zimlichman E, Henderson D, Tamir O, Franz C, Song P, Yamin CK, et al. Health care-associated infections: a meta-analysis of costs and financial impact on the US health care system. JAMA Intern Med. 2013;173:2039–46.
8. Goudie A, Dynan L, Brady PW, Rettiganti M. Attributable cost and length of stay for central line-associated bloodstream infections. Pediatrics. 2014;133:1525–32.
9. Wilson MZ, Rafferty C, Deeter D, Comito MA, Hollenbeak CS. Attributable costs of central line-associated bloodstream infections in a pediatric hematology/oncology population. Am J Infect Control. 2014;42:1157–60.
10. Wagner M, Bonhoeffer J, Erb TO, Glanzmann R, Hacker FM, Paulussen M, et al. Prospective study on central venous line associated bloodstream infections. Arch Dis Child. 2011;96:827–31.
11. Coco I, Casale F, Indolfi P. Infections from CVC in the pediatric neoplastic patient. Single institution experience. Minerva Pediatr. 2012;64:385–94.
12. Pinon M, Bezzio S, Tovo PA, Fagioli F, Farinasso L, Calabrese L, et al. A prospective 7-year survey on central venous catheter-related complications at a single pediatric hospital. Eur J Pediatr. 2009;168:1505–12.
13. Bezzio S, Scolfaro C, Broglia R, Calabrese R, Mignone F, Abruzzese PA, et al. Prospective incidence study of bloodstream infection in infants and children with central venous catheters after cardiac surgery in Italy. Infect Control Hosp Epidemiol. 2009;30:698–701.
14. Ciofi Degli Atti ML, Cuttini M, Ravà L, Ceradini J, Paolini V, Ciliento G, et al. Trend of healthcare-associated infections in children: annual prevalence surveys in a research hospital in Italy, 2007–2010. J Hosp Infect. 2012;80:6–12.
15. Centers of Disease Control and Prevention. Bloodstream Infection Event (Central Line-Associated Bloodstream Infection and Non-central line-associated Bloodstream Infection). 2015. www.cdc.gov/nhsn/PDFs/pscManual/4PSC_CLABScurrent.pdf. Accessed 27 Jun 2016.
16. Galli L, Becciani S, Anziati M, et al. Incidence study on central line associated bloodstream infections (CLABSI) and on ventilation associated pneumonia (VAP). Poster presentation. ESPID 2014, Dublin.
17. European Centre for Disease Control and Prevention. Point prevalence survey of healthcare-associated infections and antimicrobial use in European acute care hospitals, 2011–2012. http://ecdc.europa.eu/en/publications/Publications/healthcare-associated-infections-antimicrobial-use-PPS.pdf. Accessed 27 Jun 2016.
18. Advani S, Reich NG, Sengupta A, Gosey L, Milstone AM. Central line-associated bloodstream infection in hospitalized children with peripherally inserted central venous catheters: extending risk analyses outside the intensive care unit. Clin Infect Dis. 2011;52:1108–15.
19. Barrier A, Williams DJ, Connelly M, Creech CB. Frequency of peripherally inserted central catheter complications in children. Pediatr Infect Dis J. 2012;31:519–21.
20. Jumani K, Advani S, Reich NG, Gosey L, Milstone AM. Risk factors for peripherally inserted central venous catheter complications in children. JAMA Pediatr. 2013;167:429–35.
21. Levy I, Bendet M, Samra Z, Shalit I, Katz J. Infectious complications of peripherally inserted central venous catheters in children. Pediatr Infect Dis J. 2010;29:426–9.
22. Goes-Silva E, Abreu TF, Frota AC, Pessoa-Silva CL, Cunha AJ, Hofer CB. Use of peripherally inserted central catheters to prevent catheter-associated bloodstream infection in children. Infect Control Hosp Epidemiol. 2009;30:1024–6.
23. Westergaard B, Classen V, Walther-Larsen S. Peripherally inserted central catheters in infants and children - indications, techniques, complications and clinical recommendations. Acta Anaesthesiol Scand. 2013;57:278–87.
24. Logan LK. Carbapenem-resistant enterobacteriaceae: an emerging problem in children. Clin Infect Dis. 2012;55:852–9.
25. European Centre for Disease Prevention and Control. Antimicrobial resistance interactive database (EARS-Net). http://ecdc.europa.eu/en/healthtopics/antimicrobial_resistance/database/Pages/database.aspx. Accessed on 27 Jun 2016.
26. Montagnani C, Prato M, Scolfaro C, Colombo S, Esposito S, Tagliabue C, et al. Carbapenem-resistant Enterobacteriaceae infections in children: an Italian retrospective multicenter study. Pediatr Infect Dis J. 2016;35:862–8. [Epub ahead of print].

16

Trends in the annual incidence of carbapenem-resistant *Klebsiella pneumoniae* bloodstream infections: a 8-year retrospective study in a large teaching hospital in northern Italy

Cristiano Alicino[1†], Daniele Roberto Giacobbe[2*†], Andrea Orsi[1], Federico Tassinari[1], Cecilia Trucchi[1], Giovanni Sarteschi[2], Francesco Copello[3], Valerio Del Bono[2], Claudio Viscoli[2] and Giancarlo Icardi[1]

Abstract

Background: Bloodstream infections (BSI) due to carbapenem-resistant (C-R) *Klebsiella pneumoniae* (Kp) are of global concern from both clinical and public health standpoints. This retrospective study aimed to describe C-R Kp BSI epidemiology in a large teaching hospital in northern Italy.

Methods: Between 1 January 2007 and 31 December 2014, annual incidences both of C-R Kp BSI and of carbapenem-susceptible (C-S) Kp BSI were calculated as the number of events per 10,000 patient-days. A Chi square test for linear trend was used to assess the change in the incidence of C-R Kp BSI and C-S Kp BSI over the study period. Crude 30-day mortality rates were provided both for C-R Kp BSI and for C-S Kp BSI.

Results: From 2007 to 2014, we observed 511 episodes of Kp BSI, 349 of which were caused by C-R Kp (68.3 %). The incidence of C-R Kp BSI considerably increased from 0.04/10,000 patient-days in 2007 to 1.77/10,000 patient-days in 2014 (Chi square for trend $p < 0.001$). The highest incidence of C-R Kp BSI was observed in intensive care units (ICUs), with a peak of 22.01 C-R Kp BSI/10,000 patient-days in 2012. A less marked but significant increase of C-S Kp BSI was also observed (Chi square for trend $p = 0.004$). Crude 30-day mortality was 36.1 % in patients with C-R Kp BSI and 23.5 % in those with C-S Kp BSI.

Conclusions: During the study period, we observed a dramatic increase in the incidence of C-R Kp BSI in our hospital. More concerted infection-control efforts are needed to contain this alarming C-R Kp diffusion.

Keywords: Incidence, Bloodstream infection, Carbapenem-resistant *Klebsiella pneumoniae*

Background

Bloodstream infections (BSI) due to carbapenem-resistant (C-R) *Klebsiella pneumoniae* (Kp) are of global concern from both clinical and public health standpoints. Indeed, these severe infections are caused by rapidly spreading clones that are frequently resistant to almost all the antibiotics used in the everyday clinical practice [1–6].

Occurring especially across Southern Europe, the rapid diffusion of C-R Kp has worryingly impressed the medical community, and several guidelines have been recently developed to reduce the spread of these difficult-to-treat gram-negative rods [7–9]. In Italy, carbapenem resistance among blood Kp isolates has dramatically increased from 1.3 % in 2009 to 29.1 % in 2012, and even higher rates of 34.3 % have been reported in 2013 [10, 11]. With the aim of more clearly investigate this alarming C-R Kp diffusion, we retrospectively assessed the epidemiology of C-R Kp BSI in a large teaching hospital in northern Italy over a 8-year period.

* Correspondence: daniele.roberto.giacobbe@gmail.com
†Equal contributors
[2]Department of Health Sciences, University of Genoa and Infectious Diseases Unit, IRCCS AOU San Martino-IST teaching Hospital, L.go R. Benzi, 10-16132 Genoa, Italy
Full list of author information is available at the end of the article

Methods

Data collection and definitions

We performed a retrospective study in IRCCS AOU San Martino – IST, a 1,300-beds tertiary adult acute-care teaching hospital in Genoa, Italy. Between 1 January 2007 and 31 December 2014, numbers of hospital patient-days were obtained from the digital archives of patients' clinical charts. Then, numbers of both carbapenem-susceptible (C-S) BSI and C-R Kp BSI were identified through the computerized microbiology laboratory database. The completeness and quality of laboratory data was successfully assessed by matching the hospital admission code with data obtained by clinical charts.

Only health-care associated C-R Kp BSI were considered for the analysis. According to the European Center for Disease Control and prevention (ECDC) definitions, a health-care associated C-R Kp BSI was defined as a positive blood culture collected at least 48 h after hospital admission, or within 48 h from hospital admission in those patients who had been discharged in the preceding two days [12]. For patients with multiple episodes of C-R Kp BSI, a novel event was considered as independent if occurring at least 30 days after the last positive blood culture [12].

This epidemiological analysis was performed within the Institutional surveillance of C-R Kp BSI that is periodically reported to the Regional Health Authority as a component of the Regional Plan for the Healthcare-associated infections Prevention and Control, approved by regional and national laws [13, 14]. The study involved the analysis of existing anonymized clinical and laboratory data. An informed consent for the use of anonymized data for scientific purposes is signed by all patients admitted to IRCCS AOU San Martino – IST and included in surveillance databases. The study has been approved by the Regional Ethics Committee of Liguria Region.

Microbiology

The Vitek 2 system (bioMérieux, Marcy l'Etoile, France) was used for Kp identification and antimicrobial susceptibility testing. The interpretative breakpoints were based on the European Committee on Antimicrobial Susceptibility Testing (EUCAST) criteria (EUCAST breakpoint tables for interpretation of MICs and zone diameters, version 4.0, 2014; http://www.eucast.org). For the analysis of data, Kp isolates which were resistant to one or more carbapenems tested in our institution (i.e., ertapenem, imipenem, or meropenem) were considered to be C-R, while isolates showing full or intermediate susceptibility to all tested carbapenems were classified as C-S.

Statistical analysis

The primary study analysis aimed to establish the annual incidences of C-R Kp BSI during the study period. Annual incidences of C-R Kp BSI with their 95 % confidence intervals (CI) were calculated as the number of events per 10,000 patient-days. In addition, annual incidences of C-R Kp BSI were also stratified by subgroups according to the ward where the diagnosis of C-R Kp BSI was made (i.e., intensive care units [ICUs], medical wards, surgical wards, or rehabilitation wards). A Chi square test for linear trend was used to assess the change in the incidence of C-R Kp BSI in our hospital over the study period.

An additional aim was to detail the overall trends in the incidence of Kp BSI. Therefore, annual incidences of health-care associated C-S Kp BSI were also calculated, by means of the methods described above. Finally, crude 30-day mortality rates were assessed both for C-R Kp BSI and for C-S Kp BSI.

All the analyses were performed using Epi-Info 7.0 (Centers for Disease Control and Prevention, CDC, Atlanta, GA, USA) and the SPSS Statistics version 20.0 (IBM Corp., Armonk, NY, USA).

Results

Between January 2007 and December 2014, we identified 511 episodes of Kp BSI, 349 of which were caused by C-R Kp (68.3 %). These episodes occurred in 327 patients, of whom 19 had recurrent infections (5.8 %). The median age of patients was 68 years (interquartile range [IQR] 57–76). As many as 231/349 C-R Kp BSI occurred in males (66.2 %), thus defining a 2:1 male to female ratio. The median time to C-R Kp BSI diagnosis from hospital admission was 24 days (IQR 12–45), and the median length of hospital stay was 52 days (IQR 30–90).

During the study period, the overall incidence of C-R Kp BSI was 0.92/10,000 patient-days, increasing from 0.04/10,000 patient-days in 2007 to 1.77/10,000 patient-days in 2014 (Chi square for trend $p < 0.001$). Detailed year-by-year incidences of C-R Kp BSI are outlined in Table 1, which also reports annual incidences of C-R Kp BSI according to wards' subgroups. As shown in the table, C-R Kp BSI were first observed in 2007, reflecting a limited cluster in ICUs. No C-R Kp BSI occurred in 2008, while they reappeared since 2009, with annual incidences increasing from 0.56/10,000 patient-days in 2009 to 1.75/10,000 patient-days in 2012. After a temporary decrease in 2013, the incidence of C-R Kp BSI rose again to 1.77/10,000 patient-days in 2014.

Overall, the incidence of Kp BSI (C-R plus C-S) increased from 0.50/10,000 patient-days in 2007 to 2.42/10,000 patient-days in 2014 (Chi square for trend $p < 0.001$). The singular trends of C-R Kp BSI and C-S Kp BSI over the study period are depicted in Fig. 1. As shown in the figure, the overall increase in the incidence of Kp BSI was mostly due to C-R Kp BSI, although a less

Table 1 Annual incidences of health-care associated carbapenem-resistant *Klebsiella pneumoniae* bloodstream infections

Year	No. of episodes	Incidence per 10,000 patient-days (95 % CI)				
		Ward where the diagnosis of C-R Kp BSI was made				
		Overall	ICU	Surgical wards	Medical wards	Rehabilitation wards
2007	2	0.04 (0.01 – 0.17)	1.15 (0.29 – 4.59)	-	-	-
2008	0	-	-	-	-	-
2009	27	0.56 (0.38 -0.82)	12.70 (8.44 – 19.1)	0.14 (0.04 – 0.57)	0.04 (0 – 0.28)	0.60 (0.09-4.27)
2010	39	0.83 (0.60-1.13)	17.18 (11.94 – 24.71)	0.08 (0.01 – 0.55)	0.32 (0.16 – 0.64)	0.44 (0.06 – 3.12)
2011	59	1.22 (0.94-1.57)	21.06 (15.40-28.81)	0.69 (0.36-1.32)	0.36 (0.19 – 0.69)	0.60 (0.02 – 2.39)
2012	83	1.75 (1.41-2.17)	22.01 (16.09 – 30.11)	1.55 (0.99-2.43)	0.96 (0.64 -1.44)	0.44 (0.11 – 1.76)
2013	60	1.30 (1.01 – 1.68)	18.17 (12.98 – 25.42)	0.61 (0.29 – 1.29)	0.72 (0.44 – 1.17)	0.48 (0.15 – 1.48)
2014	79	1.77 (1.42 – 2.20)	18.79 (13.62 – 25.93)	0.66 (0.31 – 1.37)	1.32 (0.92 – 1.89)	0.98 (0.41 – 2.36)

C-R Kp BSI carbapenem-resistant *Klebsiella pneumoniae* bloodstream infections, *ICU* intensive care unit

marked but significant increase of C-S Kp BSI was also observed (Chi square for trend $p = 0.004$).

Finally, crude 30-day mortality was higher in patients with C-R Kp BSI than in those with C-S Kp BSI (36.1 vs. 23.5 %, respectively). However, this comparison was not further considered in our analyses, since it could not be adjusted for some important clinical confounders (e.g., severity of illness, type of antibiotic therapy) that were not explored in this epidemiologic study.

Discussion

From 2007 to 2014 we noticed an impressive increase of more than 300 % in the incidence of Kp BSI in our hospital, that was mostly driven by C-R strains. This finding is of particular concern, since C-R Kp BSI carry a heavy burden in terms of morbidity and mortality [3–6].

A worrisome and persistent increase of carbapenem-resistance among Kp isolates has been reported in Italy since 2005, with current national rates being as high as 34 % [11, 12]. Our experience confirms this picture, since we observed a rapid increase in the incidence of C-R Kp BSI starting from 2007, that peaked at 1.75/10,000 patient-days in 2012. A temporary decrease was then observed in 2013, possibly because of the intensification of our hospital-based infection control measures (i.e., rapid identification of colonized and/or infected patients trough a centralized and computerized laboratory-based alert system, patient dedicated use of gowns and gloves) that occurred at that time. Starting from the same period, an active surveillance of colonized patients and their contacts was also implemented, by means of rectal swab and according to European guidelines [9].

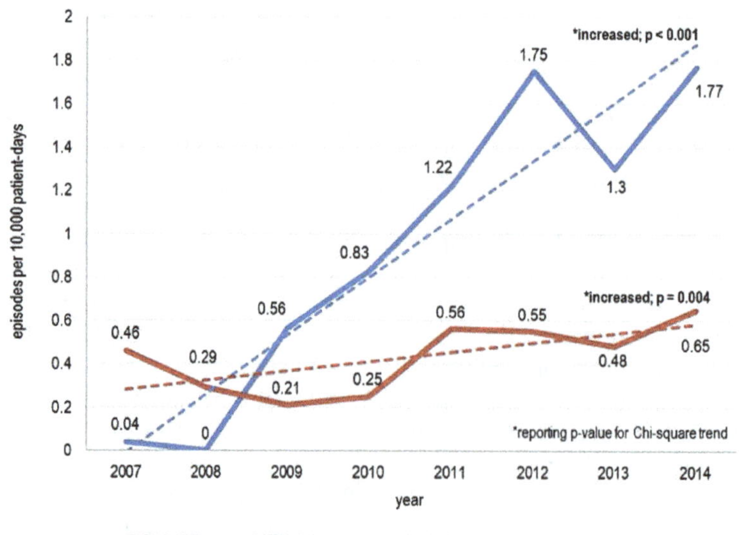

Fig. 1 Annual incidences of health-care associated *Klebsiella pneumoniae* bloodstream infections (C-R and C-S)

All these measures have been already proven to reduce the incidence of infections due to multidrug resistant gram negatives, including C-R Kp [15–19]. However, after the temporary decrease mentioned above, the incidence of C-R Kp BSI in our hospital rose again to 1.77/10,000 patient-days in 2014. Although a lack of adherence to contention measures might have occurred in some cases, another factor possibly underlie this increase that mostly occurred outside the ICU. Indeed, we recently observed that some C-R Kp intestinal carriers in low risk wards (i.e., wards other than ICU or cancer wards) might not be considered at risk (and thus not screened) even if all recommended infection-control protocols are adopted [20]. This finding suggests that a considerable number of unknown carriers might be circulating in our hospital that are not subjected to contact precautions because of the unawareness of their status. This possibility is rather worrisome, since it could lead to an uncontrolled C-R Kp diffusion, thus fueling the reservoir of patients who possibly develop C-R Kp BSI [20, 21]. In such an uncontrolled endemic setting, further infection-control efforts (e.g., a dynamic redefinition of wards to adopt universal screening through regular point-prevalence surveys) might be necessary to successfully counteract the alarming spread of C-R Kp.

The present study has some important limitations. First, we could not depict the true pattern of C-R Kp diffusion, since only blood C-R Kp isolates were considered. However, C-R Kp BSI can provide a reliable picture of this diffusion, since blood cultures are collected from nearly all patients with C-R Kp BSI because of the symptomatic nature of the infection. Conversely, any possible estimation based on colonized patients would have been affected by an important selection bias due to the differences in the number of screened patients across the study years. Second, the retrospective nature of the study prevented us from investigating the degree of compliance to infection-control measures during the study period, as well as the molecular characteristics of C-R Kp isolates. In this regard, a major limitation is the lack of information about both the clonal type of Kp isolates and their mechanisms of resistance to carbapenems. Finally, this was a single center study, and incidences of C-R Kp BSI may differ significantly across centers. Therefore, any extrapolation of our findings to other settings should be made with due caution.

Conclusions

In our hospital a dramatic increase in the incidence of C-R Kp BSI occurred from 2007 to 2014 that appeared to be only temporarily arrested by the intensification of hospital-based infection-control measures. More concerted efforts are necessary to tackle this alarming C-R Kp diffusion. Because of the dramatic shortage in antibiotics active against C-R Kp, further improvements in our infection-control protocols are also of paramount importance to curtail the high number of deaths due to C-R Kp BSI.

Abbreviations

BSI: Bloodstream infections; C-R: Carbapenem-resistant; C-S: Carbapenem-susceptible; CI: Confidence intervals; ECDC: European Center for Disease Control and prevention; EUCAST: European Committee on Antimicrobial Susceptibility Testing; Kp: *Klebsiella pneumoniae*; ICUs: Intensive care units; IQR: Interquartile range; MICs: Minimum inhibitory concentrations.

Competing interest

All authors report no conflicts of interest relevant to this article.

Authors' contributions

CA and DRG conceived and designed the research, collected data, cleaned and analyzed the data, and drafted and revised the paper. AO conceived and designed the research and drafted and revised the paper. FT collected and cleaned the data and revised the paper. CT revised the paper. GS collected and cleaned the data and revised the paper. FC collected the data and revised the paper. VDB revised the paper. CV conceived and designed the research and revised the paper. GI conceived and designed the research and revised the paper. All authors read and approved the final manuscript.

Acknowledgments

Financial support

None reported.

Author details

[1]Department of Health Sciences, University of Genoa and Hygiene and Infection Control Unit, IRCCS AOU San Martino-IST teaching Hospital, Genoa, Italy. [2]Department of Health Sciences, University of Genoa and Infectious Diseases Unit, IRCCS AOU San Martino-IST teaching Hospital, L.go R. Benzi, 10-16132 Genoa, Italy. [3]Occupational Medicine Unit, IRCCS AOU San Martino-IST teaching Hospital, Genoa, Italy.

References

1. Munoz-Price LS, Poirel L, Bonomo RA, Schwaber MJ, Daikos GL, Cormican M, et al. Clinical epidemiology of the global expansion of Klebsiella pneumoniae carbapenemases. Lancet Infect Dis. 2013;13:785–96.
2. Nordmann P, Dortet L, Poirel L. Carbapenem resistance in Enterobacteriaceae: here is the storm! Trends Mol Med. 2012;18:263–72.
3. Qureshi ZA, Paterson DL, Potoski BA, Kilayko MC, Sandovsky G, Sordillo E, et al. Treatment outcome of bacteremia due to KPC-producing Klebsiella pneumoniae: superiority of combination antimicrobial regimens. Antimicrob Agents Chemother. 2012;56:2108–13.
4. Tumbarello M, Viale P, Viscoli C, Trecarichi EM, Tumietto F, Marchese A, et al. Predictors of mortality in bloodstream infections caused by Klebsiella pneumoniae carbapenemase-producing K. pneumoniae: importance of combination therapy. Clin Infect Dis. 2012;55:943–50.
5. Zarkotou O, Pournaras S, Tselioti P, Dragoumanos V, Pitiriga V, Ranellou K, et al. Predictors of mortality in patients with bloodstream infections caused by KPC-producing Klebsiella pneumoniae and impact of appropriate antimicrobial treatment. Clin Microbiol Infect. 2011;17:1798–803.
6. Tumbarello M, Trecarichi EM, De Rosa FG, Giannella M, Giacobbe DR, Bassetti M, et al. Infections caused by KPC-producing Klebsiella pneumoniae: differences in therapy and mortality in a multicentre study. J Antimicrob Chemother. 2015;70:2133–43.
7. Centers for Disease Control and Prevention (CDC). Guidance for control of infections with carbapenem-resistant or carbapenemase-producing Enterobacteriaceae in acute care facilities. MMWR Morb Mortal Wkly Rep. 2009;58:256–60.
8. European Centre for Disease Prevention and Control. Risk assessment on the spread of carbapenemase-producing Enterobacteriaceae (CPE) through patient transfer between healthcare facilities, with special emphasis on cross-border transfer. Stockholm: ECDC; 2011.

9. Tacconelli E, Cataldo MA, Dancer SJ, De Angelis G, Falcone M, Frank U, et al. ESCMID guidelines for the management of the infection control measures to reduce transmission of multidrug-resistant Gram-negative bacteria in hospitalized patients. Clin Microbiol Infect. 2014;20:1–55.
10. European Centre for Disease Prevention and Control. Antimicrobial resistance surveillance in Europe 2013. Annual Report of the European Antimicrobial Resistance Surveillance Network (EARS-Net). Stockholm: ECDC; 2014.
11. European Centre for Disease Prevention and Control. Antimicrobial resistance surveillance in Europe 2012. Annual Report of the European Antimicrobial Resistance Surveillance Network (EARS-Net). Stockholm: ECDC; 2013.
12. HELICS Surveillance of Nosocomial Infections in Intensive Care Units protocol, version 6.1, September 2004. Available from http://ecdc.europa.eu/en/activities/surveillance/HAI/Documents/0409_IPSE_ICU_protocol.pdf. Accessed date October 1, 2015.
13. Agenzia Regionale Sanitaria della Regione Liguria. Determina del Direttore Generale n. 125 del 19/12/2014 "Gestione di Enterobacteriaceae resistenti ai carbapeneminelle Strutture Sanitarie". Available from http://www.arsliguria.it/index.php?option=com_docman&task=doc_download&gid=1284&Itemid=240.
14. Ministero della Salute. Circolare del Ministero della Salute n. 4968 del 26/02/2013 "Sorveglianza, e controllo delle infezioni da batteri produttori di carbapenemasi (CPE). Available from http://www.trovanorme.salute.gov.it/norme/renderNormsanPdf;jsessionid=f7-y3XA5uvri021r5t2+Kw__.sgc3-prd-sal?anno=0&codLeg=45499&parte=1%20&serie=.
15. Gbaguidi-Haore H, Legast S, Thouverez M, Bertrand X, Talon D. Ecological study of the effectiveness of isolation precautions in the management of hospitalized patients colonized or infected with Acinetobacter baumannii. Infect Control Hosp Epidemiol. 2008;29:1118–23.
16. Kochar S, Sheard T, Sharma R, Hui A, Tolentino E, Allen G, et al. Success of an infection control program to reduce the spread of carbapenem-resistant Klebsiella pneumoniae. Infect Control Hosp Epidemiol. 2009;30:447–52.
17. Vonberg RP, Wolter A, Chaberny IF, Kola A, Ziesing S, Suerbaum S, et al. Epidemiology of multi-drug-resistant gram-negative bacteria: data from an university hospital over a 36-month period. Int J Hyg Environ Health. 2008;211:251–57.
18. Viale P, Tumietto F, Giannella M, Bartoletti M, Tedeschi S, Ambretti S, et al. Impact of a hospital-wide multifaceted programme for reducing carbapenem-resistant Enterobacteriaceae infections in a large teaching hospital in northern Italy. Clin Microbiol Infect. 2015;21:242–7.
19. Hayden MK, Lin MY, Lolans K, Weiner S, Blom D, Moore NM, et al. Prevention of Colonization and Infection by Klebsiella pneumoniae Carbapenemase-Producing Enterobacteriaceae in Long-term Acute-Care Hospitals. Clin Infect Dis. 2015;60:1153–61.
20. Giacobbe DR, Del Bono V, Marchese A, Viscoli C. Early carbapenem-resistant Klebsiella pneumoniae bacteraemia: should we expand the screening? Clin Microbiol Infect. 2014;20:01157–8.
21. Giannella M, Trecarichi EM, De Rosa FG, Del Bono V, Bassetti M, Lewis RE, et al. Risk factors for carbapenem-resistant Klebsiella pneumoniae bloodstream infection among rectal carriers: a prospective observational multicenter study. Clin Microbiol Infect. 2014;20:1357–62.

17

Peripheral venous catheter-related bloodstream infection is associated with severe complications and potential death

Akihiro Sato[1,2], Itaru Nakamura[1*], Hiroaki Fujita[1,3], Ayaka Tsukimori[1,3], Takehito Kobayashi[1,3], Shinji Fukushima[1], Takeshi Fujii[2] and Tetsuya Matsumoto[3]

Abstract

Background: The purpose of this study was to identify the clinical characteristics and outcomes of peripheral vascular catheter-related bloodstream infections (PVC-BSIs) and determine the risk of severe complications or death.

Methods: We performed a retrospective observational study from June 2010 to April 2015 at two regional university-affiliated hospitals in Tokyo. We studied the clinical manifestations, underlying diseases, laboratory results, treatment methods, recurrence rates, and complications in 62 hospitalized patients diagnosed with PVC-BSIs by positive blood cultures.

Results: The median time from admission to bacteremia was 17 days (range, 3–142 days) and that from catheter insertion to bacteremia diagnosis was 6 days (range, 2–15 days). Catheter insertion sites were in the arm in 48 (77.4%) patients, in the foot in 3 (4.8%) patients, and in an unrecorded location in 11 (17.7%) patients. Additionally, the causative pathogens were Gram-positive microorganisms in 58.0% of cases, Gram-negative microorganisms in 35.8% of cases, Candida spp. in 6.2% of cases, and polymicrobials in 25.8% of cases. Eight (12.9%) patients died within 30 days of their blood culture becoming positive. Patients who died of PVC-BSIs had a higher proportion of *Staphylococcus aureus* infection than patients who survived (odds ratio, 8.33; $p = 0.004$).

Conclusions: PVC-BSIs are a significant cause of health care-associated infection. We observed cases of severe PVC-BSI requiring intensive and long-term care along with lengthy durations of antibiotic treatment due to hematogenous complications, and some patients died. For patients with PVC-BSIs, *S. aureus* bacteremia remains a major problem that may influence the prognosis.

Keywords: Peripheral venous catheter-related bloodstream infection, Catheter-related bloodstream infection, Sepsis, *Staphylococcus aureus*

Background

Reported nosocomial infection sites include the urinary tract (34%), surgical wounds (17%), bloodstream (14%), and lower respiratory tract (13%) [1]. The catheter retained in a blood vessel is the most common cause of bloodstream infections, and catheter-related bloodstream infection (CRBSI) has been the subject of extensive surveillance and research. However, although intravenous devices are indispensable in modern-day medical practice and are used in most hospitalized patients, many such reports involve central venous CRBSIs (CVC-BSIs), not peripheral vascular CRBSIs (PVC-BSIs), and clinical and epidemiological data on PVC-BSI are lacking [2–5]. A previous study reported an incidence of 0.5 and 2.7 episodes per 1000 patient-days for PVC-BSI and CVC-BSI, respectively. The reported incidence of PVC-BSIs is lower than that of CVC-BSIs, but the cumulative duration of PVC insertion

* Correspondence: task300@tokyo-med.ac.jp
[1]Department of Infection Prevention and Control, Tokyo Medical University Hospital, 6-7-1 Nishishinjuku, Shinjuku-ku, Tokyo 160-0023, Japan
Full list of author information is available at the end of the article

is 15 times that of CVC insertion because PVCs are inserted in 30 to 80% of inpatients [6]. Although the frequency of infection is low, the number of PVC-BSIs is high because of the high number of patients undergoing PVC insertion.

In the clinical setting, we sometimes observe PVC-BSI cases that subsequently cause local and systemic complications, suppurative thrombophlebitis, and osteomyelitis. These complications may become severe, necessitating admission to the intensive care unit and resulting in death in some cases. In particular, superficial thrombophlebitis occurs at a frequency ranging from 6.8 to 21.7% [7, 8]. Risk factors for thrombophlebitis are numerous but depend mainly on the type of infusion and duration of peripheral catheter use [9]. Local infection occurs in 0.08–6.90% of cases, but its course is usually mild [10]. Severe infection is much less frequent (0.036–0.100% of cases) but is responsible for high morbidity and mortality rates [11]. Moreover, these severe complications lengthen the treatment period and worsen the prognosis. We must, therefore, recognize that in addition to CVC-BSIs, PVC-BSIs are also important nosocomial infections.

The objective of our study was to describe the clinical characteristics and outcomes of PVC-BSIs and elucidate their associated risk of severe complications or death.

Methods

We retrospectively studied the clinical manifestations, underlying diseases, laboratory results, treatment methods, recurrence rates, and complications in 62 patients diagnosed with PVC-BSIs by positive blood cultures from 1 June 2010 to 30 April 2015 at two regional hospitals in Tokyo: Tokyo Medical University Hospital (a 1015-bed university-affiliated hospital) and Tokyo Medical University Hachioji Medical Center (a 610-bed university-affiliated hospital). The study population included all hospitalized patients.

The diagnostic criteria for PVC-BSIs were as follows: I) growth of concordant bacterial species in a semi-quantitative tip culture and percutaneously drawn blood cultures without another apparent source of bacteremia, or II) catheter tip culture was not performed but bacteremia was present with one of the following conditions: (i) phlebitis (including redness, swelling, pain, or purulent discharge) or (ii) clear resolution of clinical symptoms upon catheter withdrawal and careful exclusion of an alternative explanation for the bacteremia. The infectious disease specialists in our hospitals personally examined all patients at the time when blood cultures began showing positive results and excluded any other apparent sources of bacteremia. Overall mortality was defined as the death of the patient within 30 days of hospitalization after the BSI.

PVCs were usually inserted by doctors and maintained by ward nurses using aseptic techniques. During the 5 years of this study, there were not any policy or protocol changes that affected the way in which PVCs were inserted. The skin was prepared with a single-patient applicator containing 76.9 vol% to 81.4 vol% ethanol and allowed to dry. The physician's hands were decontaminated using an established hand hygiene procedure before and after contact with each patient. Hands were cleaned immediately before donning and after removing gloves. Gloves were single-use and were removed and discarded immediately after use. A sterile, transparent, semipermeable dressing was used to allow for daily observation of the insertion site. PVCs were re-sited every week or sooner if there was evidence of phlebitis.

Blood specimens were inoculated in BACTEC Culture Media (Becton, Dickinson and Company, Tokyo, Japan). Blood was cultured with the BACTEC 9240 system (Becton, Dickinson and Company), and strains were identified with the MicroScan WalkAway-96 (Beckman Coulter, Inc., Brea, CA, USA). Breakpoints of each antibiotic were in accordance with Clinical and Laboratory Standards Institute breakpoints. We calculated the percentage of each category of causative pathogen, including duplicate polymicrobials.

Statistical analysis was performed using SPSS for Windows, version 24 (IBM SPSS, Inc., Chicago, IL, USA). Mean values were compared using the two-sample t-test for independent samples and the chi-squared test or Fisher's exact test as appropriate. For continuous variables, Student's t test or the Mann–Whitney U test was performed depending on the distribution of the respective variable. Statistical significance was defined as $p < 0.05$.

Results

The case characteristics are summarized in Table 1. The causative pathogens were Gram-positive microorganisms in 58.0%, Gram-negative microorganisms in 35.8%, Candida spp. in 6.2%, and polymicrobials in 25.8% of cases; the calculated percentages of each causative pathogen type included the duplicate polymicrobials. The 13 catheter tip cultures that were able to be analyzed became positive, but the catheter had already been removed at the time of PVC-BSI diagnosis in all 49 other cases, so those catheter tips could not be cultured. A total of 23 cases had blood cultures turn positive more than twice: 16 (25.8%) cases turned positive twice, 4 (6.5%) cases turned positive three times, and 3 (4.8%) cases turned positive five times.

Twenty-three (37.1%) patients with complications required a longer duration of antibiotic treatment than the other 39 patients (average, 33.5 vs. 15.8 days, respectively; p = 0.004). All 39 of these patients had

Table 1 Comparison between patients who died within 30 days of bacteremia diagnosis and patients who survived

	Full cohort *n*(%)	Died within 30 days *n* (%)	Survived *n* (%)	Odds ratio	95% CI	*P*
Total	62	8(100)	54(100)			
Gender (male)	40 (64.5)	6 (75.0)	34 (63.0)			0.512
Age, median (years)	69 (range; 1–92)	76 (range; 52–86)	69 (range; 1–92)			0.126
Duration from admission to bacteremia, median (days)	17 (range; 3–142)	33(range; 9–142)	16(range; 3–86)			0.089
Duration of antibiotic therapy from diagnosis of PVC-BSI, median (days)	16 (range; 5–100)	17(range; 7–46)	16(range; 3–100)			0.737
Time from catheter insertion to bacteremia, median (days)	6 (range; 2–15)	7 (range; 2–9)	7 (range; 3–15)			0.526
Unknown	26 (41.9)	2 (25.0)	24 (44.4)	0.42	0.08–2.25	0.298
< 3 days	4 (11.1)	2 (25.0)	2 (3.7)	8.67	1.03–73.25	0.022
4–7 days	19 (52.8)	1(16.7)	18 (66.7)	0.29	0.03–2.50	0.232
> 8 days	13 (36.1)	3(50.0)	10 (30.0)	2.64	0.54–12.91	0.218
Causative microorganism (including duplicate polymicrobials)						
Gram-positive microorganisms	47(58.0)	7(77.8)	40(54.8)	2.45	0.28–21.72	0.408
S.aureus	14(17.3)	5(62.5)	9(16.7)	8.33	1.68–41.29	**0.004**
MSSA	10(71.4)	3(37.5)	7(12.7)	4.03	0.78–20.70	0.078
MRSA	4(28.6)	2(25.0)	2(3.7)	8.67	1.03–73.25	0.022
CNS	21(25.9)	2(25.0)	16(29.6)	0.79	0.14–4.35	0.788
Bacillus spp.	6(7.4)	0	6(11.1)	0.44	0.02–8.53	0.576
Enterococcus spp.	6(7.4)	0	6(11.1)	0.44	0.02–8.53	0.576
Gram-negative microorganisms	30(35.8)	2(22.2)	28(38.4)	0.31	0.06–1.67	0.156
Enterobacter spp.	9(11.1)	0	6(11.1)	0.44	0.02–8.53	0.576
Klebsiella spp.	5(6.2)	1(12.5)	4(7.4)	1.79	0.17–18.35	0.621
Pseudomonus spp.	4(4.9)	1(12.5)	3(5.6)	2.43	0.22–26.69	0.455
Acinetobacter spp.	4(4.9)	0	4(7.4)	0.66	0.03–13.40	0.785
Serratia spp.	4(4.9)	0	4(7.4)	0.66	0.03–13.40	0.785
E.coli	3(3.7)	0	3(5.6)	0.87	0.04–18.29	0.926
Citrobacter spp.	1(1.2)	0	1(1.9)	2.10	0.08–55.84	0.651
Candida spp.	5(6.2)	0(0.0)	5(6.8)	0.53	0.03–10.48	0.671
Polymicrobial	16(25.8)	1(12.5)	15(27.8)	0.37	0.04–3.28	0.357
Underlying diseases (including duplicate)						
Malignancy	33 (53.2)	4(50.0)	26(48.1)	1.08	0.24–4.76	0.922
Hypertension	14 (22.6)	0	14	0.16	0.01–0.03	0.172
Diabetes mellitus	11 (17.7)	0	11	0.22	0.01–4.15	0.274
Cerebral infarction	7 (11.3)	2(25.0)	5(9.3)	3.27	0.52–20.69	0.189
Orthopedic disorder	3 (4.8)	0	3 (5.6)	0.87	0.04–18.29	0.926
Department						
Surgery	35 (56.5)	3(37.5)	32(59.3)	0.41	0.09–1.91	0.247
Internal medicine	21 (33.9)	5(62.5)	16(29.6)	3.96	0.84–18.57	0.067
Obstetrics and Gynecology	5 (8.1)	0	5 (9.3)	0.53	0.03–10.48	0.672
Pediatrics	1 (1.6)	0	1 (1.9)	2.10	0.08–55.84	0.651

Table 1 Comparison between patients who died within 30 days of bacteremia diagnosis and patients who survived *(Continued)*

Place of insertion						
Arm	48 (77.4)	7 (87.5)	41 (75.9)	2.22	0.25–19.76	0.465
Foot	3 (4.8)	1(12.5)	2 (3.7)	3.71	0.30–46.48	0.279
Unknown	11 (17.7)	0	11 (20.4)	0.22	0.01–4.15	0.274
Complication						
Suppurative thrombophlebitis	18 (29.0)	3(37.5)	15(27.8)	1.56	0.33–7.35	0.572
Bacterial cellulitis	3 (4.8)	2 (25.0)	1 (1.8)	17.67	1.39–225.05	0.004
Osteomyelitis	2 (3.2)	0	2 (3.7)	1.24	0.05–28.02	0.894

Abbreviations: *S. aureus*, *Staphylococcus aureus*; MSSA, Methicillin-sensitive *S. aureus*; MRSA, Methicillin-resistant *S. aureus*; CNS, coagulase-negative *Staphylococcus*; *P. aeruginosa*, *Pseudomonus aeruginosa*; *E. coli*, *Escherichia coli*

Footnote: Some of the patients included in our study had multiple diseases. When we calculated the incidence of each underlying disease, we included the patients with multiple underlying diseases in all relevant calculations, so some patients were counted more than once

phlebitis, but only 11 underwent vascular ultrasonography. None of the patients had infective endocarditis. Nine (14.5%) patients required admission to the intensive care unit because of changes in vital signs and multiple organ failure secondary to PVC-BSIs.

Eight (12.9%) patients died within 30 days of the blood culture becoming positive (Table 2). All of these patients had an underlying immunodeficiency caused by conditions such as malignancy or leukemia.

We compared two groups: patients who died within 30 days of their blood culture becoming positive and patients who survived. *S. aureus* was the primary causative organism in five of the eight fatal cases. Patients who died of PVC-BSIs had a higher proportion of *S. aureus* infection than did patients who survived (odds ratio, 8.33; $p = 0.004$). A < 3-day duration from catheter insertion to bacteremia (odds ratio, 8.67; $p = 0.022$) and bacterial cellulitis (odds ratio, 17.67; $p = 0.004$) were each associated with a high 30-day mortality rate. No differences were observed in other pathogens, underlying diseases, department (surgery vs. internal medicine), or catheter insertion site (Table 1).

Discussion

Among patients who died within 30 days, the time from catheter insertion to bacteremia ranged from 2 to 9 days, and the time from bacteremia to death ranged from 5 to 23 days. Of the 14 patients with *S. aureus* bacteremia, five (35.8%) died within 30 days of its diagnosis. We found that *S. aureus* was the pathogen most commonly associated with PVC-BSI-related death in this study (Table 1).

Catheter removal is warranted when a CRBSI is suspected. The Infectious Diseases Society of America recommends diagnosing CRBSI when the same organism is grown in at least one percutaneous blood culture and catheter tip culture [12]. However, the diagnosis of PVC-BSIs using this criterion may be difficult because the catheter has often already been removed when clinicians suspect a PVC-BSI. Only 13 (21.0%) patients underwent catheter tip culture in the present study; the catheter tips from the other 49 (79.0%) were not available to be tested. This indicates the possibility that PVC-BSIs are under-diagnosed and under-reported. We recommend culturing both the blood and catheter tip to ensure the correct diagnosis according to the IDSA

Table 2 Clinical and epidemiological data of patients who died

Case no.	Time from hospitalization to bacteremia (days)	Time from catheter insertion to bacteremia (days)	Time from bacteremia to death (days)	Complication	Microbiology
1	44	Unknown	20	Suppurative thrombophlebitis	*S. aureus* *P. aeruginosa*
2	33	Unknown	12	None	CNS
3	13	2	10	Cellulitis	*S. aureus*
4	18	9	23	Cellulitis	CNS
5	9	3	5	Suppurative thrombophlebitis	*K. oxytoca*
6	44	7	19	None	*S. aureus*
7	42	8	14	None	*S. aureus*
8	142	9	25	Suppurative thrombophlebitis	*S. aureus*

Abbreviations: *S. aureus*, *Staphylococcus aureus*; CNS, coagulase-negative *Staphylococcus*; *P. aeruginosa*, *Pseudomonus aeruginosa*; *K. oxytoca*, *Klebsiella oxytoca*

guideline as soon as signs of infection, such as redness and swelling, are observed at the insertion site and the patient has a fever of unknown origin or a high C-reactive protein concentration. When two blood samples, one drawn from the catheter hub and the other from a peripheral vein, are cultured and they meet the CRBSI criteria for differential time to positivity, this can also be used for diagnosing CRBSI [12]; however, this criterion cannot be used for PVC-BSI diagnosis. Furthermore, the incidence of redness, tenderness, and pus at the catheter insertion site in patients with either type of CRBSI is only about 3% [12–14]; due to the low incidence of these symptoms, some clinicians may inadvertently overlook CRBSI. Diagnosis of PVC-BSIs is more difficult than diagnosis of CVC-BSIs for these reasons. It is important not only to examine the catheter insertion site but also to take aggressive measures to diagnose PVC-BSIs by performing blood and catheter tip cultures.

For PVC-BSI diagnosis, clinicians must both recognize the presence of PVC-BSIs and rule out other foci of infection. This study is focused only on cases in which the infections progressed to bacteremia and did not include cases with only localized infection. It is likely that the overall incidence of PVC infections is much greater than what is suggested by the number of total PVC-BSI cases in our study because the incidence of infections that remain localized is probably much greater than that of those that progress to bacteremia. It is imperative to carefully examine the insertion site daily to prevent PVC-BSIs from developing into bacteremia and to use assessment tools, such as the Visual Infusion Phlebitis score [15].

The patients in the present study were given antibiotics to treat PVC-BSIs for 5–100 days. The course of treatment, duration of antibiotics, and need for catheter removal depend on the causative organism. We recommend that primary physicians institute a therapeutic regimen according to the Infectious Diseases Society of America guidelines [12]. Patients with hematogenous complications tend to require longer durations of therapy and hospitalization. The average duration of antibiotic treatment in cases with hematogenous complications was 33.5 days, while that in cases with only phlebitis was 15.8 days (p = 0.004).

According to a previous study, the risk factors for hematogenous complications of *S. aureus* infection are failure to remove the catheter (relative risk, 2.28; 95% confidence interval, 1.22–4.27) and, among patients for whom the catheter has been removed, a longer mean duration from symptom onset to catheter removal (5 vs. 2 days; $p < 0.001$) [16]. The risk of increased disease severity is also higher among patients with persistent bacteremia; the interval in days between antibiotic initiation and the last positive blood culture tended to be longer in patients with delayed catheter removal than in patients with prompt removal, but this difference did not reach statistical significance in this small study (p = 0.07) [17]. These results might be explained in part by the failure to carefully examine the insertion site; thorough examination is imperative to prevent hematogenous complications. While there are no reports on the average cost of PVC-BSIs, treating CVC-BSIs is quite expensive and it is likely that treating PVC-BSIs infections is also costly [18, 19]. Furthermore, both the potential harm to patients and the additional costs resulting from extended hospitalization are serious problems.

With respect to microbiological data, a previous study reported that patients with PVC-BSIs had a higher proportion of *S. aureus* infections than did patients with CVC-BSIs (53% vs. 33%) [20]. When PVC-related bacteremia caused by *S. aureus* was compared with PVC-related bacteremia due to other pathogens, no differences were observed in age, sex, insertion site, time from catheter insertion to BSI, or complications.

In another study, the overall mortality rate was 29% among patients with nosocomial *S. aureus* bacteremia admitted to two hospitals in Oxford, UK [21]; however, we found a higher overall mortality rate (35.8%) among patients with *S. aureus* bacteremia in the present study. The high mortality rate observed in our study could be related to several factors, such as severe underlying disease, older age, and the presence of metastatic complications. Unfortunately, the retrospective nature of this study precluded our ability to distinguish between all-cause 30-day mortality and 30-day mortality related to PVC-BSIs.

Our study has a number of limitations, such as its retrospective nature and the lack of record concerning the infection site in 11 (17.7%) cases or the duration of catheter insertion in 26 (41.9%) cases. Furthermore, we were not able to identify cases in which only localized infection occurred at the insertion site and did not lead to bacteremia. Additional research is needed to reveal how many PVC infection cases only have a localized infection that does not lead to bacteremia. Moreover, the currently available information regarding the causative organisms of PVC-BSIs is inadequate because of a lack of surveillance data, making comparison of our data difficult. Furthermore, there is the possibility that our study had confounding factors; however, our sample size was not adequate to determine potential confounders. Future work will aim to adjust the data for the time from catheter insertion to bacteremia, department, and complications. Further investigation of these findings is warranted.

Conclusions

PVC-BSIs are a significant cause of health care-associated infection. Here, we observed severe cases of PVC-BSI requiring intensive and long-term care along with lengthy durations of antibiotic treatment due to hematogenous complications, and some patients died. For patients with PVC-BSIs, *S. aureus* bacteremia remains a major problem that may influence the prognosis. For *S. aureus* bacteremia of unknown focus, catheter removal may prevent hematogenous complications and death. Importantly, isolated assessments of the PVC-BSI risk at medical facilities using information such as prevalence, duration of catheter insertion, and dressing management are insufficient because of a lack of surveillance data. More cases and data must be collected for further analyses on this important subject.

Abbreviations

CRBSI: Catheter-related bloodstream infection; CVC-BSIs: Central venous catheter-related bloodstream infections; PVC-BSIs: Peripheral vascular catheter-related bloodstream infections

Acknowledgements

Edanz Group Ltd. provided assistance in preparing and editing the manuscript.

Funding

None.

Authors' contributions

AS, IN, TF, and TM conceived and designed the study. AS, IN, HF, AT, TK, and SF collected the data. AS analyzed the data and wrote the paper. All authors read and approved the final manuscript.

Competing interests

The authors declare that they have no competing interests.

Consent for publication

Not applicable.

Author details

[1]Department of Infection Prevention and Control, Tokyo Medical University Hospital, 6-7-1 Nishishinjuku, Shinjuku-ku, Tokyo 160-0023, Japan. [2]Department of Infection Prevention and Control, Tokyo Medical University Hachioji Medical Center, 1163 Tatemachi, Hachioujishi, Tokyo 193-0998, Japan. [3]Department of Microbiology, Tokyo Medical University, 6-1-1 Shinjuku, Shinjuku-ku, Tokyo 160-8402, Japan.

References

1. Weinstein RA. Nosocomial infection update. Emerg Infect Dis. 1998;4:416–20.
2. Tager IB, Ginsberg MB, Ellis SE, Walsh NE, Dupont I, Simchen E, et al. An epidemiologic study of the risks associated with peripheral intravenous catheters. Am J Epidemiol. 1983;118:839–51.
3. Pronovost P, Needham D, Berenholtz S, Sinopoli D, Chu H, Cosgrove S, et al. An intervention to decrease catheter-related bloodstream infections in the ICU. N Engl J Med. 2006;355:2725–32.
4. Schulman J, Stricof R, Stevens TP, Horgan M, Gase K, Holzman IR, et al. Statewide NICU central-line-associated bloodstream infection rates decline after bundles and checklists. Pediatrics. 2011;127:436–44.
5. Mermel LA. Prevention of intravascular catheter-related infections. Ann Intern Med. 2000;132:391–402.
6. Maki DG, Kluger DM, Crnich CJ. The risk of bloodstream infection in adults with different intravascular devices: a systematic review of 200 published prospective studies. Mayo Clin Proc. 2006;81:1159–71.
7. Soifer NE, Borzak S, Edlin BR, Weinstein RA. Prevention of peripheral venous catheter complications with an intravenous therapy team: a randomized controlled trial. Arch Intern Med. 1998;158:473–7.
8. Lai KK. Safety of prolonging peripheral cannula and i.V. Tubing use from 72 hours to 96 hours. Am J Infect Control. 1998;26:66–70.
9. Maki DG, Ringer M. Risk factors for infusion-related phlebitis with small peripheral venous catheters. A randomized controlled trial. Ann Intern Med. 1991;114:845–54.
10. Bregenzer T, Conen D, Sakmann P, Widmer AF. Is routine replacement of peripheral intravenous catheters necessary? Arch Intern Med. 1998;158:151–6.
11. Collignon PJ. Intravascular catheter associated sepsis: a common problem. The Australian study on intravascular catheter associated sepsis. Med J Aust. 1994;161:374–8.
12. Mermel LA, Allon M, Bouza E, Craven DE, Flynn P, O'Grady NP, et al. Clinical practice guidelines for the diagnosis and management of intravascular catheter-related infection: 2009 update by the Infectious Diseases Society of America. Clin Infect Dis. 2009;49:1–45.
13. Mermel LA, Farr BM, Sherertz RJ, Raad I, O'Grady N, Harris JS, et al. Guidelines for the management of intravascular catheter-related infections. J Intraven Nurs. 2001;24:180–205.
14. Safdar N, Maki DG. Inflammation at the insertion site is not predictive of catheter-related bloodstream infection with short-term, noncuffed central venous catheters. Crit Care Med. 2002;30:2632–5.
15. IVTEAM: VIP score website. http://www.vipscore.net (2012). Accessed 20 Oct 2015.
16. Fowler VG Jr, Justice A, Moore C, Benjamin DK Jr, Woods CW, Campbell S, et al. Risk factors for hematogenous complications of intravascular catheter-associated Staphylococcus Aureus bacteremia. Clin Infect Dis. 2005;40:695–703.
17. Malanoski GJ, Samore MH, Pefanis A, Karchmer AW. Staphylococcus Aureus catheter-associated bacteremia. Minimal effective therapy and unusual infectious complications associated with arterial sheath catheters. Arch Intern Med. 1995;155:1161–6.
18. Fukuda H, Lee J, Imanaka Y. Costs of hospital-acquired infection and transferability of the estimates: a systematic review. Infection. 2011;39:185–99.
19. Nakamura I, Fukushima S, Hayakawa T, Sekiya K, Matsumoto T. The additional costs of catheter-related bloodstream infections in intensive care units. Am J Infect Control. 2015;43:1046–9.
20. Pujol M, Hornero A, Saballs M, Argerich MJ, Verdaguer R, Cisnal M, et al. Clinical epidemiology and outcomes of peripheral venous catheter-related bloodstream infections at a university-affiliated hospital. J Hosp Infect. 2007; 67:22–9.
21. Wyllie DH, Crook DW, Peto TE. Mortality after Staphylococcus Aureus bacteraemia in two hospitals in Oxfordshire, 1997-2003: cohort study. BMJ. 2006;333:281.

18

Risk factors for carbapenem-resistant *K. pneumoniae* bloodstream infection and predictors of mortality in Chinese paediatric patients

Ye Zhang[1], Ling-Yun Guo[1], Wen-Qi Song[2], Yan Wang[2], Fang Dong[2*] and Gang Liu[1*]

Abstract

Background: Bloodstream infections (BSI) caused by carbapenem-resistant *K. pneumoniae* (CRKP) are associated with high rates of morbidity and mortality. Early identification of patients at highest risk is very important. The aim of this study was to describe the clinical characteristics and mortality of *K. pneumoniae* BSI and to identify risk factors associated with CRKP BSI among paediatric patients.

Methods: From January 2011 to December 2014, a retrospective case-control study was conducted at Beijing Children's Hospital, China. Risk factors for CRKP BSI and for *K. pneumoniae* BSI-related death were evaluated. Patients with BSI caused by *K. pneumoniae* were identified from the microbiology laboratory database. Data regarding demographic, microbiological and clinical characteristics, therapy and outcome were collected from the medical records.

Results: A total of 138 patients with *K. pneumoniae* BSI were enrolled, including 54 patients with CRKP BSI and 84 patients with carbapenem-susceptible *K. pneumoniae* (CSKP) BSI. Most of the BSI (114; 82.6%) were healthcare-associated, while the rest (24; 17.4%) were community-acquired. Hematologic malignancies (odds ratio (OR):4.712, [95% CI: 2.181–10.180], $P < 0.001$) and previous cephalosporin administration (OR: 3.427, [95% CI: 1.513–7.766], $P = 0.003$) were found to be associated with the development of CRKP BSI. 28-day mortality of *K. pneumoniae* BSI was 8.7%. Mechanical ventilation (OR:9.502, [95% CI: 2.098–43.033], $P = 0.003$), septic shock (OR:6.418, [95% CI: 1.342–30.686], $P = 0.020$), and isolation of CRKP (OR:9.171, [95% CI: 1.546–54.416], $P = 0.015$) were independent risk factors for 28-day mortality of *K. pneumoniae* BSI.

Conclusion: Hematologic malignancies and previous cephalosporin administration were associated with the development of CRKP BSI, while mechanical ventilation, septic shock and CRKP infection were independent mortality predictors for *K. pneumoniae* BSI. More attention should be paid to CRKP BSI in the paediatric population.

Keywords: Carbapenem-resistant *K. pneumoniae*, Bloodstream infection, Risk factor, Children

* Correspondence: fangd32@163.com; liugangbch@sina.com
[2]Department of Laboratory Medicine, Beijing Children's Hospital, Capital Medical University, No. 56 Nanlishi Road, Xi Cheng District, Beijing 100045, People's Republic of China
[1]Department of Infectious Disease, Beijing Children's Hospital, Capital Medical University, No. 56 Nanlishi Road, Xi Cheng District, Beijing 100045, People's Republic of China

Background

During the last decade, carbapenem resistant *K. pneumoniae* (CRKP) has spread worldwide, including to China [1, 2]. This organism is rapidly becoming a major threat to public health because of the limited therapeutic options and the high morbidity and mortality. Previous studies found that mortality rates ranged from 30 to 50% for infections caused by CRKP [3–6]. In China, this pathogen became endemic in many regions; the data from CHINET (an antimicrobial resistance surveillance network in China) surveillance regarding bacterial resistance demonstrated a marked increasing trend of CRKP between 2005 and 2014, with the rate rising from 2.4 to 13.4% [7].

CRKP can cause many types of infections, including pneumonia, urinary tract infections, bloodstream and intra-abdominal infections [8, 9]. Bloodstream infection (BSI) is the most important infection, with a high risk of mortality [10]. At its worst, with broad-spectrum antibiotic resistance, treatment options for BSI caused by CRKP are very limited [11, 12].

Because there are fewer therapeutic options in children [13, 14], the treatment of CRKP BSI is a real challenge for the paediatrician. The keys to success in preventing and treating CRKP infections are the implementation of infection control measures and early detection of patients at highest risk [14]. In this context, recognizing the risk factors associated with the development of CRKP BSI is of great importance when considering treatment options. Many studies have explored risk factors associated with carbapenem resistance among adults, including use of medical devices, previous antibiotic exposure, and ICU admission [14–16]. However, data regarding risk factors among children remain limited. Thus, the purpose of this study was to evaluate risk factors associated with CRKP BSI and mortality of *K. pneumoniae* BSI among paediatric patients as well as to describe clinical characteristics of *K. pneumoniae* BSI.

Methods

Study design and patients

This study was conducted at Beijing Children's Hospital (a 970-bed tertiary paediatric hospital in China with an average of 70,000 admissions per year) between January 2011 and December 2014. Patients (from birth to 18 years of age) with confirmed *K. pneumoniae* BSI were included. A *K. pneumoniae* BSI was defined as the presence of at least once positive blood culture with concomitant signs and symptoms of infection according to established criteria [17, 18]. *K. pneumoniae* BSI cases were identified from the microbiology laboratory database. Only the first episode of *K. pneumoniae* BSI was included. Patients with polymicrobial BSIs or whose medical records were incomplete were excluded. CRKP was defined as minimal inhibition concentration (MIC) for imipenem or meropenem ≥ 4 μg/mL, or isolates were confirmed to produce carbapenemase (https://www.cdc.gov/hai/pdfs/cre/cre-guidance-508.pdf). To assess risk factors for CRKP BSI, a retrospective case-control study was performed. The CRKP group (case group) consisted of patients with CRKP BSI. Patients with BSI due to carbapenem-susceptible *K. pneumoniae* (CSKP) were defined as the CSKP group (control group).

The study was approved by the Ethics Committee of Beijing Children's Hospital, Capital Medical University. Informed consent was waived because this study did not cause injury to patients.

Data collection and definitions

The data collected included information regarding demographics, underlying diseases, hospitalization, intensive care unit (ICU) admission, antibiotic therapy, intravascular catheter use, bacterial infections, and immunosuppressive therapy in the 90 days prior to the date of BSI onset; length of hospitalization, microbiological data, antimicrobial therapies, and patient outcomes were also collected.

BSI onset was defined as the collection date of a positive blood culture. BSI was classified as healthcare-related (HCR) or community-acquired (CA). Positive blood cultures obtained from patients who were hospitalized ≥ 48 h, or positive blood cultures obtained from patients who were hospitalized < 48 h but had been hospitalized in the previous six months, were defined as HCR-BSI; CA-BSI were defined as positive blood cultures obtained from patients who were hospitalized < 48 h without having been hospitalized in the previous six months [17]. Neutropenia was defined as absolute neutrophil count (ANC) lower than 500 cells/mm^3 [18]. Therapy with one or more antimicrobial drugs within ≤ 24 h from BSI onset was defined as empirical antimicrobial therapy; treatment with antimicrobials after the susceptibility results became available was defined as definitive therapy [17]. The active antibiotic agent was defined as MIC within the susceptible range [19]. Appropriate antimicrobial therapy refers to the administration of the in vitro active agent, while inappropriate therapy was defined as treatment without active drugs [20]. The final outcome was determined as survival and all-cause death at 28 days after the date of BSI onset.

Microbiological methods

The Vitek 2 system (bioMérieux, Marcy l'Etoile, France) and the Phoenix100 automated system (Becton Dickinson, Spark, MD, USA) were used for isolate identification. The MIC values for tested antimicrobial agents were determined by an automated broth microdilution method (Becton Dickinson, Spark, MD, USA). The results were interpreted according to CLSI criteria (CLSI2014) [20].

For colistin, the results were interpreted in accordance with European Committee on Antimicrobial Susceptibility Testing (EUCAST) clinical breakpoints (version 6.0). Polymerase chain reaction (PCR) testing was performed for detection of carbapenemase genes using a previously described method [21].

Statistical analysis

Categorical variables were presented as numbers and percentages. Continuous variables were presented as the mean and standard deviation (SD) (normally distributed) or median and interquartile range(IQR) (non-normally distributed). Categorical variables were compared using the chi-square or Fisher's exact tests. Continuous variables were compared by Student's t test or Mann–Whitney U test according to their distribution.

For univariate analysis, the results were presented as odds ratios (ORs), 95% confidence intervals (CIs) and *P* values. Significant variables with *P* value of < 0.1 were then selected into a logistic regression model for multivariate analysis to evaluate risk factors for CRKP BSIs and for *K. pneumoniae* BSI-related mortality. The discrimination ability of the logistic regression model was assessed by estimating the area under the receiver operating characteristic (ROC) curve. Calibration of the model was assessed using the Hosmer-Lemeshow test for goodness of fit. Two-tailed *P* value of < 0.05 was considered statistically significant. All statistical analyses were performed with SPSS 17.0 software (IBM Corporation).

Results

Characteristics of patients

We identified a total of 161 unique cases of bloodstream infections with *K. pneumoniae* during the study period. After excluding 23 cases (polymicrobial BSIs [$n = 14$]; incomplete medical records [$n = 9$]), 138 patients with *K. pneumoniae* BSIs fulfilled the inclusion criteria and were enrolled in this study. Fifty-four cases (39.1%) were identified as CRKP, and 84 (60.9%) were identified as CSKP.

The median patient age was 24.8 months (range, 0 to 204.3 months; interquartile range [IQR], 1.1 to 101.6 months). Patients in the CSKP group were younger than those in CRKP group (10.9 vs. 46.3 months, $P = 0.021$). Eighty (58.0%) were male, and 58 (42.0%) were female. Most of the BSI (114; 82.6%) were healthcare-associated, while the rest (24; 17.4%) were community-acquired. Most children (118; 85.5%) had at least one underlying disease, including hematologic malignancies (66; 55.9%), congenital anomalies (19; 16.1%), premature at birth (13; 11.0%), solid tumours (8; 6.8%), malnutrition (7; 5.9%), and immunodeficiency (6; 5.1%). One hundred and one patients (73.2%) had a hospitalization history within 90 days prior to the onset of BSIs, and the majority of these (69; 68.3%) had been admitted to hematology-oncology department. The median duration of hospitalization was 21 days (IQR, 15 to 32 days), and the median duration of hospital stay before the onset of BSI was 10 days (IQR, 1 to 15 days). The demographic and clinical data of patients with *K. pneumoniae* BSI according to CSKP and CRKP are shown in Table 1.

Microbiological characteristics of *K. pneumoniae* strains

Fifty-four isolates were identified as CRKP. Fifty-one isolates had a meropenem/imipenem MIC ≥ 4 μg/mL. Most of them (40/51, 78.4%) were tested for carbapenemase. The most frequently detected carbapenemase was NDM-1 (23/40, 57.5%) followed by IMP-4 (13/40, 32.5%) and KPC-2 (4/40, 10.0%). Three isolates that were susceptible to meropenem (MIC ≤ 1 μg/mL) and intermediate to imipenem (MIC = 2 μg/mL) were bla_{IMP-4} harboring. As shown in Table 2, CRKP isolates showed higher rates of resistance than did CSKP isolates. In the CRKP group, resistance to imipenem and meropenem was 94.4 and 85.2%, respectively. The most active drugs were amikacin (susceptibility of 90.7%, 49/54) and ciprofloxacin (susceptibility of 90.7%, 49/54). MIC of meropenem > 8 μg/ml was associated with higher mortality compared with MIC ≤ 1 μg/ml (Fig. 1).

Risk factors for CRKP BSI

To identify risk factors associated with CRKP BSI, we conducted a retrospective case-control study. On univariate analysis, the following factors were most associated with the development of CRKP BSI: age, underlying disease, hematologic malignancies, number of previous hospitalizations, prior presence of intravascular catheter, previous immunosuppressive therapy, previous neutropenia, previous antibiotic therapy, and number of antibiotic agents. Prior exposure to cephalosporin, antifungal agents and glycopeptides were also significant risk factors.

The results of the multivariate analysis are shown in Table 3: the independent risk factors for CRKP BSI were hematologic malignancies (OR:4.712, [95% CI: 2.181–10.180], $P < 0.001$) and previous cephalosporin administration (OR: 3.427, [95%CI: 1.513–7.766], $P = 0.003$). The result of Hosmer-Lemeshow chi-square testing ($X^2 = 0.588$; $P = 0.745$) was indicative of good calibration. The ROC area under the curve was 0.729, suggesting that the multivariate model had good predictive ability.

Treatment and outcome

Antibiotic treatments and outcomes of patients with *K. pneumoniae* BSI are shown in Table 1 and Fig. 2. Patients with CRKP BSI were less likely to receive active antibiotic agents as empirical treatment than were patients with CSKP BSI (19/54 vs. 63/84, $P < 0.001$). Empiric therapy was given to all patients with CRKP BSI: 70.4% (38) received meropenem or imipenem,

Table 1 Characteristics of 138 patients with KP BSI according to CSKP or CRKP isolates

Variable	Total (n = 138)	CSKP (n = 84)	CRKP (n = 54)	P
Age (months)	24.8 (1.1–101.6)	10.9 (0.5–98.9)	46.3 (14.1–107.6)	***0.021***
Male	80 (58.0)	49 (58.3)	31 (57.4)	0.914
Underlying disease	118 (85.5)	67 (79.8)	51 (94.4)	***0.032***
Hematologic malignancies	66 (55.9)	29 (43.3)	37 (72.5)	***0.003***
Congenital anomalies	19 (16.1)	15 (22.4)	4 (7.8)	***0.043***
Prematurity	13 (11.0)	10 (14.9)	3 (5.9)	0.147
Solid tumors	8 (6.8)	6 (9.0)	2 (3.9)	0.463
Malnutrition	7 (5.9)	5 (7.5)	2 (3.9)	0.697
Immunodeficiencies	6 (5.1)	5 (7.5)	1 (2.0)	0.233
Departments				
Hematology-oncology	74 (53.6)	35 (41.7)	39 (72.2)	***< 0.001***
General medical	32 (23.2)	25 (29.8)	7 (13.0)	***0.024***
NICU	14 (10.1)	13 (15.5)	1 (1.9)	***0.009***
PICU	6 (4.3)	2 (2.4)	4 (7.4)	0.210
Surgical	12 (8.7)	9 (10.7)	3 (5.6)	0.366
Healthcare-related infection	114 (82.6)	66 (78.6)	48 (88.9)	0.119
Length of hospitalization	21 (15–32)	21 (15–31.75)	22.5 (12–32.25)	0.825
Length of hospitalization before the onset of BSI	10 (1–15)	8.5 (0–15)	12 (3–15.25)	0.091
Intravascular catheter	108 (78.3)	57 (67.9)	51 (94.4)	***< 0.001***
Mechanical ventilation	17 (12.3)	7 (8.3)	10 (18.5)	0.076
Fever	122 (88.4)	74 (88.1)	48 (88.9)	0.887
Organ disfunction (any)	53 (38.4)	32 (38.1)	21 (38.9)	0.925
Septic shock	15 (10.9)	6 (7.1)	9 (16.7)	0.079
Leukocytes (cells/mm^3)	690 (200–6170)	4180 (300–6790)	295 (120–3887.5)	***< 0.001***
Neutrophils (cells/mm^3)	100 (0–2237.5)	935 (0–2960)	10 (0–367.5)	***0.002***
< 500 cells/mm^3	77 (55.8)	36 (42.9)	41 (75.9)	***< 0.001***
Empirical antibiotic treatment (n = 138)				***< 0.001***
No active antibiotic	56 (40.6)	21 (25.0)	35 (64.8)	–
≥ 1 active antibiotic	82 (59.4)	63 (75.0)	19 (35.2)	–
Change in antibiotic treatment after the positive culture	57 (41.3)	29 (34.5)	28 (51.9)	***0.044***
Definitive antibiotic treatment (n = 134)				***< 0.001***
No active antibiotic	29 (21.6)	9 (10.8)	20 (39.2)	–
≥ 1 active antibiotic	105 (78.4)	74 (89.1)	31 (60.8)	–
Carbapenem-including treatment(n = 134)	95 (70.9)	59 (71.1)	36 (70.6)	0.951
Length of antibiotic treatment	13 (9–18)	14 (9.25–18)	12 (7–18.25)	0.079
Outcome				
7-day mortality	10 (7.2)	1 (1.2)	9 (16.7)	***0.002***
28-day mortality	12 (8.7)	2 (2.4)	10 (18.5)	***0.003***
Hospital mortality	17 (12.3)	7 (8.3)	10 (18.5)	0.076

Data are n (%) or median (IQR)
P value in bold italic shows that the variables are statistically significant

18.5% (10) received amikacin, and 16.7% (9) received cephalosporins or β-lactam-β-lactamase inhibitors. Thirty-nine patients received one drug as empiric treatment, while nine received in vitro active drug. Only 27.8% (15) patients received a combination of two or more drugs, while 10 received appropriate empiric therapy. Compared with those

Table 2 Resistance of *K. pneumoniae* strains to specific antimicrobials

Antibiotic (N)	All	CSKP	CRKP	*P* value
Ampicillin (131)	99.2%	100.0%	97.9%	0.359
Ceftazidime (130)	65.4%	47.6%	97.8%	< 0.001
Cefepime (137)	66.4%	45.8%	98.1%	< 0.001
Meropenem (138)	33.3%	0.0%	85.2%	< 0.001
Imipenem (138)	37.0%	0.0%	94.4%	< 0.001
Gentamicin (138)	48.6%	34.5%	70.4%	< 0.001
Amikacin (137)	3.6%	0.0%	9.3%	0.008
Ciprofloxacin (138)	7.2%	6.0%	9.3%	0.465
Trimethoprim-sulfamethoxazole (138)	72.5%	61.9%	88.9%	0.001
Colistin (138)	0.0%	0.0%	0.0%	-

of other departments, patients in the hematology-oncology ward received a higher proportion of appropriate empiric therapy (17/39 vs. 2/15, $P = 0.056$). After detection of CRKP BSI, three patients died before antibiotic susceptibility results were available, one of whom had received active antibiotic.

Mortality was significantly higher in patients with CRKP BSI than in those with CSKP BSI (7-day mortality: 16.7% vs. 1.2%, $P = 0.001$; 28-day mortality: 18.5% vs. 2.4%, $P = 0.003$). In the CRKP BSI group, 28-day mortality of patients who received at least one active antibiotic agent as empirical treatment was not significantly different from the mortality of patients who did not receive active antibiotic agent (4/19 vs. 6/35, $P = 0.728$). Carbapenem-including treatment was administered to 39 patients, and their mortality was similar to that of patients who did not receive carbapenem-including treatment (7/39 vs. 3/15, $P = 1.0$). Overall, 28-day mortality was lower among patients in the hematology-oncology ward (6/39, 15.4%) than in patients in other wards (4/15, 26.7%, $P = 0.438$).

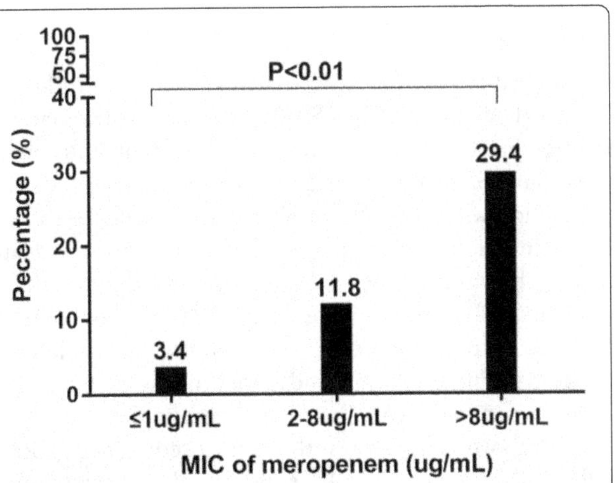

Fig. 1 The relationship between mortality and the meropenem MIC of KP isolates

Univariate analysis indicated that organ dysfunction, septic shock, mechanical ventilation and isolation of CRKP were associated with 28-day mortality. On multivariate analysis, the independent risk factors for 28-day mortality were mechanical ventilation (OR:9.502, [95% CI: 2.098–43.033], $P = 0.003$), septic shock (OR:6.418, [95% CI: 1.342–30.686], $P = 0.020$), and isolation of CRKP (OR:9.171, [95% CI: 1.546–54.416], $P = 0.015$) (Table 4). The area under the ROC curve for this model was 0.878, and the Hosmer-Lemeshow goodness-of-fit *P*-value was 0.346.

Discussion

CRKP infections are becoming a serious problem in children and are of great concern because of the limited treatment options and unfavourable impact on prognosis [14, 22]. According to previous studies, children with risk factors appear to be more vulnerable to CRKP infections [14]. In the present study, we described the clinical characteristics, risk factors and outcome of BSI due to *K. pneumoniae* in the paediatric population.

In our study, the predominant carbapenemase was NDM-1. In China, the main factor causing carbapenem resistance was KPC-2 among adults [23]; however, NDM-1- producing *K. pneumoniae* was most common in children [21]. Three isolates that were susceptible to meropenem and intermediate to imipenem were $bla_{IMP\text{-}4}$ harboring, suggesting that some CRKP may test as susceptible or intermediate to carbapenems [14]. Patients with CRKP BSI were older than those with CSKP; this may be because the majority of them came from the hematology-oncology ward.

Previous studies have identified several risk factors associated with development of CRKP BSI, including exposure to healthcare, previous ICU stay or admission, presence of indwelling devices and exposure to antibiotics (such as cephalosporins, fluoroquinolones and carbapenems) [14–16]. We showed that CRKP BSI was associated with several factors including age, underlying disease, number of previous hospitalizations, prior presence of intravascular catheter, previous immunosuppressive therapy, and previous antibiotic therapy. However, only hematologic malignancies and previous cephalosporin administration were independent risk factors for CRKP BSI. Patients with hematologic malignancies usually undergo more frequent exposure to healthcare, longer duration of antibiotic therapy, more invasive procedures and have pre-existing immunosuppression. All of these factors can increase the risk for infections [10, 24]. According to Kwak et al., prior use of carbapenem and cephalosporin were risk factors for acquisition of CRKP

Table 3 Univariate and multi-variate analysis of risk factor for BSI caused by CRKP compared with patients with BSI caused by CSKP

Variable	CSKP (*n* = 84)	CRKP (*n* = 54)	Univariate analysis		Multi-variate analysis	
			OR (95% CI)	*P*	OR (95% CI)	
Age (months)	10.9 (0.5–98.9)	46.3 (14.1–107.6)	–	0.021	–	0.067
Male	49 (58.3)	31 (57.4)	–	0.914	–	–
Underlying disease	67 (79.8)	51 (60.7)	–	0.032	–	0.873
Hematologic malignancies	29 (43.3)	37 (72.5)	4.128 (1.990–8.561)	< 0.001	4.712 (2.181–10.180)	***< 0.001***
Congenital anomalies	15 (22.4)	4 (7.8)	–	0.137	–	–
Prematurity	10 (14.9)	3 (5.9)	–	0.343	–	–
Solid tumors	6 (9.0)	2 (3.9)	–	0.638	–	–
Malnutrition	5 (7.5)	2 (3.9)	–	0.849	–	–
Immunodeficiencies	5 (7.5)	1 (2)	–	0.468	–	–
Prior hospitalization	58 (69.0)	43 (79.6)	–	0.171	–	–
Number of previous hospitalizations	1 (0–4)	3 (1–5)	–	0.023	–	0.873
Previous ICU admission	11 (13.1)	5 (9.3)	–	0.492	–	–
Previous surgery	9 (10.7)	8 (14.8)	–	0.474	–	–
Previous presence of intravascular catheter	41 (48.8)	37 (68.5)	2.283 (1.115–4.671)	0.023	–	0.859
Previous bacterial infections	9 (10.7)	10 (18.5)	–	0.194	–	–
Previous immunosuppressive therapy	33 (39.3)	33 (61.1)	2.429 (1.205–4.894)	0.012	–	0.551
Previous neutropenia	21 (25.0)	30 (55.6)	3.750 (1.808–7.777)	< 0.001	–	0.161
Previous antibiotic therapy	61 (72.6)	49 (90.7)	3.695 (1.309–10.429)	0.006	–	0.067
Number of antibiotic agent	2 (0–3)	3 (2–5)		0.001	–	0.537
Cephalosporins	44 (52.4)	41 (75.9)	2.867 (1.345–6.110)	0.006	3.427 (1.513–7.766)	***0.003***
Penicillins	17 (20.2)	8 (14.8)	–	0.420	–	–
β-Lactam-β-lactamase inhibitor	23 (27.4)	21 (38.9)	–	0.157	–	–
Carbapenems	26 (31)	22 (40.7)	–	0.239	–	–
Aminoglycosides	6 (7.1)	5 (9.3)	–	0.654	–	–
Fluoroquinolones	0 (0.0)	2 (3.7)	–	0.151	–	–
Antifungal agents	22 (26.2)	28 (51.9)	3.035 (1.474–6.249)	0.002	–	0.271
Glycopeptides	24 (28.6)	30 (55.6)	3.125 (1.528–6.392)	0.002	–	0.346
Others	11 (13.1)	10 (18.5)	–	0.387	–	–

Data are n (%) or median (IQR).
P-values in bold italic shows variables with evidence of association in univariate and multi-variate analysis

[25]. Liu et al. and Orsi et al. found that previous cephalosporin exposure was an independent risk factor ertapenem-resistant *K. pneumoniae* infections [26, 27]. Our study also suggested that previous cephalosporin administration was associated with CRKP BSI. The carbapenems, fluoroquinolones and glycopeptides were independent risk factors for CRKP infections, according to the previous studies [16, 25, 28]; however, the present study did not show an association between these agents and the development of CRKP BSI.

The overall hospital mortality was 12.3%, lower than that reported in previous paediatric studies [29, 30]. The 28-day mortality in the CRKP group (18.5%) was also lower than that of previous reports, where mortality for CRKP BSI ranged from 39 to 82% [31]. Most recently, Montagnani et al. reported that 4 of 9 children (44.4%) in Italy died from CRKP BSI [22]. Another study demonstrated that the rate of carbapenem-resistant Enterobacteriaceae BSI-related mortality in the Indian paediatric population was 52% [32]. Previous studies suggested that ICU admission was an independent risk factor for death [6, 10]; however, compared with this Indian study (38% were in ICU), there were only 9.3% in our cohort. Patients with hematologic malignancies have relatively better baseline condition and undergo less invasive procedures compare with these who admitted to the ICU. All the above factors were the main predictors of CRKP infection mortality [32]. We supposed that these reasons may explain our low mortality rate. On the other hand, 72.5% patients with CRKP BSI had hematologic

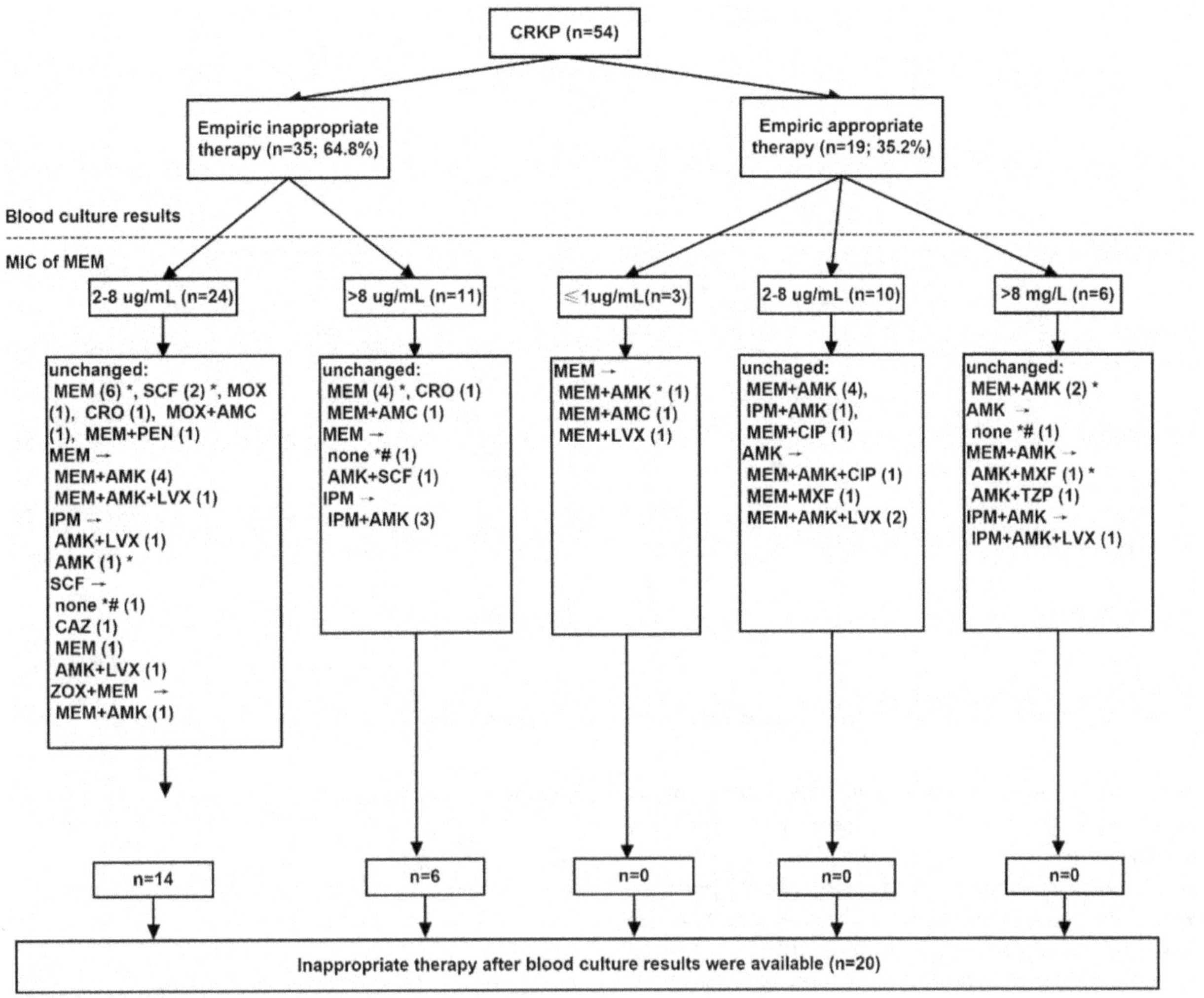

Fig. 2 Antibiotic therapy and outcome for patients with CRKP BSIs. AMK, Amikacin; AMC, Amoxycillin/clavulanic acid; CAZ, Ceftazidime; CIP, Ciprofloxacin; CRO, Ceftriaxone; LVX, Levofloxacin; MEM, Meropenem; MOX, Latamoxef; MXF, Moxifloxacin; PEN, Penicillin; SCF, Cefoperazone/sulbactam; TZP, Piperacillin/tazobactam; ZOX, Ceftizoxme. * Died. *# Patients died before blood culture results were available

malignancies in our cohort. Patients with hematologic malignancies often received more effective empirical treatment due to high clinical suspicion for multidrug-resistant gram-negative bacteria in our hematology-oncology ward. It has been shown that appropriate antimicrobial treatment can help to improve the survival rate [32, 33]. Our study also demonstrated that 28-day mortality was lower among patients in the hematology-oncology ward than in patients in other wards.

Consistently with previous studies [10, 33, 34], the mortality appeared to be higher in CRKP BSI than in CSKP BSI (18.5% vs. 2.4%) in our study, and isolation of CRKP was the independent risk factor for 28-day mortality. A review also suggested that the isolation of CRKP was the main risk factor for mortality from BSI [35]. This finding could be explained by the limited CRKP treatment options. Several studies also indicated that empirical therapy with non-active antibiotics may contribute to unfavourable outcomes [36, 37]. In our study, both the proportions of active empirical and definitive antibiotic treatment were significantly lower in patients with CRKP BSI. However, we did not identify an association between active antibiotic agents and mortality. This may be explained by the small number of cases in this cohort.

We also found mechanical ventilation and septic shock were associated with higher 28-day mortality, consistent with the findings of previous studies [38, 39]. Several reports suggested that age and the seriousness of patients' conditions (including septic shock) were independent risk factors for mortality [16, 31]. Villegas and colleagues also found that critical illness was a statistically

Table 4 Univariate and multi-variate analysis of risk factor associated with 28-day mortality among patients with KP BSI

Variable	Survived (*n* = 126)	Died (*n* = 12)	Univariate analysis		Multi-variate analysis	
			OR (95% CI)	*P*	OR (95% CI)	*P*
Age (months), median (IQR)	24.23 (0.91–107.55)	32.41 (3.54–52.99)	–	0.919	–	–
Male	72 (57.1)	8 (66.7)	–	0.739	–	–
Underlying disease	106 (84.1)	12 (100)	–	0.214	–	–
Hematologic malignancies	60 (47.6)	6 (50.0)	–	0.875	–	–
Congenital anomalies	16 (12.7)	3 (25.0)	–	0.457	–	–
Prematurity	12 (9.5)	1 (8.3)	–	1.000	–	–
Malnutrition	6 (4.8)	1 (8.3)	–	1.000	–	–
Immunodeficiencies	6 (4.8)	0 (0)	–	1.000	–	–
Deep venous catheterization	97 (77.0)	11 (91.7)	–	0.417	–	–
Mechanical ventilation	10 (7.9)	7 (58.3)	16.240 (4.352–60.607)	< 0.001	9.502 (2.098–43.033)	***0.003***
Organ dysfunction	44 (34.9)	9 (75.0)	5.591 (1.439–21.718)	0.016	–	–
Septic shock	9 (7.1)	6 (50.0)	13.000 (3.476–48.623)	< 0.001	6.418 (1.342–30.686)	***0.020***
Empirical treatment active in vitro	76 (60.3)	5 (41.7)	–	0.233	–	–
Definitive treatment active in vitro [a]	100 (79.4)	5 (62.5)	–	0.370	–	–
Carbapenem-including treatment [a]	90 (71.4)	5 (62.5)	–	0.691	–	–
Isolation of CRKP	44 (34.9)	10 (83.3)	9.318 (1.955–44.421)	0.003	9.171 (1.546–54.416)	***0.015***

[a] Four patients had died before blood culture results were available.
P-values in bold italic shows variables with evidence of association in univariate and multi-variate analysis

significant factor associated with mortality among patients with BSI caused by carbapenemase-producing Enterobacteriaceae [40]. Xu et al. conducted a meta-analysis of mortality of patients infected with *K. pneumoniae* and concluded that patients' physical condition had a close relationship with their survival [10].

There were some limitations in this study. Firstly, it was a retrospective study and was conducted in a single centre, including 138 paediatric patients. This may have influenced the power of the analysis to identify risk factors. Further prospective, multicentre studies are needed. Secondly, we did not test all the CRKP isolates to determine the carbapenem resistance mechanisms; therefore, it is possible for us to overestimate or underestimate the prevalence of NDM-1.

Conclusion

Hematologic malignancies and previous cephalosporin administration were associated with the development of CRKP BSI. We also found low mortality caused by *K. pneumoniae* BSI in children. Isolation of CRKP was the independent risk factor for mortality, while patients with serious baseline conditions (including septic shock) had higher mortality. Thus, more attention should be paid to CRKP BSI in the paediatric population, especially in patients with a poor state of health.

Abbreviations

ANC: Absolute neutrophil count; BSI: Bloodstream infection; CA: Healthcare-related (HCR) or community-acquired; CRKP: Carbapenem-resistant *K. pneumoniae*; CSKP: Carbapenem-susceptible *K. pneumoniae*; ICU: Intensive care unit; MIC: Minimal inhibition concentration

Acknowledgements

The abstract has been previously published as a conference abstract and accepted as the poster presentation in 10th World Congress of the World Society for Pediatric Infectious Diseases (WSPID 2017) Session "Clinical Infectious Disease" Shenzhen, China in December 2- December 5, 2017.

Authors' contributions

All authors contributed to this work. All authors read and approved the final manuscript. GL, FD, LYG, YW and WQS designed the study. YZ collected the data. GL, FD and YZ interpreted the data. YZ wrote the first draft of the paper. GL, FD and LYG reviewed and approved the final report.

Competing interests

The authors declare that they have no competing interests.

References

1. Chen S, Feng W, Chen J, Wei L, He N, Wang Q, Sun F, Xia P. Spread of Carbapenemase-producing Enterobacteria in a southwest Hospital in China. Ann Clin Microb Anti. 2014;13(1):42.
2. Kumarasamy KK, Toleman MA, Walsh TR, Bagaria J, Butt F, Balakrishnan R, Chaudhary U, Doumith M, Giske CG, Irfan S. Emergence of a new antibiotic resistance mechanism in India, Pakistan, and the UK: a molecular, biological, and epidemiological study. Lancet Infect Dis. 2010;10(9):597–602.

3. Patel G, Huprikar S, Factor SH, Jenkins SG, Calfee DP. Outcomes of Carbapenem-ResistantKlebsiella pneumoniaeInfection and the impact of antimicrobial and adjunctive therapies. Infection Control & Hospital Epidemiology. 2008;29(12):1099–106.
4. Schwaber MJ, Klarfeld-Lidji S, Navon-Venezia S, Schwartz D, Leavitt A, Carmeli AY. Predictors of carbapenem-resistant Klebsiella pneumoniae acquisition among hospitalized adults and effect of acquisition on mortality. Antimicrobial Agents & Chemotherapy. 2008;52(3):1028.
5. Falagas ME, Rafailidis PI, Kofteridis D, Virtzili S, Chelvatzoglou FC, Papaioannou V, Maraki S, Samonis G, Michalopoulos A. Risk factors of carbapenem-resistant Klebsiella pneumoniae infections: a matched case control study. J Antimicrob Chemoth. 2007;60(5):1124.
6. Borer A, Saidelodes L, Riesenberg K, Eskira S, Peled N, Nativ R. Attributable mortality rate for Carbapenem-resistant Klebsiella pneumoniae bacteremia. Infection Control & Hospital Epidemiology. 2009;30(10):972–6.
7. Hu FP, Guo Y, Zhu DM, Wang F, Jiang XF, Xu YC, Zhang XJ, Zhang CX, Ji P, Xie Y. Resistance trends among clinical isolates in China reported from CHINET surveillance of bacterial resistance, 2005-2014. Clinical Microbiology & Infection the Official Publication of the European Society of Clinical Microbiology & Infectious Diseases 2016, 22 Suppl 1:S9.
8. Daikos GL, Markogiannakis A, Souli M, Tzouvelekis LS. Bloodstream infections caused by carbapenemase-producing Klebsiella pneumoniae: a clinical perspective. Expert Rev Anti-Infect Ther. 2012;10(12):1393–404.
9. Broberg CA, Palacios M, Miller VL. Klebsiella: a long way to go towards understanding this enigmatic jet-setter. F1000Prime Rep. 2014;6:64.
10. Xu L, Sun X, Ma X. Systematic review and meta-analysis of mortality of patients infected with carbapenem-resistant Klebsiella pneumoniae. Ann Clin Microbiol Antimicrob. 2017;16(1):18.
11. Bowers DR, Huang V. Emerging issues and treatment strategies in Carbapenem-resistant Enterobacteriaceae (CRE). Curr Infect Dis Rep. 2016;18(12):48.
12. Morrill HJ, Pogue JM, Kaye KS, LaPlante KL. Treatment options for Carbapenem-resistant Enterobacteriaceae infections. Open Forum Infect Dis. 2015;2(2):v50.
13. Maltezou HC, Kontopidou F, Katerelos P, Daikos G, Roilides E, Theodoridou M. Infections caused by carbapenem-resistant gram-negative pathogens in hospitalized children. Pediatr Infect Dis J. 2013;32(4):151–4.
14. Logan LK. Carbapenem-resistant Enterobacteriaceae: an emerging problem in children. Clin Infect Dis. 2012;55(6):852.
15. Tian L, Tan R, Chen Y, Sun J, Liu J, Qu H, Wang X. Epidemiology of Klebsiella pneumoniae bloodstream infections in a teaching hospital: factors related to the carbapenem resistance and patient mortality. Antimicrob Resist Infect Control. 2016;5:48.
16. Jiao Y, Qin Y, Liu J, Li Q, Dong Y, Shang Y, Huang Y, Liu R. Risk factors for carbapenem-resistant Klebsiella pneumoniae infection/colonization and predictors of mortality: a retrospective study. Pathog Glob Health. 2015;109(2):68–74.
17. Hussein K, Raz-Pasteur A, Finkelstein R, Neuberger A, Shachor-Meyouhas Y, Oren I, Kassis I. Impact of carbapenem resistance on the outcome of patients' hospital-acquired bacteraemia caused by Klebsiella pneumoniae. J Hosp Infect. 2013;83(4):307–13.
18. Freifeld AG, Bow EJ, Sepkowitz KA, Boeckh MJ, Ito JI, Mullen CA, Raad II, Rolston KV, Young JA, Wingard JR. Clinical practice guideline for the use of antimicrobial agents in neutropenic patients with cancer: 2010 update by the infectious diseases society of america. Clin Infect Dis. 2011;52(4):e56-e93.
19. Navarro-San FC, Mora-Rillo M, Romero-Gomez MP, Moreno-Ramos F, Rico-Nieto A, Ruiz-Carrascoso G, Gomez-Gil R, Arribas-Lopez JR, Mingorance J, Pano-Pardo JR. Bacteraemia due to OXA-48-carbapenemase-producing Enterobacteriaceae: a major clinical challenge. Clin Microbiol Infect. 2013;19(2):E72–9.
20. CLSI. Performance standards for antimicrobial susceptibility testing; 24th informational supplement, M100-S24. PA: Wayne; 2014.
21. Wang S, SUN J, SU W, HU Z, YANG J, Wang Y. Epidemiological analysis of NDM-1-positive bacteria in China. Military Medical Sciences. 2015;39(11):825–30.
22. Montagnani C, Prato M, Scolfaro C, Colombo S, Esposito S, Tagliabue C, Lo VA, Bruzzese E, Loy A, Cursi L, et al. Carbapenem-resistant Enterobacteriaceae infections in children: an Italian retrospective multicenter study. Pediatr Infect Dis J. 2016;35(8):862–8.
23. Zheng B, Dai Y, Liu Y, Shi W, Dai E, Han Y, Zheng D, Yu Y, Li M. Molecular epidemiology and risk factors of Carbapenem-resistant Klebsiella pneumoniae infections in eastern China. Front Microbiol. 2017;8
24. Micozzi A, Gentile G, Minotti C, Cartoni C, Capria S, Ballaro D, Santilli S, Pacetti E, Grammatico S, Bucaneve G, et al. Carbapenem-resistant Klebsiella pneumoniae in high-risk haematological patients: factors favouring spread, risk factors and outcome of carbapenem-resistant Klebsiella pneumoniae bacteremias. BMC Infect Dis. 2017;17(1):203.
25. Kwak YG, Choi SH, Choo EJ, Chung JW, Jeong JY, Kim NJ, Woo JH, Ryu J, Kim YS. Risk factors for the acquisition of carbapenem-resistant Klebsiella pneumoniae among hospitalized patients. Microb Drug Resist. 2005;11(2):165–9.
26. Orsi GB, Garcia-Fernandez A, Giordano A, Venditti C, Bencardino A, Gianfreda R, Falcone M, Carattoli A, Venditti M. Risk factors and clinical significance of ertapenem-resistant Klebsiella pneumoniae in hospitalised patients. J Hosp Infect. 2011;78(1):54–8.
27. Liu SW, Chang HJ, Chia JH, Kuo AJ, Wu TL, Lee MH. Outcomes and characteristics of ertapenem-nonsusceptible Klebsiella pneumoniae bacteremia at a university hospital in northern Taiwan: a matched case-control study. J Microbiol Immunol Infect. 2012;45(2):113–9.
28. Gomez RV, Zuleta TJ. Risk factors for infection with carbapenem-resistant Klebsiella pneumoniae: a case-case-control study. Colomb Med (Cali). 2014;45(2):54–60.
29. Zaoutis TE, Goyal M, Chu JH, Coffin SE, Bell LM, Nachamkin I, McGowan KL, Bilker WB, Lautenbach E. Risk factors for and outcomes of bloodstream infection caused by extended-spectrum beta-lactamase-producing Escherichia coli and Klebsiella species in children. Pediatrics. 2005;115(4):942–9.
30. Kim YK, Pai H, Lee HJ, Park SE, Choi EH, Kim J, Kim JH, Kim EC. Bloodstream infections by extended-spectrum beta-lactamase-producing Escherichia coli and Klebsiella pneumoniae in children: epidemiology and clinical outcome. Antimicrob Agents Chemother. 2002;46(5):1481–91.
31. de Maio CC, de Oliveira LM, Gaudereto J, Perozin JS, Urbano MR, Camargo CH, Grion CM, Levin AS, Costa SF. A prospective study of treatment of carbapenem-resistant Enterobacteriaceae infections and risk factors associated with outcome. BMC Infect Dis. 2016;16(1):629.
32. Nabarro LE, Shankar C, Prakasam A, Mathew G, Jeyaseelan V, Veeraraghavan B, Verghese VP. Clinical and bacterial risk factors for mortality in children with Carbapenem- resistant Enterobacteriaceae bloodstream infections in India. Pediatr Infect Dis J. 2017;36(6):e161-e166.
33. Zarkotou O, Pournaras S, Tselioti P, Dragoumanos V, Pitiriga V, Ranellou K, Prekates A, Themeli-Digalaki K, Tsakris A. Predictors of mortality in patients with bloodstream infections caused by KPC-producing Klebsiella pneumoniae and impact of appropriate antimicrobial treatment. Clin Microbiol Infect. 2011;17(12):1798–803.
34. Tumbarello M, Trecarichi EM, De Rosa FG, Giannella M, Giacobbe DR, Bassetti M, Losito AR, Bartoletti M, Del BV, Corcione S, et al. Infections caused by KPC-producing Klebsiella pneumoniae: differences in therapy and mortality in a multicentre study. J Antimicrob Chemother. 2015;70(7):2133–43.
35. Viale P, Giannella M, Lewis R, Trecarichi EM, Petrosillo N, Tumbarello M. Predictors of mortality in multidrug-resistant Klebsiella pneumoniae bloodstream infections. Expert Rev Anti-Infect Ther. 2013;11(10):1053–63.
36. Akturk H, Sutcu M, Somer A, Aydin D, Cihan R, Ozdemir A, Coban A, Ince Z, Citak A, Salman N. Carbapenem-resistant Klebsiella pneumoniae colonization in pediatric and neonatal intensive care units: risk factors for progression to infection. Braz J Infect Dis. 2016;20(2):134–40.
37. Satlin MJ, Cohen N, Ma KC, Gedrimaite Z, Soave R, Askin G, Chen L, Kreiswirth BN, Walsh TJ, Seo SK. Bacteremia due to carbapenem-resistant Enterobacteriaceae in neutropenic patients with hematologic malignancies. J Inf Secur. 2016;73(4):336–45.
38. Mariappan S, Sekar U, Kamalanathan A. Carbapenemase-producing Enterobacteriaceae: risk factors for infection and impact of resistance on outcomes. Int J Appl Basic Med Res. 2017;7(1):32–9.

39. Chang YY, Chuang YC, Siu LK, Wu TL, Lin JC, Lu PL, Wang JT, Wang LS, Lin YT, Huang LJ, et al. Clinical features of patients with carbapenem nonsusceptible Klebsiella pneumoniae and Escherichia coli in intensive care units: a nationwide multicenter study in Taiwan. J Microbiol Immunol Infect. 2015;48(2):219–25.
40. Villegas MV, Pallares CJ, Escandon-Vargas K, Hernandez-Gomez C, Correa A, Alvarez C, Rosso F, Matta L, Luna C, Zurita J, et al. Characterization and clinical impact of bloodstream infection caused by Carbapenemase-producing Enterobacteriaceae in seven Latin American countries. PLoS One. 2016;11(4):e154092.

19

Peripherally inserted central catheter-related bloodstream infection due to *Tsukamurella pulmonis*

Jun Suzuki[1], Teppei Sasahara[1,2*], Masaki Toshima[1] and Yuji Morisawa[1]

Abstract

Background: *Tsukamurella pulmonis* is an aerobic gram-positive and rod-shaped organism that causes central catheter-related bloodstream infections in immunocompromised hosts. However, peripherally inserted central catheter (PICC)-related bloodstream infections due to this organism have not been reported.

Case presentation: We describe a case of a 48-year-old man with acquired immunodeficiency syndrome and diffuse large B cell lymphoma who received five courses of chemotherapy including rituximab, cyclophosphamide, doxorubicin hydrochloride, vincristine, and prednisone via a PICC. Five days after the last chemotherapy course, he presented with a high fever and shaking chills. His absolute neutrophil count was 4200/μL. Cultures obtained from blood and PICC culture revealed *T. pulmonis*. The colony count of *T. pulmonis* grown from PICC culture was 10^3 colony-forming units. Therefore, he was diagnosed with *T. pulmonis* bacteremia resulting from PICC-related bloodstream infection. The patient's condition improved and he became afebrile within 48 h after intravenous administration of cefozopran hydrochloride, which is a fourth generation cephalosporin.

Conclusions: PICCs can be associated with *T. pulmonis* bacteremia, and fourth generation cephalosporins may be effective treatment.

Keywords: *Tsukamurella pulmonis*, Acquired immunodeficiency syndrome (AIDS), Diffuse large B cell lymphoma (DLBCL), Peripherally inserted central catheters (PICCs), Catheter-line associated bloodstream infection (CLABSI)

Background

Tsukamurella species are aerobic gram-positive and rod-shaped organisms with a specific cell wall chemistry that separates them from aerobic actinomycetes [1]. Although infections caused by *Tsukamurella* species are rare, these species can cause nosocomial infections in immunocompromised hosts [2]. A report from 1996 described isolation of *Tsukamurella pulmonis* from the sputum of a 92-year-old woman with lung mycobacterium infection [3]. *T. pulmonis* infections are associated with hematological and immunosuppressed patients, and the reported observations of the infection include conjunctivitis [4], keratitis [5], pneumonia [6], and central catheter-related bloodstream infections [7].

Peripherally inserted central catheters (PICCs) have been popular because of their safety, easy insertion, and lower rates of infection [8–10]. Although the use of central venous catheters (CVCs) and Hickman catheters is a reported cause of catheter-line associated bloodstream infection (CLABSI) due to *T. pulmonis* [7], PICC-related bloodstream infections with this organism have not been reported.

Here, we present the case of 48-year-old patient with acquired immunodeficiency syndrome (AIDS) who was diagnosed with PICC-related bloodstream infection due to *T. pulmonis*.

* Correspondence: protozoa@jichi.ac.jp
[1]Division of Infectious Diseases, Jichi Medical University Hospital, 3311-1 Yakushiji, Shimotsuke, Tochigi 329-0498, Japan
[2]Department of Infection and Immunity, School of Medicine, Jichi Medical University, 3311-1 Yakushiji, Shimotsuke, Tochigi 329-0498, Japan

Case presentation

A 48-year-old Japanese man presented with symptoms of right-sided facial asymmetry and right hand palsy that had lasted for 10 days. He had a past medical history of syphilis, gonorrhea, varicella, hepatitis B viral infection, and chronic use of tobacco (1–2 packs of cigarettes per day for 28 years). Laboratory examinations revealed positivity for human immunodeficiency virus (HIV) antigen/antibody, a CD4 positive lymphocyte count of 84 cells/μL, and an HIV-1 RNA viral load of 180,000 copies/mL. Contrast-enhanced magnetic resonance imaging of the head showed three mass lesions in the brain, and the specimen biopsy from these lesions revealed diffuse large B cell lymphoma. He was diagnosed with AIDS-associated primary brain malignant lymphoma. The patient was administered emtricitabine/tenofovir disoproxil combination therapy and raltegravir as the antiretroviral therapy. Atovaquone and azithromycin were also used for prophylaxis of pneumocystis pneumonia and nontuberculous mycobacterial infections.

A PICC was implanted, and he received five courses of R-CHOP chemotherapy (rituximab, cyclophosphamide, doxorubicin hydrochloride, vincristine, and prednisone). Five days after the last R-CHOP chemotherapy course, he suddenly developed a fever with shivering chills. His white blood cell count was 4300/μL, and his neutrophil count was 4200/μL. The CD4-positive lymphocyte cell count was 228 cells/μL, and the HIV-1 RNA viral load was 20 copies/mL. We administered 2 g cefozopran hydrochloride, which is a fourth generation cephalosporin, and vancomycin on day 1 (every 12 h) and on day 3, respectively, and the PICC was removed. The patient's condition improved and become afebrile within 48 h after the initiation of cefozopran hydrochloride. Cultures obtained from blood and revealed gram-positive rods, which were identified as *T. pulmonis* using 16S ribosomal RNA gene sequencing. The colony count of *T. pulmonis* grown from PICC culture was 10^3 colony-forming units. Thus, he was diagnosed with *T. pulmonis* bacteremia resulting from a PICC-related bloodstream infection. Because of the results of the susceptibility test (Table 1), we continued cefozopran hydrochloride for 16 days. Follow up blood culture on 5 days after treatment was negative and clinical relapse was not observed. He remains in complete remission as of this report.

Discussion and conclusions

Although *T. pulmonis* generally causes CLABSI from CVCs and Hickman catheters, we report a case of PICC-related bloodstream infection due to this microorganism and review the related literature.

Table 2 summarizes the seven reported cases of *T. pulmonis* bacteremia in the literature [2, 7, 11–14]. Three

Table 1 Minimum inhibitory concentrations (MICs) of the *Tsukamurella pulmonis* strain in the present case

Antibiotics	MIC (mg/mL)	Antibiotics	MIC (mg/mL)
Penicillin G	8	Gentamicin	2
Ampicillin	≥16	Amikacin	≤4
Ceftriaxone	0.5	Minomycin	≤0.5
Cefozopran	1	Clindamycin	≥2
Cefepime	≤1	Vancomycin	2
Imipenem	≤1	Levofloxacin	≤0.25
Meropenem	0.5		

patients had severe immunodeficiency combined with bone marrow transplantation, IgA nephropathy, or metastatic breast cancer as the underlying disease [7]. Another three cases had hematological malignancy. One patient had an intracerebral hemorrhage and CLABSI [14]. CVCs or Hickman-catheters were implanted in all of these cases. Therefore, a relationship between CVCs or Hickman-catheters and the presence of *T. pulmonis* bacteremia exists; however, the risk of *T. pulmonis* bacteremia has not been reported with PICCs.

However, a recent systematic review and meta-analysis showed that the reduced risk of CLABSI with PICCs in comparison to CVCs was greatest for outpatients (RR, 0.22; 95% CI, 0.18–0.27) than for hospitalized patients (RR 0.73; 95% CI, 0.54–0.98) and PICC-associated CLABSI occurred as frequently as CVC-associated CLABSI in hospitalized patients (incidence rate ratio 0.91; 95% CI, 0.46–1.79) [15]. Thus, PICCs may also be a risk factor for CLABSI due to *T. pulmonis* bacteremia.

The appropriate treatment for *T. pulmonis* bacteremia remains unknown because standard susceptibility methods for this organism have not been established. There have been a few reports describing various treatments based on susceptibility methods (Table 2), including the E-test using Mueller-Hinton agar plates [13] and the disk diffusion technique [12]. In the present case, minimum inhibitory concentration (MIC) results using the broth dilution method showed susceptibility to vancomycin and cefozopran hydrochloride (Table 1). We continued cefozopran hydrochloride only because of the relatively high MIC for vancomycin. Although further studies are needed to confirm the standard susceptibility methods and optimal susceptibility interpretations, fourth generation cephalosporins including cefozopran hydrochloride and cefepime may be effective against *T. pulmonis* and may represent appropriate treatment for *T. pulmonis* bacteremia.

The relation between AIDS and the incidence of *T. pulmonis* bacteremia is unknown. *T. pulmonis* bacteremia has not been previously reported in AIDS patients, although an advanced-stage AIDS patient with *Tsukamurella* spp.

Table 2 Summary of case reports of *Tsukamurella pulmonis* bacteremia

Age (years)	Sex	Diseases	Catheter	Transplantation	Antibiotics	Outcome	Reference
1.5	M	SCID	Hickman	+	Amikacin, clarithromycin, ceftriaxone, vancomycin	Survived	[7]
3	F	ALL	CVC	–	Cefixime, ertapenem, ciprofloxacin, amikacin oral clarithromycin	Survived	[13]
38	F	High-grade Burkitt-like lymphoma	Hickman	+	Teicoplanin	Survived	[12]
39	M	ALL	Hickman	No data	Vancomycin, meropenem, amphotericin B	No data	[11]
48	F	IgA nephropathy	CVC	–	Ciprofloxacin, gentamicin, vancomycin	No data	[7]
48	M	Intracerebral hemorrhage	CVC	–	Ceftazidime, vancomycin	Survived	[14]
67	F	Metastatic breast cancer	CVC	–	Sulfamethoxazole-trimethoprim	No data	[7]

SCID severe combined immune deficiency, *ALL* acute lymphocytic leukemia, *CVC* central venous catheter

pneumonia was reported by Alcaide et al. [16]. When the CD4-positive lymphocyte cell count is over 200 cells/μL, the defect in cell mediated immunity is mild to moderate, not severe, and it is not clear if this defect is sufficient to explain the predisposition to *Tsukamurella* infection.

In conclusion, we encountered a case of PICC-related bloodstream infection due to *T. pulmonis*. The present case suggests that PICCs may be a risk factor for developing *T. pulmonis* bacteremia, and fourth-generation cephalosporins may be effective treatment.

Abbreviations
AIDS: Acquired Immunodeficiency Syndrome; ALL: Acute lymphocytic leukemia; CI: confidence interval; CLABSI: catheter-line associated bloodstream infection; DLBCL: diffuse large B cell lymphoma; HIV: human immunodeficiency virus; PICCs: peripherally inserted central catheters; RR: relative risk; SCID: severe combined immune deficiency

Acknowledgements
Not applicable.

Funding
All data containing relevant information to support the study findings are included in the manuscript.

Authors' contributions
JS drafted the manuscript. TS helped and revised the manuscript. MT and YM participated in manuscript writing. All authors read and approved the final manuscript.

Consent for publication
The patient provided informed consent for publication of this report. A copy of written consent is available for review by the Editor of this journal.

Competing interests
The authors declare that they have no competing interests.

References

1. Stackebrandt E, Rainey FA, Ward-Rainey NL. Proposal for a new hierarchic classification system, Actinobacteria classis nov. Int J Syst Evol Microbiol. 1997;47:479–91.
2. Bouza E, Pérez-Parra A, Rosal M, Martín-Rabadán P, Rodríguez-Créixems M, Marín M. Tsukamurella: a cause of catheter-related bloodstream infections. Eur J Clin Microbiol Infect Dis. 2009;28:203–10.
3. Yassin AF, Rainey FA, Brzezinka H, Burghardt J, Rifai M, Seifert P, Feldmann K, Schaal KP. Tsukamurella pulmonis sp. nov. Int J Syst Bacteriol. 1996;46:429–36.
4. Woo PC, Ngan AH, Lau SK, Yuen KY. Tsukamurella conjunctivitis: a novel clinical syndrome. J Clin Microbiol. 2003;41:3368–71.
5. Woo PC, Fong AH, Ngan AH, Tam DM, Teng JL, Lau SK, Yuen KY. First report of Tsukamurella keratitis: association between T. Tyrosinosolvens and T. Pulmonis and ophthalmologic infections. J Clin Microbiol. 2009;47:1953–6.
6. Xue XY, Zhou M, Fu WF, Pan YG, Zhao J. Colonic metastasis from primary lung adenocarcinoma: case report and review of the literature. Med Oncol. 2012;29:644–7.
7. Schwartz MA, Tabet SR, Collier AC, Wallis CK, Carlson LC, Nguyen TT, Kattar MM, Coyle MB. Central venous catheter-related bacteremia due to Tsukamurella species in the immunocompromised host: a case series and review of the literature. Clin Infect Dis. 2002;35:e72–7.
8. Gunst M, Matsushima K, Vanek S, Gunst R, Shafi S, Frankel H. Peripherally inserted central catheters may lower the incidence of catheter-related blood stream infections in patients in surgical intensive care units. Surg Infect. 2011;12:279–82.
9. Al Raiy B, Fakih MG, Bryan-Nomides N, Hopfner D, Riegel E, Nenninger T, Rey J, Szpunar S, Kale P, Khatib R. Peripherally inserted central venous catheters in the acute care setting: a safe alternative to high-risk short-term central venous catheters. Am J Infect Control. 2010;38:149–53.
10. Kim-Saechao SJ, Almario E, Rubin ZA, Warren DK. Impact of a surgeon-led peripherally inserted central venous catheter team on peripherally inserted central venous catheter-related complications and costs. Surg Infect. 2016; 17:352–6.
11. Shim HE, Sung H, Baek SM, Namgung S, Kim MN, Kim YG, Lee GH. A case of catheter-related bacteremia of Tsukamurella pulmonis. Korean J Lab Med. 2009;29:41–7.
12. Maertens J, Wattiau P, Verhaegen J, Boogaerts M, Verbist L, Wauters G. Catheter-related bacteremia due to Tsukamurella pulmonis. Clin Microbiol Infect. 1998;4:51–3.
13. Pérez Del Molino Bernal IC, Cano ME, García de la Fuente C, Martínez-Martínez L, López M, Fernández-Mazarrasa C, Agüero J. Tsukamurella pulmonis bloodstream infection identified by secA1 gene sequencing. J Clin Microbiol. 2015;53:743–5.
14. Cho AR, Kim HR, Lee M-K, Choi SH, Yun SW. A case report of Tsukamurella pulmonis infection misidentified as atypical mycobacteria. Korean J Clin Microbiol. 2010;13:93–7.

Bloodstream infections at a tertiary level paediatric hospital in South Africa

Harsha Lochan[1], Vashini Pillay[1], Colleen Bamford[2], James Nuttall[1] and Brian Eley[1*]

Abstract

Background: Bloodstream infection (BSI) in children causes significant morbidity and mortality. There are few studies describing the epidemiology of BSI in South African children.

Methods: A retrospective descriptive cohort study was conducted at a paediatric referral hospital in Cape Town, South Africa. The National Health Laboratory Service (NHLS) microbiology database was accessed to identify positive blood culture specimens during the period 2011–2012. Demographic and clinical details, antimicrobial management and patient outcome information were extracted from medical and laboratory records. Antibiotic susceptibility results of identified organisms were obtained from the NHLS database.

Results: Of the 693 unique bacterial and fungal BSI episodes identified during the study period, 248 (35.8%) were community-acquired (CA), 371 (53.5%) hospital-acquired (HA) and 74 (10.7%) healthcare-associated (HCA). The overall risk was 6.7 BSI episodes per 1000 admissions. *Escherichia coli, Staphylococcus aureus* and *Streptococcus pneumoniae* were the most frequent causes of CA-BSI and *Klebsiella pneumoniae, Acinetobacter baumanii* and *S. aureus* were most commonly isolated in HA-BSI. On multivariable analysis, severe underweight, severe anaemia at the time of BSI, admission in the ICU at the time of BSI, and requiring ICU admission after BSI was diagnosed were significantly associated with 14-day mortality.

Conclusion: This study adds to the limited literature describing BSI in children in Africa. Further studies are required to understand the impact that BSI has on the paediatric population in sub-Saharan Africa.

Keywords: Bloodstream infections, Children, Africa, Antimicrobial resistance

Background

Bloodstream infection (BSI) causes significant morbidity and mortality in children and increase healthcare expenditure [1, 2]. In Africa, community-acquired (CA)-BSI was identified in 5.8% of children presenting to hospital in Tanzania and up to 19.9% in rural Ghana [3, 4], while hospital-acquired (HA) BSI was less frequently described. In a recent study among children hospitalised in a Kenyan district hospital, the overall risk of acquiring a nosocomial BSI was 5.9 per 1000 admissions. [5]. South Africa has a paucity of literature describing BSI in children. In one study, the risk of CA-BSI and HA-BSI was 16 and 5 per 1000 admissions, respectively [6]. More recent studies have documented lower pathogen yields and high contamination rates in blood culture specimens. The spectrum of pathogens described was similar to elsewhere in Africa with the exception of lower rates of infection caused by non-typhoidal *Salmonella species* [7, 8].

Clinical manifestations of childhood BSI in sub-Saharan Africa (SSA) are also poorly documented. Fever may be the only manifestation of childhood invasive infection. In SSA with the added burden of malaria, HIV-infection, tuberculosis and malnutrition, the treatment of fever is often syndromic, targeting multiple possible aetiologies, without necessarily considering BSI as a potential cause [9]. Not all fever is due to malaria, as shown in a recent Tanzanian study where viruses and bacteria caused more than 90% of childhood fevers. In that study only 6.4% of fever episodes were caused by malaria [10]. In HIV-infected children treated with antiretroviral therapy (ART), the risk of BSI is highest in the

* Correspondence: Brian.eley@uct.ac.za
[1]Paediatric Infectious Diseases Unit, Red Cross War Memorial Children's Hospital and the Department of Paediatrics and Child Health, University of Cape Town, Cape Town, South Africa

first 3 months after ART initiation with a steady decline thereafter [11].

Antimicrobial resistance is an important global public health threat. A systematic review on antimicrobial resistance among gram-negative bacteria in developing countries including 15 studies from Africa showed that in children, 50% and 11% of *Escherichia coli* isolates were resistant to ampicillin and gentamicin, respectively and 30% of *Klebsiella pneumoniae* isolates were resistant to ceftriaxone [12]. These antimicrobials are used empirically to treat ill children with invasive infection. None of the studies in this review included children from South Africa but Dramowski and colleagues recently showed that more than 75% of *K. pneumoniae* isolates at their hospital in Cape Town were extended spectrum beta-lactamase (ESBL) producing organisms [7].

Despite the growing body of literature there remains many gaps in our knowledge about the clinical and laboratory aspects of BSI in SSA. To address some of these aspects of BSI in SSA we conducted an observational study aimed at describing the epidemiology, clinical manifestations and antimicrobial management of BSI at Red Cross War Memorial Children's Hospital (RCWMCH).

Methods

Study design and setting

This retrospective descriptive cohort study was completed at RCWMCH on children with culture-confirmed BSI, diagnosed between 1 January 2011 and 31 December 2012. RCWMCH is a 273-bed tertiary level paediatric hospital in Cape Town, Western Cape province, South Africa. The hospital has emergency, general paediatric, specialised paediatric, surgical, burns, trauma and intensive care facilities serving as a referral centre for the Western Cape and surrounding provinces. Dedicated early neonatal care linked to obstetric services is provided by other hospitals in Cape Town. However, neonates requiring immediate surgical care, or medical care after the first 7 days of life are admitted to RCWMCH.

Study population

Most children hospitalised in RCWMCH originate from poor, peri-urban communities in the Western Cape. During the study period there were 43,663 admissions to the hospital and 16,951 blood culture specimens were processed from patients with suspected invasive infection, i.e. 1 blood culture specimen per 2.6 hospital admissions. The medical microbiology database of the National Health Laboratory Service (NHLS) was accessed, and 2084 positive blood culture results of children hospitalised at RCWMCH during the study period were identified. Organisms isolated from these blood cultures were stratified into pathogens and non-pathogens. Coagulase-negative staphylococci, *Staphylococcus epidermidis*, *Bacillus* spp., *Micrococcus* spp., viridans streptococci, and coryneform bacteria were regarded as contaminants and excluded from the analysis unless they were isolated in two or more independent blood culture specimens from the same patient within a 48-h period, in which case they were included as a pathogen [13]. Within this group of blood culture results, repeat blood cultures within 14 days of the initial blood culture and yielding an identical pathogen were regarded as part of the same potential BSI episode, and therefore excluded. A recurrent BSI episode was defined as the isolation of the same or different organism on blood culture more than 14 days after the initial/previous BSI episode. To verify each BSI episode (new or recurrent) identified during this laboratory review, the medical records of all patients linked to these events were reviewed. During this process 20 episodes were excluded as they had been misclassified as BSI episodes. Thus the study population comprised 548 children who experienced 693 unique bacterial or fungal BSI episodes (Fig. 1).

Data collection

Paper-based medical records of patients with BSI episodes were reviewed and relevant data was extracted and manually transferred onto standardised data collection forms. HIV status was determined using HIV test results obtained from patient medical and laboratory records. Microbiological results obtained from the NHLS database were also entered on the data collection forms.

Microbiological procedures

All microbiology testing was conducted at the Groote Schuur National Health Laboratory Service (NHLS) microbiology laboratory. The laboratory uses the BACTEC™ 9240 automated blood culture system (Becton Dickinson, Sparks, Maryland). For blood culture bottles flagging positive with mono-morphic Gram-negative bacilli seen on Gram stain, a locally validated method of direct inoculation into the automated Vitek®2 system (bioMérieux, Inc., France) was employed, using Vitek®2 ID-GNB and AST-N133 cards for identification and susceptibility testing respectively. This direct method was supplemented, where necessary with repeat testing from bacterial colonies subcultured onto agar plates, using either Vitek®2, disk diffusion or gradient diffusion E-test (bioMérieux, Marcy l'Etoile, France) methods. Standard biochemical methods and disk diffusion and gradient diffusion antibiotic susceptibility tests were used to evaluate Gram-positive organisms, while yeasts were tested with the Vitek®2's YST identification and AST-YS07 cards.

Susceptibility results were interpreted according to the Clinical Laboratory Standards Institute (CLSI)

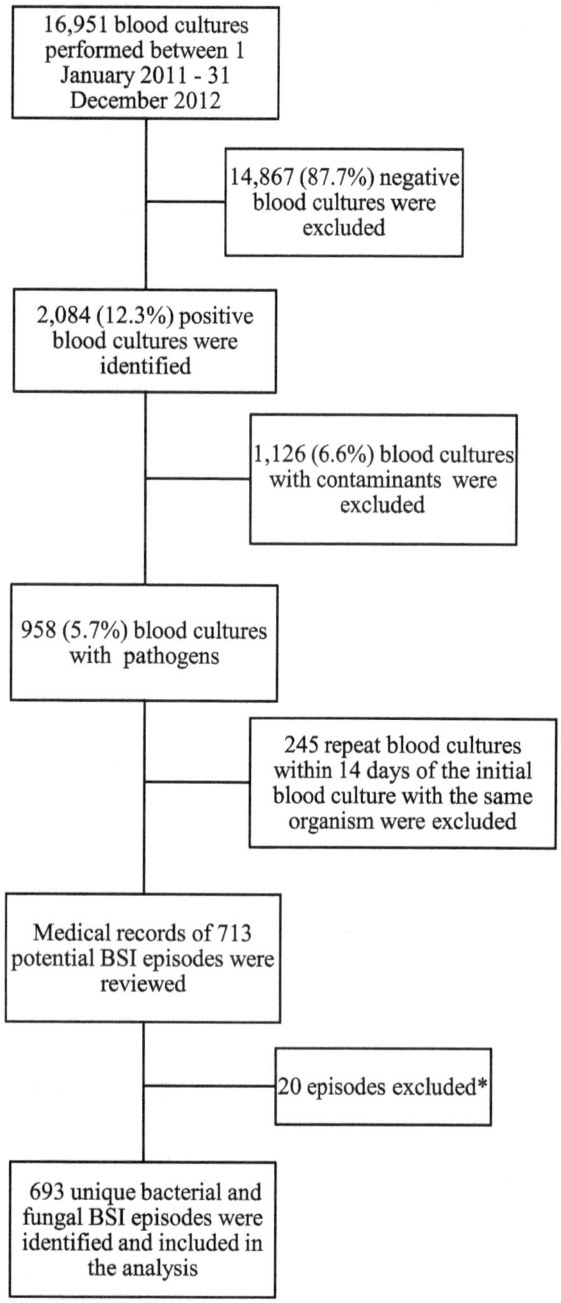

Fig. 1 Selection of BSI episodes for data analysis at Red Cross War Memorial Children's Hospital (RCWMCH). *14 post-mortem specimens and 6 non-blood specimens (peritoneal fluid [3], eye fluid aspirate [1], pus [1] and lymph node aspirate [1]) inoculated in blood culture bottles

criteria for 2011 and 2012 [14, 15]. Ertapenem minimum inhibitory concentration (MIC) breakpoints for Gram-negative organisms were revised in 2012, as were the ciprofloxacin breakpoints for *Salmonella* species. For *Pseudomonas* species, the breakpoints for meropenem, imipenem and piperacillin-tazobactam were revised in 2012.

ESBLs were detected by the Vitek®2 Advanced Expert system or by the double disk synergy method if using disk diffusion testing. Despite the changes to reporting of cephalosporin susceptibility in ESBL-producing organisms introduced by CLSI in 2010, the laboratory, in line with the contemporary national practice, continued to report ESBL- producing *Enterobacteriaceae* as resistant to all cephalosporins.

Study definitions

BSI was classified as (1) *community-acquired* (CA) if the pathogen was isolated within the first 48 h after admission and did not meet the definition of healthcare-associated infection, (2) *hospital-acquired* (HA) if the pathogen was isolated from a blood culture obtained more than 48 h after hospitalisation without the patient having been a resident of a long-term care facility or hospitalised during the preceding 28 days, or (3) *healthcare-associated* (HCA) if the pathogen was isolated in a patient within the first 48 h of being hospitalised from a long-term care facility, or readmitted within 28 days of discharge from a hospital or birth facility [5, 13]. BSI with a clinical focus refers to a laboratory confirmed BSI event accompanied by one of more clinical sites of infection such as pneumonia, meningitis, soft tissue infection or line infection as extracted from the patient's medical records.

The HIV status was defined as follows: (1) *HIV-infected*: a child < 18 months old with a positive HIV DNA PCR result confirmed by either a quantitative HIV RNA PCR or repeat HIV DNA PCR test, or a child ≥ 18 months old with 2 positive serological test results (HIV ELISA or HIV Rapid test) or a positive HIV DNA PCR result confirmed by either a quantitative HIV RNA PCR or repeat HIV DNA PCR test, (2) *HIV-uninfected*: a child with a negative HIV serological or HIV DNA PCR result and (3) *Unknown HIV status:* a child with unknown maternal HIV status and who was not tested for HIV infection.

Moderate and severe underweight for age (UWFA) were defined as weight-for-age z score (WAZ) between −2 and −3 standard deviations (SD) below the median World Health Organisation (WHO) growth reference standards, and a WAZ < −3 SD respectively [16].

Antimicrobial management at the time of the BSI was considered to be effective if the organism isolated was susceptible to the prescribed antimicrobial agent.

Statistical analysis

All data was entered anonymously into an Excel spreadsheet and analysed using Stata release 12.0 statistical software package (STATACorp, College Station, Texas). Continuous variables were expressed as medians (interquartile range, IQR). Frequencies and proportions were used to describe categorical variables. Chi-squared and Kruskal-Wallis tests of association were used to assess associations between categorical and numerical variables across the type of BSI for the baseline patient characteristics and BSI with or without a clinical focus for blood marker variables. Cox proportional hazards regression was used to assess factors associated with 14-day mortality, adjusting for the baseline demographic, clinical and blood marker variables. *P*-values < 0.05 were considered significant.

Results

Classification and risk of bloodstream infection

Overall, 248 (35.8%) CA-, 371 (53.5%) HA- and 74 (10.7%) HCA-BSI episodes were identified. Fewer blood cultures were processed and fewer BSI episodes occurred in 2012 compared to 2011. The overall risk of CA-BSI, HA-BSI and HCA-BSI was 5.7, 8.5 and 1.7 episodes per 1000 admissions, respectively (Table 1).

Baseline characteristics of study participants

Table 2 describes the baseline characteristics of the study participants at the time of each BSI episode and disaggregates the information according to the type of BSI. The median age at the time of BSI was 11.5 months (IQR 3.6–50). Furthermore, 40.7% (273/670) of episodes occurred in children who were moderately or severely underweight. Of the 524 children (75.6%) whose HIV status was known at the BSI event, 13.4% (70/524) were HIV-infected.

Clinical spectrum of bloodstream infections

A clinical site of infection in addition to the bloodstream was identified in 481/663 (72.5%) of the BSI episodes, of which 327/481(68.0%) had a single identifiable site of infection. Two or more clinical sites of infection were identified in the remaining 154 BSI episodes (Table 3). Pneumonia and gastroenteritis were commonly diagnosed at the time of the BSI episode. There was no significant difference in the proportions of BSI episodes with and without a clinical focus associated with a temperature ≥ 38° C; 60% (270/450) vs 62.8% (108/172), RR = 0.99 (95% CI: 0.86–1.14).

Table 1 Classification and risk of bloodstream infection (BSI), 2011–2012

	2011	2012	2011–2012
Hospital admissions	22,685	20,978	43,663
Blood cultures processed	9108	7843	16,951
Classification of bloodstream infection (n/N(%))			
Community-acquired	151/413 (36.6)	97/280 (34.6)	248/693 (35.8)
Hospital-acquired	214/413 (51.8)	157/280 (56.1)	371/693 (53.5)
Healthcare-associated	48/413 (11.6)	26/280 (9.3)	74/693 (10.7)
Risk of BSI per 1000 hospital admissions			
Community-acquired	6.7	4.6	5.7
Hospital-acquired	9.4	7.5	8.5
Healthcare-associated	2.1	1.2	1.7

Spectrum of organisms

Fifty two different organisms were isolated from the 693 BSI episodes including 11 fungi. Fifty eight percent of the BSI episodes were caused by gram-negative bacteria, 36% by gram-positive bacteria and 6% by fungi. *Candida albicans* (19/42) was the dominant fungal isolate. *Cryptococcus neoformans* was isolated in one HIV-infected child with severe immunodeficiency i.e. an absolute CD4 count of < 20 × 10^9/L and a CD4 percentage of < 1% (Table 4).

Susceptibility to antimicrobial agents

The majority of *Staphylococcus aureus* isolates 81/103 (78.6%) were susceptible to cloxacillin. The remaining 22 isolates were methicillin-resistant of which 17 were HA- BSI, accounting for 17/371 (5%) of all HA-BSI. Of the 57 *S. pneumoniae* isolates, 26.3% (15/57) were resistant to penicillin according to meningitis criteria with MIC > 0.06 μg/ml. Susceptibility testing for ceftriaxone and vancomycin was conducted in 52 and 21of the *S. pneumoniae* isolates, respectively with100% susceptibility for both antimicrobials. Of the 48 *Enterococcus* isolates, 54.2% (26/48) were susceptible to ampicillin and all were susceptible to vancomycin.

Table 5 describes antimicrobial susceptibility of the most commonly isolated Gram-negative organisms. Only 9.9% (9/91) of *E.coli* isolates were susceptible to ampicillin while 70.3% (64/91) were susceptible to gentamicin. Thirty four percent (31/92) of all *E.coli* isolates were extended-spectrum beta lactamase (ESBL)-producing organisms of which 10 and 16 were community-acquired and hospital-acquired respectively, accounting for 4% (10/248) and 4.3% (16/371) of CA- and HA-BSI, respectively. By contrast, 77.3% (68/88) of *K. pneumoniae* isolates were ESBL producers which accounted for 16.7% (62/371) of HA-BSI. No carbapenem-resistant *Enterobacteriacae* (CRE) isolates were identified on blood culture during the study period. Resistance to both aminoglycosides and carbapenems was present in 22% (13/59) of *A. baumanii* isolates. All *A. baumanii* isolates were susceptible to colistin. All non-typhoidal *Salmonella ssp.* isolates were susceptible to ceftriaxone, with only a single isolate not susceptible to ampicillin and ciprofloxacin. *Candida albicans* and *parapsilosis* isolates showed a 100% susceptibility to fluconazole.

Antimicrobial therapy

Information on antimicrobial therapy was available for 92% (638/693) of BSI episodes. The median (IQR) time

Table 2 Baseline patient characteristics

	CA-BSI (N = 248[a])	HA-BSI (N = 371[a])	HCA-BSI (N = 74)	Total BSIs (N = 693[a])
Age median (IQR)	9.3 (3.1–39.3)	13.0 (4.0–59.7)	7.1 (1.4–67.0)	11.5 (3.6–50.0)
Age categories, n/N(%)				
0–28 days	31 (12.5)	28 (7.5)	16 (21.6)	75 (10.8)
1 - < 2 months	17 (6.9)	17 (4.6)	6 (8.1)	40 (5.8)
2 - < 12 months	88 (35.5)	132 (35.6)	22 (29.7)	242 (34.9)
12 months – < 5 years	67 (27)	106 (28.6)	11 (14.9)	184 (26.5)
> 5 years	45 (18.1)	88 (23.7)	19 (25.7)	152 (21.9)
WAZ median (IQR)	−1.2 (−2.5–0.1)	−1.8 (−3.4–0.6)	−1.9 (−3.3–1.0)	−1.6 (−3–0.3)
WAZ categories, n/N (%)				
Severe underweight	44/240 (18.3)	103/361 (28.5)	22/69 (31.9)	169/670 (25.2)
Moderate underweight	33/240 (13.8)	60/361 (16.6)	11/69 (15.9)	104/670 (15.5)
Mild-normal	163,240 (67.9)	198/361 (54.8)	36/69 (52.2)	397/670 (59.3)
HIV-infected, n/N (%)	33 (13.3)	33 (8.9)	4 (5.4)	70 (10.1)
HIV-uninfected, n/N (%)	172 (69.3)	232 (62.5)	49 (66.2)	454 (65.5)
HIV not tested, n/N (%)	43 (6.2)	106 (28.6)	21 (28.4)	169 (24.4)
Receiving ART at the time of the BSI in HIV infected child, n/N(%)	11/33 (33.3)	29/33 (87.9)	3/4 (75)	43/70 (61.4)

[a]*N* denominator used unless otherwise stated, *IQR* interquartertile range, *BSI* bloodstream infection, *CA-BSI* community-acquired bloodstream infection, *HA-BSI* hospital-acquired bloodstream infection, *HCA-BSI* healthcare-associated bloodstream infection, *WAZ* weight-for-age z-score, *HIV-infected* human immunodeficiency virus infected, *ART* antiretroviral therapy

Table 3 Clinical classification of bloodstream infection (BSI)

	CA-BSI (N = 242[a]) n/N (%))	HA-BSI (N = 353[a]) n/N (%)	HCA-BSI (N = 68[a]) n/N (%)	Total BSIs (N = 663[a]) n/N (%)
BSI with no clinical focus	28 (11.6)	131(37.1)	23 (33.8)	182 (27.5)
Hypothermia[b]	5/28 (17.9)	2/131 (1.5)	0/23 (0)	7/182 (3.8)
Fever[c]	14/28 (50)	77/131 (58.8)	17/23 (74)	108/182 (59.3)
BSI with a clinical focus	214(88.4)	222(62.9)	45(66.2)	481 (72.5)
Hypothermia[b]	11/214 (5.1)	4/222 (1.8)	5/45 (11.1)	20/481 (4.2)
Fever[c]	112/214 (52.3)	136/222 (61.3)	22/45 (48.9)	270/481 (56.1)
Pneumonia	65/214 (30.4)	91/222 (41)	16/45 (35.6)	172/481 (35.8)
Gastroenteritis	67/214 (31.3)	28/222 (12.6)	10/45 (22.2)	105/481 (21.8)
Soft tissue infection[d]	18/214 (8.4)	50/222 (22.5)	4/45 (8.9)	72/481 (15)
Meningitis	39/214 (18.2)	1/222 (0.5)	13/45 (28.9)	53/481 (11)
UTI	29/214 (13.6)	20/222 (9)	4/45 (8.9)	53/481 (11)
Line sepsis	4/214 (1.9)	29/222 (13.1)	3/45 (6.7)	36/481 (7.4)
URTI	20/214 (9.3)	8/222 (3.6)	3/45 (6.7)	31/481 (6.4)
Empyema	4/214 (1.9)	5/222 (2.3)	–	9/481 (1.9)
Septic arthritis	6/214 (2.8)	3/222 (1.4)	–	9/481 (1.9)
Bronchiolitis	4/214 (1.9)	–	1/45 (2.2)	5/481 (1)
Pleural effusion	–	3/222 (1.4)	–	3/481 (0.6)

BSI bloodstream infection, *CA-BSI* community-acquired bloodstream infection, *HA-BSI* hospital-acquired bloodstream infection, *HCA-BSI* healthcare-associated bloodstream infection, [a]N = denominator used unless otherwise stated; [b]Body temperature ≤ 35.5 ° C around the time of BSI; [c]Body temperature ≥ 38 °C around the time of BSI; [d]Soft tissue infection includes skin abscesses, burn wound infections, wound sepsis and infected eczema or scabies, *UTI* urinary tract infection, *URTI* upper respiratory tract infection

Table 4 Spectrum of organisms identified during the study period 2011–2012

	CA-BSI n/N (%) (*N* = 248)	HA-BSI n/N (%) (*N* = 371)	HCA-BSI n/N (%) (*N* = 74)	Total BSIs n/N (%) (*N* = 693)
Gram-negative bacteria	117 (47.2)	240 (64.7)	43 (58.1)	400 (57.7)
Escherichia coli	49 (19.8)	33 (8.9)	10 (13.5)	92 (13.3)
Klebsiella pneumoniae	5 (2)	78 (21)	9 (12.2)	92 (13.3)
Acinetobacter baumanii	4 (1.6)	54 (14.6)	1 (1.4)	59 (8.5)
Pseudomonas aeruginosa	3 (1.2)	19 (5.1)	4 (5.4)	26 (3.8)
Non-typhoidal *Salmonella*	11 (4.4)	6 (1.6)	3 (4.1)	20 (2.9)
Enterobacter cloacae	3 (1.2)	12 (3.2)	3 (4.1)	18 (2.6)
Serratia marcescens	0 (0)	17 (4.6)	1 (1.4)	18 (2.6)
Neisseria meningitidis	12 (4.8)	0 (0)	1 (1.4)	13 (1.9)
Haemophilus influenza B	6 (2.4)	1 (0.3)	2 (2.7)	9 (1.3)
Salmonella typhi	4 (1.6)	0 (0)	0 (0)	4 (0.6)
Other	20 (8.1)	20 (5.4)	9 (12.2)	49 (7.1)
Gram-positive bacteria	124 (50)	97 (26.1)	28 (37.8)	249 (35.9)
Staphylococcus aureus	55 (22.2)	37 (10)	11 (14.9)	103 (14.9)
Streptococcus pneumoniae	45 (18.1)	6 (1.6)	6 (8.1)	57 (8.2)
Enterococcus faecalis	4 (1.6)	23 (6.2)	5 (6.8)	32 (4.6)
Streptococcus group B	13 (5.2)	0 (0)	4 (5.4)	17 (2.5)
Enterococcus faecium	2 (0.8)	14 (3.8)	0 (0)	16 (2.3)
Other	5 (2)	17 (4.6)	2 (2.7)	24 (3.5)
Mycobacterium tuberculosis	1 (0.4)	1 (0.3)	0 (0)	2 (0.3)
Fungi	6 (2.4)	33 (8.9)	3 (4.1)	42 (6.1)
Candida albicans	1 (0.4)	16 (4.3)	2 (2.7)	19 (2.7)
Candida parapsilosis	1 (0.4)	9 (2.4)	1 (1.4)	11 (1.6)
Other *Candida* species	4 (1.6)	8 (2.2)	0 (0)	12 (1.7)

N = denominator used unless otherwise stated

to effective antibiotic therapy for bacterial isolates of CA-, HA- and HCA- BSI was 0 (0–1) day, 1 (0–2) day and 1 (0–3) day, respectively. The median (IQR) time to effective antifungal therapy for fungal isolates was 4.5 (4–5) days, 3 (0.5–4) days and 2.5 (2–3) days for CA-, HA- and HCA-BSI, respectively. Of the 638 episodes, 592 (92.8%) received effective antimicrobial therapy based on the susceptibility profile of the isolate. In the remaining 46 episodes, 42 were treated with an ineffective antimicrobial, and 4 fungal BSI episodes did not receive antifungal therapy. Of the 42 bacterial episodes not treated with an effective antimicrobial, 10 (23.8%) resulted in a fatal outcome with the median (IQR) time to death of 4 (2–9) days, and the remaining 32 (76.2%) episodes resolved on ineffective antibiotic therapy. In 2 of the 4 fungal episodes that were not treated with antifungal therapy the patients died before the culture results were known. The remaining 2 children recovered uneventfully.

Outcomes

85 % (590/693) of BSI episodes were successfully treated and the children were discharged from hospital after these episodes. During the study period, 103 (14.9%) children died during or after a BSI episode prior to hospital discharge. Seventy of these deaths occurred within 14 days as a direct result of the BSI and were included in the survival analysis as there was a high chance of correctly identifying relevant risk factors in these children. The median time (IQR) to death of these 70 children was 3 (1–8) days. Of the 33 deaths that occurred after 14 days, the median time (IQR) to death was 46 (23–67) days.

Table 6 describes risk factors associated with 14-day inpatient mortality in children with BSI. On multivariable analysis, severe UWFA, severe anaemia at the time of BSI, admission in the ICU at the time of BSI, and requiring ICU admission after BSI was diagnosed were significantly associated with 14-day mortality. HIV-infection was not associated with increased mortality risk.

Discussion

The current study describes the aetiology and quantifies the risk of BSI at our hospital. Gram-negative organisms were the predominant cause of BSI. The risk was lower for CA-BSI but higher for HA-BSI than rates obtained in a previous South African study conducted 20 years previously [6]. The isolation of 5.7% pathogens from blood culture specimens in the present study is similar to that from another referral hospital in Cape Town [7]. Possible reasons for the low pathogen yield in our setting may include inadequate volumes of blood inoculated into blood culture specimen bottles, lack of clear clinical indications for performing blood cultures potentially inflating the number of negative cultures and the prior use of antimicrobials, particularly ceftriaxone, as part of the syndromic case management of sick children at primary health care facilities [5, 9, 17]. The contaminant prevalence of 6.6% from 16,951 blood cultures is more than double the internationally acceptable contamination rate of 2–3%, suggesting that urgent attention is needed to improve aseptic measures when obtaining specimens for blood culture [18, 19]. A previous analysis of blood culture results over a 5-year period (2008–2012) from the same institution highlighted problems of high contamination rates particularly in the less than one-year age group and low pathogen yield, and also documented the predominance of gram-negative pathogens. [8].

S. aureus, E.coli, K. pneumoniae and *A. baumanii* predominated in our study. This spectrum of organisms is similar to that documented in other African studies [5–7]. Non-typhoidal *Salmonella* is a much more frequent cause of BSI in African countries to the north of South Africa, especially those in malaria-endemic areas,

Table 5 Rates of antimicrobial susceptibility for the common gram-negative organisms identified

	Acinetobacter baumanii (*N* = 59)		*Escherichia coli* (*N* = 92)		*Klebsiella pneumoniae* (*N* = 92)		*Pseudomonas aeruginosa* (*N* = 26)		Non-typhoidal *Salmonella* (*N* = 20)	
Antimicrobial	No isolates tested	No (%) Susceptible	No isolates tested	No (%) Susceptible	No isolates tested	*N* (%) Susceptible	No isolates tested	N (%) Susceptible	No isolates tested	*N* (%) Susceptible
Ampicillin	–	–	91	9 (9.9)	92	–	–	–	20	19 (95)
Co-amoxyclav[a]	–	–	89	43 (48.3)	91	27 (29.7)	–	–	1	1 (100)
Ceftriaxone	–	–	90	59 (65.6)	88	20 (22.7)	–	–	20	20 (100)
Ceftazidime	59	24 (40.7)	91	60 (65.9)	91	20 (22)	26	23 (88.5)	1	1 (100)
Ciprofloxacin	59	45 (76.3)	87	70 (80.5)	85	52 (61.2)	26	15 (57.7)	19	18 (94.7)
Piperacillin-tazobactam	58	10 (17.2)	6[$]	5 (83.3)	49[$]	34 (69.4)	7[$]	1 (14.3)	1[$]	1 (100)
Gentamicin	59	27 (45.8)	91	64 (70.3)	89	25 (28.1)	25	15 (60)	–	–
Amikacin	58	26 (44.8)	92	77 (83.7)	91	70 (76.9)	26	16 (61.5)	–	–
Meropenem	56	26 (46.4)	92	92 (100)	92	92 (100)	26	22 (84.6)	20	20 (100)
Imipenem	49	27 (55.1)	90	90 (100)	90	90 (100)	26	21 (80.8)	20	20 (100)
Ertapenem			92	92 (100)	91	91 (100)	–	–	20	20 (100)
Colistin	59	59 (100)	90	90 (100)	89	89 (100)	26	23 (88.5)	–	–

[a]Co-amoxyclav = Amoxycillin-clavulanic acid co-formulation $ due to technical limitations with the Vitek®2 AST card piperacillin-tazobactam was infrequently reported in 2011–2012; *No* number

but has been reported as an important cause of BSI in an early South African study [20].

At the time of BSI, 27.5% of the episodes were not associated with a clinical focus of infection and 65.1% had fever (≥ 38 °C) or hypothermia (< 35.5 °C). A study done in Guinea-Bissau showed that the sensitivity of fever for detecting BSI was low at 54% with a positive predictive value (PPV) of 12% [21]. However, a Tanzanian study showed that temperature ≥ 38.5 °C was a strong predictor of BSI (odds ratio (OR) 7, 95% CI: 2.2–14.8, $P = 0.0001$) although the number of patients enrolled in that study was small [22]. Furthermore, a Malawian study of 225 hospitalised children found that the presence of at least one of five clinical features (oral thrush, malnutrition, chronic cough, lethargy on history and lethargy on examination) predicted BSI with a sensitivity of 69% [23].

Severe underweight was present in 25.2% of children in our study and was a significant predictor of 14-day mortality. These findings are in agreement with previous African studies showing that severe malnutrition significantly increases the risk of BSI, and that nutritional status is a significant determinant of survival in children with BSI [5, 24]. Although HIV infection was known to be present in 13.4% of the study cohort it did not influence 14-day mortality. Approximately 60% of the HIV-infected group was on ART at the time of BSI. This may partly explain why HIV infection did not influence mortality.

Our results show that ESBL-producing *K. pneumoniae* and *E. coli* have become important causes of CA- and HA-BSI. Of particular concern was that 30% of *E.coli* isolates in the CA-BSI group were ESBL-producing organisms. A recent study from another Cape Town hospital documented lower prevalence of CA-BSI caused by ESBL-producing *E.coli* (11.2%) and HA-BSI caused by ESBL-producing *K.pneumoniae* (78.3%) [7]. Although carbapenem-resistant *Enterobacteriaceae* infection was not observed during the study period, carbapenem overutilisation as observed in the present study (data not shown) may with time lead to the emergence of carbapenem resistant BSI isolates.

Study strengths and limitations

The study describes the spectrum of organisms causing BSI in children. The results obtained highlight the growing concern of antibiotic resistance developing particularly in CA–BSI. One limitation was the lack of susceptibility data for piperacillin-tazobactam due to technical limitations at the time of the study. With ongoing surveillance of organisms causing BSI and their susceptibility patterns, empiric antimicrobial choices may need to be altered in the future. Subsequent to the study period, updated definitions of reporting laboratory confirmed BSI were release by the CDC [25]. These definitions were not utilised in the current study and as a result, few of the HA-BSI episodes may have been misclassified. Organisms implicated in mucosal barrier injury BSI were also not stratified.

Due to the retrospective study design, there are limitations in the completeness and availability of clinical and laboratory data. The true burden of community-acquired BSI may have been underestimated. Before sick children are referred from primary and secondary health facilities to our hospital, they are often administered broad-spectrum antibiotics. This practice is consistent

Table 6 Risk factors associated with 14-day inpatient mortality in children with BSI

Factor	Univariate HR (95% CI)	*P* value	Adjusted HR (95%CI)	*P* value
Age	*N* = 693			
0–28 days	0.9 (0.4–2)	0.834	1	
1 - < 2 months	2.2 (1.1–4.6)	0.035	1	
2 - < 12 months	1.2 (0.8–2)	0.376	1	
12 months – 5 years	0.7 (0.4–1.2)	0.219	1	
> 5 years	1		1	
Nutritional status	*N* = 693			
Severe underweight for age	2.4 (1.5–3.9)	0.0001	2.0 (1.2–3.3)	0.007
Moderate underweight for age	1.1 (0.6–2)	0.851	1	
Mild-normal weight for age	1		1	
Weight not recorded	2.4 (1–5.9)	0.060	4.9 (1.2–20.8)	0.029
Haemoglobin	*N* = 693			
Severe anaemia (< 7 g/dL)	3.3 (1.7–6.4)	0.001	2.7 (1.3–5.6)	0.006
Mild anaemia (7–11 g/dL)	1 (0.6–1.7)	0.909	1	
No anaemia (≥ 11 g/dL)	1		1	
Result not available	3.7 (1.2–11.9)	0.025	4.2 (1.3–13.7)	0.018
ICU management	*N* = 693			
ICU resident at time of BSI	1.5 (0.89–2.7)	0.124	6.5 (3.7–11.6)	0.0001
BSI requiring ICU management	5.2 (3.3–8.4)	0.0001	3.5 (1.8–6.7)	0.0001
BSI not requiring ICU management	1		1	
Type of BSI	*N* = 693			
CA	1		1	
HA	1.2 (0.8–2)	0.377	1	
HCA	0.9 (0.4–1.9)	0.806	1	
HIV infection	*N* = 693			
Yes	1.5 (0.8–2.9)	0.221	1	
No	1		1	
Unknown status	0.8 (0.5–1.5)	0.523	1	

with the World Health Organization Integrated Management of Childhood Illness guidelines that have been implemented in South Africa, and frequently results in no growth on blood culture [9]. Even though the study cohort included neonates, the results obtained would not be an accurate reflection of the burden of BSI in this special group of infants. We were only able to explore a limited number of potential risk factors of BSI mortality. Further studies with larger sample sizes are required to provide a more in depth understanding of this aspect of BSI. Furthermore, it was not possible to explore risk factors associated with the acquisition of a BSI due to the lack of a suitable control group of children without BSI.

Conclusion

Our study provides insights about the risk, aetiology, clinical manifestations, antimicrobial therapy and outcomes of BSI in a sub-Saharan African setting characterized by high HIV prevalence. Further studies are required to gain a comprehensive understanding of the impact of BSI on the childhood population in SSA.

Abbreviations

ART: Antiretroviral therapy; BSI: Bloodstream infection; CA: Community-acquired; CLSI: Clinical Laboratory standards institute; CRE: Carbapenem-resistant *Enterobacteriacae*; CRP: C-reactive protein; ESBL: Extended-spectrum beta lactamase; FBC: Full blood count; HA: Hospital-acquired; HCA: Healthcare-associated; HIV infection: Human immunodeficiency virus infection; IQR: Interquartile range; NHLS: National health laboratory service; PCT: Procalcitonin; SSA: Sub-Saharan Africa; UWFA: Underweight for age; WAZ: Weight for age z-score; WCC: White cell count

Acknowledgements

Spasina King is acknowledged for assisting with data collection from the medical records.

Funding

No funding was required for the completion of this study.

Authors' contributions

HL, BE and JN conceived and designed the study. CB was responsible for the overseeing the microbiological analysis at the NHLS and interpreting susceptibility results. VP contributed to the statistical analysis of the results. HL wrote the paper with contributions from BE, CB and JN. All authors read and approved the final manuscript.

Consent for publication

Not applicable

Competing interests

The authors declare that they have no competing interests.

Author details

[1]Paediatric Infectious Diseases Unit, Red Cross War Memorial Children's Hospital and the Department of Paediatrics and Child Health, University of Cape Town, Cape Town, South Africa. [2]Division of Medical Microbiology, University of Cape Town and the National Health Laboratory Service, Groote Schuur Hospital, Cape Town, South Africa.

References

1. Berkley JA, Lowe BS, Mwangi I, Williams T, Bauni E, Mwarumba S, et al. Bacteremia among children admitted to a rural hospital in Kenya. N Engl J Med. 2005;352:39–47.
2. Reddy EA, Shaw AV, Crump JA. Community-acquired bloodstream infections in Africa. Lancet Infect Dis. 2010;10:417–32. https://doi.org/10.1016/S1473-3099(10)70072-4.
3. Crump JA, Ramadhani HO, Morrissey AB, Msuya LJ, Yang L-Y, Chow S-C, et al. Invasive bacterial and fungal infections among hospitalised HIV-infected and HIV-uninfected children and infants in northern Tanzania. Tropical Med and International health. 2011;16(7):830–7. https://doi.org/10.1111/j.1365-3156.2011.02774x.
4. Nielsen MV, Sarpong N, Krumkamp R, Dekker D, Loag W, Amemasor S, et al. Incidence and characteristics of bacteremia among children in rural Ghana. PLoSONE. 2012;7(9):e44063. https://doi.org/10.1371/journal.pone.0044063.
5. Aiken AM, Mturi N, Njuguna P, Mohammed S, Berkley JA, Mwangi I, et al. Risk and causes of paediatric hospital-acquired bacteraemia in Kilifi District Hopsital, Kenya: a prospective cohort study. Lancet. 2011;378:2021–7. https://doi.org/10.1016/S0140-6736(11)61622-X.
6. Cotton MF, Burger PJ, Bodenstein WJM. Bacteraemia in children in the south-western cape. A hospital-based survey. S Afr MJ. 1992;81:87–90.
7. Dramowski A, Cotton MF, Rabie H, Whitelaw A. Trends in paediatric bloodstream infections at a south African referral hospital. BMC Paediatrics. 2015;15:33–44. https://doi.org/10.1186/s12887-015-0354-3.
8. Lochan H, Bamford C, Eley B. Blood cultures in sick children. S Afr Med J. 2013;103(12):918–20. https://doi.org/10.7196/SAMJ.6979.
9. WHO/UNICEF. Integrated Management of Childhood Illness Chart Booklet. Geneva: WHO/UNICEF; 2008.
10. D'Acremont V, Kilowoko M, Kyungu E, Philipina S, Sangu W, Kahama-Moro J, et al. Beyond malaria – causes of fever in outpatient Tanzanian children. N Engl J Med. 2014;370:809–14. https://doi.org/10.1056/NEJMoa1214482.
11. Musiime V, Cook A, Bakeera-Kitaka S, Vhembo T, Lutakome J, Keishanyu R, et al. Bacteremia, causative agents and antimicrobial susceptibility among HIV-1–infected children on antiretroviral therapy in Uganda and Zimbabwe. Pediatr Infect Dis J. 2013;32:856–62. https://doi.org/10.1097/INF.0b013e31828c3991.
12. Le Doare K, Bielicki J, Heath PT, Sharland M. Systematic review of antibiotic resistance rates among gram-negative bacteria in children with sepsis in resource-limited countries. J Pediatric Infect Dis Society. 2015;4(1):11–20. https://doi.org/10.1093/jpids/piu014.
13. Centres for Disease Control and Prevention and the National Healthcare Safety Network. CDC/NHSN Surveillance Definitions for Specific Types of Infections. Atlanta: CDC, 2014. http://www.socinorte.com/wpcontent/uploads/2014/06/17pscNosInfDef_current.pdf. Accessed 1 Dec 2017.
14. Clinical and Laboratory Standards Institute. Performance Standards for Antimicrobial Susceptibility Testing; Twenty-First Infromational Supplement. CLSI document M100-S21. Wayne, PA. Clinical and Laboratory Standards Institute; 2011
15. Clinical and Laboratory Standards Institute. Performance Standards for Antimicrobial Susceptibility Testing; Approved Standard - Eleventh Edition. CLSI document M02-A11. Wayne, PA. Clinical and Laboratory Standards Institute; 2012
16. World Health Organization. The WHO child growth standards. Geneva: World Health Organization 2006. http://apps.who.int/gho/data/imr.jsp?id=72/RefSource> Accessed 7 July 2014.
17. Connell TG, Rele M, Cowley D, Buttery JP, Curtis N. How reliable is a negative blood culture result? Volume of blood submitted for culture in routine practice in a children's hospital. Pediatrics. 2007;119(5):891–6.
18. Hall KK, Lyman JA. Updated review of blood culture contamination. Clin Microbiol Rev. 2006;19(4):788–802. https://doi.org/10.1128/CMR.00062-05
19. Pavlovsky M, Press J, Peled N, Yagupsky P. Blood culture contamination in pediatric patients: young children and young doctors. Pediatr Infect Dis. 2006;25(7):611–4. https://doi.org/10.1097/01.inf.0000220228.01382.88
20. Berkowitz FE. Bacteraemia in hospitalised black south African children. Am J Dis Child. 1984;138:551–6.
21. Isendahl J, Manjuba C, Rodrigues A, Xu W, Henriques-Normack B, Giske CG, et al. Prevalence of community-acquired bacteraemia in Guinea-Bissau: an observational study. BMC Infect Dis. 2014;14:3859. https://doi.org/10.1186/s12879-014-0715-9.
22. Christopher A, Mshana SE, Kidenya BR, Hokororo A, Morona D. Bacteremia and resistant gram-negative pathogens among under-fives in Tanzania. Ital J Pediatr. 2013;39:27–36. https://doi.org/10.1186/1824-7288-39-27.
23. Norton EB, Archibald LK, Nwanyanwu OC, Kazembe PN, Dobbie H, Reller B, et al. Clinical predictors of bloodstream infections and mortality in hospitalized Malawian children. Paediatr Infect Dis J 2004;23:145-151.https://doi.org/10.1542/peds.2006-0440 Accessed 23 November 2016.
24. Sigaúque B, Roca A, Mandomando I, Morais L, Quintó L, Sacarlal J, et al. Community-acquired bacteraemia among children admitted to a rural hospital in Mozambique. Pediatr Infect Dis J. 2009;28:108–13. https://doi.org/10.1097/INF.0b013e318187a87d.
25. Centers for Disease Control and prevention and the National Healthcare safety Network. CDC/NHSH Surveillance. Bloodstream Infection Event (Central Line-Associated Bloodstream Infection and non-central line-associated Bloodstream Infection. CDC January 2017. https://www.cdc.gov/nhsn/pdfs/pscmanual/4psc_clabscurrent.pdf. Accessed 18 June 2017.

21

Evaluation of Candida bloodstream infection and antifungal utilization in a tertiary care hospital

Tatiana Aporta Marins[1*], Alexandre R. Marra[2,3], Michael B. Edmond[3,4], Marines Dalla Valle Martino[5], Paula Kiyomi Onaga Yokota[2], Ana Carolina Cintra Nunes Mafra[6] and Marcelino Souza Durão Junior[2]

Abstract

Background: Candida bloodstream infections carry a significant mortality risk, justifying the importance of adequate antifungal therapy. This study describes trends in antifungal consumption using the Defined Daily Dose (DDD) and Days of Therapy (DOT) metrics, identifies the microbiological profile, the time to initiation of empirical therapy, the adjustment after positive blood culture results for *Candida*, and the impact on in-hospital mortality rate in patients with candidemia.

Methods: An analysis of antifungal consumption from 2008 to 2016, and of candidemia cases from 2012 to 2016 was carried out in a private tertiary hospital.

Results: A total of 11,273 admissions were identified with a prescription for at least one type of antifungal therapy. Fluconazole was the most prescribed antifungal drug in terms of general consumption. Through the DDD and DOT metrics, we observed that over time, there was an increase in the consumption of liposomal amphotericin B, micafungin and voriconazole. *Candida albicans* was the most isolated species in blood cultures. Regarding candidemia, we analyzed samples from 115 patients. Empirical therapy was started within 24 h of blood culture in 44.3% of the cases, and in 81.7% of the cases, the antifungal was deemed to be adequate based in antifungal susceptibility testing, both of which were not associated with the in-hospital mortality rate.

Conclusions: Our study reinforces the importance of monitoring the consumption of antifungal agents, which helps in proposing actions that lead to their rational use and, consequently, reduces the appearance of resistant strains.

Keywords: Antifungal, Candidemia, Consumption, Defined daily dose, Days of therapy

Background

Since the 1980s, candidemia cases have increased substantially in different regions of the world and, in Brazilian hospitals, it is one of the highest incidence infections [1, 2]. In a recently published Brazilian study, *Candida spp.* was the seventh most prevalent agent in analyzed bloodstream infections [3]. *Candida albicans* remains the most commonly isolated microorganism among *Candida*, however, candidemia caused by non-*albicans* species has increased worldwide, particularly *C. tropicalis*, *C. glabrata*, *C. parapsilosis* and *C. krusei* [4, 5].

The severity of these infections poses a significant morbidity and mortality risk [6]. They are often expensive and difficult to treat, so adequate antifungal therapy is necessary [7–10]. Regarding the timing of initiation of empiric treatment, studies are still controversial, with some showing that mortality was lower in patients who received the antifungal early [10, 11] and others indicating that there was no significant difference in in-hospital mortality [12, 13].

In order to provide adequate antifungal therapy, it is important to know the consumption pattern and the microbiological profile of your institution and, with the obtained information, to implement opportunities for improvement that lead to the rational use of these drugs

* Correspondence: tatiana.marins@einstein.br
[1]Hospital Israelita Albert Einstein, São Paulo, Brazil

and consequently achieve therapeutic success and increase patient safety.

Despite the advances in antifungal development in the previous decade, the therapeutic arsenal available on the market, and validated for the treatment of systemic fungal infections, is still limited and candidemia and other forms of invasive candidiasis remain potentially fatal infections, justifying the careful choice of treatments [14, 15]. Currently, there are four classes of systemic antifungal drugs that are effective: polyenes, azoles, echinocandins, and flucytosine [16]. Consumption of these drugs should be monitored over the years to control overuse, measure improvements, and obtain parameters for future internal and external comparisons. Monitoring is also important to prevent resistant microorganism species in the future.

This monitoring should be performed through quantitative analysis [17, 18]. There are already well established metrics for the consumption of antimicrobials, the most common being the Defined Daily Dose (DDD), but there are others such as: days of therapy (DOT), Prescribed Daily Dose (PDD), and Recommended Daily Dose (RDD), which are also being used for the calculation of antifungal consumption [19–22]. There is still no consensus as to what is the best metric to quantify the use of these drugs. The World Health Organization (WHO) recommends consumption calculation using DDD [22], but other authors suggest DOT, since this methodology is not influenced by changes in the recommended individual dose and by dose adjustment in cases of kidney failure [23, 24].

The goal of this study is to describe and analyze antifungal consumption trends through the DDD and DOT metrics in patients who were admitted to Hospital Israelita Albert Einstein, and also identify the microbiological profile, time of onset of empirical antifungal therapy, antifungal adequacy and the impact on in-hospital mortality in patients with candidemia.

Methods

The study was conducted in a 670-bed private, tertiary hospital focused on high complexity treatments including solid organ and bone marrow transplantation, located in the city of São Paulo, Brazil. This is a descriptive and retrospective observational study that identified the global consumption of antifungal drugs in all the patients who were hospitalized from January 1, 2008 to December 31, 2016. Adult inpatients with candidemia from January 1, 2012 to December 31, 2016 were also analyzed. This study was submitted and approved by the Institution's Research Ethics Committee and informed consent was not required.

The report of inpatient antifungal medicines was generated through the hospital's electronic inventory management system. The analyzed drugs were: fluconazole, voriconazole, itraconazole, posaconazole, caspofungin, micafungin, anidulafungin, liposomal amphotericin B and amphotericin B deoxycholate. Hospital nursing units include Adult Medical and Surgical Wards (MSW, n = 14), Oncology (ONCO), Bone Marrow Transplantation (BMT), Solid Organ Transplantation (SOT), Adult Intensive Care Unit (AICU), Pediatrics (PED) and Neonatal Intensive Care Unit (NICU).

The impact of bed occupancy variation was minimized by reporting the antifungal consumption per 1000 patient-days. Two consumption metrics were used, DDD and DOT. We chose these metrics because they are the most commonly used and are recommended by health agencies [20, 22].

DDD is defined as the mean maintenance dose per day for a drug used in its primary indication in an adult patient [22]. The DOT metric measures the number of days that a patient is on a specific drug, regardless of the number of doses administered or dosing [25]. One DOT is assigned for each drug administered each day. To assess consumption in Pediatrics and Neonatology, only the DOT was calculated. DDD and DOT were calculated annually for general consumption data, and data by specialty. The formulas used for the DDD and DOT calculations were:

$$\text{DDD 1000 patient-days} = \frac{\text{drug consumption in grams for period} \times 1000}{\text{IDD} \times \text{number of patient-days in the period}}$$

$$\text{DOT 1000 patient-days} = \frac{\text{days of therapy in the period} \times 1000}{\text{number of patient-days in the period}}$$

For the DDD calculation, the anatomical therapeutic chemical (ATC)/DDD system, recognized by the World Health Organization as an international standard for drug use studies, was used. The Defined Daily Doses used were 200 mg for fluconazole, 400 mg for voriconazole, 200 mg for itraconazole, 300 mg for posaconazole, 50 mg for caspofungin, 100 mg for micafungin, 100 mg for anidulafungin and 35 mg for amphotericin B deoxycholate and liposomal amphotericin B [22].

In analyzing the medical records for hospitalized patients diagnosed with candidemia in the period between 2012 and 2016, patients under the age of 18 years, outpatients and those who had incomplete data in their medical records were excluded. The data gathered followed a standard form including the following variables: age, gender, admission weight, admission date, hospitalization time, antifungal used in the treatment, dose, time of treatment, date of collection and date of blood culture result, type of microbiological agent, antifungal sensitivity test, time of starting empiric therapy, adequacy based on antifungal susceptibility testing, prescribed dose as recommended by the institutional protocol for invasive fungal infections, and in-hospital outcome.

Patients' primary comorbidities were identified, as well as the presence of risk factors for candidemia (intensive care unit admission, mechanical ventilation, hemodialysis, blood transfusion, neutropenia (total neutrophil count $< 500/mm^3$), use of vasoactive drugs, antimicrobial agents, corticosteroids, chemotherapy drugs, parenteral nutrition, surgical procedure, presence of central venous catheter). *Breakthrough* cases were also identified, defined as a positive blood culture during antifungal therapy of at least three days duration. These *breakthrough* cases were also included in our analysis [26, 27].

A candidemia episode was defined as the isolation of *Candida* in blood culture. For all patients, the first episode of candidemia was the episode analyzed. Polymicrobial blood cultures, that are where there was growth of other microorganisms in addition to *Candida* species, were excluded from the analysis.

Empirical therapy was defined as the initiation of an antifungal drug without knowledge of the infection-causing microorganism species, and targeted therapy was defined as treatment with an antifungal drug after the culture result was reported.

Empirical therapy was considered inadequate when no intravenous antifungal agent was administered within 24 h of blood culture [11, 28]. After obtaining the blood culture result identifying the microorganism and the antifungal susceptibility testing, therapy was considered inadequate if the isolated organism was resistant to the antifungal agent in use (for example, fluconazole for *Candida krusei*), if the antifungal agent was used in inadequate doses (e.g. fluconazole doses of less than 400 mg per day) or if no antifungal agent was initiated [10, 11, 29].

The hospital has an institutional protocol to guide the clinical staff based on international antifungal guidelines. Doses recommended by the institutional protocol were as follows: liposomal amphotericin B 3 to 5 mg/kg/day, fluconazole 400 to 800 mg/day orally or intravenously, voriconazole 6 mg/kg IV every 12 h on day 1 followed by 4 mg/kg/day intravenously or orally, caspofungin loading dose of 70 mg followed by 50 mg/day thereafter, anidulafungin 200 mg loading dose followed by 100 mg/day thereafter, and micafungin 100 mg/day [16, 30].

Microbiological analysis

All positive samples were identified using BACTEC FX equipment (BD Diagnostic Systems, Franklin Lakes, NJ, USA), an automated method used to detect microorganisms in blood cultures. After yeast were identified by gram stain, the chromogenic agar ChromID CPS (bioMérieux) was used, allowing identification of yeasts by the colors produced in the medium. Until 2013, species identification was carried out by VITEK® 2 (bioMérieux) and from then on, to the present date, mass spectrometry VITEK MS (bioMérieux, Marcy l'Etoile, France) and Maldi-TOF (Bruker Microflex LT Biotyper 3.1) was used.

The antifungal susceptibility test profile was carried out for all blood culture samples positive for *Candida,* using the broth microdilution method according to CLSI document M27-A3, using current CLSI MIC interpretative criteria as M27-S4 [31, 32]. *Candida parapsilosis* ATCC22019 and *Candida krusei* ATCC6258 were used as quality controls. Commonly tested drugs were amphotericin B, fluconazole, voriconazole, anidulafungin (or caspofungin, depending on laboratory availability). Micafungin susceptibility testing was not performed because the laboratory did not have the specific test supplies for this drug during the study period.

Statistical analysis

In order to compare the DDD and DOT measurements, and to assess possible trends over time, Spearman correlation coefficients were used. In the comparison between hospitalization units in terms of antifungal consumption metrics, Kruskal-Wallis hypothesis tests were used, with post-tests corrected by the Steel [33] method, considering the medical and surgical clinic as a reference category.

Anidulafungin was introduced in the hospital formulary in 2010, micafungin in 2011 and posaconazole in 2016. These periods without consumption of these drugs were considered missing in the analysis. For the analysis of variations over time and for comparisons between units, if a unit had not consumed a certain antifungal in any valid year, the DDD and DOT values were considered zero. For correlations between DDD and DOT, zero values were not considered, but only the values or the years in which there was some antifungal consumption.

In order to investigate the in-hospital mortality associated factors, simple and multiple logistic regression models were fitted. For the multiple model, a stepwise variable selection process was conducted in both directions, considering information on the patient's profile, clinical history, antifungal treatment and hospitalization. The criterion for selection of variables was Akaike information (AIC). Model results are represented by p values, odds ratios (OR) and their 95% confidence intervals (95% CI). The analyses were performed using R 3.1.3 (R Core Team, 2015). The significance level adopted was 5%.

Results

We found high correlation between the DDD and the study period indicating that there was a significant increase in the consumption of amphotericin B (rho_{DDD} = 0.87) over time, particularly the liposomal formulation (rho_{DDD} = 0.83), micafungin (rho_{DDD} = 0.89), and intravenous voriconazole (rho_{DDD} = 0.80). There was a significant reduction in the consumption of caspofungin (rho_{DDD} = – 0.80) and intravenous fluconazole (rho_{DDD} = – 0.88) over time. The temporal DOT trends followed along the same DDD lines, but with some differences in intensity and significance. Figure 1 shows the antifungal consumption using DOT throughout the study period from 2008 to 2016.

In investigating the correlation between DDD and DOT, the values of the correlation coefficients indicated positive correlations: the higher the DDD, the higher the DOT, but the correlation was not significant for all drugs.

Table 1 shows there was a significant difference between the utilization of all antifungal agents studied in the different hospitalization units, both according to DDD and DOT measurements. The consumption of posaconazole was not analyzed because it had only one measure in 2016.

The most commonly used antifungal drug was fluconazole, followed by liposomal amphotericin B, and the units with the highest consumption of these drugs were the Bone Marrow Transplantation, Oncology, Adult Intensive Care, and Solid Organ Transplantation Units (Table 1).

In the period between 2008 and 2016 there were 11,273 hospitalizations with at least one antifungal prescribed to 6779 patients who had one to 25 admissions within the study period. In 64.9% of admissions with antifungal prescriptions, a blood culture test was requested, which was positive for *Candida* in 3.2% of cases.

One hundred fifteen patients developed candidemia between 2012 and 2016. The majority (61.7%) were men and the mean age was 68 years (SD: 17.9). Half of the patients died (51.3%) and mean length of stay of 36 days. Table 2 also shows the risk factors associated with candidemia present during hospitalization and the clinical outcomes.

In 13.9% (16/115) of patients with candidemia antifungals were not used. Eight of these cases died before blood cultures were obtained, four were discharged from the hospital before the results of blood culture returned (two of which were readmitted), and for the others we did not find reasons in the patient's records for not treating the candidemia.

The duration of treatment with antifungals ranged from less than a full day to 149 days with a median of 14 days. The most commonly used antifungal agents were fluconazole (42.6%, 49/115), followed by micafungin (35.7%, 41/115) and caspofungin (24.3%, 28/115). The most heavily used class of antifungals was echinocandins (62.6%, 72/115). Each patient may have consumed more than one type of antifungal; there were cases of antifungal substitution during the same treatment, and in one patient there was a combination of two antifungals administered at the same time without justification in the medical record. As a result, 28.7% (33/115) of the patients received echinocandins only, 19. 1% (22/115) azoles only and 4.3% (5/115) liposomal amphotericin B only. The *Candida* species most prevalent in blood cultures was *C. albicans* (36.5%, 42/115), followed by *C. parapsilosis* (22.6%, 26/115), *C. glabrata* (21.7%, 25/115), *C. tropicalis* (11.3%, 13/115), *C. krusei* (4.3%, 5/115), *C. guilliermondii* (1.7% /115). Two only species accounted for one case each.

Empiric therapy with antifungal drugs after blood cultures were drawn was started within 24 h in only 44.3% of the cases (Table 3). In 81.7% of cases (94/115), the empiric treatment was determined to be adequate after antifungal susceptibility tests were reviewed. The antifungal agent was changed in 36.5% of the cases. The first choice, in general, was fluconazole (44.4%, 44/99), caspofungin (22.2%, 22/99) or micafungin (22.2%, 22/99), and the most commonly used antifungal after switching was

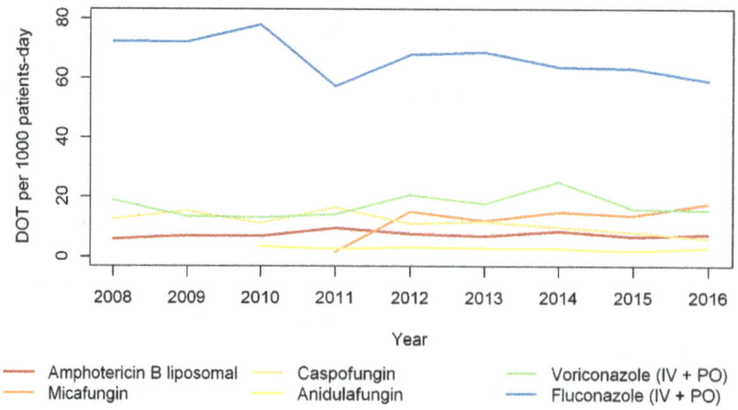

Fig. 1 Days of Therapy (DOT) per 1000 patient-days from 2008 to 2016. IV: intravenous; PO: oral

Table 1 Median antifungal consumption in hospital units between 2008 and 2016

Drug\Unit	MSC	Onco	Ped	AICU	BMT	TX	NICU	*P* Value*
DDD per 1000 patient-days								
Amphotericin B (lipos + deox)	14.2	190.9		239.4	359.0	79.2		< 0.001
P Value		0.002		0.002	0.002	0.045		
Amphotericin B liposomal	13.8	190.9		237.5	351.3	78.9		< 0.001
P Value		0.002		0.002	0.002	0.110		
Amphotericin B deoxycholate	0.4	0.0		3.2	0.0	7.9		0.012
P Value		0.904		0.110	0.940	0.135		
Anidulafugin (2010–2016)	1.4	11.6		20.0	6.2	0.0		0.002
P Value		0.009		0.009	0.995	0.568		
Caspofungin	7.2	28.1		73.3	46.7	2.0		< 0.001
P Value		0.007		0.002	0.057	0.110		
Fluconazole (IV + PO)	35.7	257.9		160.7	625.6	159.2		< 0.001
P Value		0.002		0.002	0.002	0.002		
Fluconazole L IV	25.3	163.3		150.7	382.3	52.6		< 0.001
P Value		0.002		0.002	0.002	0.002		
Fluconazole PO	11.4	124.9		14.3	134.2	102.8		< 0.001
P Value		0.002		0.035	0.002	0.002		
Itraconazole	0.7	2.7		0.6	0.00	14.7		0.001
P Value		0.625		0.690	0.006	0.324		
Micafungina (2011–2016)	3.7	41.8		71.7	153.6	21.2		0.001
P Value		0.020		0.077	0.020	0.224		
Posaconazole (2016)	0.0	44.4		6.9	87.3	0.0		–
Voriconazole (IV + PO)	3.1	82.6		22.2	174.4	7.1		< 0.001
P Value		0.002		0.002	0.002	0.495		
Voriconazole IV	1.7	44.4		16.0	83.0	3.7		< 0.001
P Value		0.002		0.002	0.002	0.993		
Voriconazole PO	1.4	42.4		5.4	80.6	3.4		< 0.001
P Value		0.002		0.007	0.002	0.324		
DOT per 1000 patient-days								
Amphotericin B (lipos + deox)	3.2	29.8	20.2	38.9	85.2	16.0	2.6	< 0.001
P Value		0.002	0.016	0.002	0.002	0.016	0.943	
Amphotericin B liposomal	2.5	29.8	19.7	36.0	82.8	10.8	0.5	< 0.001
P Value		0.002	0.004	0.002	0.002	0.134	0.069	
Amphotericin B deoxycholate	0.4	0.0	0.0	1.6	0.0	5.2	1.1	< 0.001
P Value		0.745	0.100	0.045	0.966	0.028	0.434	
Anidulafugin (2010–2016)	1.3	11.2	0.0	18.4	5.4	0.0	0.0	< 0.001
P Value		0.009	0.377	0.009	0.995	0.568	0.005	
Caspofungin	7.0	27.0	15.0	65.4	45.9	1.8	0.0	< 0.001
P Value		0.007	0.057	0.002	0.089	0.057	0.001	
Fluconazole (IV + PO)	42.9	237.0	41.5	147.7	420.1	174.4	1.1	< 0.001
P Value		0.002	0.984	0.002	0.002	0.002	0.002	
Fluconazole L IV	23.4	102.0	29.8	126.7	259.4	51.1	1.1	< 0.001
P Value		0.002	0.690	0.002	0.002	0.002	0.002	

Table 1 Median antifungal consumption in hospital units between 2008 and 2016 *(Continued)*

Drug\Unit	MSC	Onco	Ped	AICU	BMT	TX	NICU	*P* Value*
Fluconazole PO	20.1	130.4	13.2	23.6	160.6	119.7	0.0	< 0.001
P Value		0.002	0.057	0.434	0.002	0.002	0.001	
Itraconazole	0.8	1.2	1.0	0.8	0.0	11.8	0.0	< 0.001
P Value		0.753	1.000	0.812	0.008	0.324	0.001	
Micafungina (2011–2016)	3.9	45.3	8.5	73.5	225.5	21.8	0.0	< 0.001
P Value		0.020	0.624	0.077	0.020	0.224	0.024	
Posaconazole (2016)	0.0	3.1	0.0	0.5	6.2	0.0	0.0	–
Voriconazole (IV + PO)	5.4	130.1	35.0	25.4	322.3	10.1	0.00	< 0.001
P Value		0.002	0.002	0.002	0.002	0.559	0.001	
Voriconazole IV	2.6	57.2	14.0	20.1	142.7	4.7	0.00	< 0.001
P Value		0.002	0.002	0.002	0.002	0.984	0.001	
Voriconazole PO	2.2	73.7	17.7	7.1	147.7	5.6	0.00	< 0.001
P Value		0.002	0.028	0.002	0.002	0.276	0.001	

DDD Defined Daily Dose, *DOT* Days of Therapy, *IV* Intravenous, *PO* Oral, *MSW* Medical and Surgical Wards, *Onco* Oncology, *Ped* Pediatrics, *AICU* Adult Intensive Care Unit, *BTM* Bone marrow transplant, *SOT* Solid organ transplant, *NICU* Neonatal Intensive Care Unit **P* values for Kruskal-Wallis tests to test whether in at least one of the units the consumption was different from the others. Other *p*-values for post-tests with Steel correction that compare each unit with the Medical and Surgical Wards

micafungin (17.4%, 20/115), followed by liposomal amphotericin B (13%, 15/115). Table 3 also shows cases where the dose was adequate according to institutional protocol.

As for the clinical history, 59.1% (68/115) of patients suffered from cardiac disease, 27.8% (32/115) from diabetes mellitus, 23.5% (27/115) from nephropathy, 22.6% (26/115) from cancer, and 19.1% (22/115) were bone marrow and solid organ transplant patients.

In Table 4 are the variables that were evaluated by simple logistic regression analysis. In Table 5, after the construction of multiple logistic regression analysis, the factors that remained significant and associated with death risk were: age, length of stay in the ICU, use of vasoactive drugs, use of chemotherapy, hemodialysis and positive blood culture while on antifungal therapy (breakthrough candidemia).

Discussion

Analyzing the data, it was possible to identify a wide use of antifungal drugs, which may be related to the characteristics of the hospital, because it is large tertiary care facility This study is similar to a study carried out in Spain, where antifungal consumption was higher in large university hospitals [34].

In our study we observed a significant increase over time in the consumption of liposomal amphotericin B, micafungin and voriconazole, and a significant reduction in the consumption of caspofungin and fluconazole (Fig. 1). The increased use of liposomal amphotericin B and voriconazole is probably related to the empirical and prophylactic treatments used in the onco-hematology unit, and the increase of micafungin is due to its lower cost. We also suspect that the reduction of fluconazole usage may be related to the predominance of *C.* non-*albicans* species in our institution, and the reduction in the use of caspofungin due to the higher cost of this drug and the standardization of use of micafungin, which has lower cost and equivalent effectiveness. We believe that introducing an agent of the same class at a lower cost into the hospital formulary has caused this change in the pattern of echinocandin prescriptions in our institution over the years. Since studies do not show significant differences in efficacy among these drugs, cost may become a differential point in decision making over which drug to choose. Our findings were different from the Spanish study, where there was an increase in fluconazole consumption, followed by a smaller scale increase in voriconazole, and a reduction in itraconazole consumption [34]. In the same study, the consumption of echinocandins was more apparent in the ICU; we also observed in our study that the adult ICU had the highest consumption of caspofungin and anidulafungin (Table 1). In another study conducted in ICUs, a decrease in the use of fluconazole and an increase in echinocandin consumption also became evident over time [35]. In a Brazilian university hospital, the highest consumption was of the azole class, first fluconazole, followed by voriconazole and the third most consumed was amphotericin B deoxycholate, a fact that can be explained by the limitations in resources, since it is a public hospital, and this deoxycholate formulation is cheaper, with greater control over the use of liposomal amphotericin B and echinocandins, requiring

Table 2 Hospital admission data and risk factors for patients with candidemia ($N = 115$)

Variables	Descriptions
Sex *n*(%)	
Female	44 (38.3)
Male	71 (61.7)
Age (years)	
Mean (SD)	68 (17.9)
Median (1st quartile - 3rd quartile)	70 [56–84]
Minimum maximum	26–100
Length of stay (days)	
Mean (SD)	69.8 (138.4)
Median (1st quartile - 3rd quartile)	36 [21–62.5]
Minimum maximum	1–1003
Use of antimicrobial	113 (98.3)
Use of chemotherapy drugs	12 (10.4)
Use of corticosteroids	95 (82.6)
Use of parenteral nutrition	46 (40.0)
Presence of some type of central venous catheter	86 (74.8)
Had any type of surgery	79 (68.7)
Admission to the intensive care unit	94 (81.7)
Length of ICU stay (days) ($n = 94$)	
Mean (SD)	23.3 (23.3)
Median (1st quartile - 3rd quartile)	15 (6–32)
Minimum maximum	1–100
Neutropenia	6 (5.2)
Use of vasoactive drug	86 (74.8)
Use of mechanical ventilation	82 (71.3)
Hemodialysis	38 (33.0)
Had hemotherapy	27 (23.5)
Positive blood culture even when using antifungal therapy	35 (30.4)
Clinical outcome	
Discharge from hospital	56 (48.7)
In-hospital mortality	59 (51.3)

Category variables presented by absolute and relative frequencies. *SD* standard deviation

Table 3 Empiric therapy in patients with candidemia ($N = 115$)

Variables	*n*(%)
Time to start empiric therapy with antifungal after blood culture obtained (hours)	
24	51 (44.3)
48	20 (17.4)
72	16 (13.9)
96	7 (6.1)
120	5 (4.3)
No use of antifungal drug	16 (13.9)
Appropriate empirical antifungal treatment according to antifungal susceptibility test result	
No	21 (18.3)
Yes	94 (81.7)
Adequate dose according to institutional protocol[a]	
Caspofungin	28/28 (100.0)
Micafungin	31/41 (75.6)
Anidulafungin	5/8 (62.5)
Fluconazole	12/49 (24.5)
Amphotericin B liposomal	20/21 (95.2)
Voriconazole	4/5 (80.0)

Category variables presented by absolute and relative frequencies
[a]number of cases observed/number of cases using antifungal drug

authorization prior to the prescription of these high-cost drugs [36].

Two other German studies used different metrics, one Recommended Daily Dose (RDD) and the other Prescribed Daily Dose (PDD), and both showed a higher consumption of antifungal drugs in the ICU and Hematology/Oncology service [37, 38]. Our study shows that these units also have a high consumption of antifungal agents (Table 1), since antifungal prophylaxis is included in the treatment profile of these patients and the use of empiric therapy is quite common [38, 39].

When comparing our work with an earlier study performed at the same institution [1], where the DDD of antifungal drugs was calculated from 1997 to 2007, we can observe that, in general, there was an increase in the consumption of these drugs, but there was also an increase in the therapeutic arsenal available in our formulary. In 2010, anidulafungin was added, micafungin was added in 2011, and posaconazole in 2016. Fluconazole consumption remained stable, mean use 61.5 (range from 32.7 to 101.2) DDD/1000 patient-days in the first study, and mean use 62.14 (range from 50.11 to 70.66) DDD/1000 patient-days in the second study. Observation demonstrated that the use of amphotericin B deoxycholate continued to be reduced in our study, as in the previous one, due to the higher risk of nephrotoxicity associated with this formulation, which led to an increase in the prescription of liposomal amphotericin B and echinocandins.

For most drugs there was a positive correlation between DDD and DOT values, but not all of them were strong and significant. A different pattern was observed for amphotericins, which we believe to be due to the fact that when the dose administered exceeds the Individualized Daily Dose (IDD), the DDD significantly exceeds the DOT. For drugs such as caspofungin and micafungin, there is usually no significant difference between DDD and DOT per 1000 patient-days, as the daily administered dose is close to the IDD equivalent [23].

Table 4 Data for hospitalization and risk factors, by type of discharge ($N = 115$)

	Discharge ($N = 56$)	In-hospital mortality ($N = 59$)	OR (95% CI)	*P* value
Gender				
Female	23 (41.1)	21 (35.6)	1.00	
Male	33 (58.9)	38 (64.4)	1.26 (0.59; 2.69)	0.546
Age (years)			1.03 (1.01; 1.05)	0.015
Mean (SD)	63.80 (19.33)	72.03 (15.53)		
Median [1st Q - 3rd Q]	65.00 [50–81.50]	76.00 [60–85]		
Length of stay (days)			1.00 (1.00; 1.00)	0.952
Mean (SD)	69.02 (140.67)	70.58 (137.32)		
Median [1st Q - 3rd Q]	32 [20.25–64.25]	36 [23.50–56]		
Time to start empiric therapy with antifungal after blood culture				
Within 24 h	23 (41.1)	28 (47.5)	1.00	
More than 24 h	27 (48.2)	21 (35.6)	0.64 (0.29; 1.41)	0.268
No use of antifungal drug	6 (10.7)	10 (16.9)	1.37 (0.44; 4.56)	0.593
Used antimicrobial				
No	1 (1.8)	1 (1.7)	1.00	
Yes	55 (98.2)	58 (98.3)	- 11-22-2016 17:19:0 s2	0.970
Used chemotherapy				
No	52 (92.9)	51 (86.4)	1.00	
Yes	4 (7.1)	8 (13.6)	2.04 (0.60; 8.03)	0.268
Used corticosteroid				
No	15 (26.8)	5 (8.5)	1.00	
Yes	41 (73.2)	54 (91.5)	3.95 (1.40; 12.96)	0.014
Used parenteral nutrition				
No	37 (66.1)	32 (54.2)	1.00	
Yes	19 (33.9)	27 (45.8)	1.64 (0.78; 3.53)	0.197
Used some type of central venous catheter				
No	22 (39.3)	7 (11.9)	1.00	
Yes	34 (60.7)	52 (88.1)	4.81 (1.93; 13.30)	0.001
Had any type of surgery				
No	20 (35.7)	16 (27.1)	1.00	
Yes	36 (64.3)	43 (72.9)	1.49 (0.68; 3.33)	0.322
Stayed at the intensive care unit				
No	17 (30.4)	4 (6.8)	1.00	
Yes	39 (69.6)	55 (93.2)	5.99 (2.04; 22.07)	0.003
Length of stay in the intensive care unit (days) ($n = 94$)			1.04 (1.02; 1.06)	0.001
Mean (SD)	16.03 (16.86)	28.42 (25.86)		
Median [1st Q - 3rd Q]	10.00 (5.00–17.50)	23.00 (7.50–36.00)		
Neutropenia				
No	54 (96.4)	55 (93.2)	1.00	
Yes	2 (3.6)	4 (6.8)	1.96 (0.37; 14.59)	0.447
Used vasoactive drug				
No	23 (41.1)	6 (10.2)	1.00	
Yes	33 (58.9)	53 (89.8)	6.16 (2.39; 18.12)	< 0.001

Table 4 Data for hospitalization and risk factors, by type of discharge ($N = 115$) *(Continued)*

	Discharge ($N = 56$)	In-hospital mortality ($N = 59$)	OR (95% CI)	*P* value
Used mechanical ventilation				
No	26 (46.4)	7 (11.9)	1.00	
Yes	30 (53.6)	52 (88.1)	6.44 (2.61; 17.74)	< 0.001
Hemodialysis				
No	45 (80.4)	32 (54.2)	1.00	
Yes	11 (19.6)	27 (45.8)	3.45 (1.53; 8.21)	0.004
Blood transfusion				
No	48 (85.7)	40 (67.8)	1.00	
Yes	8 (14.3)	19 (32.2)	2.85 (1.16; 7.55)	0.027
Positive blood culture even when using antifungal therapy				
No	44 (78.6)	36 (61.0)	1.00	
Yes	12 (21.4)	23 (39.0)	2.34 (1.04; 5.48)	0.043

Category variables presented by absolute and relative frequencies. *Q* quartile *SD* standard deviation, *OR* odds ratio obtained by simple logistic regression model (values, 1.00 for the reference categories) and, in parentheses, the 95% Confidence Interval (95% CI)

The ideal metric to measure drug consumption is still not well defined in the literature. The two metrics used in this study have both advantages and disadvantages, and most studies involve the consumption of antibacterial drugs. A primary concern with this class of drugs is bacterial resistance, which is increasing while the development of new agents is slow. The emergence of antifungal resistance should prompt the monitoring of utilization of these drugs.

DDD allows the comparison of utilization in different hospitals, regions and countries. It can be calculated even when a computerized pharmacy data system is not available, although electronic systems aids in optimizing the calculation time by the pharmacist in both metrics [23, 25]. Disadvantages of DDD are its inaccuracy in drugs that require dose adjustment for renal function or weight-based drugs. IDD values may change with the approval of new doses for existing drugs, which can create confusion when comparisons of use are made over time [23–25, 40]. The advantages of the DOT metric are greater accuracy than DDD, it can be used to measure utilization in children (weight-based regimens), is not influenced in case of changes in recommended doses of IDD, is not influenced by discrepancies between IDD and preferred daily doses or usual daily doses, which may vary between hospitals [23, 38]. The disadvantages of DOT are: calculation is more difficult without computerized systems and there is a lack of accuracy in populations with renal failure, although the values obtained with DOT calculation are more accurate than when calculating DDD in this population [23, 25].

Table 5 Factors associated with death risk in patients with candidemia (N = 115)

Factors	OR (95% CI)	*P* value
Age (years)	1.04 (1.01; 1.08)	0.005
Treatment with antifungal (days)	0.95 (0.91; 0.99)	0.022
Time in ICU (days)	1.03 (1.01; 1.07)	0.020
Use of vasoactive drugs (Yes)	3.90 (1.18; 14.43)	0.031
Use of chemotherapy (Yes)	6.88 (1.37; 40.17)	0.023
Hemodialysis (Yes)	3.19 (1.11; 9.86)	0.035
Positive blood culture even when using antifungal drug (Yes)	4.20 (1.25; 15.86)	0.026

In parentheses, the 95% Confidence Interval (95% CI). *OR* odds ratio obtained by multiple logistic regression model

The literature recognizes the limitations regarding the use of DDD in pediatric patients, so some authors believe that DOT is more appropriate for this population, particularly for low weight patients [17, 23, 40].

Regarding microbiological characteristics, the Brazilian study published in 2016 [3] also showed an increase in the occurrence *Candida* non-*albicans*, corresponding to 65.7% of the cases, although in isolation *C. albicans* still remains as the predominant species at 34.3%, followed by *C. parapsilosis* (24.1%), *C. tropicalis* (15.3%) and *C. glabrata* (10.2%). These results are similar to those of our study, where *C. albicans* the most isolated species corresponded 36.5% of the cases, followed by *C. parapsilosis* (22.6%), *C. glabrata* (21.7%) and *C. tropicalis* (11.3%), differing only in the rank order and percentages for *C. tropicalis* and *C. glabrata.* In the prior study carried out in our institution from 1997 to 2007, *C. albicans* was the most isolated species in blood cultures (44%), followed by *C. parapsilosis* (22%), *C. tropicalis* (15%) and *C. glabrata* (9%) [1]. In view of these data, over the years we can see the increase of *C.* non-*albicans* species in our institution as well, as reported in other studies [5, 41, 42].

We did not analyze the change in antifungal susceptibilities over the years in this study, but we could make a comparison with a prior study carried out in this institution from 1997 to 2007 whose susceptibility testing data are from mid-2002 to 2007 [1]. This showed that the resistance profile remained proportionally the same, with 100% of strains susceptible to amphotericin B and 91.4% (n = 96/105) of the strains susceptible to fluconazole, compared to 82.3% in the prior study (n = 42/51). Table 6 shows the susceptibility tests of *Candida* species isolates found in the first study conducted at our institution, data from mid-2002 to 2007 [1] and the findings in our study from 2012 to 2016. Among the resistant and intermediate species (susceptible dose-dependent) are *C. krusei* and *C. glabrata*, respectively. Until 2007, we only had caspofungin on formulary at our institution, and until then no susceptibility tests were found with intermediate results for this drug. However, in the current study, we have already seen the appearance of intermediate susceptibility to echinocandins, although it is a small percentage of strains, we can consider this as a warning sign to prompt increased monitoring of the use of these class of drugs, since the use of antifungal drugs affects the susceptibility of *Candida* species [43] and the selection of resistant strains may be responsible for failures in treatment [44].

In a study carried out in Costa Rica [43], 19% of adult patients with candidemia did not receive antifungal drugs and these patients had a significantly higher risk of death within the next 30 days when compared to patients receiving antifungal drugs (OR: 2.9, 95% CI 1.8 to 4.6, $p < 0.001$). In our study, 13.9% of patients who had candidemia did not receive antifungal drugs; however, treatment with antifungals was associated with reduced mortality in multivariate analysis. In the Costa Rican study [45], 82% of candidemic patients started antifungal therapy more than 24 h after the blood culture was obtained. In our study the proportion was much smaller (41.7%) and no significant association was found between the timing of empiric therapy and mortality. In a European study, the proportion of patients receiving adequate antifungal therapy in the first 24 h after blood culture was high, and the delay in initiating antifungal therapy was not a risk factor for death [46].

In another study, which involved patients in septic shock, no differences were found in mortality regarding the timing of the beginning of antifungal therapy, but they identified a higher mortality in the group of patients where antifungal therapy was not adequate (p < 0.001) [12]. In our study, for most patients antifungal doses were in accordance with the institutional protocol but to our surprise the fluconazole dose was only adequate in 24.5% of the cases, with the majority being prescribed in suboptimal doses for the treatment of candidemia. The AmarCAND2 group study [47] also showed that the dose of fluconazole was not adequate in most patients. In view of these numbers, we can

Table 6 Comparison of microbiological data susceptibility tests between our study and Camargo et al. study [1]

Variables	*n*(%)
2002 a 2007*	
Candida albicans (*n* = 27)	
Amphotericin B (*n* = 27)	
Susceptible	27 (100.0)
Fluconazole (*n* = 27)	
Susceptible	27 (100.0)
Candida non-*albicans* (*n* = 51)	
Amphotericin B (*n* = 51)	
Susceptible	51 (100.0)
Fluconazole (*n* = 51)	
Susceptible	42 (82.3)
2012 a 2016**	
Candida albicans (*n* = 42)	
Amphotericin B (*n* = 40)	
Susceptible	40 (100.0)
Fluconazole (*n* = 41)	
Susceptible	41 (100.0)
Voriconazole (*n* = 41)	
Susceptible	41 (100.0)
Caspofungin (*n* = 1)	
Susceptible	1 (100.0)
Anidulafungin (*n* = 3)	
Susceptible	3 (100.0)
Candida non-*albicans* (*n* = 73)	
Amphotericin B (*n* = 72)	
Susceptible	72 (100.0)
Fluconazole (*n* = 64)	
Susceptible	55 (85.9)
Resistant	3 (4.7)
Intermediate	6 (9.4)
Voriconazole (*n* = 64)	
Susceptible	63 (98.4)
Intermediate	1 (1.6)
Caspofungin (*n* = 10)	
Susceptible	9 (90.0)
ntermediate	1 (10.0)
Anidulafungin (*n* = 11)	
Susceptible	8 (72.7)
Intermediate	3 (27.3)

Category variables presented by absolute and relative frequencies
*Data from Camargo TZS, et al. study [1]. **Data from our current study

conclude that the pharmacist's performance in the verification of the medical prescription by checking the doses and frequencies of the medications is very important, since treatment with inadequate doses may lead to unfavorable clinical outcomes.

In another study there was no correlation between the reduction of in-hospital mortality and the time of initiation of the therapy or initial choice of agents; instead they observed that risk factors, such as age, admission to the ICU or diabetes mellitus, have a strong impact on outcomes [13]. On the other hand, another study identified that mortality was lower when fluconazole therapy was started on the same day the culture was obtained [11]. We observed that there are still differences in the literature regarding whether the appropriate therapy actually impacts the risk of death, but it is clear that there are other factors that strongly influence the mortality related to candidemia, such as the severity of illness and the presence of comorbidities [13, 48].

An American study identified through univariate analysis that the predictors of increased mortality included the APACHE II severity of illness score, intensive care unit admission, corticosteroid treatment, and the use of mechanical ventilation [11]. In our study, independent predictors of mortality age, ICU length of stay, use of vasoactive drugs, chemotherapy, hemodialysis, and breakthrough candidemia.

The Eurobact study [44] identified mechanical ventilation and ICU admission as independent risk factors for death. These variables were not independent predictors in our study, but the length of ICU stay was an independent predictor of mortality.

Our study has some limitations primarily that it is single center and retrospective. The retrospective nature of the study made it impossible to identify the reason for the choice of specific antifungal drugs as initial therapy or the reason for the drug exchange during antifungal therapy, and also it was not possible to identify the number of cases where the antifungal was used as prophylaxis. To reduce bias, we chose to include only microbiological data from blood cultures to evaluate adequacy of antifungal therapy, since for a positive culture is highly predictive of infection and requires intervention, which is not characteristic of other sites, such as the urinary or respiratory tracts, where positivity may be due to colonization, which makes results difficult to interpret.

Conclusion

The high utilization of antifungal drugs reinforces the need for ongoing monitoring, the implementation of stewardship interventions, and the key role of the pharmacist to increase rational use and thus improve patient safety.

Abbreviations

AIC: Akaike information; AICU: Adult intensive care unit; APACHE II: Acute physiology and chronic health evaluation II; ATC: Anatomical therapeutic chemical; BMT: Bone marrow transplantation; CI: Confidence intervals; DDD: Defined daily dose; IDD: Individualized daily dose; DOT: Days of therapy; ICU: Intensive care unit; MSW: Medical and surgical wards; NICU: Neonatal intensive care unit; ONCO: Oncology; OR: Odds ratios; PDD: Prescribed daily dose; PED: Pediatrics; RDD: Recommended daily dose; SOT: Solid organ transplantation; WHO: World Health Organization

Acknowledgements

We are grateful to the Hospital Israelita Albert Einstein mainly for the Pharmacy Service and the Microbiology Laboratory for support this work.

Authors' contributions

TAM, PKOY, MDVM participated in the data collected. TAM, ARM, MBE, MSDJ, ACCNM participated in the data analysis. TAM, ARM, MBE, MSDJ participated in the design and coordination. TAM, ARM, MBE, MDVM, PKOY, ACCNM, MSDJ helped to draft the manuscript and to provide critical review to the manuscript. All authors read and approved the final manuscript.

Competing interests

The authors declare that they have no competing interests. This research received no specific grant from any funding agency in the public, commercial, or not-for-profit sectors.

Author details

[1]Hospital Israelita Albert Einstein, São Paulo, Brazil. [2]Division of Medical Practice, Hospital Israelita Albert Einstein, São Paulo, Brazil. [3]Office of Clinical Quality, Safety and Performance Improvement, University of Iowa Hospitals and Clinics, Iowa City, IA, USA. [4]Division of Infectious Diseases, Department of Internal Medicine, University of Iowa Carver College of Medicine, Iowa City, IA, USA. [5]Clinical Laboratory, Hospital Israelita Albert Einstein, São Paulo, Brazil. [6]Instituto Israelita de Ensino e Pesquisa Albert Einstein, Hospital Israelita Albert Einstein, São Paulo, Brazil.

References

1. Camargo TZS, Marra AR, Silva CV, Cardoso MFS, Martino MDV, Camargo LFA, Correa L. Secular trends of candidemia in a tertiary care hospital. Am J Infect Control. 2010;38:546–51.
2. Wisplinghoff H, Bischoff T, Tallent SM, Seifert H, Wenzel RP, Edmond MB. Nosocomial bloodstream infections in US hospitals: analysis of 24,179 cases from a prospective nationwide surveillance study. Clin Infect Dis. 2004;39: 309–17. Erratum in: 2005,40:1077
3. Doi AM, Pignatari ACC, Edmond MB, Marra AR, Camargo LFA, Siqueira RA, da Mota VP, Colombo AL. Epidemiology and microbiologic characterization of nosocomial Candidemia from a Brazilian National Surveillance Program. PLoS One. 2016;11:1.
4. Colombo AL, Ngai AL, Bourque M, Bradshaw SK, Strohmaier KM, Taylor AF, et al. Caspofungin use in patients with invasive candidiasis caused by common non-albicans Candida species: review of the Caspofungin database. Antimicrob Agents Chemother. 2010;54:1864–71.
5. Arendrup MC, Dzajic E, Jensen RH, Johansen HK, Kjaeldgaard P, Knudsen JD, et al. Epidemiological changes with potential implication for antifungal prescription recommendations for fungaemia: data from a nationwide fungaemia surveillance programme. Clin Microbiol Infect. 2013;19:343–53.
6. Colombo AL, Nucci M, Park BJ, Nouer SA, Arthington-Skaggs B, da Matta DA, Warnock D, Morgan J. Brazilian network Candidemia S: epidemiology of candidemia in Brazil: a nationwide sentinel surveillance of candidemia in eleven medical centers. J Clin Microbiol. 2006;44:2816–23.

7. Garnacho-Montero J, Diaz-Martin A, Garcia-Cabrera E, de Pipaon MRP, Hernandez-Caballero C, Lepe-Jimenez JA. Impact on hospital mortality of catheter removal and adequate antifungal therapy in Candida spp. bloodstream infections. J Antimicrob Chemother. 2013;68:206–13.
8. Ibrahim EH, Sherman G, Ward S, Fraser VJ, Kollef MH. The influence of inadequate antimicrobial treatment of bloodstream infections on patient outcomes in the ICU setting. Chest. 2000;118:146–55.
9. Kollef MH. Inadequate antimicrobial treatment: an important determinant of outcome for hospitalized patients. Clin Infect Dis. 2000;31:131–8.
10. Morrell M, Fraser VJ, Kollef MH. Delaying the empiric treatment of Candida bloodstream infection until positive blood culture results are obtained: a potential risk factor for hospital mortality. Antimicrob Agents Chemother. 2005;49:3640–5.
11. Garey KW, Rege M, Pai MP, Mingo DE, Suda KJ, Turpin RS, Bearden DT. Time to initiation of fluconazole therapy impacts mortality in patients with candidemia: a multi-institutional study. Clin Infect Dis. 2006;43:25–31.
12. Bassetti M, Righi E, Ansaldi F, Merelli M, Cecilia T, De Pascale G, Diaz-Martin A, Luzzati R, Rosin C, Lagunes L, et al. A multicenter study of septic shock due to candidemia: outcomes and predictors of mortality. Intensive Care Med. 2014;40:839–45.
13. Kludze-Forson M, Eschenauer GA, Kubin CJ, Della-Latta P, Lam SW. The impact of delaying the initiation of appropriate antifungal treatment for Candida bloodstream infection. Med Mycol. 2010;48:436–9.
14. Neoh CF, Liew D, Slavin M, Marriott D, Chen SCA, Morrissey O, et al. Cost-effectiveness analysis of anidulafungin versus fluconazole for the treatment of invasive candidiasis. J Antimicrob Chemother. 2011;66:1906–15.
15. Auzinger G, Playford EG, Graham CN, Knox HN, Weinstein D, Kantecki M, et al. Cost-effectiveness analysis of anidulafungin for the treatment of candidaemia and other forms of invasive candidiasis. BMC Infect Dis. 2015;15:463.
16. Pappas PG, Kauffman CA, Andes DR, Clancy CJ, Marr KA, Ostrosky-Zeichner L, Reboli AC, Schuster MG, Vazquez JA, Walsh TJ, et al. Clinical practice guideline for the Management of Candidiasis: 2016 update by the Infectious Diseases Society of America. Clin Infect Dis. 2016;62:409–17.
17. Guillot J, Lebel D, Roy H, Ovetchkine P, Bussieres JF. Usefulness of defined daily dose and days of therapy in pediatrics and obstetrics-gynecology: a comparative analysis of antifungal drugs (2000-2001, 2005-2006, and 2010-2011). J Pediatr Pharmacol Ther. 2014;19:196–201.
18. Kuster SP, Ruef C, Ledergerber B, Hintermann A, Deplazes C, Neuber L, et al. Quantitative antibiotic use in hospitals: comparison of measurements, literature review, and recommendations for a standard of reporting. Infection. 2008;36:549–59.
19. Morris AM, Brener S, Dresser L, Daneman N, Dellit TH, Avdic E, et al. Use of a structured panel process to define quality metrics for antimicrobial stewardship programs. Infect Control Hosp Epidemiol. 2012;33:500–6.
20. Barlam TF, Cosgrove SE, Abbo LM, MacDougall C, Schuetz AN, Septimus EJ, et al. Implementing an antibiotic stewardship program: guidelines by the Infectious Diseases Society of America and the Society for Healthcare Epidemiology of America. Clin Infect Dis. 2016;62:1197–202.
21. Ibrahim OM, Polk RE. Antimicrobial use metrics and benchmarking to improve stewardship outcomes methodology, opportunities, and challenges. Infect Dis Clin N Am. 2014;28:195.
22. World Health Organization. Collaborating Centre for Drug Statistics Methodology [Anatomical therapeutic chemical (ATC) Classification and defined daily doses (DDD)] http://www.whocc.no/atc_ddd_index Accessed 20 Jan 2017.
23. Polk RE, Fox C, Mahoney A, Letcavage J, MacDougall C. Measurement of adult antibacterial drug use in 130 US hospitals: comparison of defined daily dose and days of therapy. Clin Infect Dis. 2007;44:664–70.
24. Zagorski BM, Trick WE, Schwartz DN, Wisniewski MF, Hershow RC, Fridkin SK, et al. The effect of renal dysfunction on antimicrobial use measurements. Clin Infect Dis. 2002;35:1491–7.
25. Public Health Ontario. Antimicrobial Stewardship: Metrics and evaluation 2014. http://www.publichealthontario.ca/ Accessed 16 Jan 2017.
26. Puig-Asensio M, Fernandez-Ruiz M, Aguado JM, Merino P, Lora-Pablos D, Guinea J, et al. Propensity score analysis of the role of initial antifungal therapy in the outcome of Candida glabrata bloodstream infections. Antimicrob Agents Chemother. 2016;60:3291–300.
27. Nucci M, Colombo AL. Risk factors for breakthrough candidemia. Eur J Clin Microbiol Infect Dis. 2002;21:209–11.
28. Savage RD, Fowler RA, Rishu AH, Bagshaw SM, Cook D, Dodek P, et al. The effect of inadequate initial empiric antimicrobial treatment on mortality in critically ill patients with bloodstream infections: a multi-Centre retrospective cohort study. PLoS One. 2016;11:5.
29. Das I, Nightingale P, Patel M, Jumaa P. Epidemiology, clinical characteristics, and outcome of candidemia: experience in a tertiary referral center in the UK. Int J Infect Dis. 2011;15:759–63.
30. Colombo AL, Guimaraes T, Camargo LFA, Richtmann R, de Queiroz-Telles F, Salles MJC, et al. Brazilian guidelines for the management of candidiasis - a joint meeting report of three medical societies: Sociedade Brasileira de Infectologia, Sociedade Paulista de Infectologia and Sociedade Brasileira de Medicina tropical. Braz J Infect Dis. 2013;17:283–312.
31. Clinical and Laboratory Standards Institute. Reference method for broth dilution antifungal susceptibility testing of yeasts: approved standard. In: CLSI document M27-A3. 3rd ed. Wayne, PA, USA: CLSI; 2008.
32. Clinical and Laboratory Standards Institute. Reference method for broth dilution antifungal susceptibility testing of yeasts: fourth informational supplement. CLSI document M27-S4. Wayne, PA, USA: CLSI; 2012. p. 33.
33. Steel RG. Some rank sum multiple comparisons tests. Biometrics. 1961;17:539–52.
34. Fondevilla E, Grau S, Mojal S, Palomar M, Matas L, Gudiol F, Grp VI. Consumption of systemic antifungal agents among acute care hospitals in Catalonia (Spain), 2008-2013. Expert Rev Anti-Infect Ther. 2016;14:137–44.
35. Olaechea-Astigarraga PM, Alvarez-Lerma F, Palomar-Martinez M, Insausti-Ordenana J, Lopez-Pueyo MJ, Seijas-Betolaza I, Otal-Entraigas JJ, Gimeno-Costa R, Gracia-Arnillas MP, Grp E-H. Trends in systemic antifungal use in critically ill patients. Multicenter observational study, 2006-2010. Enfermedades Infecciosas Y Microbiologia Clinica. 2012;30:435–40.
36. de Souza MCP, dos Santos AG, Reis AMM. Drug utilization study of systemic antifungal agents in a Brazilian tertiary care hospital. Int J Clin Pharm. 2016; 38:1398–406.
37. Gross BN, Steib-Bauert M, Kern WV, Knoth H, Borde JP, Krebs S, et al. Hospital use of systemic antifungal drugs: a multi-center surveillance update from Germany. Infection. 2015;43:423–9.
38. Kd W, Steib-Bauert M, Knoth H, Fr D, Strehl E, Rothe U, et al. Hospital use of systemic antifungal drugs. BMC Clin Pharmacol. 2005;5:1.
39. Zarb P, Amadeo B, Muller A, Drapier N, Vankerckhoven V, Davey P, et al. Antifungal therapy in European hospitals: data from the ESAC point-prevalence surveys 2008 and 2009. Clin Microbiol Infect. 2012;18:389–95.
40. Bansal D, Mangla S, Undela K, Gudala K, D'Cruz S, Sachdev A, Tiwari P. Measurement of adult antimicrobial drug use in tertiary care hospital using defined daily dose and days of therapy. Indian J Pharm Sci. 2014;76:211–7.
41. Bailly S, Maubon D, Fournier P, Pelloux H, Schwebel C, Chapuis C, et al. Impact of antifungal prescription on relative distribution and susceptibility of Candida spp. - trends over 10 years. J Infect. 2016;72:103–11.
42. Colombo AL, Garnica M, Camargo LFA, Da Cunha CA, Bandeira AC, Borghi D, et al. Candida glabrata: an emerging pathogen in Brazilian tertiary care hospitals. Med Mycol. 2013;51:38–44.
43. Fournier P, Schwebel C, Maubon D, Vesin A, Lebeau B, Foroni L, et al. Antifungal use influences Candida species distribution and susceptibility in the intensive care unit. J Antimicrob Chemother. 2011;66(12):2880–6.
44. Alexander BD, Johnson MD, Pfeiffer CD, Jiménez-Ortigosa C, Catania J, Booker R, et al. Increasing echinocandin resistance in Candida glabrata: clinical failure correlates with presence of FKS mutations and elevated minimum inhibitory concentrations. Clin Infect Dis. 2013;56(12):1724–32.
45. Villalobos JM, Castro JA, Aviles A, Pelaez MC, Somogyi T, Sandoval L. Candida parapsilosis: a major cause of bloodstream infection in a tertiary care hospital in Costa Rica. Revista Chilena De Infectologia. 2016;33:159–65.
46. Paiva JA, Pereira JM, Tabah A, Mikstacki A, de Carvalho FB, Koulenti D, Ruckly S, Cakar N, Misset B, Dimopoulos G, Antonelli M, Rello J, Ma X, Tamowicz B, Timsit JF. Characteristics and risk factors for 28-day mortality of hospital acquired fungemias in ICUs: data from the EUROBACT study. Crit Care. 2016;20:53.

22

Relationship between day 1 and day 2 Vancomycin area under the curve values and emergence of heterogeneous Vancomycin-intermediate *Staphylococcus aureus* (hVISA) by Etest® macromethod among patients with MRSA bloodstream infections

Dmitriy M. Martirosov[1], Monique R. Bidell[1], Manjunath P. Pai[1], Marc H. Scheetz[2,3], Susan L. Rosenkranz[4], Corey Faragon[1], M. Malik[1], R. E. Mendes[5], R. N. Jones[5], Louise-Anne McNutt[6] and Thomas P. Lodise[1*]

Abstract

Background: In vitro data suggests that suboptimal initial vancomycin exposure may select for heterogeneous vancomycin-intermediate *Staphylococcus aureus* (hVISA) infections. However, no clinical studies have evaluated the relationship between initial vancomycin exposure and emergence of hVISA. This pilot study seeks to assess the relationship between day 1 and day 2 vancomycin area under the curve (AUC) and emergence of hVISA bloodstream infections (BSIs) by Etest® macromethod among patients with a non-hVISA BSI at baseline.

Methods: This was a retrospective cohort study of patients with methicillin-resistant *Staphylococcus aureus* (MRSA) BSIs at Albany Medical Center Hospital (AMCH) between January 2005 and June 2009. The vancomycin AUC exposure variables on day 1 ($AUC_{0\text{-}24h}$) and day 2 ($AUC_{24\text{-}48h}$) were estimated using the maximal a posteriori probability (MAP) procedure in ADAPT 5.

Results: There were 238 unique episodes of MRSA BSIs during the study period, 119 of which met inclusion criteria. Overall, hVISA emerged in 7/119 (5.9%) of patients. All 7 cases of hVISA involved patients who did not achieve area under the curve over broth microdilution minimum inhibitory concentration ($AUC_{0\text{-}24h}/MIC_{BMD}$) ratio of 521 or an $AUC_{24\text{-}48h}/MIC_{BMD}$ ratio of 650. No associations between other day 1 and day 2 AUC variables and emergence of hVISA were noted.

Conclusions: Although more data are needed to draw definitive conclusions, these findings suggest that hVISA emergence among patients with non-hVISA MRSA BSIs at baseline may be partially explained by suboptimal exposure to vancomycin in the first 1 to 2 days of therapy. At a minimum, these findings support further study of the relationship between initial vancomycin exposure and hVISA emergence among patients with MRSA BSIs in a well-powered, multi-center, prospective trial.

Keywords: Vancomycin, Heteroresistance, *Staphylococcus aureus*, MRSA

* Correspondence: thomas.lodise@acphs.edu
[1]Albany College of Pharmacy and Health Sciences, Albany, NY 12208-3492, USA
Full list of author information is available at the end of the article

Background

Vancomycin is often employed as a first-line treatment of serious infections due to methicillin-resistant *Staphylococcus aureus* (MRSA) [1]. While susceptibility to vancomycin among MRSA remains near 100%, there are growing report of vancomycin-susceptible strains that exhibit a "heteroresistant" phenotype. Heterogeneous vancomycin-intermediate methicillin-resistant *S. aureus* (hVISA) is defined by the presence of an intermediate-resistant subpopulation at a frequency of 10^{-5}–10^{-6} CFU in a susceptible isolate with an $MIC_{BMD} \leq 2$ mg/L [2]. Laboratory studies suggest that suboptimal vancomycin exposure early in the course of therapy may select for hVISA during or shortly after completion of therapy [3]. This in vitro finding is concerning as data suggest that patients with hVISA infections are less responsive to vancomycin [4]. Despite this potential association between suboptimal exposure to vancomycin and hVISA emergence, clinical studies evaluating the relationship between initial vancomycin exposure and emergence of hVISA are largely nonexistent. This pilot study seeks to assess the relationship between day 1 and day 2 vancomycin area under the curve (AUC) and emergence of hVISA bloodstream infections (BSIs) by Etest® macromethod among patients with a non-hVISA BSI at baseline. Bayesian techniques were used to estimate the vancomycin concentration-time profile for each patient and the relationships between area under the curve (AUC), AUC/MIC, minimum concentration (Cmin), and AUC/MIC and hVISA emergence were examined. The Bayesian approach used to estimate exposure profiles in this study has recently been validated as a method to estimate vancomycin exposure values with low bias and high precision in situations where trough-only PK data are available.

Methods

This was a retrospective cohort study of patients with MRSA BSIs at Albany Medical Center Hospital (AMCH) between January 2005 and June 2009 performed in accordance with the AMCH Institutional Review Board. The study was approved by expedited review by the Institutional Review Board of AMCH and a HIPAA waiver was obtained. Patients were included if they met the following criteria: (1) age ≥ 18 years; (2) absolute neutrophil count ≥1000 cells/mm^3; (3) not receiving renal replacement therapy; (4) MRSA blood culture met the Centers for Disease Control and Prevention (CDC) criteria for BSI [5]; (5) index and at least 1 subsequent MRSA bloodstream isolates were available for phenotypic characterization; (6) index MRSA isolate was negative for hVISA by Etest® macromethod [6]; (7) received vancomycin within 48 h of index blood culture; (8) received at least 2 days of vancomycin; and (9) had at least one vancomycin level collected within 5 days of starting treatment.

The study methods are comparable to our recently published study [7]. Isolates were identified as *S. aureus* according to standard methods. Initial susceptibility testing for oxacillin resistance was performed according to CLSI guidelines [8]. Isolates were stored in trypticase soy broth with 20% glycerol at −70 °C. All MRSA bloodstream isolates obtained from the patient were shipped to JMI Laboratories (North Liberty, IA) for hVISA screening and determination of MIC through broth microdilution method (BMD) and Etest® strips (lot# BJ0469) according to the manufacturer's instructions (bioMérieux, Marcy l'Etoile, France). BMD and Etest® MICs were performed for MRSA using *S. aureus* ATCC 29213 and *Enterococcus faecalis* ATCC 29212 as quality control strains. Screening for hVISA was performed by Etest® macromethod using Mu 3 as a control strain as described by Wootton et al. [6].

All inpatient antibiotic treatment and vancomycin concentration data during the study period were collected. The vancomycin area under the curve exposure variables on day 1 ($AUC_{0\text{-}24h}$) and day 2 ($AUC_{24\text{-}48h}$) were estimated using the maximal a posteriori probability (MAP) procedure in ADAPT 5 as previously described [7, 9, 10]. This method has been validated to estimate AUC values with low bias and high precision utilizing trough-only sampling [10]. With the Bayesian posterior PK information for a given individual, ADAPT 5 was also used to estimate $Cmin_{24h}$ and $Cmin_{48h}$. The primary vancomycin exposure variables considered in the analyses included: (1) $AUC_{0\text{-}24h}$; (2) $AUC_{0\text{-}24h}/MIC_{BMD}$; (3) $AUC_{0\text{-}24h}/MIC_{Etest}$; (4) $AUC_{24\text{-}48h}$; (5) $AUC_{24\text{-}48h}/MIC_{BMD}$; (6) $AUC_{24\text{-}48h}/MIC_{Etest}$; (7) C_{min24h}; and (8) $Cmin_{48h}$. We assessed both $AUC_{0\text{-}24h}$ and $AUC_{24\text{-}48h}$, as $AUC_{0\text{-}24h}$ reflects initial exposure conditions and is consistent with the exposure profile evaluated in animal model studies [11, 12], while $AUC_{24\text{-}48h}$ represents a near steady-state exposure profile associated with a maintenance vancomycin regimen.

The primary outcome of the study was emergence of hVISA, defined as the documentation of a hVISA bloodstream isolate after 24 h of vancomycin treatment and up to 60 days after completion of therapy among patients with a non-hVISA BSI at baseline. Classification and Regression Tree (CART) analysis was used to identify vancomycin day 1 and day 2 AUC exposure variables associated with an increased probability of hVISA emergence. Bivariate comparisons were assessed using Fisher's exact test, Student's t test, and Mann-Whitney *U* test. Poisson regression with robust variance estimates analyses were performed to identify variables independently associated with hVISA emergence. Each CART-derived vancomycin AUC exposure variable was evaluated in a separate regression analysis. All baseline variables associated with emergence of hVISA at a *P*-

value <0.2 were considered at model entry and a stepwise approach was employed to identify independent variables. Calculations were performed using SAS version 9.3 (Cary, North Carolina) and CART software (Salford Systems, San Diego, California).

Results

There were 238 unique episodes of MRSA BSIs during the study period, 119 of which met inclusion criteria. Emergence of hVISA by Etest® macromethod was observed in 7 (5.9%) patients. Nearly all hVISA isolates emerged during vancomycin treatment and 4 of 7 appeared within 15 days of the index MRSA blood culture (Table 1). One case of hVISA emerged after therapy discontinuation. There was a documented intervention in the medical record related to source control in >95% of cases when warranted. In the CART analysis, patients failing to achieve an $AUC_{0\text{-}24h}/MIC_{BMD}$ ratio of 521 and an $AUC_{24\text{-}48h}/MIC_{BMD}$ ratio of 650 had increased incidences of hVISA emergence. Among the 61 patients who did not achieve an $AUC_{0\text{-}24h}/MIC_{BMD}$ ratio of 521 or an $AUC_{24\text{-}48h}/MIC_{BMD}$ ratio of 650, 11.5% had emergence of hVISA. All 7 cases of hVISA emerged in patients who did not achieve $AUC_{0\text{-}24h}/MIC_{BMD}$ ratio of 521 or an $AUC_{24\text{-}48h}/MIC_{BMD}$ ratio of 650; variables were not completely mutually exclusive (Table 1). No associations between other day 1 and day 2 AUC variables and emergence of hVISA were noted (data not shown). No association between $Cmin_{24h}$ and $Cmin_{48h}$ was noted. Among patients with hVISA, the mean (SD) $Cmin_{24h}$ and $Cmin_{48h}$ were 7.3 (3.4) and 13.4 (5.1), respectively. Similar mean (SD) $Cmin_{24h}$ and $Cmin_{48h}$ were observed among non-hVISA patients (8.7 (4.8) and 11.3 (6.0), respectively).

Comparisons between baseline characteristics and emergence of hVISA and day 1 and day 2 AUC/MIC $_{BMD}$ ratio groups and hVISA emergence are shown in Table 2. Compared to their non-hVISA counterparts, hVISA patients were entirely male, had lower baseline mean renal function, and were more likely to have infective endocarditis and receiving immunosuppressive therapy. Relative to patients with an $AUC_{0\text{-}24h}/MIC_{BMD}$ ratio < 521, patients with an $AUC_{0\text{-}24h}/MIC_{BMD}$ ratio of ≥521 were significantly more likely to be older and have heart failure, but less likely to have a $MIC_{BMD} \geq 1$ mg/L. Patients with an $AUC_{24\text{-}48h}/MIC_{BMD}$ ratio ≥ 650 were more likely to have recent surgery in the previous 30 days and less likely to have $MIC_{BMD} \geq 1$ mg/L relative to those with an $AUC_{24\text{-}48h}/MIC_{BMD}$ ratio < 650.

Results of the Poisson regression analyses are shown in Table 3. When controlling for all baseline variables associated with emergence of hVISA at a P-value <0.2, patients with a $AUC_{0\text{-}24h}/MIC_{BMD} \geq 521$ had a lower risk of hVISA emergence (relative risk (RR) = 0.14, 95% confidence interval (CI): 0.03–0.60) in the day 1 model. Presence of infective endocarditis, CL_{CR}, and skin and soft tissue source of infection were also found to be independently associated with hVISA emergence. In the day 2 model, $AUC_{24\text{-}48h}/MIC_{BMD}$ ratio ≥ 650 was found to be associated with lower risk of hVISA emergence but the associated p-value was 0.08 (R = 0.16, 95% CI: 0.02–1.28). Other variables associated with hVISA emergence in the day 2 model included CL_{CR} and presence of infective endocarditis.

Discussion

This pilot study evaluated the relationship between vancomycin exposure and emergence of hVISA by Etest® macromethod in patients with non-hVISA MRSA BSIs at baseline. Nearly all 7 cases of hVISA emerged during vancomycin treatment and 4 of 7 appeared within 15 days of the index MRSA blood culture (Table 1). One case of hVISA emerged after therapy discontinuation. Using a validated Bayesian technique to estimate each patient's $AUC_{0\text{-}24h}$ and $AUC_{24\text{-}48h}$ values with limited PK sampling [10], we found that failure to achieve an $AUC_{0\text{-}24h}/MIC_{BMD}$ ratio of 521 and an $AUC_{24\text{-}48h}/MIC_{BMD}$ ratio of 650 was associated with an increased risk of hVISA emergence. Of the 7 patients for which hVISA emerged, 6 occurred in patients with $AUC_{0\text{-}24h}/MIC_{BMD}$ ratio less than 521 and $AUC_{24\text{-}48h}/MIC_{BMD}$ ratio less than 650. Interestingly, all 7 cases of hVISA emerged in

Table 1 Clinical characteristics of patients in whom hVISA population was detected

	Patient Number						
	1	2	3	4	5	6	7
$AUC0_{0\text{-}24h}/MIC_{BMD}$ ratio	420.8	226.4	358.6	519.5	251.9	302.6	759.6
$AUC_{24\text{-}48h}/MIC_{BMD}$ ratio	506.6	600.9	505.6	806.6	534.7	442.1	545.3
Creatinine clearance (mL/min)	34.2	22.8	34.5	22.1	65.7	25.3	8.4
Days from index MRSA blood culture to emergence of hVISA	62	2	2	14	15	62	23
Days from start of vancomycin to emergence of hVISA	62	2	1	14	13	61	22
hVISA emergence on treatment	Y	Y	Y	Y	Y	N	Y

Abbreviations: *hVISA* heterogeneous vancomycin-intermediate *Staphylococcus aureus*, *$AUC_{0\text{-}24h}/MIC_{BMD}$* area under the curve from 0 to 24 h over broth microdilution minimum inhibitory concentration, *$AUC_{24\text{-}48h}/MIC_{BMD}$*, area under the curve from 24 to 48 h over broth microdilution minimum inhibitory concentration, *Y* yes, *N*, no

Table 2 Associations between baseline characteristics and (a) CART-derived $AUC_{0\text{-}24h}/MIC_{BMD}$ and $AUC_{24\text{-}48h}/MIC_{BMD}$ groups and (b) emergence of hVISA

	$AUC_{0\text{-}24h}/MIC_{BMD}$ < 521 (*N* = 52)	$AUC_{24\text{-}48h}/MIC_{BMD}$ ≥ 521 (*N* = 67)	$AUC_{24\text{-}48h}/MIC_{BMD}$ < 650 (*N* = 54)	$AUC_{24\text{-}48h}/MIC_{BMD}$ ≥ 650 (*N* = 65)	Non-hVISA (*N* = 112)	hVISA (*N* = 7)
Age in years, mean (SD)	57.1 (15.6)**	64.5 (14.6)**	58.0 (17.1)*	64.0 (14.4)*	60.8 (15.6)	68.4 (10.9)
Sex-male	34 (65.4)	49 (73.1)	39 (72.2)	44 (67.7)	76 (67.9)1*	7 (100)*
Weight in kg, mean (SD)	86.5 (28.3)	82.6 (31.7)	84.7 (27.9)	84.4 (33.0)	84.0 (30.7)	89.5 (20.5)
Recent residence in healthcare institution in previous 6 months	30 (57.5)	43 (64.2)	27 (50.0)	40 (61.5)	68 (60.7)	5 (71.4)
Diabetes mellitus	19 (36.5)	33 (49.3)*	21 (38.9)	31 (47.7)	48 (42.9)	4 (57.1)
Heart failure	11 (21.2)	27 (40.3)**	13 (24.1)*	25 (38.5)*	37 (33.0)	1 (2.6)
COPD	12 (23.1)	26 (38.8)*	17 (31.5)	21 (32.3)	35 (31.3)	3 (42.9)
Hepatic dysfunction	1 (1.9)	4 (6.0)	1 (1.9)	4 (6.2)	5 (4.5)	0 (0.0)
Malignancy	19 (36.5)	14 (20.9)*	17 (31.5)	16 (24.6)	30 (26.8)	3 (42.9)
Decubitus ulcers	11 (21.2)	14 (20.9)	12 (22.2)	13 (20.0)	24 (21.4)	1 (14.3)
Immunosuppressants	13 (25.0)	10 (14.9)	12 (22.2)	11 (16.9)	20 (17.9)*	3 (42.9)*
HIV	3 (5.8)	1 (1.5)	3 (5.6)	1 (1.5)	4 (3.6)	0 (0.0)
History of cerebrovascular event	5 (9.6)	8 (11.9)	5 (9.3)	8 (12.3)	13 (11.6)	0 (0.0)
Recent surgery in previous 30 days	21 (40.4)	19 (28.4)*	26 (48.1)**	14 (21.5)**	36 (32.1)	4 (57.1)
Recent antibiotics in previous 30 days	29 (55.8)	36 (53.7)	29 (53.7)	36 (55.4)	62 (55.4)	3 (42.9)
Prior vancomycin in past 30 days	11 (21.2)	9 (13.4)	10 (18.5)	10 (15.4)	20 (17.9)	0 (0.0)
Length of stay in days prior to index culture collection, median (IQR) days	2 (0–14)	1 (0–12)	3 (0–19)	1 (0–13)	3 (0–14)*	0 (0–0)*
Intensive care unit at onset	15 (28.8)	26 (38.8)	18 (33.3)	23 (35.4)	40 (35.7)	1 (14.3)
Baseline CL_{CR} in mL/min, mean (SD)	77.8 (56.8)	71.1 (46.9)	80.1 (58.4)	69.8 (47.0)	76.7 (51.5)**	30.4 (17.8)**
APACHE-II Score, mean (SD)	13.3 (5.6)	14.4 (6.5)	14.2 (6.2)	14.1 (6.0)	13.7 (6.1)*	17.7 (4.5)*
MIC_{BMD} ≥ 1 mg/L	16 (30.8)**	8 (9.0)**	16 (29.6)**	6 (9.2)**	18 (16.1)**	4 (57.1)**
MIC_{Etest} ≥ 1.5 mg/L	35 (67.3)*	35 (52.2)*	35 (64.8)	35 (53.8)	65 (58.0)	5 (71.4)
Source of bloodstream infection						
• Intravenous catheter	25 (48.1)*	24 (35.8)*	23 (42.6)	26 (40.0)	48 (42.9)	1 (14.3)
• Skin and soft tissue	13 (25.0)	14 (20.9)	15 (27.8)	12 (18.5)	23 (20.5)**	4 (57.1)**
• Bone and joint	2 (3.8)	6 (9.0)	2 (3.7)	6 (9.2)	8 (7.1)	0 (0.0)
• Respiratory tract	2 (3.8)	7 (10.4)	2 (3.7)*	7 (10.8)*	9 (8.0)	0 (0.0)
• Intra-abdominal	3 (5.8)	4 (6.0)	4 (7.4)	3 (4.6)	6 (5.4)	1 (14.3)
• Urinary tract	1 (1.9)	1 (1.5)	1 (1.9)	1 (1.5)	2 (1.8)	0 (0.0)
• Infected graft/device	2 (3.8)	5 (7.5)	2 (3.7)	5 (7.7)	5 (5.4)	1 (14.3)
• Unknown	4 (7.7)	6 (9.0)	5 (9.3)	5 (7.7)	10 (8.9)	0 (0.0)
Presence of Infective Endocarditis	9 (17.3)	8 (11.9)	9 (16.7)	8 (12.3)	14 (12.6)*	3 (42.9)*

All data presented as number (percent) unless otherwise indicated

**P-value < 0.2*

***P-value < 0.05*

Abbreviations: *hVISA* heterogeneous vancomycin-intermediate *Staphylococcus aureus*, *SD* standard deviation, *COPD* chronic obstructive pulmonary disease, *HIV* human immunodeficiency virus *IQR* interquartile range, CL_{CR} creatinine clearance, *APACHE-II* Acute Physiology and Chronic Health Evaluation II, MIC_{BMD} broth microdilution minimum inhibitory concentration, MIC_{Etest} Etest® minimum inhibitory concentration

patients who did not achieve $AUC_{0\text{-}24h}/MIC_{BMD}$ ratio of 521 or an $AUC_{24\text{-}48h}/MIC_{BMD}$ ratio of 650 (Table 1), suggesting the dual importance of both day 1 and day 2 vancomycin AUC exposures and cumulative vancomycin exposure over the first 2 days of therapy. Presence of infective endocarditis was also found to be associated with an increased risk of hVISA emergence in the multivariate analyses. This is consistent with a meta-analysis from van Hal and Paterson [13] which described an association between high-inoculum infections (e.g.

Table 3 Variables associated with emergence of hVISA in the multivariate analyses

	Variable	Relative Risk	95% confidence interval	*P-value*
Day 1	$AUC_{0\text{-}24h}/MIC_{BMD} \geq 521$	0.14	0.03–0.60	0.008
	CL_{CR}	0.93	0.88–0.98	0.004
	Presence of IE	4.94	1.67–14.68	0.004
	Skin and soft tissue source	4.89	1.43–16.71	0.01
Day 2	$AUC_{24\text{-}48h}/MIC_{BMD} \geq 650$	0.16	0.02–1.28	0.08
	CL_{CR}	0.95	0.91–0.98	0.007
	Presence of IE	4.62	1.67–12.77	0.003

Abbreviations: *hVISA* heterogeneous vancomycin-intermediate *Staphylococcus aureus*, $AUC_{0\text{-}24h}/MIC_{BMD}$ area under the curve from 0 to 24 h over broth microdilution minimum inhibitory concentration, $AUC_{24\text{-}48h}/MIC_{BMD}$ area under the curve from 24–48 h over broth microdilution minimum inhibitory concentration, *IE* infective endocarditis

infective endocarditis) and hVISA. Future studies should aim to better elucidate these findings, including the possibility that an alternative exposure threshold may exist for these patients. The observed associations between decreased baseline creatinine clearance and hVISA infection in the multivariate analyses are also not surprising given the number of reports of resistance emergence in this population throughout the literature [14].

Several things should be considered when interpreting these results. This study is subject to limitations inherent to the study design, namely confounding and selection bias. However, the comparable distribution of baseline characteristics between the CART-derived $AUC_{24\text{-}48h}/MIC_{BMD}$ groups and persistence of findings in the multivariate analysis suggest that confounding is unlikely to contribute to the exposure-response observed findings. Results may not be applicable to neutropenic and dialysis patients as these patients were excluded from this study; AMCH does not have an appreciable neutropenic population, and exposure variables are numerous and difficult to characterize for hemodialysis-dependent patients (e.g. sporadic dosing, inconsistent removal volumes due to variable durations and filters). Both of these excluded populations are frequently identified at risk for resistance emergence [14] and the incidence of hVISA emergence may be higher in these populations than that observed in our study population. Two study patients had emergence of hVISA within 2 days of vancomycin therapy. It is unclear if suboptimal exposure to vancomycin selected for these isolates or if they were present in a sufficient density for detection at baseline. Clear delineation between exposure accrual and subsequent resistance emergence should be an important consideration in future studies as well.

Our CART-derived AUC_h/MIC_{BMD} ratio breakpoints for defining hVISA emergence can only be considered a rough estimation due to the small sample size. While vancomycin dose and concentration collections used to generate estimates of vancomycin PK parameters for each individual patient occurred within the first 5 days of therapy, most were obtained on days 1–3. Limiting collection to days 1 and 2 to estimate $AUC_{0\text{-}24h}$ and $AUC_{24\text{-}48h}$ would have been preferred, but this would have severely restricted our already small study sample. For this reason, we employed a vancomycin population PK model as the Bayesian prior that included creatinine clearance as a covariate to account for potential changes in renal function during the first few days of therapy. As previously described, use of a vancomycin population PK model including creatinine clearance ensured a good fit of the model to the observed vancomycin concentrations collected over the first few days of therapy relative to predicted concentrations in our study population [7]. Future studies should consider intensive PK collections on the day the exposure profile is estimated.

Lastly, hVISA phenotypes were not confirmed by population analysis profile (PAP)-area under the curve (AUC). However, the macrodilution Etest® used in the study has been shown to be a viable screening method with a specificity ranging from 89–98% with few false positives [6]. The presence of hVISA by macrodilution Etest® has also shown to be predictive of patient outcomes across of a number of studies, further highlighting the importance of findings from our pilot investigation and need for further study [13]. Finally, future hypothesis analyzing studies should include DNA fingerprinting of the first isolate and subsequent isolates to ensure that isolates are the same.

Conclusion

In conclusion, the findings from this pilot suggest that in patients with non-hVISA MRSA BSIs at baseline, failure to achieve an $AUC_{0\text{-}24h}/MIC_{BMD}$ ratio of 521 or an $AUC_{24\text{-}48h}/MIC_{BMD}$ ratio of 650 is associated with hVISA emergence by macrodilution Etest®. Though we acknowledge that many factors contribute to emergence of hVISA, and that the occurrence of all outcomes are multi-factorial, our pilot findings strongly suggest that day 1 and day 2 vancomycin AUC profiles may be contributory. Definitive conclusions are limited by the retrospective and exploratory nature of the study and its small sample size. However, these data contribute to existing literature in support of AUC monitoring during the first 48 h of vancomycin therapy in patients with MRSA BSIs [7]. Prospective validation in a larger-scale, multi-center clinical trial is necessary to determine the vancomycin pharmacokinetic/pharmacodynamic profile associated with hVISA emergence given its potentially critical importance for defining early optimal vancomycin therapy.

Abbreviations

AMCH: Albany Medical Center Hospital; AUC: Area under the curve; AUC_{0-24h}/MIC_{BMD}: Area under the curve from 0–24 h over broth microdilution minimum inhibitory concentration; AUC_{24-48h}/MIC_{BMD}: Area under the curve from 24–48 h over broth microdilution minimum inhibitory concentration; BSIs: Bloodstream infections; CART: Classification and Regression Tree; hVISA: Heterogeneous vancomycin-intermediate *Staphylococcus aureus*; IE: Infective endocarditis; MAP: Maximal a posteriori; MRSA: Methicillin resistant *Staphylococcus aureus*

Acknowledgements

None.

Funding

This work was supported in part by the National Institute of Allergy and Infectious Diseases (grant number AI105742) to (TPL and MHS). Its contents are solely the responsibility of the authors and do not necessarily represent the official views of the NIAID.

Authors' contributions

DMM substantially contributed to the conception and design of the study, acquisition and analysis of data and interpretation of results, writing and critical review of the manuscript, gave approval of the final version of the manuscript to be published, and agreed to be accountable for the integrity of the data and the accuracy of the work. MRB substantially contributed to the conception and design of the study, acquisition and analysis of data and interpretation of results, writing and critical review of the manuscript, gave approval of the final version of the manuscript to be published, and agreed to be accountable for the integrity of the data and the accuracy of the work. MPP substantially contributed to the conception and design of the study, acquisition and analysis of data and interpretation of results, writing and critical review of the manuscript, gave approval of the final version of the manuscript to be published, and agreed to be accountable for the integrity of the data and the accuracy of the work. MHS substantially contributed to the conception and design of the study, acquisition and analysis of data and interpretation of results, writing and critical review of the manuscript, gave approval of the final version of the manuscript to be published, and agreed to be accountable for the integrity of the data and the accuracy of the work. SLR substantially contributed to the conception and design of the study, acquisition and analysis of data and interpretation of results, writing and critical review of the manuscript, gave approval of the final version of the manuscript to be published, and agreed to be accountable for the integrity of the data and the accuracy of the work. CF substantially contributed to the conception and design of the study, acquisition and analysis of data and interpretation of results, writing and critical review of the manuscript, gave approval of the final version of the manuscript to be published, and agreed to be accountable for the integrity of the data and the accuracy of the work. MM substantially contributed to the conception and design of the study, acquisition and analysis of data and interpretation of results, writing and critical review of the manuscript, gave approval of the final version of the manuscript to be published, and agreed to be accountable for the integrity of the data and the accuracy of the work. REM substantially contributed to the conception and design of the study, acquisition and analysis of data and interpretation of results, writing and critical review of the manuscript, gave approval of the final version of the manuscript to be published, and agreed to be accountable for the integrity of the data and the accuracy of the work. RNJ substantially contributed to the conception and design of the study, acquisition and analysis of data and interpretation of results, writing and critical review of the manuscript, gave approval of the final version of the manuscript to be published, and agreed to be accountable for the integrity of the data and the accuracy of the work. LM substantially contributed to the conception and design of the study, acquisition and analysis of data and interpretation of results, writing and critical review of the manuscript, gave approval of the final version of the manuscript to be published, and agreed to be accountable for the integrity of the data and the accuracy of the work. TPL substantially contributed to the conception and design of the study, acquisition and analysis of data and interpretation of results, writing and critical review of the manuscript, gave approval of the final version of the manuscript to be published, and agreed to be accountable for the integrity of the data and the accuracy of the work. All authors read and approved the final manuscript.

Consent for publication

Not applicable.

Competing interests

T.P.L. is a consultant for Cubist. M.H.S. has served on a consulting board for Trius Pharmaceuticals with all proceeds being donated to Midwestern University. He is a grant-funded investigator for Cubist Pharmaceutical for an antimicrobial stewardship study. All other authors: none to declare.

Author details

[1]Albany College of Pharmacy and Health Sciences, Albany, NY 12208-3492, USA. [2]Midwestern University Chicago College of Pharmacy, Downers Grove, IL, USA. [3]Northwestern Medicine, Chicago, IL, USA. [4]Harvard School of Public Health, Boston, MA, USA. [5]JMI Laboratories, North Liberty, IA, USA. [6]University at Albany, State University of New York, Albany, NY, USA.

References

1. Liu C, Bayer A, Cosgrove SE, et al. Clinical practice guidelines by the infectious diseases society of america for the treatment of methicillin-resistant Staphylococcus Aureus infections in adults and children: executive summary. Clin Infect Dis. 2011;52(3):285–92.
2. Wootton M, Howe RA, Hillman R, Walsh TR, Bennett PM, MacGowan AP. A modified population analysis profile (PAP) method to detect hetero-resistance to vancomycin in Staphylococcus Aureus in a UK hospital. J Antimicrob Chemother. 2001;47(4):399–403.
3. Charles PG, Ward PB, Johnson PD, Howden BP, Grayson ML. Clinical features associated with bacteremia due to heterogeneous vancomycin-intermediate Staphylococcus Aureus. Clin Infect Dis. 2004;38:448–51.
4. Casapao AM, Leonard SN, Davis SL, Lodise TP, Patel N, Goff DA, et al. Clinical outcomes in patients with heterogeneous vancomycin-intermediate Staphylococcus Aureus (hVISA) bloodstream infection. Antimicrob Agents Chemother. 2013;57:4252–9.
5. Garner JS, Jarvis WR, Emori TG, Horan TC, Hughes JM. CDC definitions for nosocomial infections, 1988. Am J Infect Control. 1988;16:128–40.
6. Wootton M, MacGowan AP, Walsh TR, Howe RA. A multicenter study evaluating the current strategies for isolating Staphylococcus Aureus strains with reduced susceptibility to glycopeptides. J Clin Microbiol. 2007;45:329–32.
7. Lodise TP, Drusano GL, Zasowski E, Dihmess A, Lazariu V, Cosler L, et al. Vancomycin exposure in patients with Methicillin-resistant Staphylococcus Aureus bloodstream infections: how much is enough? Clin Infect Dis. 2014; 59:666–75.
8. Clinical and Laboratory Standards Institute. Methods for Dilution Antimicrobial Susceptibility Tests for Bacteria That Grow Aerobically; Approved Standard—Ninth Edition M07-A9. Wayne: CLSI; 2012.
9. D'Argenio DZ, Schumitzky A, Wang X. ADAPT 5 User's guide: pharmacokinetic/Pharmacodynamic systems analysis software. Los Angeles: Biomedical Simulations Resource; 2009.
10. Neely MN, Youn G, Jones B, Jelliffe RW, Drusano GL, Rodvold KA, et al. Are vancomycin trough concentrations adequate for optimal dosing? Antimicrob Agents Chemother. 2014;58:309–16.
11. Craig WA. Basic pharmacodynamics of antibacterials with clinical applications to the use of beta-lactams, glycopeptides, and linezolid. Infect Dis Clin N Am. 2003;17:479–501.

12. Craig WA, Andes DA. Abstracts of the forty-sixth annual meeting of the Interscience conference on antimicrobial agents and chemotherapy, San Francisco, CA, 2006. Abstract A-644. In: In vivo pharmacodynamics of vancomycin against VISA, heteroresistant VISA (hVISA) and VSSA in the neutropenic murine thigh-infection model. Washington: American Society for Microbiology.
13. van Hal SJ, Paterson DL. Systematic review and meta-analysis of the significance of heterogeneous vancomycin-intermediate Staphylococcus Aureus isolates. Antimicrob Agents Chemother. 2011;55:405–10.
14. Centers for Disease Control and Prevention. Antibiotic Resistance Threats in the United States. Department of Health and Human Services; 2013. http://www.cdc.gov/drugresistance/threat-report-2013/pdf/ar-threats-2013-508.pdf. Accessed 6 Feb 2017

Efficacy of introducing a checklist to reduce central venous line associated bloodstream infections in the ICU caring for adult patients

Dominic Wichmann[1*], Cristina E. Belmar Campos[2], Stephan Ehrhardt[3], Timo Kock[1], Claudia Weber[4], Holger Rohde[2] and Stefan Kluge[1]

Abstract

Background: Central line-associated bloodstream infections (CLABSI) are a major source of sepsis in modern intensive care medicine. Some years ago bundle interventions have been introduced to reduce CLABSI. The use of checklists may be an additional tool to improve the effect of these bundles even in highly specialized institutions. In this study we investigate if the introduction of a checklist reduces the frequency of CLABSI.

Methods: During the study period from October 2011 to September 2012, we investigated the effect of implementing a checklist for the placement of central venous lines (CVL). Patients were allocated either to the checklist group or to the control group, roughly in a 1:2 ratio. The frequency of CLABSI was compared between the two groups.

Results: During the study period 4416 CVL were inserted; 1518 in the checklist group and 2898 in the control group. The use of the checklist during CVL placement resulted in a lower CLABSI frequency. The incidence in the checklist group was 3.8 per 1000 catheter days as compared to 5.9 per 1000 catheter days in the control group (IRR = 0.57; $p = 0.001$). The use of the checklist also reduced the frequency of catheter colonisation significantly, 36.3 per 1000 catheter days in the checklist group vs 21.2 per 1000 catheter days in the control group, respectively (IRR = 0.58; $p < 0.001$).

Conclusion: The introduction of a checklist to improve the adherence to hygiene standards while placement of central venous lines reduced the frequency of infections significantly.

Background

Central line-associated blood stream infections (CLABSI) are a major source of hospital acquired infections and an important contributor to the medical and financial burden in modern intensive care medicine [1–4].

Costs for a single blood stream infection are estimated at 16,500 US$ and the mortality of patients with CLABSI is 2–4 fold higher than that of similar patients without [4, 5]. Rigorous hygiene standards for placement and handling of central venous lines (CVL) are needed to prevent infections [6].

In high risk environments like aviation or nuclear power plants, checklists are standard tools to improve safety and prevent system breakdowns [7]. Knowledge transfer is not the primary intention of checklists. Pilots are trained to fly and physicians in an intensive care unit (ICU) are trained to place a CVL, thus the effect of checklists is to focus the attention of the persons involved on the actual task [7]. The use of checklists has been advocated by the World Health Organization to improve the safety of surgery and initial studies demonstrated a benefit [8]. Yet, some studies have questioned the general applicability of this approach [9]. Highly trained personnel and well established backup systems in place (e.g. blood banks, extra personnel on site, interdisciplinary support), have been put forward to explain these findings.

We aimed to assess the effect of introducing a checklist for the placement of a CVL on the frequency of CLABSI

* Correspondence: d.wichmann@uke.de
[1]Department of Intensive Care Medicine, University Medical Center Hamburg-Eppendorf, Martinistrasse 52, 20246 Hamburg, Germany

in ICU-patients in a setting of highly trained personnel in a large university hospital.

Methods

Setting and study design

This was an observational, prospective, single-center study at the Department of Intensive Care Medicine at the University Medical Center Hamburg–Eppendorf, Hamburg, Germany from 1st October 2011 to 30th September 2012. The department consists of 11 wards with a total of 132 ICU beds for adult patients. Each ward consists of 12 beds and is operated by a fixed team of two to three supervising senior physicians, 34 specialized nursing staff and eight assistant physicians. The department is serving for all medical and surgical specialities in need of intensive care medicine. Due to logistic reasons some wards are specialized on certain patients groups (e.g. cardiac surgery, stem cell transplantation, neurosurgery) but all teams adhere to the same standard operating procedures and there is frequent exchange of knowledge and patients between the wards. All these wards are operated on the first floor of the university campus.

To improve compliance with the Institute of Healthcare Improvement recommendations for CVL placement [10], we chose a two-step approach. In brief the measures recommended by the institute were a) hand disinfection b) full barrier nursing c) sterile disinfection of the insertion site d) avoidance of the femoral vein and e) strict indication for CVL. Physicians and nurses handling CVL placements were experienced ICU staff and intensively trained on these hygienic procedures. Training started in July 2011 with a department wide kick-off event introducing the study and theoretical backgrounds. Followed by frequent additional reminders during staff meetings on the wards to improve awareness. During the study period the decision whether or not to use the checklist for CVL placement, was made by the individual team. A ward-based team consisted of the assistant physician in charge (responsible for placing the CVL) and the assigned nursing staff (responsible for filling the checklist).

Primary outcome

The frequency of CLABSI in both patient CVL was placed with or without the use of the checklist.

Checklist

An English version of the checklist used in this study can be found in the (Additional file 1). In addition to the bundle components the checklist contained two formal parts for the evaluation of the study. The first part allowed to identify the setting, in detail: catheter site (jugular vs subclavian vs femoral), type (dialysis vs cvl) and urgency of placement (routine vs emergency), whereas the second part was used to document the duration of the procedure and the members of the team performing the procedure.

Catheter types

During the study Certofix® trio-catheters (Braun, Melsungen, Germany) andMARHUKAR™ triple-lumen dialysis-catheters (Covidien™, Neustadt/Donau, Germany) were implanted.

Patients

Data of all patients treated during the study period in one of the ICU wards with a central venous line or a temporary dialysis catheter were analyzed.

Microbiological methods

In patients with a new episode of sepsis [11, 12] and a CVL as potential focus of sepsis, a pair of blood-cultures was taken from a peripheral site, the catheter was explanted and the tip was sent for microbiological testing. The microbiologists who had to evaluate the microbiological results had no information of the patients' exposure status (checklist used or not used).

Blood cultures (BD Bactec PLUS Aerob/F and Bactec PLUS Anaerobe /F, Becton Dickinson, Cockeysville, USA) were incubated in a Bactec FX 40 machine for a total of five days. Material from flagged bottles was streaked onto appropriate agar media and incubated overnight at 37 °C. In parallel, aliquots taken from positive bottles were analyzed by Gram straining. All cultivated microorganisms were further differentiated to the species level by MALDI-ToF mass spectronomy (MALDI Biotyper, Bruker Daltonics, Bremen, Germany). If necessary, additional methods for species identification according to routine microbiological procedures were applied.

Explanted catheter tips were placed into 5 ml of trypticase soy broth and incubated at 37 °C without shaking. Cultures were visually inspected for growth on a daily basis. Any cultures suspected for microbial growth was streaked onto agar media (Columbia agar containing sheep blood [5% *v*/v]; McConkey agar; Sabouraud agar, all Oxoid, Basingstoke, UK). Microorganisms were further differentiated as outlined above.

The broad use of antimicrobial substances in an ICU setting reduces the sensitivity of blood cultures by about 36% [12–14]. Therefore statistical analyses were performed stratified by CLABSI and colonized CVL.

Definition of CLABSI

Corresponding positive microbiological cultures from the catheter tip and a blood culture taken from a peripheral site at the time of the device explantation in a patient with a new onset of sepsis and a CVL as potential sepsis focus [15].

Definition of colonized CVL

A positive microbiological culture from the catheter tip but no corresponding blood culture taken from a peripheral site at the time of the device explantation in a patient with a new onset of sepsis and a CVL as potential sepsis focus [15].

Definition of sepsis

Sepsis was defined according to the international guidelines of the Surviving Sepsis Campaign [16].

Statistical methods

We first computed descriptive statistics like counts, frequencies, and incidences per 1000 catheter days. Incidence rate ratios (IRRs), 95% confidence intervals (CIs) and *P*-values were calculated using STATA 12.1.

Results

During the study period 4416 CVL were implanted, 1518 in the checklist group and 2898 in the control group. Patient characteristics in both groups did not differ significantly with respect to age (64.7 ± 14.4 checklist group; 64.8 ± 14.8 control group), male to female ratio (2:1), patient type (surgical, medical), disease severity, or length of ICU stay.

We identified CLABSI in 39 of 1518 patients contributing 11,540 catheter days (3.8 per 1000 catheter days) in the checklist group and in 127 of 2898 patients contributing 21,349 catheter days (5.9 per 1000 catheter days) in the control group (IRR 0.57, 95% CI 0.39–0.82, $P = 0.001$).

When analyzing colonized CVL, we detected 245 events in 1518 patients (11,540 catheter days; 21.2 per 1000 catheter days) in the checklist group and 776 events in 2898 patients (21,349 catheter days; 36.3 per 1000 catheter days) in the control group (IRR 0.58, 95% CI 0.50–0.68, $P < 0.001$).

When analyzing the formal aspects of the checklist we identified 267 checklists (17.6%), where at least one of the paragraphs was filled out incompletely, suggesting incomplete compliance. An example for a checklist obviously filled out after the procedure, is available in the (Additional file 2). Nevertheless patients with incomplete checklists had the same reduction in CLABSI as patients with complete checklists. These effects were consistent over all types of ICUs (surgical, medical, neurological); data not shown. In two ICUs patients had a much below average length of stay (< 3 days), with very few newly placed CVLs. Thus here a statistical evaluation of the adherence to the checklist was not possible.

For CLABSI the majority of pathogens isolates were Coagulase negative *Staphylococci* (CoNS) (79%), *Enterococci* (5%), *S. aureus* (3%) and yeasts (7%) in the checklist group and CoNS (76%), *Enterococci* (7%), *S. aureus* (6%) and yeast (6%) in the control group. For colonized CVL the distribution was CoNS (63%), *Enterococci* (18%), *S. aureus* (3%) and yeasts (5%) in the checklist group and CoNS (61%), *Enterococci* (17%), *S. aureus* (4%) and yeasts (5%) in the control group (Fig. 1). When analyzing the CLABSI

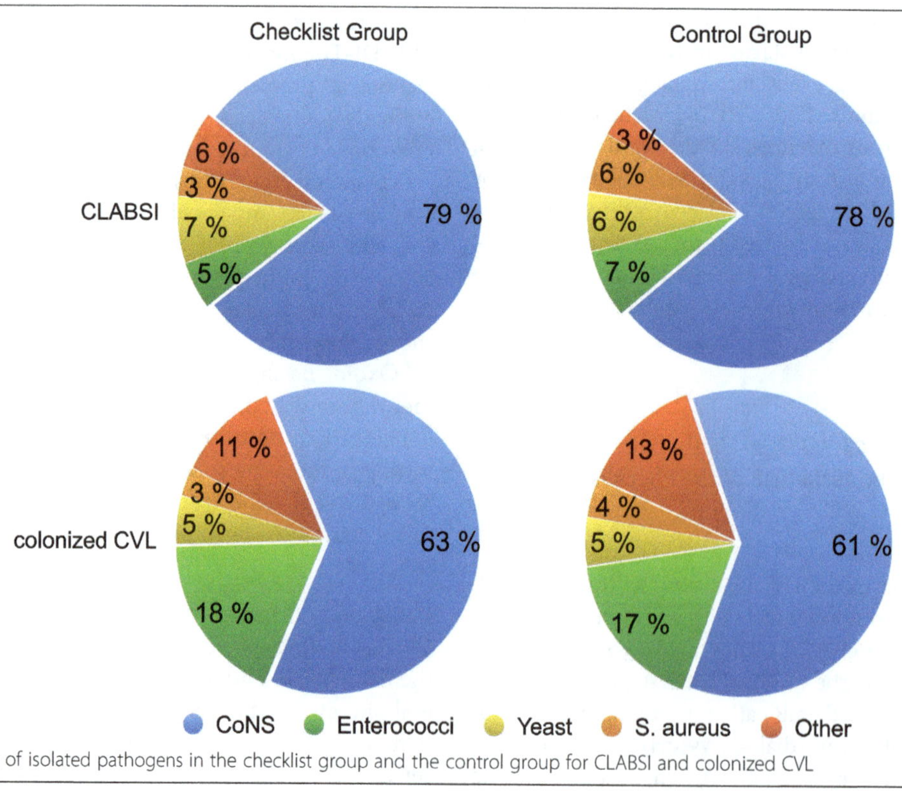

Fig. 1 Distribution of isolated pathogens in the checklist group and the control group for CLABSI and colonized CVL

no significant differences were detected for the site of catheter insertion. Data for the site of insertion were available for $n = 1249$ catheters; jugular vein ($n = 710$), subclavian vein ($n = 272$), femoral vein ($n = 267$). Catheters placed in the jugular vein had an infection rate of 3.6 per 1000 catheter days compared to 2.7 per 1000 catheter days for all other sites (IRR 1.33, 95% CI 0.60–3.02, P 0.23). Subclavian vein catheters had an infection rate of 1.3 per 1000 catheter days compared to 3.4 per 1000 catheter days for all other sites (IRR 1.04, 95% CI 0.40–2.43, $P = 0.45$). Femoral vein catheters had an infection rate of 2.0 per 1000 catheter days compared to 7.8 per 1000 catheter days for all other sites (IRR 0.58, 95% CI 0.15–1.67, $P = 0.16$).

For colonized CVL a protective effect for catheters placed in the subclavian vein was seen (infection rate 5.1 per 1000 catheter days vs 23.5 per 1000 catheter days compared to other sites; IRR 0.52, 95% CI 0.34–0.76, $P = 0.0001$). When analyzing potential effects of the setting in which the catheter was placed (emergency vs routine) no significant differences were detected for both CLABSI definitions (Fig. 2).

Discussion

Introduction of a checklist to improve compliance with hygiene standards for CVL placement in a high volume intensive care setting lead to a significant reduction in CLABSI. Benchmarking with other German hospitals in 2010/11 demonstrated that we ranked in the upper half for CLABSI-incidence in the ICU before introducing the checklist. CLABSI contribute substantially to healthcare cost [2]. The reduction of hospital acquired infections has been found cost effective [17, 18]. According to conservative estimates, the cost of a single CLABSI-episode is about 16,500 US$ [5]. Use of the checklist would thus have resulted in savings of more than 0.9 Mio US$ per year in our study population. Although our study was not designed to demonstrate an effect on mortality it seems a reasonable assumption that the reduction in CLABSI frequency of about 40% would have resulted in a notable improvement of patient safety and outcomes [4, 5]. Thus our study demonstrates that checklists may improve the quality of standard tasks associated with a relatively high proportion of complications. All team members were constantly educated on advantages of checklists as well as the special content and intention of our checklist and the aim of our study in particular. Interestingly, completing the checklist for a standard ICU task had a significant effect on the reduction of CLABSI, even if the checklist was used with incomplete compliance. For example a checklist obviously filled out after the procedure had the same effect on reducing the CLABSI rates as a checklist filled out correctly. One might speculate that the team is focusing on the task if they are aware of the existence of the checklist even if they do not actually use it during the task itself. This may explain why checklists have generally been shown to improve the performance of even highly trained personnel when performing tasks under stress [7]. The Institute of Healthcare Improvement has promoted recommendations for CVL placement to prevent CLABSI [10]. Checklists have been used in various settings (pediatric/surgical ICUs, developed) with generally positive results [19–21]. Yet, the use of checklists in highly developed and high volume health care settings has been questioned by recent data from Urbach and colleagues [9]. Failure to demonstrate an advantage of checklists may, however, be due to the endpoint mortality. Differences in mortality may be difficult to demonstrate in a well developed health care system, when rescue measures are in place to deal with potentially hazardous situations like bleeding, shock, or infections. For the prevention of CLABSI the results of our study are in line

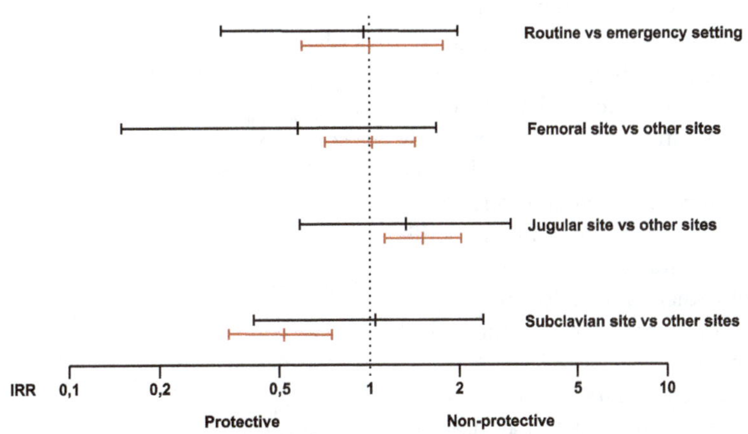

Fig. 2 Incidence rate ratios (central vertical line) and 95% confidence intervals (horizontal lines) for various catheter placement sites compared to their comparators. Values for CLABSI are displayed in black, values for colonized CVL in red. Values smaller "1" demonstrate a protective effect, larger "1" a non-protective. Incidence rate ratios for emergency vs routine setting are shown accordingly

with findings of other groups [19, 22]. Pronovost and colleagues used a multicenter approach together with the state health system of Michigan. Each participating ICU chose a nurse and a physician as multipliers to distribute the information to the ICU staff, local infection control teams gave monthly feedback about infection rates and measures to improve a safety culture were implemented by periodic team meetings and conferences. The adherence to the infection-control practices was supported by the use of checklist [22]. A similar project reported by DePalo and colleagues from ICUs in Rhode Island highlights the need for the implementation of a local safety culture and the designation of local team leaders and the commitment for ongoing improvement by quality improvement cycles (Engagement, Education, Execute and Evaluate) [19].

In clinical practice the decision whether or not to treat inconclusive microbiological results (colonized CVL) is often difficult, particularly if common skin flora like CoNS, *S. aureus* or yeasts are isolated [23, 24]. Contamination of the catheter tip during explantation might be one explanation, inoculation during catheter placement with concomitant colonization and infection the other. Most of our patients were critical ill patients and received antibiotic treatment for various reasons (secondary/tertiary peritonitis after abdominal surgery, hematological/oncological patients with sepsis, patients with neurological diseases and hospital acquired pneumonia). Pazin and colleagues showed that the sensitivity of blood cultures drops significantly in a setting like this [13].

In our study the catheter site (jugular/subclavian/femoral) had no effect on the frequency of CALBSI episodes. This is in contrast to older studies and current guidelines [6]. Meta-analyses however [25], suggested that site-specific effects may be due to two studies with extreme results [26, 27]. When excluding these studies from the analysis no effect of the insertion site with regard to infection frequency was observed [25, 28].

On the other hand we could demonstrate a protective effect for the subclavain vein insertion site compared to all other sites in the stratum of colonized CVL, which has also been shown by Parienti [29]. This is most likely explained by the fact that the subclavian route has the longest subcutaneous distance between skin and vessel entry. However regarding this issue our results are difficult to interpret because of unstable estimates due to the relatively low numbers of catheters included in this analysis and a large number of catheters where the site of placement was not documented.

Our study has limitations. First, the lack of randomization in this observational study may have introduced confounding. On the other hand all participants were instructed on the content of the checklist even if the CVL was implanted without using it. This may have resulted in an underestimation of the effect of the intervention. Second, this was a single center experience of a high-volume ICU without specialized "CVL teams". Thus, while we believe our setting is not unusual, caution is needed when generalizing our findings to other settings.

Conclusion

Our data suggest that a checklist is a valuable tool to prevent CLABSI in ICU patients, may improve patient safety, and subsequently reduce costs for hospital acquired infections. The implementation of checklists for CVL placement should be encouraged even when performed by highly trained ICU personnel.

Abbreviations

CLABSI: Central line-associated blood stream infection; CoNS: coagulase negative staphylococci; CVL: Central venous line; ICU: Intensive care unit; IRR: Incidence rate ratio; MALDI-TOF: Matrix assisted laser desorption ionization - time of flight

Acknowledgements

We very much appreciate the help of all participating staff members of the department of intensive care medicine and the department of microbiology for supporting this study.

Authors' contribution

Study design: DW and CW; data collection: TK, DW and CEB-C; data analysis DW and TK; statistical analysis: SE; drafting the manuscript DW, HR and SK. All authors have read and approved the final version of the manuscript.

Funding

This study was funded by internal grands of the University Medical Center Hamburg-Eppendorf. No funding bodies had any role in study design, data collection and analysis, decision to publish, or preparation of the manuscript.

Competing interests

The authors declare that they have no competing interests.

Author details

[1]Department of Intensive Care Medicine, University Medical Center Hamburg-Eppendorf, Martinistrasse 52, 20246 Hamburg, Germany. [2]Institute for Medical Microbiology, Virology and Hygiene, University Medical Center Hamburg-Eppendorf, Martinistrasse 52, 20246 Hamburg, Germany. [3]Department of Epidemiology, Johns Hopkins Bloomberg School of Public Health, 615 North Wolfe Street, Baltimore, MD 21205, USA. [4]Schoen-Klinik Hamburg Eilbek, Dehnhaide 120, 22081 Hamburg, Germany.

References

1. Mayr FB, Yende S, Angus DC. Epidemiology of severe sepsis. Virulence. 2014;5:4–11.
2. Magill SS, Edwards JR, Bamberg W, Beldavs ZG, Dumyati G, Kainer MA, Lynfield R, Maloney M, McAllister-Hollod L, Nadle J, et al. Multistate point-prevalence survey of health care-associated infections. N Engl J Med. 2014;370:1198–208.
3. Malacarne P, Boccalatte D, Acquarolo A, Agostini F, Anghileri A, Giardino M, Giudici D, Langer M, Livigni S, Nascimben E, et al. Epidemiology of nosocomial infection in 125 Italian intensive care units. Minerva Anestesiol. 2010;76:13–23.

4. Ziegler MJ, Pellegrini DC, Safdar N. Attributable mortality of central line associated bloodstream infection: systematic review and meta-analysis. Infection. 2015;43:29–36.
5. (CDC) CfDCaP: Vital signs: central line-associated blood stream infections–United States, 2001, 2008, and 2009. MMWR Morb Mortal Wkly Rep 2011, 60: 243–248.
6. O'Grady NP, Alexander M, Burns LA, Dellinger EP, Garland J, Heard SO, Lipsett PA, Masur H, Mermel LA, Pearson ML, et al. Guidelines for the prevention of intravascular catheter-related infections. Clin Infect Dis. 2011; 52:e162–93.
7. Kerber CW. Changing our culture: adopting the military aviation safety system. J Neurointerv Surg. 2014;6:332–41.
8. Haynes AB, Weiser TG, Berry WR, Lipsitz SR, Breizat A-HS, Dellinger EP, Herbosa T, Joseph S, Kibatala PL, Lapitan MCM, et al. A surgical safety checklist to reduce morbidity and mortality in a global population. N Engl J Med. 2009;360:491–9.
9. Urbach DR, Govindarajan A, Saskin R, Wilton AS, Baxter NN. Introduction of surgical safety checklists in Ontario, Canada. N Engl J Med. 2014;370:1029–38.
10. How-to Guide: Prevent Central Line-Associated Bloodstream Infections (CLABSI) [http://www.ihi.org/resources/Pages/Tools/HowtoGuidePreventCentralLineAssociatedBloodstreamInfection.aspx].
11. Dellinger RP, Levy MM, Rhodes A, Annane D, Gerlach H, Opal SM, Sevransky JE, Sprung CL, Douglas IS, Jaeschke R, et al. Surviving Sepsis campaign: international guidelines for management of severe sepsis and septic shock, 2012. Intensive Care Med. 2013;39:165–228.
12. Reinhart K, Brunkhorst FM, Bone HG, Bardutzky J, Dempfle CE, Forst H, Gastmeier P, Gerlach H, Grundling M, John S, et al. Prevention, diagnosis, therapy and follow-up care of sepsis: 1st revision of S-2k guidelines of the German Sepsis society (deutsche Sepsis-Gesellschaft e.V. (DSG)) and the German interdisciplinary Association of Intensive Care and Emergency Medicine (deutsche Interdisziplinare Vereinigung fur Intensiv- und Notfallmedizin (DIVI)). Ger Med Sci. 2010;8 Doc14
13. Pazin GJ, Saul S, Thompson ME. Blood culture positivity: suppression by outpatient antibiotic therapy in patients with bacterial endocarditis. Arch Intern Med. 1982;142:263–8.
14. Cockerill FR, Wilson JW, Vetter EA, Goodman KM, Torgerson CA, Harmsen WS, Schleck CD, Ilstrup DM, Washington JA, Wilson WR. Optimal testing parameters for blood cultures. Clin Infect Dis. 2004;38:1724–30.
15. Mermel LA, Allon M, Bouza E, Craven DE, Flynn P, O'Grady NP, Raad II, Rijnders BJ, Sherertz RJ, Warren DK. Clinical practice guidelines for the diagnosis and management of intravascular catheter-related infection: 2009 update by the Infectious Diseases Society of America. Clin Infect Dis. 2009;49:1–45.
16. Bone RC, Sprung CL, Sibbald WJ. Definitions for sepsis and organ failure. Crit Care Med. 1992;20:724–6.
17. Dick AW, Perencevich EN, Pogorzelska-Maziarz M, Zwanziger J, Larson EL, Stone PW. A decade of investment in infection prevention: a cost-effectiveness analysis. Am J Infect Control. 2015;43:4–9.
18. Mutters R, Mutters NT. Hygiene and infection control measures in intensive care units. Med Klin Intensivmed Notfmed. 2016;111:261–6.
19. DePalo VA, McNicoll L, Cornell M, Rocha JM, Adams L, Pronovost PJ. The Rhode Island ICU collaborative: a model for reducing central line-associated bloodstream infection and ventilator-associated pneumonia statewide. Qual Saf Health Care. 2010;19:555–61.
20. Sacks GD, Diggs BS, Hadjizacharia P, Green D, Salim A, Malinoski DJ. Reducing the rate of catheter-associated bloodstream infections in a surgical intensive care unit using the Institute for Healthcare Improvement Central Line Bundle. Am J Surg. 2014;207:817–23.
21. Zachariah P, Furuya EY, Edwards J, Dick A, Liu H, Herzig CT, Pogorzelska-Maziarz M, Stone PW, Saiman L. Compliance with prevention practices and their association with central line-associated bloodstream infections in neonatal intensive care units. Am J Infect Control. 2014;42:847–51.
22. Pronovost P, Needham D, Berenholtz S, Sinopoli D, Chu H, Cosgrove S, Sexton B, Hyzy R, Welsh R, Roth G, et al. An intervention to decrease catheter-related bloodstream infections in the ICU. N Engl J Med. 2006; 355:2725–32.
23. Lutz JT, Diener IV, Freiberg K, Zillmann R, Shah-Hosseini K, Seifert H, Berger-Schreck B, Wisplinghoff H. Efficacy of two antiseptic regimens on skin colonization of insertion sites for two different catheter types: a randomized, clinical trial. Infection. 2016;44:707–12.
24. Luzzati R, Merelli M, Ansaldi F, Rosin C, Azzini A, Cavinato S, Brugnaro P, Vedovelli C, Cattelan A, Marina B, et al. Nosocomial candidemia in patients admitted to medicine wards compared to other wards: a multicentre study. Infection. 2016;44:747–55.
25. Marik PE, Flemmer M, Harrison W. The risk of catheter-related bloodstream infection with femoral venous catheters as compared to subclavian and internal jugular venous catheters: a systematic review of the literature and meta-analysis. Crit Care Med. 2012;40:2479–85.
26. Nagashima G, Kikuchi T, Tsuyuzaki H, Kawano R, Tanaka H, Nemoto H, Taguchi K, Ugajin K. To reduce catheter-related bloodstream infections: is the subclavian route better than the jugular route for central venous catheterization? J Infect Chemother. 2006;12:363–5.
27. Lorente L, Henry C, Martin MM, Jimenez A, Mora ML. Central venous catheter-related infection in a prospective and observational study of 2,595 catheters. Crit Care. 2005;9:R631–5.
28. LeMaster CH, Schuur JD, Pandya D, Pallin DJ, Silvia J, Yokoe D, Agrawal A, Hou PC. Infection and natural history of emergency department-placed central venous catheters. Ann Emerg Med. 2010;56:492–7.
29. Parienti JJ, Mongardon N, Megarbane B, Mira JP, Kalfon P, Gros A, Marque S, Thuong M, Pottier V, Ramakers M, et al. Intravascular complications of central venous catheterization by insertion site. N Engl J Med. 2015;373:1220–9.

Characterization of *Salmonella enterica* from invasive bloodstream infections and water sources in rural Ghana

Denise Dekker[1,2*], Ralf Krumkamp[1,2], Daniel Eibach[1,2], Nimako Sarpong[3], Kennedy Gyau Boahen[3], Michael Frimpong[3], Elina Fechtner[1], Sven Poppert[1], Ralf Matthias Hagen[4], Norbert Georg Schwarz[1], Yaw Adu-Sarkodie[5], Ellis Owusu-Dabo[3], Justin Im[6], Florian Marks[6,7], Hagen Frickmann[4,8] and Jürgen May[1,2]

Abstract

Background: Non-typhoidal *Salmonella* (NTS) cause the majority of bloodstream infections in Ghana, however the mode of transmission and source of invasive NTS in Africa are poorly understood. This study compares NTS from water sources and invasive bloodstream infections in rural Ghana.

Methods: Blood from hospitalised, febrile children and samples from drinking water sources were analysed for *Salmonella* spp. Strains were serotyped to trace possible epidemiological links between human and water-derived isolates.. Antibiotic susceptibility testing was performed,

Results: In 2720 blood culture samples, 165 (6%) NTS were isolated. *S.* Typhimurium (70%) was the most common serovar followed by *S.* Enteritidis (8%) and *S.* Dublin (8%). Multidrug resistance (MDR) was found in 95 (58%) NTS isolates, including five *S.* Enteritidis. One *S.* Typhimurium showed reduced fluroquinolone susceptibility. In 511 water samples, 19 (4%) tested positive for *S. enterica* with two isolates being resistant to ampicillin and one isolate being resistant to cotrimoxazole. Serovars from water samples were not encountered in any of the clinical specimens.

Conclusion: Water analyses demonstrated that common drinking water sources were contaminated with *S. enterica* posing a potential risk for transmission. However, a link between *S. enterica* from water sources and patients could not be established, questioning the ability of water-derived serovars to cause invasive bloodstream infections.

Keywords: invasive non-typhoidal *Salmonella*, water sources, transmission reservoir

Background

S. enterica causes more than 1.2 million annual deaths worldwide, the majority occurring in resource-poor countries [1]. *Salmonella* infections other than typhoid fever, so-called non-typhoidal *Salmonella* (NTS), are usually limited to gastrointestinal disease in industrialized countries. In contrast, in sub-Saharan Africa (SSA), NTS are one of the most frequent causes of bacterial bloodstream infections in both adults and children, associated with high case fatality rates of 20 to 47%, also in Ghana [2–5]. In industrialized countries, infections with NTS are typically of zoonotic origin with regular food-borne outbreaks being described [6–8]. A broad spectrum of animal products such as poultry, beef, pork and eggs as well as contact to farm animals have been associated with infections [9–11]. The *Salmonella* serovar Enteritidis has been strongly linked to poultry farming and egg production [12].

So far, studies from SSA on *S. enterica* isolated from livestock and animal products demonstrate a broad *Salmonella* serovar distribution of types not commonly associated with human infections hence suggesting other transmission routes [13–15]. Despite the disease burden caused, the exact mode of transmission of invasive non-typhoidal *Salmonella* (iNTS) is largely unknown.

Residents in many SSA regions often do not have access to safe drinking water, but use water from sources such as rivers, lakes, wells and boreholes, which may be contaminated

* Correspondence: dekker@bnitm.de
[1]Infectious Disease Epidemiology, Bernhard Nocht Institute for Tropical Medicine (BNITM), Bernhard-Nocht-Str. 74, D-20359 Hamburg, Germany
[2]German Center for Infection Research (DZIF), Hamburg-Borstel, Lübeck, Germany
Full list of author information is available at the end of the article

with bacteria from environmental sources, such as sewage wastewater in the absence of good sanitary facilities.

There is evidence that *Salmonella* serovars are specifically adapted to the human host with no or limited potential to be transmitted beyond this reservoir, suggesting anthroponotic transmission as a major route of recently evolved African strains [16–18]. So far, comparisons on serovar level of human and environmental *Salmonella* isolates from SSA have rarely been conducted. This information is important to understand reservoirs, and potential transmission routes of iNTS in order to institute efficient management and control strategies.

In the rural Asante Akyem district in Ghana, we investigated contamination of drinking water with *S. enterica* to identify a potential source for strains causing invasive blood stream infections in hospitalized febrile children.

Methods

Study site and laboratory procedures

The study was conducted in the rural Asante Akyem District in Ghana, which is the catchment area of the Agogo Presbyterian Hospital (APH), a district hospital with 250 beds. The municipal area has an estimated population of 142,400 inhabitants, spread over an area of 1160 km^2. The region has a tropical climate with two rainy seasons from March to June and from September to October and is mainly covered by secondary rain forest and cultivated land. Malaria is highly endemic in this area.

Blood was taken from children aged ≤15 years attending APH with fever (≥38 °C) between September 2007 and November 2012. For microbiological analysis, 1–3 ml venous blood was injected into vials for paediatric blood cultures (Becton Dickinson, NJ 07417, USA) and incubated in an automated BACTEC 9050 instrument (Becton Dickinson). Broth from positive blood culture bottles was examined microscopically (Gram stain) and plated on MacConkey agar, Columbia agar enriched with 5% sheep blood, and chocolate agar (Oxoid, Hampshire, United Kingdom). The following organisms were classified as contaminants: coagulase-negative *Staphylococcus* spp., *Micrococcus* spp., *Propionibacterium* spp., coryneform bacteria and *Bacillus* spp.

Water samples were collected from 69 villages within the Asante Akyem from October 2009 until December 2009. Water sources considered for sampling were those commonly used by the village populations to collect drinking water, namely wells, rivers, boreholes, outdoor pipes and container-stored water from unknown origin. From the collected water samples, 100 ml was filtered with a 0.45 μm pore cellulose membrane filter (Millipore, Cork, Ireland). The filter was placed into an enrichment broth (Selenite F broth, Oxoid), which was further sub-cultured onto a chromogenic medium (Brilliance *Salmonella* agar, Oxoid) after 18–24 h incubation at 35–37 °C in normal atmosphere. For the identification of *Salmonella* spp., the Analytical Profile Index (API 20E) test (bioMerieux, Durham, North Carolina) was performed and confirmed by a *Salmonella* Latex Test (Oxoid). Serotyping was carried out with standard antisera (SIFIN, Berlin, Germany) according to the White Kauffmann le Minor Scheme. For *Salmonella* positive samples, two colonies were selected to increase the chance for detecting multiple serovars per sample.

Antibiotic susceptibility testing

Susceptibility testing was performed using the disk diffusion method (Kirby Bauer) and interpreted using current Clinical and Laboratory Standards Institute (CLSI) guidelines (www.clsi.org). *Salmonella* isolates were tested for the following antibiotics: ampicillin, ampicillin/sulbactam, ceftriaxone, chloramphenicol, nalidixic acid, cotrimoxazole and tetracycline. Minimum inhibitory concentrations (MICs) for ciprofloxacin were determined by E-test (Oxoid). Isolates were interpreted as ciprofloxacin susceptible with an MIC ≤0.06 μg/mL, as intermediate (reduced susceptibility) with an MIC < 1 μg/mL and > 0.06 μg/mL and as resistant with an MIC ≥1 μg/mL. Ceftriaxone was used as a screening drug for the detection of extended spectrum beta lactamase (ESBL) producing strains. *Salmonella* isolates exhibiting resistance to ampicillin, cotrimoxazole, and chloramphenicol were classified as multidrug resistant (MDR).

Statistical analysis

Descriptive statistics were applied to show variable distribution amongst blood and water samples. Observations with missing values were not excluded from the analysis, thus possibly resulting in different denominators. Results were presented for blood and water samples separately and were finally compared. All analyses were conducted using Stata Statistical Software 14 (College Station, TX: StataCorp LP).

Results

Bacterial bloodstream infections

Blood culture samples were collected from 2720 patients of whom 1255 (45%) were females. Median age of all study children was 2 years (IQR: 0–4) and children positive for *S. enterica* had a median age of 2 (IQR: 1–3). Two hundred forty-one (9%) positive blood cultures were classified as contaminants and excluded from the analysis. Pathogenic bacteria were isolated from the remaining 382 (14%) positive blood cultures, with *S. enterica* being the most frequently detected bacterial species ($n = 222$, 58%). Within *S. enterica,* 165 (43%) NTS and 57 (15%) *S.* Typhi were isolated. The three most common NTS serovars were *S.* Typhimurium ($n = 115$; 70%), *S.* Enteritidis ($n = 13$; 8%) and *S.* Dublin ($n = 8$; 5%; Table 1).

Antimicrobial susceptibility

Ninety-five (58%) NTS strains exhibited MDR (Table 2). All strains were sensitive to ceftriaxone, thus testing for

Table 1 Non-typhoidal *Salmonella* serovars and multidrug resistance in children attending Agogo Presbyterian Hospital, Ghana

NTS serovars	Frequency (%) *N* = 165	MDR n/N (%)
S. Typhimurium	115 (70)	76/113 (67)
S. Enteritidis	13 (8)	0/12 (0)
S. Dublin	8 (5)	1/6 (17)
S. Heidelberg	1 (1)	0/1 (0)
S. Rostock	1 (1)	0/1 (0)
S. Stanleyville	1 (1)	0/1 (0)
S. Virchow	1 (1)	0/1 (0)
Other serovars[a]	25 (15)	18/28 (64)

Abbreviations: *NTS* non-typhoidal *Salmonella*, *MDR n/N* Multi-drug resistance in ampicillin, cotrimoxazole and chloramphenicol (data not available for all samples)
[a]serovar unknown due to loss of isolate

ESBL-producing *Salmonella* strains was not performed. Reduced ciprofloxacin susceptibility was confined to five *S.* Enteritidis and one *S.* Typhimurium strain.

Water analysis

The majority of water samples were collected from wells ($n = 249$; 49%), followed by container-stored water of unknown sources ($n = 136$; 27%) (Table 2).

S. enterica was isolated from 19 (4%) water samples. While samples from rivers had the highest *Salmonella* contamination (n = 8; 15%), no *Salmonella* were isolated from pipe or borehole samples. Amongst the 19 *Salmonella* positive water samples, 22 *Salmonella* isolates were identified. Three of the samples contained two different *Salmonella* serovars. In total, 14 different serovars were found including the following: *S.* Ajiobo (n = 1), *S.* Colindale (n = 2), *S. Corvallis* (n = 1), *S.* Duisburg ($n = 3$), *S.* Georgia (n = 1), *S.* Kingston (n = 1), *S.* Mim (n = 1), *S.* Poona (n = 1), *S.* Pramiso (n = 1), *S.* Rovaniemi (n = 1), *S.* Pasing (n = 1) *S.* Rubislaw (n = 3), *S.* Santander ($n = 4$), and *S.* Stanleyville (n = 1). Apart from two ampicillin and one cotrimoxazole resistant isolate, all isolates were susceptible to all tested antibiotics.

There was no overlap between the water-derived *Salmonella* serovars and the iNTS serovars.

Table 2 Contamination of water samples with *Salmonella enterica* collected in the Asante Akyem district, Ghana

Water Source	Samples analysed	*Salmonella* contamination (%)[a]
Well	249	10 (4.0)
Household[b]	136	1 (0.7)
Borehole	60	0 (0.0)
River	55	8 (14.5)
Pipe	11	0 (0.0)

[a]percentage per samples analysed
[b]container-stored water of unknown origin in households

Discussion

The results highlight the significance of MDR *S. enterica* as a major cause of bacterial bloodstream infections in children in rural Ghana and emerging FQ resistance primarily related to *S.* Enteritidis. The study demonstrates a distinct distribution of *Salmonella* serovars with no overlaps between human and water-derived samples. Hence, *Salmonella* frequently found in drinking water are probably not a major source for invasive bloodstream infections in humans. Recent studies from SSA, using Whole Genome Sequencing methods, strongly suggest that *Salmonella* serovars causing invasive infections in humans have evolved and adapted within specific hosts [16–19]. These data support the hypothesis that invasive *Salmonella* infections are rather transmitted within the human population and not originate from zoonotic sources and are therefore less frequently found in the environment.

In addition, improved awareness of gastrointestinal infections and hygiene practices in the study area, might explain the infrequent environmental contamination with human *Salmonella* strains.

Currently, little information is available from resource poor countries on contamination of *Salmonella* serovars in water sources, although studies have shown the presence of a large diversity of different serovars in the aquatic environment [20–23]. The data correlates well with previous studies showing that rather unusual serovars, not-typically encountered in clinical specimens, colonise drinking water sources. This study indicates that contamination with *S. enterica* is frequent in the Asante Akyem District especially in dug well and river water. Animals such as reptiles may play an important role in the contamination of water sources, as these are known to be carriers of a vast variety and of uncommon serovars [24]. Overall, data on the potential of such strains to cause disease is scarce and was not investigated in this study. However, environmental *S. enterica* strains might play a significant role in self-limiting gastrointestinal infections not resulting in invasive disease with hospital admissions. Nonetheless, as no stool samples were assessed, this hypothesis remains speculative. Still, it is known that *S. enterica* found in drinking water may constitute a risk to human health because almost all serovars of *S. enterica* have the potential to cause illness in man [20].

Furthermore, resistance to locally administered antibiotics was high amongst *S. enterica* from blood cultures but almost absent amongst isolates from water. This suggests that *S. enterica* from water samples were not previously or repeatedly exposed to selective drug pressure as a result of previous antimicrobial treatment.

As for *Salmonella* blood culture isolates, reports across the African continent from studies with similar inclusion criteria have been published, in which the predominance of MDR *S. enterica*, in particular infections with NTS have been reported [25, 26]. The high frequency of MDR *S.* Typhimurium and *S.* Enteritidis in the study presented here confirms the distribution described in the review by Reddy and colleagues [3].

Drawbacks of the study include different collection times of water and blood culture samples complicating interpretation of transmission pathways. In addition, only two individual colonies were selected per sample while several distinct serovars may colonize one water source at the same time. This may have decreased the chance of detecting multiple serovars in one source and hence possible associations. Also, the overall test sensitivity would have increased by testing larger amounts of water and by longitudinal testing. Nevertheless, the *Salmonella* isolates found in the water samples give a crude estimation of the serovar composition of prevailing strains in the aquatic environment in the study area. Although the sampling strategy cannot be considered as representative, the exemplarily testing at least demonstrates that serovars found in invasive human disease do not play a quantitatively dominating role in local water sources. It, however, remains speculative where the *Salmonella* serovars found in the water sources predominantly come from and what their potential to cause disease is. These are important questions to be further investigated.

Conclusion

Quantitative relevance of water-associated transmission of iNTS seems unlikely in this study area. Nevertheless, water contamination with *S. enterica* might play a role in gastrointestinal infections, which should be further examined.

There is an important information gap, which needs to be filled to understand infection reservoirs and transmission pathways of iNTS in order to devise effective management and control strategies. Future studies are required that focus on genome comparisons of human and zoonotic iNTS isolates in order to investigate *Salmonella* adaptation to the host more thoroughly and possible anthroponotic transmission.

Also MDR and emerging fluorquinolone resistance in *S. enterica* associated bloodstream infections in children from SSA urge to investigate evidence-based preventive interventions, like hygiene and sanitation measures or vaccines for high-risk populations.

Abbreviations

APH: Agogo Presbyterian Hospital; API: Analytical Profile Index; BNITM: Bernhard Nocht Institute for Tropical Medicine; CLSI: Clinical Laboratory Standards Institute; DNA: Deoxyribonucleic Acid; ESBL: Extended spectrum beta lactamase; FQ: Fluorquinolone; iNTS: invasive nontyphoidal *Salmonella*; IVI: International Vaccine Institute; KCCR: Kumasi Centre for Collaborative Research in Tropical Medicine; KNUST: Kwame Nkrumah University of Science and Technology; MDR: multidrug resistance; MICs: minimum inhibitory concentrations (MICs); NTS: non-typhoidal *Salmonella*; PFGE: Pulsed-field gel electrophoressis; SSA: sub-Saharan Africa

Acknowledgements

We are grateful to all the children and their guardians who participated in this study and to the personnel at the Agogo Presbyterian Hospital in particular Richard Afrey and the villagers for the provision of water samples. Without their efforts, this research study would not have been possible.

Funding

The publication is based on research funded by the UBS Optimus Foundation and the Bill & Melinda Gates Foundation (OPPGH5231). Serotyping of the clinical *Salmonella* isolates was funded by the German armed forces, scientific project number 03 K2-S-450709.

Consent to publish

Not applicable.

Authors' contributions

DD and JM designed and managed this study. DE supported writing and revising this manuscript. HF, RH, SP helped coordinating serotyping and contributed in writing the manuscript. KYB and MF were involved in water sample collection and performed the preliminary identification of isolates. RK, NGS prepared and analysed the data. NS, JI, FM, EOD and YAS and EF supported planning and managing the study in Ghana. All authors critically reviewed and approved the final manuscript.

Ethics approval and consent to participate

All participants were informed about the study's purpose and procedures. Prior to sample collection, written informed consent was obtained from the parents or guardians of the participating children. Ethical approval for the study was attained from the Committee on Human Research, Publications and Ethics, School of Medical Science, Kwame Nkrumah University of Science and Technology, Kumasi, Ghana and the Institutional Review Board of the International Vaccine Institute (IVI), Seoul, Korea.

Competing interests

The authors declare that they have no competing interests.

Author details

[1]Infectious Disease Epidemiology, Bernhard Nocht Institute for Tropical Medicine (BNITM), Bernhard-Nocht-Str. 74, D-20359 Hamburg, Germany. [2]German Center for Infection Research (DZIF), Hamburg-Borstel, Lübeck, Germany. [3]Kumasi Centre for Collaborative Research in Tropical Medicine (KCCR), Kumasi, Ghana. [4]Bundeswehr Hospital of Hamburg, Germany, Department of Tropical Medicine at the Bernhard Nocht Institute, Bernhard-Nocht-Str. 74, D-20359 Hamburg, Germany. [5]Kwame Nkrumah University of Science and Technology (KNUST), Kumasi, Ghana. [6]Epidemiology Unit, International Vaccine Institute (IVI), Seoul, Republic of Korea. [7]The Department of Medicine, The University of Cambridge, Cambridge, UK. [8]Institute for Medical Microbiology, Virology and Hygiene, University Medicine Rostock, Schillingallee 70, 18055 Rostock, Germany.

References

1. Lokken KL, Walker GT, Tsolis RM. Disseminated infections with antibiotic-resistant non-typhoidal *Salmonella* strains: contributions of host and pathogen factors. Pathogens and Diseases. 2016;74(8):fttw103.
2. Crump JA, Luby SP, Mintz ED: The global burden of typhoid fever. Bulletin World Health Organization 2004, 82(5)346–353.
3. Reddy EA, Shaw AV, Crump JA. Community-acquired bloodstream infections in Africa: a systematic review and meta-analysis. Lancet Infect Dis. 2010;10(6):417–32.
4. Morpeth SC, Ramadhani HO, Crump JA. Invasive non-Typhi *Salmonella* disease in Africa. Clin Infect Dis. 2009;49(4):606–11.
5. Feasey NA, Dougan G, Kingsley RA, Heyderman RS, Gordon MA. Invasive non-typhoid *Salmonella* disease: an emerging and neglected tropical disease in Africa. Lancet. 2012;379(9835):2489–99.
6. Laufer AS, Grass J, Holt K, Whichard JM, Griffin PM, Gould LH. Outbreaks of *Salmonella* infections attributed to beef-US. Epidemiol Infect. 2015;143(9): 2003–13.
7. De Knegt LV, Pires SM, Hald T. Attributing foodborne salmonellosis in

humans to animal reservoirs in the European Union using a multi country stochastic model. Epidemiol Infect. 2015;143(6):1175–86.
8. EFSA. EU summary report on zoonoses, zoonotic agents and food-borne outbreaks 2014. *EFSA J.* 2015;13(12):4329.
9. Mazurek J, Salehi E, Propes D, Holt J, Bannerman T, Nicholson LM, Bunesen M, Duffy R, Moolenaa RL. A multistate outbreak of *Salmonella* enterica serotype typhimurium infection linked to raw milk consumption-Ohio 2003. J Food Prot. 2004;67(10):2165–70.
10. Varma JK, Greene KD, Ovitt J, Barrett TJ, Medalla F, Angulo FJ. Hospitalization and antimicrobial resistance in *Salmonella* outbreaks. Emerg Infect Dis. 2005;11:943–6.
11. Wall PG, Threlfall EJ, Ward LR, Rowe B. Multiresistant *Salmonella* typhimurium DT104 in cats. A public health problem. Lancet. 1996;17:348–471.
12. Ward LR, Thelfall J, Smith HR, O'Brien SJ. *Salmonella* Enteritidis epidemic. *Science.* 2000;10(287):1753–4.
13. Kikuvi GM, Ombui JN, Mitema ES. Serotypes and antimicrobial resistance profiles of *Salmonella* isolates from pigs at slaughter in Kenya. J Infect Dev Ctries. 2010;1;4(4):243–8.
14. Sibhat B, Molla ZB, Zerhin A, Muckle A, Cole L, Boerlin P, Wilkie E, Perets A, Mistry K, gebreyes WA. *Salmonella* serovars and antimicrobial resistance profiles in beef cattle, slaughterhouse personnel and slaughterhouse environment in Ethiopia. Zoonoses Public Health. 2011;58(2):102–9.
15. Tadesse G, Gebremedhin EZ. Prevalence of *Salmonella* in raw animal products in Ethiopia: a meta-analysis. BMC Research Notes. 2015;8(163)
16. Okoro CK, Barquist L, Connor TR, Harris SR, Clare S, Stevens MP, Arends MJ, Hale C, Kane L, Pickard DJ, et al. Signatures of adaptation in human invasive *Salmonella* typhimurium ST313 populations from sub-Sahara Africa. PLoS Negl Trop Dis. 2015;9:e0003611.
17. Ramachandran G, Perkins DJ, Schmidlein PJ, Tulapurkar ME, Tennant SM. Invasive *Salmonella* typhimurium ST313 with naturally attenuated flagellin elicits reduced inflammation and replicates within macrophages. PLoS Negl Trop Dis. 2015;9:e3394.
18. Feasey NA, Hadfield J, Keddy KH, Dallman DJ, Jacobs J, Deng X, Wigley P, Barquist L, Langridge GC, Feltwell T, et al. Distinct *Salmonella* Enteritidis lineages associated with enterocolitis in high-income settings and invasive disease in low-income countries. Nat Genet. 2016;48:1211–7. https://doi.org/10.1038/ng.3644.
19. Kingsley RA, Msefula CL, Thomson NR, Kariuki S, Holt KE, Gordon MA, Harris D, Clarke L, Whitehead S, Sangal V, et al. Epidemic multiple drug resistant *Salmonella* typhimurium causing invasive disease in sub-Saharan Africa have distinct genotype. Genome Research (letter). 2009;19(12):2279–87.
20. Catalao-Dionisio LP, Joao M, Ferreiro VS, Fidalgo ML, Garcia Rosado ME, Borrego JJ. Occurrence of *Salmonella* spp. in estuarine and coastal waters of Portugal. Antonie Van Leeuwenhoek. 2000;78(1):99–106.
21. Baudart J, Lemarchand K, Brisabois A, Lebaron P. Diversity of *Salmonella* strains isolated from the aquatic environment as determined by serotyping and amplification of the ribosomal DNA spacer regions. Appl Environ Microbiol. 2000;66(4):1544–52.
22. Arvanitidou M, Stathopoulos GA, Constantinidis TC, Katsouyannopoulos V. The occurrence of *Salmonella*, *Campylobacter* and *Yersinia* spp. in river and lake waters. Microbiol Res. 1995;150(2):153–8.
23. Dekker DM, Krumkamp R, Sarpong N, Frickmann H, Boahen KG, Frimpong M, Asare R, Larbi R, Hagen RM, Poppert S, et al. Drinking water from dug wells in rural Ghana-*Salmonella* contamination, environmental factors, and genotypes. Int J Environ Res Public Health. 2015;27;12(4):3535–46.
24. Pedersen K, Lassen-Nielsen AM, Nordentoft S, Hammer AS. Serovars of *Salmonella* from captive reptiles. Zoonoses Public Health. 2009;56(5):238–42.
25. Bronzan RN, Taylor TE, Mwenechanya J, Tembo M, Kayira K, Bwanaisa L, Njobvu A, Kondowe W, Chalira C, Walsh AL, et al. Bacteremia in Malawian children with severe malaria: prevalence, etiology, HIV coinfection, and outcome. J Infect Dis. 2007;195(6):895–904.
26. Mtove G, Amos B, von Seidlein L, Hendriksen I, Mwambuli A, Kimera J, Mallahiyo R, Kim DR, Ochiai RL, Clemens JD, Reyburn H, et al. Invasive salmonellosis among children admitted to a rural Tanzanian hospital and a comparison with previous studies. PLoS One. 2010;5(2):e9244.

25

Bloodstream infections caused by *Klebsiella pneumoniae*: prevalence of bla_{KPC}, virulence factors and their impacts on clinical outcome

Min Xu[1†], Yiqi Fu[2†], Haishen Kong[3], Xiao Chen[3], Yu Chen[1,3], Lanjuan Li[3] and Qing Yang[3*]

Abstract

Background: *Klebsiella pneumoniae* bloodstream infections (BSIs) occur with significant prevalence and high mortality worldwide. Antimicrobial resistance and virulence are two main factors participating in the pathogenicity of *K. pneumoniae*. Here we investigated the prevalence of bla_{KPC} and virulence factors in *K. pneumoniae* isolated from patients with BSIs and their association with clinical outcome.

Methods: The clinical data of 285 *K. pneumoniae* BSI cases diagnosed from January 2013 to December 2015 in a Chinese university hospital were retrospectively evaluated. The "string test" was performed to identify hypermucoviscous *K. pneumoniae* (HMKP). bla_{KPC}, *rmpA*, *magA* and serotype-specific genes were detected by PCR amplification. Finally, a Cox proportional hazards model was employed to determine the predictors of 14-day mortality.

Results: Of these isolates, the prevalence of bla_{KPC} and *rmpA* were 33.3% (95/285) and 31.6% (90/285) respectively. 69 isolates (24.2%, 69/285) were HMKP. *rmpA* was strongly associated with HM phenotype. The KPC-producing KP and HMKP were almost non-overlapping and only three HMKP isolates harbored bla_{KPC}. K1 (28, 40.6%) and K2 (22, 31.9%) were the most common serotypes in HMKP. 44.9% of HMKP BSIs had origin of biliary tract infection or liver abscess. The 14-day mortality was 100% in bla_{KPC}^{+}/HM^{+} subgroup (3/3), followed by bla_{KPC}^{+}/HM^{-} (39/92, 42.4%), bla_{KPC}^{-}/HM^{+} (5/66, 7.6%) and bla_{KPC}^{-}/HM^{-} (7/124, 5.6%). The 14-day cumulative survival was significantly different between bla_{KPC}^{+} and bla_{KPC}^{-} subgroup (Log-rank $p < 0.001$) but almost equal between bla_{KPC}^{-}/HM^{+} and bla_{KPC}^{-}/HM^{-} subgroup (Log-rank $p = 0.578$) under the condition of comparable illness severity between bla_{KPC}^{-}/HM^{+} and bla_{KPC}^{-}/HM^{-} subgroup. Independent risk factors for 14-day mortality were Pitt bacteremia score (HR 1.24, CI 95% 1.13–1.36, $p < 0.001$), Charlson comorbidity index (HR 1.24, CI 95% 1.09–1.41, $p = 0.001$), septic shock (HR 2.61, CI 95% 1.28–5.35, $p = 0.009$) and bla_{KPC} (HR 2.20, CI 95% 1.06–4.54, $p = 0.034$).

Conclusions: Most of HMKP were antibiotic-susceptible and people infected received appropriate antimicrobial therapy, which may explain the favorable outcome of HMKP BSIs. The KPC-producing HMKP BSIs were scarce but life-threatening. bla_{KPC} was valuable in predicting 14-day mortality.

Keywords: Bloodstream infections, *Klebsiella pneumoniae*, KPC, Hypermucoviscous, Prognosis

* Correspondence: yq721227@zju.edu.cn
†Min Xu and Yiqi Fu contributed equally to this work.
[3]State Key Laboratory for Diagnosis and Treatment of Infectious Diseases, Collaborative Innovation Center for Diagnosis and Treatment of Infectious Diseases, The First Affiliated Hospital, College of Medicine, Zhejiang University, Hangzhou, China
Full list of author information is available at the end of the article

Background

Klebsiella pneumoniae is the second most common pathogen in Enterobacteriaceae bloodstream infections (BSIs). The reported mortality rate of *K. pneumoniae* BSIs varies from 15 to 79% [1–4], which was lower than that of *Acinetobacter baumannii* BSIs (30 to 84%) [5, 6] but higher than *Escherichia coli* (5 to 22%) [7–9]. Antimicrobial resistance and virulence are generally considered as significant factors in the pathogenicity of *K. pneumoniae*. During the past years, as the increasing of antimicrobial resistance, especially the emerging of carbapenem-resistant *K. pneumoniae*, a serious dilemma has been posed to clinical therapy [10]. *K. pneumoniae* carbapenemase (KPC) is the most important genetic mechanism of carbapenem resistance [11]. Several studies that focus on KPC-producing *K. pneumoniae* (KPC-KP) BSI have found a high mortality rate [2–4]. However, similar large research in our geographical area is still missing.

Hypervirulent *K. pneumoniae* (hvKP), traditionally characterized as hypermucoviscous (HM) phenotype, has emerged as a significant pathogen since first described in 1986 [12]. The HM phenotype has been proved to be strongly associated with *rmpA* (regulator of the mucoid phenotype gene *A*) [13]. The other virulence-associated factors in hvKP include *magA* (mucoviscosity-associated gene *A*) and capsular polysaccharide, especially K1 and K2 serotypes. These factors confer *K. pneumoniae* the ability to colonize mucous surface and evade the phagocytosis of immune cells [14]. hvKP is usually associated with severe infectious diseases, such as pyogenic liver abscess, endophthalmitis, meningitis, and necrotizing fasciitis [15, 16], but only limited information is available about hvKP BSIs [1, 17, 18]. Studies in animal model have shown that both the HM phenotype and the capsular serotypes (K1 and K2) are strongly associated with death [19], but only small amounts of clinical studies with small sample size have evaluated the impact of these virulence factors in the outcome of *K. pneumoniae* BSIs hitherto, and the results are still controversial [1, 18, 20].

Generally, most HMKP are only resistant to ampicillin. There is largely non-overlapping between antimicrobial-resistant and HM phenotype, but recent study shows the antimicrobial resistant rate of HMKP is increasing [20]. Some cases of KPC-producing HMKP infections have been already reported in China [21, 22]. More surveillance is needed to illustrate the prevalence of KPC-producing HMKP strains. Therefore, we conducted this three-year period study of *K. pneumoniae* BSIs in a Chinese university hospital for two main objects: investigate microbial characteristics including the prevalence of bla_{KPC} responsible for carbapenem resistance, and several virulence-associated factors; and analyze their impact on clinical outcomes.

Methods

Setting and design

This retrospective cohort study was conducted in The First Affiliated Hospital, College of Medicine, Zhejiang University, Hangzhou, China, a 2500-bed tertiary hospital having approximately 131,000 admissions each year, and three intensive care units (ICU): a 29-bed medical ICU, a 29-bed surgical ICU and a 15-bed emergency ICU. There is infectious diseases service at this hospital.

The patients aged over 18 years and developed *K. pneumoniae* BSIs during hospitalization were identified between January 2013 and December 2015. Only the first episode for each patient was included in our analysis. Patients with polymicrobial bacteremia were excluded. The relevant clinical and microbiological data we needed were extracted from the electronic or paper medical records and microbiologic database. In present study, the data was de-identified and hence informed consent was waived. Ethical approval was granted from the Ethics Committees and review board of the First Affiliated Hospital, College of Medicine, Zhejiang University.

Variables and definitions

A *K. pneumoniae* BSIs were defined as an infection confirmed by blood culture positive for *K. pneumoniae* and clinical signs of the systemic inflammatory response syndrome [23].

The following data were collected: demographics (sex, age), date and unit of hospitalization; infections acquisition categorized as either nosocomial or community-acquired [20]; baseline severity of illness estimated by the Acute Physiology and Chronic Health Evaluation (APACHE) II score; comorbidities and severity of underlying diseases assessed by the Charlson comorbidity index [24]; severity of bacteremia calculated using Pitt bacteremia score [25]; and source of bacteremia. Immunosuppressive state (chemotherapy, radiotherapy and/or immunosuppressive drugs), septic shock and multiple organ dysfunction syndrome (MODS) at the onset of BSI were also documented. Empirical antibiotics therapy was defined as therapy given within 24 h of the culture being taken, while definitive antimicrobial therapy was considered the administration of antibiotics for at least 48 h. Antibiotics therapy was considered appropriate if it include at least on antimicrobial agent to which the causative pathogen displayed in vitro susceptibility [26].

Assessment of the resistance profile and bla_{KPC}

The isolate identification and antimicrobial susceptibility testing were conducted by Vitek 2 automated system (bioMérieux, France). Minimum inhibitory concentrations (MICs) were categories according to the breakpoints defined by Clinical and Laboratory Standards Institute (CLSI, 2016). For tigecycline, disk diffusion method was used and the results were interpreted according to the U. S. Food and Drug Administration criteria (susceptible ≥19 mm, resistant < 14 mm).

The presence of the bla_{KPC} was investigated by PCR and sequencing [27].

Detection of the HM phenotype, capsular serotype and virulence genes

The "string test" was used to identify HM phenotype. A positive string test was defined as the generation of a viscous string of > 5 mm in length, when using a bacteriology loop to stretch bacterial colony cultured on an agar plate overnight at 37 °C. [14].

The virulence genes *magA*, *rmpA*, and serotype-specific genes for the K1, K2, K5, K20, K54 and K57 capsular serotype were amplified by PCR as described previously [20].

Multilocus sequence typing (MLST)

In order to identify prevalent high-risk clones, MLST of the isolates from the non-survivors subgroup was performed. It was done with seven housekeeping genes (*gapA*, *infB*, *mdh*, *phoE*, *pgi*, *rpoB* and *tonB*) according to the protocol on the MLST website [28]. Sequence types (STs) that had not been described previously were submitted to the database.

Statistical analysis

Continuous variables were expressed as mean and standard deviation (SD) for normally distributed data, or as median and interquartile rang (IQR) for non-normal data. Categorical variables were presented as absolute numbers and their relative frequencies. The two-tailed t test or Mann-Whitney test was used for continuous variables, and the chi-square test or Fisher exact test was used for categorical variables, when appropriate. A Cox regression model by including the variables emerging from univariate analysis with P value < 0.1 as well as clinically important were applied to analysis the effect of different variables on 14-day mortality. In order to estimate the risk of death, survival curves were constructed with the Kaplan-Meier method and log-rank test. All the statistical analyses were two-tailed, and P value ≤0.05 was considered significant. The SPSS software (version 20.0) was used for data analysis in the present study.

Results

Microbiological characteristics

During the study period, a total of 285 *K. pneumoniae* BSI cases that met the inclusion criteria were identified. The characteristics of antimicrobial resistance and virulence-associated factors according to bla_{KPC} and HM phenotype are shown in Table 1.

34.7% isolates (99/285) displayed non-susceptibility to carbapenem, most of which (92.9%, 92/99) carried bla_{KPC}. There were another three bla_{KPC} positive isolates were carbapenem susceptible. Amikacin and tigecycline had the lowest non-susceptible rates among the studied drugs. The detailed antimicrobial non-susceptibility profiles of the 15 drugs are listed in Additional file 1: Table S1.

The HM phenotype was found in 69 (24.2%) isolates. K1 (28 isolates) and K2 (22 isolates) were the most common serotypes. PCR detected virulence gene *rmpA* in 90 isolates (31.6%) and *magA* in 24 isolates (8.4%). The detection rates of K1, K2, *rmpA* and *magA* were significantly higher in HM^+ group than HM^- group. Multivariate analysis showed *rmpA* and K2 to be the independent factor truly associated with HM phenotype (Additional file 2: Table S2).

Compared with non-KPC-KP, KPC-KP showed much more antimicrobial resistance, but less HM phenotype, capsular serotype, *magA* and *rmpA*.

The HMKP and KPC-producing KP were almost non-overlapping. Three HMKP were proved to carry bla_{KPC}, in which two isolates also harbored capsular serotype genes and *rmpA*.

Clinical characteristics according to bla_{KPC} and HM phenotype

According to bla_{KPC} and HM phenotype, the 285 KP BSI cases were divided into four subgroups, bla_{KPC}^+/HM^+, bla_{KPC}^+/HM^-, bla_{KPC}^-/HM^+, and bla_{KPC}^-/HM^-. The baseline demographic and clinical characteristics are shown in Table 2.

Due to the limited number, bla_{KPC}^+/HM^+ subgroup was not included in statistical analysis.

To compare with bla_{KPC}^-/HM^+ and bla_{KPC}^+/HM^- subgroups, bla_{KPC}^+/HM^- subgroup showed apparently distinct characterization by statistical analysis. Patients in the latter subgroup were more likely to be nosocomial acquired infection (96.7%) and have ICU hospitalization (40.2%). Respiratory tract source of BSIs was more frequent in bla_{KPC}^+/HM^- subgroup, but fewer biliary tract or liver abscess origin. This group also had much severer illness process (higher APACHE II score and Pitt bacteremia score; more incidence of MODS and septic shock), less opportunity to receive appropriate antibiotic therapy and much higher 14-day mortality.

There were no significant differences in demographic data, underlying diseases, Charlson comorbidity index, severity of illness evaluation (APACHE II score, Pitt bacteremia score, MODS and septic shock) and 14-day mortality between the bla_{KPC}^-/HM^+ and bla_{KPC}^-/HM^- subgroups. However, community acquired infection, liver abscess source of BSIs and immunocompetent state were more frequent in bla_{KPC}^-/HM^+ subgroup.

Outcomes and mortality predictors

Most fatalities occurred within 14 days after *K. pneumoniae* BSIs onset (18.9%, 54/285) and the in-hospital

Table 1 bla_{KPC} and virulence-associated factors of the 285 *K. pneumoniae* isolated from BSIs

Characteristics	Total (*n* = 285)	bla_{KPC}^{+} (*n* = 95)	bla_{KPC}^{-} (*n* = 190)	*P* value[a]	HMKP (*n* = 69)	cKP (*n* = 216)	*P* value[b]
bla_{KPC}	95 (33.3)	–	–	–	3 (4.3)	92 (42.6)	< 0.001
Virulence factors							
HM phenotype	69 (24.2)	3 (3.2)	66 (34.7)	< 0.001	–	–	–
K1	28 (9.8)	1 (1.1)	27 (14.2)	< 0.001	18 (26.1)	10 (4.6)	< 0.001
K2	22 (7.7)	0	22 (11.6)	0.001	21 (30.4)	1 (0.5)	< 0.001
K5	3 (1.1)	0	3 (1.6)	0.55	2 (2.9)	1 (0.5)	0.15
K20	3 (1.1)	1 (1.1)	2 (1.1)	0.99	2 (2.9)	1 (0.5)	0.15
K54	6 (2.1)	0	6 (3.2)	0.18	4 (5.8)	2 (0.9)	0.03
K57	3 (1.1)	0	3 (1.6)	0.55	3 (4.3)	N	0.01
K-nontypable	220 (77.2)	93 (97.9)	127 (66.8)	< 0.001	19 (27.5)	201 (93.1)	< 0.001
magA	24 (8.4)	0	24 (12.6)	< 0.001	17 (24.6)	7 (3.2)	< 0.001
rmpA	90 (31.6)	2 (2.1)	88 (46.3)	< 0.001	62 (89.9)	28 (13.0)	< 0.001

Data are presented as No. (%) unless otherwise specified
Abbreviations: *HM* hypermucoviscous, *HMKP* hypermucoviscous *K. pneumoniae*, *cKP* classic *K. pneumoniae*
[a] bla_{KPC}^{+} vs bla_{KPC}^{-}
[b] HMKP vs cKP

mortality rate was 32.6% (93/285). The 14-day mortality of three bla_{KPC}^{+}/HM^{+} KP-BSI cases was 100%, followed by bla_{KPC}^{+}/HM^{-} (42.4%), bla_{KPC}^{-}/HM^{+} (7.6%) and bla_{KPC}^{-}/HM^{-} subgroup (5.6%).

Kaplan-Meier curves were used to evaluate the impact of bla_{KPC} and HM phenotype on 14-day survival. As shown in Fig. 1a, the 14-day cumulative survival was significantly different between bla_{KPC}^{+} and bla_{KPC}^{-} group (55.8% versus 93.7%, $P < 0.001$). Although the 14-day cumulative survival of HM^{-} group (78.7%) was lower than that of HM^{+} group (88.4%), the difference was not statistically significant ($P = 0.08$, Fig. 1b). The prevalence of bla_{KPC} was significantly higher in HM^{-} group than in HM^{+} group (42.6% versus 4.3%, $P < 0.001$. Table 1), which may contribute to the relatively low survival in HM^{-} group. In order to exclude the influence of bla_{KPC}, comparison of the 14-day cumulative survival was performed between bla_{KPC}^{-}/HM^{+} and bla_{KPC}^{-}/HM^{-} subgroups. It also showed minor impact of HM phenotype on outcome (cumulative survival, 92.4% for bla_{KPC}^{-}/HM^{+} versus 94.4% for bla_{KPC}^{-}/HM^{-}; Log-rank $P = 0.578$) under the condition of comparable illness severity between bla_{KPC}^{-}/HM^{+} and bla_{KPC}^{-}/HM^{-} subgroups.

In the univariate analysis, several clinical and microbial factors were significantly associated with mortality (Table 3). Patients in nonsurvivor group were more likely to have ICU hospitalization, nosocomial acquired infection, chronic kidney disease, heart disease, and immunosuppression state. This group also had severer illness evaluation and higher prevalence of bla_{KPC}. However, biliary tract or liver abscess sourced BSI, appropriate empiric or definitive antibiotic therapy, *rmpA* positive and HM phenotype were associated with survival.

Cox regression analysis identified Charlson comorbidity index (HR 1.24, CI 95% 1.09–1.41, $P = 0.001$), septic shock (HR 2.61, CI 95% 1.28–5.35, $P = 0.009$), Pitt bacteremia score (HR 1.24, CI 95% 1.13–1.36, $P < 0.001$), and bla_{KPC} (HR 2.20, CI 95% 1.06–4.54, $P = 0.034$) as independent predictors of 14-day crude mortality (Table 3).

Molecular genotyping

MLST of the 54 isolates from the 14-day nonsurvival subgroup identified 19 sequence types (STs), as shown in Additional file 3: Figure S1. ST11 was the most prevalent ($n = 36$, 66.7%). The other STs had only one isolate each. All of the ST11 isolates were bla_{KPC} positive except one isolate. Two cases caused by ST11 were defined as community-acquired infection. However, both of the patients had been hospitalized during previous 2 months. The remaining 34 ST11 cases were unambiguous nosocomial infection. Looking at the detailed clinical epidemiological information of all the 36 ST11 cases, there was no sudden increase in incidence of the infection during this period and the patients who had a close sampling time had non-overlapping stays in the same unit, suggesting just endemicity of ST11 clone in our hospital and nil outbreak happened. Eight HMKP isolates had unique STs. Three bla_{KPC}^{+}/HM^{+} isolates were ST11, ST893 and ST15, and had apparent diversity in genetic background.

Discussion

The retrospective study involved 285 *K. pneumoniae* BSI cases occurred from January 2013 to December 2015 in a Chinese hospital. The prevalence of bla_{KPC} and several virulence-associated factors were investigated, as well as

Table 2 The clinical characteristics of *K. pneumoniae* BSIs according to bla_{KPC} and HM phenotype

Characteristics	bla_{KPC}^{+}/HM^{+} (n = 3)	bla_{KPC}^{+}/HM^{-} (n = 92)	bla_{KPC}^{-}/HM^{+} (n = 66)	bla_{KPC}^{-}/HM^{-} (n = 124)	P value[c]	P value[d]	P value[e]
Demographic data							
Age (years), mean (±SD)	68.0 ± 19.2	57.4 ± 15.3	57.1 ± 13.9	56.0 ± 17.4	0.93	0.94	0.88
Male sex	2 (66.7)	68 (73.9)	44 (66.7)	85 (68.5)	0.32	0.39	0.79
Hospitalization unit							
Medical	0	55 (59.8)	56 (84.8)	105 (84.7)	**0.001**	**< 0.001**	0.98
ICU	3 (100)	37 (40.2)	10 (15.2)	19 (15.3)			
Acquisition							
Nosocomial	2 (66.7)	89 (96.7)	29 (43.9)	86 (69.4)	**< 0.001**	**< 0.001**	**0.001**
Community	1 (33.3)	3 (3.3)	37 (56.1)	38 (30.6)			
Underlying diseases							
Diabetes	0	22 (23.9)	11 (16.7)	30 (24.2)	0.27	0.96	0.23
Hematologic malignancy	1 (33.3)	7 (7.6)	3 (4.5)	20 (16.1)	0.52	0.06	**0.02**
Solid tumor	1 (33.3)	11 (12.0)	21 (31.8)	34 (27.4)	**0.002**	**0.006**	0.52
Solid organ transplantation	0	21 (22.8)	4 (6.1)	8 (6.5)	**0.004**	**< 0.001**	0.92
Heart disease	0	16 (17.4)	8 (12.1)	11 (8.9)	0.36	0.06	0.48
Chronic lung disease	0	10 (10.9)	10 (15.2)	8 (6.5)	0.43	0.25	0.051
Chronic kidney disease	1 (33.3)	31 (33.7)	8 (12.1)	22 (17.7)	**0.002**	**0.007**	0.31
Origin of BSI							
Respiratory tract	2 (66.7)	29 (31.5)	7 (10.6)	11 (8.9)	**0.002**	**0.001**	0.14
Intraabdominal	1 (33.3)	19 (20.7)	9 (13.6)	7 (5.6)	0.26	**0.001**	0.06
Soft tissue	0	4 (4.3)	4 (6.1)	2 (1.6)	0.72	0.41	0.19
Intravenous catheter	0	6 (6.5)	0	4 (3.2)	**0.04**	0.42	0.30
Urinary tract	0	4 (4.3)	1 (1.5)	9 (7.3)	0.40	0.37	0.18
Biliary tract	0	5 (5.4)	16 (24.2)	31 (25)	**0.001**	**< 0.001**	0.91
Liver abscess	0	3 (3.3)	15 (22.7)	10 (8.1)	**< 0.001**	0.14	**0.004**
Unknown	0	14 (15.2)	12 (18.2)	46 (37.1)	0.62	**< 0.001**	**0.007**
Other(s)[a]	0	8 (8.7)	2 (3.0)	3 (2.4)	0.20	0.08	0.80
Clinical presentation							
APACHE II score, median (IQR)	25 (23.5–26.5)	23 (18–30)	14 (11–20)	15 (11–20)	**< 0.001**	**< 0.001**	0.96
Pitt bacteremia score, median (IQR)	4 (3–4.5)	7 (2–9)	1 (1–2)	1 (0–2)	**< 0.001**	**< 0.001**	0.60
Charlson comorbidity index, median (IQR)	2[b]	3 (1–4)	2 (1–3)	2 (1–4)	0.56	0.40	0.81
Septic shock	2 (66.7)	46 (50.0)	10 (15.2)	11 (8.9)	**< 0.001**	**< 0.001**	0.19
MODS	2 (66.7)	37 (40.2)	2 (3.0)	7 (5.6)	**< 0.001**	**< 0.001**	0.65
Immunosuppression state	1 (33.3)	45 (48.9)	8 (12.1)	40 (32.3)	**< 0.001**	**0.013**	**0.002**
Therapy							
Appropriate empiric therapy	0	33 (35.9)	60 (90.9)	96 (77.4)	**< 0.001**	**< 0.001**	**0.02**
Appropriate definitive therapy	0	60 (65.2)	65 (98.5)	105 (84.7)	**< 0.001**	**0.001**	**0.003**
14-day mortality	3 (100)	39 (42.4)	5 (7.6)	7 (5.6)	**< 0.001**	**< 0.001**	0.84

Data are presented as No. (%) unless otherwise specified; boldface, indicates statistical significance ($p<0.05$)

Abbreviations: *HM* hypermucoviscous, *BSIs* bloodstream infections, *CNS* central nervous system, *APACHE* Acute Physiology and Chronic Health Evaluation, *MODS* multiple organ dysfunction syndrome, *SD* standard deviation, *IQR* interquartile range

[a]Central nervous system infection, 9 cases; mediastinal infection, 1 cases; endocarditis, 3 cases

[b]The three cases had same Charlson comorbidity index

[c]bla_{KPC}^{+}/HM^{-} vs bla_{KPC}^{-}/HM^{+}

[d]bla_{KPC}^{+}/HM^{-} vs bla_{KPC}^{-}/HM^{-}

[e]bla_{KPC}^{-}/HM^{+} vs bla_{KPC}^{-}/HM^{-}

the impact of these factors on mortality. It represented one of the largest investigations of *K. pneumoniae* BSIs in Chinese hospital that focused on microbial and clinical characterization simultaneously.

In this study, the carbapenem resistant rate of *K. pneumoniae* isolated from BSIs was 34.7%, which was much higher than the result of a national investigation reported by Xu et al. in China (5.5%) [29]. The disparity

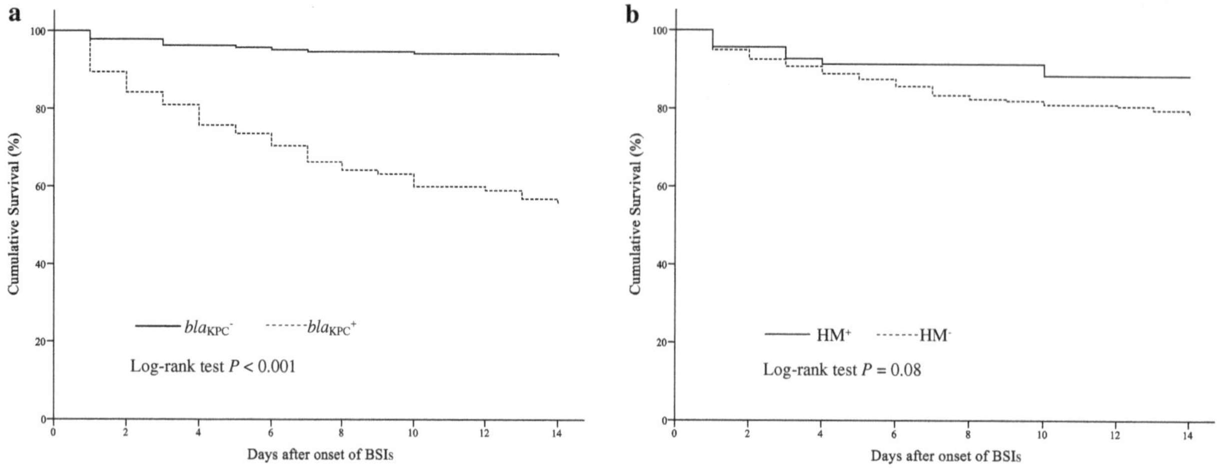

Fig. 1 Kaplan-Meier curves about impact of bla_{KPC} (**a**) and HM phenotype (**b**) on 14-day survival. HM, hypermucoviscous; BSIs, bloodstream infections

can be attributed to the variant distribution of bla_{KPC} among regions. As the most important carbapenemase gene of *K. pneumoniae*, bla_{KPC} was detected in 33.3% of 285 isolates. Although there was no information concerning the detection frequency of bla_{KPC} in *K. pneumoniae* isolated from BSIs in China hereto, this data was higher than that reported by Yedidah et al. (25.0%) in Israel [3]. MLST showed 66.7% of isolates from the 14-day nonsurvival group was ST11, which belonged to CC258, a well-known international high-risk MDR clone of *K. pneumoniae* [30]. Almost all of the ST11 isolates were bla_{KPC} positive and caused nosocomial infection in this study. It is believed that the nosocomial clonal dissemination of KPC-producing ST11 *K. pneumoniae* played a significant role in the high detection rate of bla_{KPC}. In addition, the positive rate of bla_{KPC} was 44.2% in isolates from nosocomial-acquired infection, but only 5.1% in isolates from community-acquired infection. Therefore, including of more nosocomial infection cases (72.3%) and relatively less community infection cases (27.7%) may also lead to the increased overall carbapenem resistant rate.

The study showed 24.2% (69/285) of *K. pneumoniae* BSI cases were caused by HMKP. This percentage was much higher than that recently reported by Cubero et al. in Spain (5.4%) [17], but lower than that described in other regions of China (31.4% [1] and 28% [20]). In accordance with a number of previous studies, K1 and K2 were the most common serotypes [1, 17, 20, 31]. However, the prevalence of these two serotypes in this study was lower than those reported by other Chinese researchers [1, 20]. Besides the geographic variation, the discrepancy in sample size might account for these differences.

As expected, most HMKP displayed susceptibility to carbapenem (94.2%, 65/69), which was consistent to the traditional view that HMKP is rarely resistant to antibiotics except its intrinsic resistance to ampicillin [21]. However, recent studies have indicated that the degree of antimicrobial resistance of HMKP strains increased over time [20]. Even KPC-producing HMKP isolates have been reported in China [22, 32]. In our study, 4.3% (3 isolates) isolates were identified as KPC-producing HMKP strains and they belonged to three distinctive STs (ST11, ST15 and ST893) without molecular epidemiological relationship, suggesting they were sporadic cases. The isolates of ST11 and ST15 were K-nontypable and *rmpA* and *magA* negative. Other factors may be responsible for the HM phenotype. In addition, as far as our best knowledge, it is the first report of KPC-producing HMKP ST893 co-harboring K20 serotype and *rmpA*.

When classified according to HM and bla_{KPC} phenotype, clinical characteristics were significantly different between subgroups. Besides community acquisition infections ($P = 0.001$), liver abscess ($P = 0.004$) and immune status ($P = 0.002$) were most significantly associated with HMKP (bla_{KPC}^-/HM$^+$ versus bla_{KPC}^-/HM$^-$). This feature is consistent with previous reports that HMKP usually infects immunocompetent subjects and causes liver abscess [14]. On the contrary, KPC-KP were more likely to be nosocomial acquisition, happen in patients with serious underlying diseases (solid organ transplantation, central nervous diseases and chronic kidney disease) and have respiratory tract or intraabdominal source. These differences indicate that HMKP and KPC-KP each has unique potential reservoir and pathogenicity.

Several studies have reported the mortality of HMKP BSIs was lower than that of cKP BSIs [1, 31]. Although without significant difference, the trend was also observed in this study (14-day mortality, HMKP 11.6%

Table 3 Univariate and multivariate analysis of factors associated with 14-day mortality

Characteristic	Total	Survivors	Non-survivors	*P* value	Multivariate analysis	
	(n = 285)	(*n* = 231)	(*n* = 54)		HR (95% CI)	*P* value
Demographic data						
Age (years), mean (±SD)	56.8 ± 15.9	56.7 ± 16.4	57.2 ± 14.1	0.83		
Male sex	199 (69.8)	159 (68.8)	40 (74.1)	0.45		
ICU hospitalization	69 (24.2)	48 (20.8)	21 (38.9)	**0.005**		
Nosocomial acquisition	206 (72.3)	158 (68.4)	48 (88.9)	**0.002**		
Underlying diseases						
Diabetes	63 (22.1)	52 (22.5)	11 (20.4)	0.73		
Hematologic malignancy	31 (10.9)	23 (10.0)	8 (14.8)	0.30		
Solid tumor	67 (23.5)	60 (26.0)	7 (13.0)	**0.04**		
Solid organ transplantation	33 (11.6)	24 (10.4)	9 (16.7)	0.19		
Heart disease	35 (12.3)	23 (10.0)	12 (22.2)	**0.01**		
Chronic lung disease	28 (9.8)	25 (10.8)	3 (5.6)	0.24		
Chronic kidney disease	62 (21.8)	38 (16.5)	24 (44.4)	**< 0.001**		
Origin of BSI						
Respiratory tract	49 (17.2)	28 (12.1)	21 (38.9)	**< 0.001**		
Intraabdominal	36 (12.6)	26 (11.3)	10 (18.5)	0.15		
Soft tissue	10 (3.5)	6 (2.6)	4 (7.4)	0.19		
Intravenous catheter	10 (3.5)	9 (3.9)	1 (1.9)	0.75		
Urinary tract	14 (4.9)	14 (6.1)	0	0.13		
Biliary tract	52 (18.2)	51 (22.1)	1 (1.9)	**0.001**		
Liver abscess	28 (9.8)	28 (12.1)	0	**0.007**		
Unknown	72 (25.3)	60 (26.0)	12 (22.2)	0.57		
Other(s)	13 (4.6)	8 (3.5)	5 (9.3)	0.14		
Clinical presentation						
APACHE II score, median (IQR)	18 (12–24)	15 (11–21)	26 (21–33.3)	**< 0.001**		
Pitt bacteremia score, median (IQR)	2 (1–6)	1 (0–3)	8 (4.75–10.5)	**< 0.001**	1.24 (1.13–1.36)	**< 0.001**
Charlson comorbidity index, median (IQR)	2 (1–4)	2 (1–4)	3 (2–5)	**0.02**	1.24 (1.09–1.41)	**0.001**
Septic shock	69 (24.2)	30 (13.0)	39 (72.2)	**< 0.001**	2.61 (1.28–5.35)	**0.009**
MODS	48 (16.8)	19 (8.2)	29 (53.7)	**< 0.001**		
Immunosuppression state	94 (33.0)	67 (29.0)	27 (50.0)	**0.003**		
Therapy						
Appropriate empiric therapy	189 (66.3)	163 (70.6)	26 (48.1)	**0.002**		
Appropriate definitive therapy	230 (80.7)	194 (84.0)	36 (66.7)	**0.004**		
HM phenotype	69 (24.2)	61 (26.4)	8 (14.8)	0.08		
bla$_{KPC}$	95 (33.3)	53 (22.9)	42 (77.8)	**< 0.001**	2.20 (1.06–4.54)	**0.034**
rmpA	90 (31.6)	83 (35.9)	7 (13.0)	**0.001**		

Data are presented as No. (%) unless otherwise specified; boldface, indicates statistical significance ($p<0.05$)
Abbreviations: *HM* hypermucoviscous, *BSIs* bloodstream infection, *CNS* central nervous system, *APACHE* Acute Physiology and Chronic Health Evaluation, *MODS* multiple organ dysfunction syndrome, *SD* standard deviation, *IQR* interquartile range, *CI* confidence interval, *HR* hazard ratio

versus cKP 21.3%, Log-rank $P = 0.08$). Because of low resistant rates, the empirical and definitive anti-infective therapy against HMKP BSIs could be reasonable and effective, which may explain the relatively favorable prognosis. We also performed 14-day survival analysis between *bla*$_{KPC}^{-}$/HM^{+} and *bla*$_{KPC}^{-}$/HM^{-} subgroups to exclude the interference of resistance. The result also showed HM phenotype alone had minor impact on the poor prognosis of BSIs (14-day mortality, 7.6% versus 5.6%, $P = 0.578$). However, new evidence has suggested that a HM phenotype only is not sufficient to indicate a hypervirulent state [33]. Other important virulence-associated factors such as siderophores were not performed in this study may lead to bias on identification of real hypervirulent *K. pneumoniae*.

Previous studies on KPC-KP BSIs reported mortality rates up to 79% [2]. In this study, the 14-day mortality of KPC-KP BSIs was 44.2%. Compared with patients of non-KPC-KP BSIs, patients of KPC-KP BSIs were more critical (higher APACHE II score and Pitt bacteremia score at the onset of BSIs). It might be that KPC carriage is collinear with severity of illness, and thus mortality might not be necessarily associated with KPC but rather with severity. Cox analysis subsequently showed bla_{KPC} was an independent predictor of 14-day mortality, as well as Charlson comorbidity index, Pitt bacteremia score, and septic shock. Thus, KPC-KP BSIs are associated with a poor outcome. The mortality outside the ICUs in present study was 15.3% (33/216), which although significantly lower than that of patients stayed in ICUs (15.3% vs 38.9%, $p = 0.005$) but still relative high. Among the 27 patients stayed in hepato-biliary unit suffering from liver transplantation, 9 patients had fatal outcome at day 14. So, the high mortality of these patients (33.3%) might attribute to the overall high mortality of patients outside the ICUs. Additionally, the *K. pneumoniae* strains isolated from these 9 patients were all positive for bla_{KPC}, which further confirmed that the KPC-KP BSIs were associated with a poor outcome.

The 14-day mortality of the three cases caused by KPC-producing HMKP was 100% in our study. Zhang et al. reported three cases of KPC-producing HMKP infections, in which two were survived and one unknown [32]. However, there was only one BSIs case. In another study, Zhang et al. reported five cases of KPC-producing HMKP BSIs with 100% mortality [22]. Although limited information available, it seemed KPC-producing HMKP BSIs had disastrous outcome.

Conclusions

Our study showed the resistance characteristics and clinical manifestation were significantly different between HMKP BSIs and KPC-KP BSIs. HMKP were usually antibiotic susceptible and associated with favorable outcome of BSIs. bla_{KPC} was an independent predictor of poor outcome. The emergence of KPC-producing HMKP is a potential threat of public health and must be critically monitored.

Additional files

Additional file 1: Table S1. Non-susceptible rates of 15 antimicrobial agents for 285 *K. pneumoniae* isolates from bloodstream infections according to bla_{KPC} and HM phenotype.

Additional file 2: Table S2. Factors associated with hypermucoviscosity phenotype in *K. pneumoniae* isolated from BSIs.

Additional file 3: Figure S1. Characteristics of 54 *K. pneumoniae* isolates from the non-survival subgroup.

Abbreviations

APACHE: Acute Physiology and Chronic Health Evaluation; BSIs: Bloodstream infections; CI: confidence interval; cKP: classic *K. pneumoniae*; CLSI: Clinical Laboratory Standards Institute; CNS: central nervous system; HM: hypermucoviscous; HMKP: hypermucoviscous *K. pneumoniae*; HR: hazard ratio; hvKP: hypervirulent *K. pneumoniae*; ICU: intensive care units; IQR: interquartile range; KPC: *K. pneumoniae* carbapenemase; KPC-KP: KPC-producing *K. pneumoniae*; MICs: minimum inhibitory concentrations; MLST: multilocus sequence typing; MODS: multiple organ dysfunction syndrome; SD: standard deviation

Acknowledgements

We thank the entire staff at the Department of Microbiology, The First Affiliated Hospital, College of Medicine, Zhejiang University for their daily contributions to this study. We also thank the team of curators from the Institut Pasteur MLST system (Paris, France) for importing novel alleles and profiles at http://bigsdb.pasteur.fr/klebsiella/klebsiella.html.

Funding

This work was supported by the Natural Science Foundation of Zhejiang Province (no. LQ13H190001), Medical Science and Technology Project of Zhejiang Province (no. 2014KYB096) and National Natural Science Foundation (no. 81301459).

Authors' contributions

MX and LL designed the study. MX and YF performed data analysis and drafted the manuscript. HK and YF participated in the collection of strains and clinical information. QY and XC performed the phenotypic and genotypic analysis of the clinical isolates. YC and LL reviewed the paper and provided recommendations. All authors read and approved the final manuscript.

Consent for publication

Not applicable.

Competing interests

The authors declare that they have no competing interests.

Author details

[1]Key Laboratory of Clinical In Vitro Diagnostic Techniques of Zhejiang Province, Center of Clinical Laboratory, The First Affiliated Hospital, College of Medicine, Zhejiang University, Hangzhou, China. [2]Department of Respiratory Diseases, The First Affiliated Hospital, College of Medicine, Zhejiang University, Hangzhou, China. [3]State Key Laboratory for Diagnosis and Treatment of Infectious Diseases, Collaborative Innovation Center for Diagnosis and Treatment of Infectious Diseases, The First Affiliated Hospital, College of Medicine, Zhejiang University, Hangzhou, China.

References

1. Liu YM, Li BB, Zhang YY, Zhang W, Shen H, Li H, et al. Clinical and molecular characteristics of emerging hypervirulent *Klebsiella pneumoniae* bloodstream infections in mainland China. Antimicrob Agents Chemother. 2014;58:5379–85.
2. da Silva KE, Maciel WG, Sacchi FP, Carvalhaes CG, Rodrigues-Costa F, da Silva AC, et al. Risk factors for KPC-producing *Klebsiella pneumoniae*: watch out for surgery. J Med Microbiol. 2016;65:547–53.
3. Fraenkel-Wandel Y, Raveh-Brawer D, Wiener-Well Y, Yinnon AM, Assous MV. Mortality due to bla_{KPC} *Klebsiella pneumoniae* bacteraemia. J Antimicrob Chemother. 2016;71:1083–7.

4. Falcone M, Russo A, Iacovelli A, Restuccia G, Ceccarelli G, Giordano A, et al. Predictors of outcome in ICU patients with septic shock caused by *Klebsiella pneumoniae* carbapenemase-producing *K. pneumoniae*. Clin Microbiol Infect. 2016;22:444–50.
5. Liu Q, Li W, Du X, Li W, Zhong T, Tang Y, et al. Risk and prognostic factors for multidrug-resistant *Acinetobacter Baumannii* complex bacteremia: a retrospective study in a tertiary Hospital of West China. PLoS One. 2015;10: e0130701.
6. Freire MP, de Oliveira GD, Garcia CP, Campagnari Bueno MF, Camargo CH, Kono Magri ASG, et al. Bloodstream infection caused by extensively drug-resistant *Acinetobacter baumannii* in cancer patients: high mortality associated with delayed treatment rather than with the degree of neutropenia. Clin Microbiol Infect. 2016;22:352–8.
7. Giannella M, Pascale R, Toschi A, Ferraro G, Graziano E, Furii F, et al. Treatment duration for *Escherichia coli* bloodstream infection and outcomes: retrospective single-Centre study. Clin Microbiol Infect. 2018; https://doi.org/10.1016/j.cmi.2018.01.013.
8. Abernethy JK, Johnson AP, Guy R, Hinton N, Sheridan EA, Hope RJ. Thirty day all-cause mortality in patients with *Escherichia coli* bacteraemia in England. Clin Microbiol Infect. 2015;21:251 e1–8.
9. Schwab F, Geffers C, Behnke M, Gastmeier P. ICU mortality following ICU-acquired primary bloodstream infections according to the type of pathogen: a prospective cohort study in 937 Germany ICUs (2006-2015). PLoS One. 2018;13:e0194210.
10. Nordmann P, Cuzon G, Naas T. The real threat of *Klebsiella pneumoniae* carbapenemase-producing bacteria. Lancet Infect Dis. 2009;9:228–36.
11. Munoz-Price LS, Poirel L, Bonomo RA, Schwaber MJ, Daikos GL, Cormican M, et al. Clinical epidemiology of the global expansion of *Klebsiella pneumoniae* carbapenemases. Lancet Infect Dis. 2013;13:785–96.
12. Liu YC, Cheng DL, Lin CL. *Klebsiella pneumoniae* liver abscess associated with septic endophthalmitis. Arch Intern Med. 1986;146:1913–6.
13. Yu WL, Ko WC, Cheng KC, Lee HC, Ke DS, Lee CC, et al. Association between *rmpA* and *magA* genes and clinical syndromes caused by *Klebsiella pneumoniae* in Taiwan. Clin Infect Dis. 2006;42:1351–8.
14. Shon AS, Bajwa RP, Russo TA. Hypervirulent (hypermucoviscous) *Klebsiella pneumoniae*: a new and dangerous breed. Virulence. 2013;4:107–18.
15. Fang CT, Lai SY, Yi WC, Hsueh PR, Liu KL, Chang SC. *Klebsiella pneumoniae* genotype K1: an emerging pathogen that causes septic ocular or central nervous system complications from pyogenic liver abscess. Clin Infect Dis. 2007;45:284–93.
16. Cheng NC, Yu YC, Tai HC, Hsueh PR, Chang SC, Lai SY, et al. Recent trend of necrotizing fasciitis in Taiwan: focus on monomicrobial *Klebsiella pneumoniae* necrotizing fasciitis. Clin Infect Dis. 2012;55:930–9.
17. Cubero M, Grau I, Tubau F, Pallares R, Dominguez MA, Linares J, et al. Hypervirulent *Klebsiella pneumoniae* clones causing bacteraemia in adults in a teaching hospital in Barcelona, Spain (2007-2013). Clin Microbiol Infect. 2016;22:154–60.
18. Togawa A, Toh H, Onozawa K, Yoshimura M, Tokushige C, Shimono N, et al. Influence of the bacterial phenotypes on the clinical manifestations in *Klebsiella pneumoniae* bacteremia patients: a retrospective cohort study. J Infect Chemother. 2015;21:531–7.
19. Yu VL, Hansen DS, Ko WC, Sagnimeni A, Klugman KP, von Gottberg A, et al. Virulence characteristics of Klebsiella and clinical manifestations of *K. pneumoniae* bloodstream infections. Emerg Infect Dis. 2007;13:986–93.
20. Li W, Sun G, Yu Y, Li N, Chen M, Jin R, et al. Increasing occurrence of antimicrobial-resistant hypervirulent (hypermucoviscous) *Klebsiella pneumoniae* isolates in China. Clin Infect Dis. 2014;58:225–32.
21. Yao B, Xiao X, Wang F, Zhou L, Zhang X, Zhang J. Clinical and molecular characteristics of multi-clone carbapenem-resistant hypervirulent (hypermucoviscous) *Klebsiella pneumoniae* isolates in a tertiary hospital in Beijing, China. Int J Infect Dis. 2015;37:107–12.
22. Zhang R, Lin D, Chan EW, Gu D, Chen GX, Chen S. Emergence of Carbapenem-resistant serotype K1 Hypervirulent *Klebsiella pneumoniae* strains in China. Antimicrob Agents Chemother. 2016;60:709–11.
23. Kang CI, Kim SH, Park WB, Lee KD, Kim HB, Kim EC, et al. Bloodstream infections caused by antibiotic-resistant gram-negative bacilli: risk factors for mortality and impact of inappropriate initial antimicrobial therapy on outcome. Antimicrob Agents Chemother. 2005;49:760–6.
24. Charlson ME, Pompei P, Ales KL, MacKenzie CR. A new method of classifying prognostic comorbidity in longitudinal studies: development and validation. J Chronic Dis. 1987;40:373–83.
25. Paterson DL, Ko WC, Von Gottberg A, Mohapatra S, Casellas JM, Goossens H, et al. International prospective study of *Klebsiella pneumoniae* bacteremia: implications of extended-spectrum beta-lactamase production in nosocomial infections. Ann Intern Med. 2004;140:26–32.
26. Zarkotou O, Pournaras S, Tselioti P, Dragoumanos V, Pitiriga V, Ranellou K, et al. Predictors of mortality in patients with bloodstream infections caused by KPC-producing *Klebsiella pneumoniae* and impact of appropriate antimicrobial treatment. Clin Microbiol Infect. 2011;17:1798–803.
27. Qi Y, Wei Z, Ji S, Du X, Shen P, Yu Y. ST11, the dominant clone of KPC-producing *Klebsiella pneumoniae* in China. J Antimicrob Chemother. 2011;66:307–12.
28. MLST databases. Pasteur Institute, Paris. 2017. http://bigsdb.pasteur.fr/perl/bigsdb/bigsdb.pl?db=pubmlst_klebsiella_isolates_public. Accessed 13 May 2017.
29. Xu A, Zheng B, Xu YC, Huang ZG, Zhong NS, Zhuo C. National epidemiology of carbapenem-resistant and extensively drug-resistant gram-negative bacteria isolated from blood samples in China in 2013. Clin Microbiol Infect. 2016;22(Suppl 1):S1–8.
30. Mathers AJ, Peirano G, Pitout JD. The role of epidemic resistance plasmids and international high-risk clones in the spread of multidrug-resistant *Enterobacteriaceae*. Clin Microbiol Rev. 2015;28:565–91.
31. Zhang Y, Zhao C, Wang Q, Wang X, Chen H, Li H, et al. High prevalence of hypervirulent *Klebsiella pneumoniae* infection in China: geographic distribution, clinical characteristics and antimicrobial resistance. Antimicrob Agents Chemother. 2016;60:6115–20.
32. Zhang Y, Zeng J, Liu W, Zhao F, Hu Z, Zhao C, et al. Emergence of a hypervirulent carbapenem-resistant *Klebsiella pneumoniae* isolate from clinical infections in China. J Inf Secur. 2015;71:553–60.
33. Catalan-Najera JC, Garza-Ramos U, Barrios-Camacho H. Hypervirulence and hypermucoviscosity: two different but complementary *Klebsiella* spp. phenotypes? Virulence. 2017;8:1111–23.

26

Impact of inappropriate antifungal therapy according to current susceptibility breakpoints on Candida bloodstream infection mortality

María Fernanda González-Lara[1], Pedro Torres-González[1], Patricia Cornejo-Juárez[2], Consuelo Velázquez-Acosta[2], Areli Martinez-Gamboa[1], Andrea Rangel-Cordero[1], Miriam Bobadilla-del-Valle[1], Luis Ostrosky-Zeichner[3], Alfredo Ponce-de-León[1] and José Sifuentes-Osornio[4*]

Abstract

Background: The mortality of Candida Bloodstream Infection (CBSI) remains high. Antifungal susceptibility breakpoints were recently updated for *Candida* species, the impact remains unknown. In this study we evaluated the impact of inappropriate antifungal treatment according to recent breakpoints on 30-day mortality of CBSI.

Methods: From June 2008 to July 2014, data on CBSI episodes from two tertiary-care centers, treated > 72 h were analyzed. Antifungal therapy and 30-day mortality were registered. Inappropriate antifungal treatment according to current Clinical & Laboratory Standards Institute (CLSI) breakpoints was adjusted with 30-day mortality-related co-variates.

Results: One hundred forty-nine episodes of CBSI were analyzed. The most frequent species were: *C. albicans* (40%), *C. tropicalis* (23%) and *C. glabrata* complex (20%). According to the 2012 CLSI, 10.7% received inappropriate treatment. The 30-day mortality was 38%; severe sepsis [Odds ratio (OR) 3.4; 95% CI 1.3–8.4], cirrhosis (OR 36; 95% CI 12.2–605), early central venous catheter removal (OR 0.23; 95% CI 0.08–0.66) and previous antifungal therapy (OR 0.15; 95%CI 0.03–0.62), were associated with 30-day mortality by multivariate analysis. Inappropriate antifungal treatment was not (OR 0.19; 95% CI 0.03–1.2).

Conclusions: Appropriate antifungal therapy according to CLSI 2012 did not have an impact on mortality. Mortality of CBSI remains high due to disease severity and comorbidities; early antifungal therapy and catheter removal may reduce it.

Keywords: Antifungal susceptibility testing, Candida bloodstream infections, Fluconazole resistance, Candidemia treatment

Background

Candida bloodstream infections (CBSI) represent 10% of all bloodstream infections. The CBSI incidence in North America reaches 0.3–0.9 cases per 1000 admissions, whereas in Latin America it may reach 5.3 cases per 1000 admissions [1–4]. The mortality rate of CBSI remains high (46%–75%) despite the availability of effective antifungal therapy [1]. Inappropriate antifungal therapy has been reported as a risk factor for increased mortality [5]. However, routine clinical care in many sites is not guided by antifungal susceptibility testing (AST) but selected according to the species-specific known susceptibility and the patient's clinical condition.

The Clinical and Laboratory Standards Institute (CLSI) recently defined new clinical breakpoints (CBP) for the most common *Candida* species to categorize them into resistant, intermediate and susceptible and guide antifungal therapy, these breakpoints are now drug and species specific [6]. The rationale for these modifications was the relationship between a higher minimal inhibitory concentration (MIC) and worse outcome showed in some studies, epidemiologic cutoffs values, and pharmacokinetic/pharmacodynamic studies [7]. However, the

* Correspondence: sifuentesosornio@gmail.com
[4]Department of Medicine, Instituto Nacional de Ciencias Médicas y Nutrición Salvador Zubirán, Vasco de Quiroga 15, Belisario Domínguez Sección XVI, Tlalpan, Zip Code 14080 Mexico City, Mexico
Full list of author information is available at the end of the article

impact of these modifications on mortality remains to be defined. Broth microdilution (BMD) is the reference method for *Candida* species AST; unfortunately, it is labor intensive, expensive, requires trained personnel, and is subjected to reading bias. Nowadays, antifungal susceptibility testing by automatized systems is considered reliable and may be more easily incorporated into routine clinical care [8–10].

The objective of this study was to assess the impact that the modified antifungal susceptibility breakpoints might have had on 30-day mortality of CBSI.

Methods

Study design. A retrospective laboratory-based survey was performed; patients admitted to two referral tertiary centers in Mexico City from June 2008 to July 2014 with a positive blood culture for *Candida* spp., 30-day survival was retrieved. Socio-demographic and clinical variables were recorded in a specially designed case report form. One hundred and forty-nine samples from 149 patients who received antifungal treatment ≥ 72 h were considered for this analysis. During the study period, AST was not routinely available in the study's centers, the selection of antifungal treatment was decided by the attending physician according to the patient's clinical condition and the *Candida* species isolated. For this analysis, AST was performed post hoc from the available stored isolates. Our main objective was to identify whether inappropriate antifungal therapy, considering the updated susceptibility breakpoints, was associated with an increased 30-day mortality. A secondary objective was to describe the prevalence of antifungal resistance during the study period.

Definitions

Empirical therapy was defined as the initiation of an antifungal agent at the first clinical suspicion of fungal infection [11]. Initial antifungal therapy was defined as modification of the empirical antifungal therapy or initiation of any antifungal drug after a positive blood culture with yeasts on a Gram stain, before species identification; whereas definitive treatment was the antifungal administered after species identification. Severe sepsis was defined as the presence of sepsis with any of the following: sepsis-induced hypotension, hyperlactatemia, urine output < 5 ml/Kg/h for more than 2 h following fluid resuscitation, acute lung injury with $PaO_2/FIO_2 < 250$ or < 200 in the absence and presence of pneumonia, creatinine > 2 mg/dL, bilirubin > 2 mg/dL, platelet count < 100,000 cell/mm^3 or coagulopathy [12].

Antifungal therapy was considered appropriate if the patient received an antifungal agent for which, the *Candida* isolate was susceptible according to CLSI 2012 breakpoints and inappropriate if the MIC of the isolate was in non-susceptible range [6, 13].

Laboratory procedures

All the *Candida* spp. isolates recovered from blood cultures during the study period were sent to a central laboratory for identification and AST. The isolates were cultured on Sabouraud media, underwent germ tube testing and were identified using the Vitek 2, (BioMeriéux, Lyon, France). A sample from each culture was stored as water suspension at −80 °C, until retrieved for susceptibility testing. A small aliquote was unfrozen at room temperature for 24 h, and cultured on Sabouraud agar at 30 °C for 24 h to ensure viability. AST was performed on 178 available isolates of which 149 received antifungal treatment and were included for analysis. AST was performed with Vitek 2 using the AST-YS07 card (Biomérieux, Lyon, France) and interpreted according to CLSI guidelines in document M27A3 and its updated version in M27-S4. For those isolates without a species specific clinical breakpoint, epidemiologic cutoff values were used (*C. guilliermondii, C. pelliculosa and Clavispora lusitaniae*). For species without a reported epidemiological cut off value, AST was classified according to the Vitek-2 software (Global CLSI-based + Natural Resistance) (V. 07.01) [14–16].

The reference strains *C. parapsilosis* ATCC 22019 and *C. krusei* ATCC 6258 were used as controls. Species identified as *C. parapsilosis* complex and *C. glabrata* complex refer to *C. parapsilosis* complex and *C. glabrata* complex, since phenotypic testing cannot differentiate the cryptic species within the complexes. Isolates were considered susceptible to echinocandins if the micafungin MIC was within the susceptible ranges, since anidulafungin is not available for YS07 card, and the known variability in the caspofungin MIC with Vitek2 [17, 18]. Assays to identify antifungal resistance mechanisms were not done.

Statistical analysis

Categorical data was summarized using frequency tables, and the χ^2 test was used for comparison between groups. Characteristics of patients were compared using Mann-Whitney U test for continuous variables. To evaluate 30-day mortality in multivariate analysis, we built a multiple logistic regression model including inappropriate antifungal treatment as well as variables with a *p*-value < 0.2 in univariate analysis or biological plausibility. Stratification for severe sepsis is provided in a separate analysis. Odds ratio (OR) with 95% confidence interval (CI) was reported. A *p*-value < 0.05 was considered significant for all the analysis. Stata 11.0 (Stata Corp College Station, TX) software was used for analysis.

Ethics statement

The study was reviewed and approved by the Scientific and Bioethics Committee at the Instituto Nacional de Cancerología (reference number INCAN/005/10) and the Research and Bioethics Committee at the Instituto Nacional de Ciencias Médicas y Nutrición "Salvador Zubirán" (reference number 1912). Because of the observational nature of the study, a waiver of informed consent was granted. Authors involved in data analysis could not identify individual patients since the database used numbers specific to the study.

- Availability of data and materials. The datasets used and/or analyzed during the current study are available from the corresponding author on reasonable request.

Results

During the 72 months of the study period, 83,942 blood cultures were collected in both institutions; 16.2% (13,637) yielded a positive result, and 1.7% (227) corresponded to episodes of CBSI. One hundred and seventy-eight isolates (78.4%) were available for AST at the end of the study period. Of these, 84% (149/178) were episodes treated for ≥ 72 h and were included for analysis (Fig. 1).

At the time of CBSI diagnosis, 25% (37/149) of the patients were admitted to intensive care unit (ICU), and 75% (112/149) were admitted to medical or surgical wards. Thirty percent (45/149) had diagnosis of hematologic malignancy and 17.4% (26/149) other forms of cancer. APACHE II score, to assess mortality and disease severity was available for 122 episodes with a median score of 18.9 (IQR 14–24).

The possible source of the CBSI was identified in 49% (73/149) of the episodes, 30.8% (46/149) had an intra-abdominal infection, 7.3% (11/149) catheter-relatedinfection, and 10.7% (16/149) had both. Ten percent (16/149) were diagnosed with additional forms of candidiasis (n: 5 hepatosplenic candidiasis, n: 4 skin involvement, n: 3 endocarditis, n: 2 ophthalmic candidiasis, n: 2 osteomyelitis). Forty-four percent developed severe sepsis, and 22% (34/149) had neutropenia at CBSI diagnosis of which, 17.6%% (6/34) received primary antifungal prophylaxis. Eighty-two percent (123/149) had a central venous catheter in place at the time of CBSI diagnosis. Early central venous catheter (CVC) removal (< 72 h) was achieved in 59% (73/123) of the episodes (Table 1).

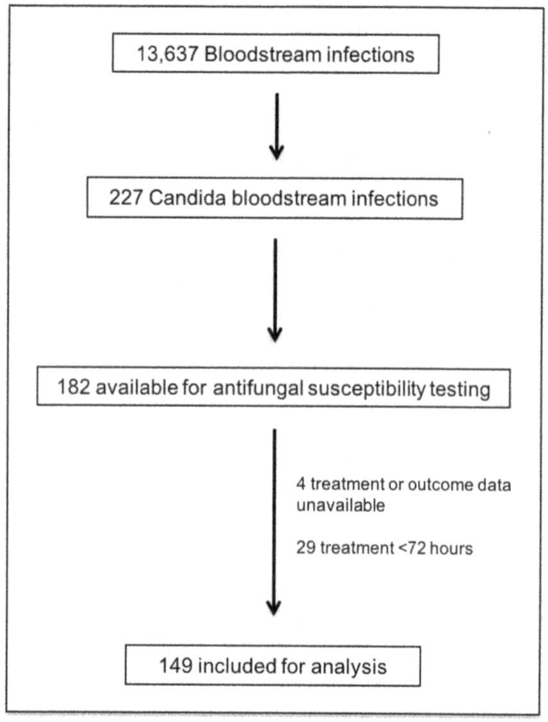

Fig. 1 Flowchart of patients during the study period

Candida species distribution and antifungal susceptibility

Blood cultures yielded a positive result for *Candida* spp. in a median of 2 days (IQR 1–3) after drawn. The most frequent isolated species were: *C. albicans* (n: 60, 40%), *C. tropicalis* (n: 34, 23%), *C. glabrata* complex (n: 30, 20%), *C. parapsilosis* complex (n: 15, 10%) and *C. guilliermondi* (n: 3, 2%). Other less frequent were: *C. krusei* (n: 2, 1.3%), *C. norvegensis* (n: 1, 0.6%), *C. inconspicua* (n: 1, 0.6%), *C. lusitaniae* (n:1, 0.6%) *C. lipolytica* (n: 1, 0.6%) and *C. pelliculosa* (n: 1, 0.6%).

According to the 2012 CLSI susceptibility breakpoints, 70% (104/149) of the isolates were susceptible to fluconazole, 95.3% (142/149) to caspofungin and, 97.3% (145/149) isolates to micafungin; and 98.6% (147/149) were susceptible to AmB (Table 2).

Overall fluconazole resistance was 6% (2 *C. albicans*, 2 *C. glabrata* complex, 2 *C. kruzei*, 1 *C. parapsilosis* complex, 1 *C. tropicalis* and 1 *C. pelliculosa*). Overall echinocandin resistance was 1.3% (1 *C. albicans* and 1 *C. glabrata*).

A single echinocandin-resistant *C. glabrata* was identified, which also was intermediate to fluconazole. One isolate of *C. albicans* showed resistance to every antifungal class (azoles, echinocandins and amphotericin B), from a patient who subsequently developed *C. glabrata* BSI secondary to a diabetic foot osteomyelitis in a 42-year-old male patient who died after 22 days of treatment with caspofungin.

Antifungal treatment

Thirty-five of 149 patients (23%) were receiving antifungal therapy at the time the CBSI was identified, in 23/35 (66%) cases the indication was empiric therapy for suspected invasive fungal infection, 15/35 (42.8%) cases were receiving antifungal therapy for another demonstrated

Table 1 Thirty-day mortality in Candida bloodstream infection. Univariate analysis

	Total, $n = 149$	30-d Survivors, $n = 93$	30-d Non-survivors $n = 56$	*p*-value
Demographics				
Female	78 (52.3)	50 (53.7)	28 (50)	0.65
Age, median (IQR)	47 (32–58)	44 (30–55)	48 (35.5–61.5)	0.23
Intensive care unit admission	37 (24.8)	15 (16.1)	22 (39.2)	< 0.001
APACHE II $n = 122$, median (IQR)	18 (14–24)	16 (12–20)	23 (18.5–28.5)	< 0.001
Severe sepsis	66 (44.3)	29 (31.1)	37 (66)	< 0.001
Comorbidities				
Hematologic neoplasia	45 (30.2)	22 (23.6)	23 (41)	0.025
Solid neoplasia	26 (17.4)	17 (18.2)	9 (16)	0.73
Cardiovascular	37 (24.8)	22 (23.6)	15 (26.7)	0.7
Chronic kidney disease	18 (12)	10 (10.7)	8 (14.2)	0.52
Cirrhosis	11 (7.3)	1 (1)	10 (17.8)	< 0.001
Diabetes mellitus	19 (12.7)	12 (12.9)	7 (12.5)	0.94
Intra-abdominal infection	62 (41.6)	45 (48.3)	17 (30.3)	0.031
Neutropenia	34 (22.8)	16 (17.2)	18 (32.1)	0.035
Cancer CT	38 (25.5)	18 (19.3)	20 (35.7)	0.026
CA-BSI	27 (18.1)	22 (23.6)	5 (8.9)	0.024
CVC	123 (82.5)	80 (86)	43 (76.7)	0.15
Early CVC removal	73 /123 (59.3)	55/80 (68.7)	18 /43 (41.8)	0.004
Total parenteral nutrition	49 (32.8)	36 (38.7)	13 (23.2)	0.034
Empiric antifungal therapy	35 (23.8)	27 (29.6)	8 (14.3)	0.033
Steroid use	40 (26.8)	20 (21.5)	20 (35.7)	0.08
Time to antifungal therapy median (IQR)	2 (1–3)	2 (1–2)	2 (1–3)	0.165
Initial treatment				
Echinocandin	64 (42.9)	42 (45.1)	22 (39.1)	0.48
Caspofungin	43 (28.8)	27 (29)	16 (28.5)	0.89
Anidulafungin	21 (14.1)	15 (16.1)	6 (11.3)	0.4
AmB-d	61 (40.9)	35 (37.6)	26 (46.4)	0.29
Azoles	25 (16.7)	16 (17.2)	9 (16)	0.85
Fluconazole	24 (16.1)	15 (16.1)	9 (16)	0.95
Voriconazole	1 (0.6)	1 (1)	–	–
Definitive treatment				
Echinocandin	56 (37.5)	36 (38.7)	20 (35.7)	0.71
Caspofungin	31 (20.8)	17 (18.2)	14 (25)	0.34
Anidulafungin	25 (16.7)	19 (20.4)	6 (10.7)	0.23
AmB-d	46 (30.8)	21 (22.5)	25 (44.6)	0.005
Azoles	47 (31.5)	36 (38.7)	11 (19.6)	0.015
Fluconazole	41 (27.5)	31 (33.3)	10 (17.8)	0.4
Voriconazole	6 (4)	5 (5.3)	1 (1.8)	0.27
Inappropriate initial antifungal treatment	13 (8.7)	9 (9.6)	4 (7.1)	0.59
Inappropriate definitive antifungal treatment	8 (5.3)	6 (6.4)	2 (3.5)	0.36
Inappropriate initial and/or definitive treatment	16 (10.7)	11 (11.8)	5 (8.9)	0.58
Non-albicans CBSI	89 (59.7)	62 (66.6)	27 (48.2)	0.026
C. tropicalis	35 (24)	19 (20)	16 (29)	0.25

Table 1 Thirty-day mortality in Candida bloodstream infection. Univariate analysis *(Continued)*

	Total, $n = 149$	30-d Survivors, $n = 93$	30-d Non-survivors $n = 56$	p-value
C. glabrata	28 (19)	19 (20.4)	9 (16)	0.5
C. parapsilosis	16 (10.7)	15 (16)	1 (1.8)	0.006

IQR interquartile range, *APACHE* acute physiology and chronic health evaluation, *CT* chemotherapy, *CA-BSI* catheter associated blood stream infection, *CVC* central venous catheter, *AmB-d* amphotericin B-deoxycholate, *CBSI* candida blood stream infection

Table 2 Antifungal susceptibility of 149 isolates and categorical agreement between CLSI 2008 and 2012

Species/ antifungal (n)	MIC range (mg/L)	MIC $_{50}$ (mg/L)	MIC $_{90}$ (mg/L)	CLSI 2008 n (%)			CLSI 2012 n (%)		
				S	I	R	S	SDD[a]/I	R
C. albicans (60)									
Fluconazole	≤ 1–8	1	1	60 (100)	–	–	56 (93.3)	2 (3.3)	2 (3.3)
Voriconazole	≤ 0.12	0.12	0.12	60 (100)	–	–	60 (100)	–	–
Caspofungin	≤ 0.25–1	0.25	0.25	60 (100)	–	–	56 (93.3)	1 (1.6)	3 (5)
Micafungin	≤ 0.06–1	0.06	0.06	60 (100)	–	–	58 (96.6)	1 (1.6)	1 (1.6)
C. tropicalis (34)									
Fluconazole	≤ 1–8	1	1	34 (100)	–	–	32 (94.1)	1 (2.9)	1 (2.9)
Voriconazole	≤ 0.12	0.12	0.12	34 (100)	–	–	34 (100)	–	–
Caspofungin	≤ 0.25–1	0.25	0.25	34 (100)	–	–	34 (100)	–	–
Micafungin	≤ 0.06–0.5	0.06	0.06	34 (100)	–	–	34 (100)	–	–
C. glabrata (30)									
Fluconazole	≤ 1–64	4	8	28 (93.3)	–	2 (6.6)	0	28 (93.3)	2 (6.6)
Caspofungin	< 0.25–1	0.25	0.25	30 (100)	–	–	29 (96.6)	–	1 (3.3)
Micafungin	< 0.06–0.5	0.06	0.06	30 (100)	–	–	29 (96.6)	–	1 (3.3)
C. parapsilosis (15)									
Fluconazole	≤ 1–8	1	8	15 (100)	–	–	13 (86.6)	1 (6.6)	1 (6.6)
Voriconazole	≤ 0.12–0.25	0.12	0.12	15 (100)	–	–	15 (100)	–	–
Caspofungin	< 0.25–1	1	1	15 (100)			15 (100)	–	–
Micafungin	< 0.06–1	0.5	1	15 (100)			15 (100)	–	–
C. guilliermondi (3)									
Fluconazole	2–8	2	8	3 (100)			–	–	–
Voriconazole	< 0.12	< 0.12	< 0.12	3 (100)			–	–	–
Caspofungin	0.25–1	0.25	1	3 (100)			–	–	–
Micafungin	0.5	0.5	0.5	3 (100)			–	–	–
C. kruzei (2)									
Voriconazole	≤ 0.12	0.12	0.12	2 (100)			2 (100)	–	–
Caspofungin	≤ 0.25–0.5	0.25	0.5	2 (100)			1	1	–
Micafungin	0.12	0.12	0.12	2 (100)			2	–	–
Other[b] (5)									
Fluconazole	≤ 1–16	2	16	3 (60)	2 (40)		–	–	–
Voriconazole	≤ 0.12	0.12	0.12	5 (100)	–	–	–	–	–
Caspofungin	≤ 0.25- > 4	0.25	4	4 (80)	–	–	–	–	–
Micafungin	< 0.06- > 4	0.12	4	4 (80)	–	–	–	–	–

MIC minimal inhibitory concentration, *S* susceptible, *I* intermediate, *R* resistant, *SDD* susceptible dose dependent, *CLSI* Clinical Laboratory Standards Institute
[a]SDD applies for fluconazole and voriconazole instead of intermediate
[b]Other species: *C. lusitaniae, C. pelliculosa, C. norvegensis, C. lypolitica, C. inconspicua*

fungal infection; 18/35 (51.4%) patients received azoles (2 voriconazole and 16 fluconazole), 9/35 (25.7%) received AmB-d and 9/35 (25.7%) received echinocandins (3 caspofungin and 6 anidulafungin). In 7/35 (20%) cases, the CBSI agent was non-susceptible to empiric therapy.

Antifungal was initiated or modified within a median of two days (IQR 1–3) after the blood culture was drawn. Echinocandins were the most frequent initial treatment (42.9%), followed by amphotericin B-deoxycholate (AmB-d) (40.2%), and fluconazole (16.1%). One patient received combination therapy with AmB-d and fluconazole, and one received voriconazole. The initial antifungal agent was modified in 37% (55/149) of the episodes. Among these 47.3% (26/55) were switched to fluconazole after species identification. Twenty-three percent (13/55) were switched to other antifungal due lack of a clinical response; 12.7% (7/55) due to a nonsusceptible isolate (according to the known species-specific susceptibility); 5.4% (3/55) due to toxicity and 5.4% (3/55) due to proven or probable invasive aspergillosis; 3.6% (2/55) to treat other molds and 3.6% (2/55) due to unspecified reasons. Definitive antifungal treatment of 149 episodes was administered with echinocandins (37.5%), AmB-d (30.2%), and fluconazole (31.5%). One patient received a combination of AmB-d and fluconazole. Among the 89 non-albicans CBSI episodes, 41 (46%) received echinocandins as definitive treatment, 29 (32%) AmB-d, and 19 (21.3%) azoles. The median time of antifungal therapy was 14 days (IQR 5–20).

Regarding the CLSI 2012 breakpoints, 8.7% (13/149) patients received inappropriate initial antifungal treatment, four of which died: one patient received 12 days of fluconazole (6 mg/Kg) for a non-susceptible fluconazole *C. albicans* isolate, was switched later to caspofungin due lack of clinical response and died a day after. Two patients received fluconazole for susceptible dose-dependent (SDD) *C. glabrata;* one died five days after CBSI diagnosis, the other was switched to caspofungin on the sixth day and died. The remainder patient had a CBSI due to a fluconazole-resistant *C. albicans* isolate, the patient was started on fluconazole, was switched to caspofungin twelve days later and died 26 days after the CBSI diagnosis. Inappropriate definitive antifungal treatment was administered in 5.3% (8/149) of the episodes (5 *C. glabrata,* 2 *C. albicans,* and 1 *C. tropicalis*), two of which died: one patient received eight days of AmB-d, was switched to fluconazole for a fluconazole –SDD *C. glabrata* and died 22 days after diagnosis.

No patient received inappropriate initial or definitive treatment according to 2008 guidelines (Table 1).

Outcome

Thirty-day mortality was 38% (56/149); non-survivors more often presented with severe sepsis and required mechanical ventilation. Non-survivors were also more likely to have hematologic neoplasia, cirrhosis, severe neutropenia and to receive definitive treatment with AmB-d. Survivors were more likely to have an intraabdominal infection, an early central-venous catheter removal, have received empirical antifungal therapy, to receive definitive treatment with azoles and to have a Non-albicans CBSI (Table 1). In multivariate analysis, severe sepsis (OR 3.4; 95% CI 1.3–8.4) and previous diagnosis of cirrhosis (OR 36 95% CI 12.2–605) were independently associated with increased 30-day mortality. Early CVC withdrawal (OR 0.23; 95% CI 0.08–0.66) and empirical antifungal therapy (OR 0.15; 95% CI 0.03–0.62) were independently associated with reduced 30-day mortality. When stratified by severe sepsis, survivors were more likely to receive empirical antifungal therapy (OR 0.05; 95% CI 0.005–0.55) and early CVC removal (OR 0.07; 95% CI 0.017–0.28) among patients without severe sepsis. Of note neither empirical antifungal therapy nor early CVC removal were associated with reduced mortality in patients with severe sepsis. Inappropriate initial or/and definitive antifungal treatment was not associated with 30-day mortality (OR 0.19; 95% CI 0.03–1.2), not even after stratification for severe sepsis (Table 3).

Persistent candidemia occurred in 21% (34/149). Inappropriate treatment was not associated with increased frequency of persistent candidemia ($p = 0.7$).

Discussion

In this observational study, we did not find an association between inappropriate antifungal therapy defined by the updated CLSI clinical breakpoints and increased mortality. Of note, severe sepsis, and cirrhosis were independently associated with increased mortality. On the contrary, modifiable factors such as empirical antifungal therapy and early CVC removal, were independently associated with decreased 30-day mortality.

The rationale of the CLSI 2012 updates was to identify the emergence of acquired mechanisms of resistance promptly. Recently IDSA treatment guidelines have advocated the testing for azoles to all bloodstream and other relevant isolates for testing, as well as echinocandin testing for those cases with previous exposure and species with known emerging resistance to these drugs, when previous expert recommendations suggested AST only when a patient was not improving [15, 19–21]. However, it is not clear if AST for CBSI should be routinely performed and the impact of routine AST for CBSI on mortality is not clear [22, 23].

In a similar study, in which AST by automatized systems (Sensititre YeastOne) was interpreted according to previous CBP, appropriate early treatment was not associated with survival in multivariate analysis. However, in a subgroup analysis excluding patients who received < 24 h of appropriate antifungal therapy, the authors

Table 3 Thirty-day mortality in Candida bloodstream infection. Multivariate analysis

Characteristic	OR (95%CI)	OR (95%CI) without severe sepsis
Age	1.01 (0.98–1.03)	1.02 (0.99–1.05)
Inappropriate antifungal treatment [a]	0.16 (0.02–1.3)	0.1 (0.009–1.05)
Severe sepsis	3.5 (1.4–8.9)	–
Cirrhosis	42.1 (2.3–744)	56 (0.06–47,908)
Early CVC withdrawal	0.22 (0.07–0.63)	0.07 (0.017–0.28)
Empirical antifungal therapy	0.15 (0.03–0.62)	0.05 (0.005–0.55)

OR Odds ratio; 95% CI: 95% confidence interval
[a]According to CLSI 2012, *CT* Chemotherapy, *CVC* central venous catheter

found a statistically significant association between survival and appropriate-early treatment [24]. No other study has reported the impact of updated breakpoints on clinical outcome. In this study, we excluded patients with less than 72 h of antifungal treatment and did not find improved survival among those patients who received appropriate antifungal therapy. However, our definition of appropriateness did not include the dosage of antifungals; this issue becomes more critical while evaluating azoles, which require weight-adjusted loading dose. Contrary to what was expected, the azole therapy showed a tendency to increased survival by univariate analysis, whereas the opposite was observed for AmB-d. This may be explained by the fact that a larger proportion of critical patients received fungicidal treatment rather than fluconazole.

After stratifying for severe sepsis, we identified variables associated with 30-day mortality for CBSI: Cirrhosis, a risk factor for infection and increased mortality due to the multifactorial immune dysfunction occurring in these patients [25–28]. and the removal of a CVC. While several retrospective analysis show increased survival and reduced duration of the CBSI when removing the CVC [29–31]. other studies have not supported these findings [32]. No trial has randomized catheter withdrawal, but a recent patient level quantitative review of 1915 patients from 7 randomized trials confirmed that CVC removal at any time during treatment was associated with a reduced 30-day mortality, clinical and microbiological succes. In our study, this finding remained significant in both, the *C. albicans* and the non-albicans *Candida* subgroups, as well as in the lowest APACHE II score quartiles [33]. Furthermore, empirical antifungal therapy was independently associated with reduced 30-day mortality. It has been previously demonstrated that mortality increases wih each subsequent day that empirical therapy is delayed [34, 35].

We found an important proportion of CBSI caused by non-albicans species, the increasing prevalence of non-albicans CBSI has been previously reported worldwide. [3, 36] The increasing rate of isolation of *C. glabrata* in Brazil and Latin America may be related to older age, geographic factors, and underlying comorbidities such as cancer, particularly in cases not related to selective pressure with fluconazole or areas with low fluconazole resistance rates; *C. parapsilosis* is related to indwelling catheters and chronic conditions and *C. tropicalis* usually occurs among patients with hematological malignancies, neutropenia and mucositis; all of which are risk factors frequently found in tertiary care centers, as in this study [1].

In this study, most *C. albicans* isolates remained susceptible to fluconazole and to echinocandins when tested through the automatized system Vitek2. These results agree with a recent report from the SENTRY study using the updated CBPs by BMD [37], and within the range reported by other studies [38–40]. Resistance to fluconazole or echinocandins among *C. glabrata* was an infrequent event, as compared to others [41].

This study has several limitations: This was an observational study thus, there was probable bias in the selection of antifungals by the attending physicians according to disease severity, hindering to predict mortality; the antifungal doses were not systematically registered, which is a sensitive issue regarding azoles; we were unable to retrieve all *Candida* isolates for performing AST, which was achieved using Vitek 2, instead of the standard of reference broth microdilution (BMD). However, AST by automatized systems is FDA approved and considered to be comparable to BMD, with the benefit of being a standardized, reproducible, easier to perform and less expensive method [8–10, 42].

Conclusion

Inappropriate antifungal treatment according with the current clinical breakpoints was not associated with mortality in this retrospective analysis. Mortality in CBSI remains high due to disease severity and comorbidities such as cirrhosis at the time of diagnosis. In addition, we identified some modifiable factors as early antifungal therapy and catheter removal which may improve the outcome of these patients. Consequently, prospective studies are needed.

Acknowledgements
Not applicable.

Funding
The study was supported by internal funding.

Authors' contributions
MFGL contributed to data acquisition, analysis and interpretation and drafting of the article. PTG contributed to conception and design, analysis and interpretation of data, drafting of the article and critical revision for important intellectual content. PCJ contributed to conception and design, analysis and interpretation of data and critical revision for important intellectual content. CVA contributed to data acquisition and critical revision for important intellectual content. AMG contributed to conception and design, analysis and interpretation of data and critical revision for important intellectual content. ARC contributed to data acquisition and critical revision for important intellectual content. MBDV contributed to conception and design, analysis and interpretation of data and critical revision for important intellectual content. LOZ contributed to conception and design, analysis and interpretation of data and critical revision for important intellectual content. APL contributed to conception and design, analysis and interpretation of data and critical revision for important intellectual content. JSO contributed to conception and design, analysis and interpretation of data and critical revision for important intellectual content. All authors read and approved the final manuscript.

Ethics approval and consent to participate
The study was reviewed and approved by the Research Ethics Committee (Comité de Ética en Investigación) at the Instituto Nacional de Ciencias Médicas y Nutrición "Salvador Zubirán" with the reference number 1912. The Scientific Committee and Bioethics Committee (Comité científico y comité de Bioética) at the Instituto Nacional de Cancerología reviewed and approved the study (Reference number INCAN/CC/005/10). Because of the observational nature of the study, a waiver of informed consent was granted.

Consent for publication
Not applicable

Competing interests
J. Sifuentes-Osornio has received research grants from Senosiain, Pfizer, Merck Sharp & Dhome, Sanofi Pasteur, AstraZeneca, and bioMérieux; personal fees from Pfizer, Merck Sharp& Dhome, and Sanofi Pasteur; and non-financial support from Pfizer,Merck Sharp & Dhome, Sanofi Pasteur, and bioMérieux. P. Torres-Gonzalez has received research grants from Pfizer and Sanofi Pasteur. A. Ponce-de-Leon has received research grants from Merck Sharp & Dhome and Pfizer; and is on the advisory board for Merck Sharp & Dhome, Pfizer, Janssen-Cilag, and Novartis. L. Ostrosky-Zeichner has received research funding and honoraria from Merck, Astellas, Pfizer, Cidara, T2 Biosystems, and Scynexis. The rest of the authors declare they have no competing interests.

Author details
[1]Department of Infectious Diseases, Instituto Nacional de Ciencias Médicas y Nutrición Salvador Zubirán, Vasco de Quiroga 15, Belisario Domínguez Sección XVI, Tlalpan, Zip Code 14080 Mexico City, Mexico. [2]Department of Infectious Diseases, Instituto Nacional de Cancerología, Ave. San Fernando 22, Belisario Dominguez Sección XVI, Zip code 14080 Mexico City, Mexico. [3]University of Texas Health Science Center at Houston, 6431 Fannin. MSB 2.112, Houston, TX 77030, USA. [4]Department of Medicine, Instituto Nacional de Ciencias Médicas y Nutrición Salvador Zubirán, Vasco de Quiroga 15, Belisario Domínguez Sección XVI, Tlalpan, Zip Code 14080 Mexico City, Mexico.

References

1. Pfaller MA, Diekema DJ. Epidemiology of invasive candidiasis: a persistent public health problem. Clin Microbiol Rev. 2007;20:1.
2. Colombo AL, Nucci M, Park BJ, Nouer SA, Arthington-Skaggs B, da Matta DA, et al. Epidemiology of candidemia in Brazil: a nationwide sentinel surveillance of candidemia in eleven medical centers. J Clin Microbiol. 2006;44:8.
3. Nucci M, Queiroz-Telles F, Alvarado-Matute T, Tiraboschi IN, Cortes J, Zurita J, et al. Epidemiology of candidemia in Latin America: a laboratory-based survey. PLoS One. 2013;8:3.
4. Sifuentes-Osornio J, Corzo-Leon DE, Ponce-de-Leon LA. Epidemiology of invasive fungal infections in Latin America. Curr Fungal Infect Rep. 2012;6:1.
5. Parkins MD, Sabuda DM, Elsayed S, Laupland KB. Adequacy of empirical antifungal therapy and effect on outcome among patients with invasive Candida species infections. J Antimicrob Chemother. 2007;60:3.
6. Shah DN, Yau R, Weston J, Lasco TM, Salazar M, Palmer HR, et al. Evaluation of antifungal therapy in patients with candidaemia based on susceptibility testing results: implications for antimicrobial stewardship programmes. J Antimicrob Chemother. 2011;66:9.
7. Fothergill AW, Sutton DA, McCarthy DI, Wiederhold NP. Impact of new antifungal breakpoints on antifungal resistance in Candida species. J Clinical Microbiol. 2014;52:3.
8. Pfaller MA, Diekema DJ, Procop GW, Rinaldi MG. Multicenter comparison of the VITEK 2 yeast susceptibility test with the CLSI broth microdilution reference method for testing fluconazole against Candida spp. J Clin Microbiol. 2007;45:3.
9. Peterson JF, Pfaller MA, Diekema DJ, Rinaldi MG, Riebe KM, Ledeboer NA. Multicenter comparison of the Vitek 2 antifungal susceptibility test with the CLSI broth microdilution reference method for testing caspofungin, micafungin, and posaconazole against Candida spp. J Clin Microbiol. 2011;49:5.
10. Pfaller MA, Diekema DJ, Procop GW, Rinaldi MG. Multicenter comparison of the VITEK 2 antifungal susceptibility test with the CLSI broth microdilution reference method for testing amphotericin B, flucytosine, and voriconazole against Candida spp. J Clin Microbiol. 2007;45:11.
11. Freifeld AG, Bow EJ, Sepkowitz KA, Boeckh MJ, Ito JI, Mullen CA, et al. Clinical practice guideline for the use of antimicrobial agents in neutropenic patients with cancer: 2010 update by the infectious diseases society of america. Clin Infect Dis. 2011;52:4.
12. Dellinger RP, Levy MM, Rhodes A, Annane D, Gerlach H, Opal SM, et al. Surviving sepsis campaign: international guidelines for management of severe sepsis and septic shock: 2012. Crit Care Med. 2013;41:2.
13. DePestel DD, Eiland EH, 3rd, Lusardi K, Destache CJ, Mercier RC, McDaneld PM, et al. Assessing appropriateness of antimicrobial therapy: in the eye of the interpreter. Clin Infect Dis. 2014;59;Suppl 3:S154-61.
14. Pfaller MA, Diekema DJ. Progress in antifungal susceptibility testing of Candida spp. by use of clinical and laboratory standards institute broth microdilution methods, 2010 to 2012. J Clin Microbiol. 2012;50:9.
15. Pfaller MA, Andes D, Diekema DJ, Espinel-Ingroff A, Sheehan D. Testing CSfAS. Wild-type MIC distributions, epidemiological cutoff values and species-specific clinical breakpoints for fluconazole and Candida: time for harmonization of CLSI and EUCAST broth microdilution methods. Drug Resist Updat. 2010;13:6.
16. Espinel-Ingroff A, Alvarez-Fernandez M, Canton E, Carver PL, Chen SC, Eschenauer G, et al. Multicenter study of epidemiological cutoff values and detection of resistance in Candida spp. to anidulafungin, caspofungin, and micafungin using the Sensititre YeastOne colorimetric method. Antimicrob Agents Chemother. 2015;59:11.
17. Arendrup MC, Perlin DS. Echinocandin resistance: an emerging clinical problem? Curr Opin Infect Dis. 2014;27:6.
18. Astvad KM, Perlin DS, Johansen HK, Jensen RH, Arendrup MC. Evaluation of caspofungin susceptibility testing by the new Vitek 2 AST-YS06 yeast card using a unique collection of FKS wild-type and hot spot mutant isolates, including the five most common candida species. Antimicrob Agents Chemother. 2013;57:1.
19. Pfaller MA, Diekema DJ, Andes D, Arendrup MC, Brown SD, Lockhart SR, et al. Clinical breakpoints for the echinocandins and Candida revisited: integration of molecular, clinical, and microbiological data to arrive at species-specific interpretive criteria. Drug resistance updat. 2011;14:3.
20. Pappas PG, Kauffman CA, Andes DR, Clancy CJ, Marr KA, Ostrosky-Zeichner L, et al. Clinical practice guideline for the Management of Candidiasis: 2016 update by the Infectious Diseases Society of America. Clin Infect Dis. 2016;62:4.
21. Nachimuthu N, Ostrosky-Zeichner L. Antifungal susceptibility testing: evolution, indications, and role in clinical practice. Curr Treat Options Infect Dis. 2015;7:3.
22. Oxman DA, Chow JK, Frendl G, Hadley S, Hershkovitz S, Ireland P, et al.

Candidaemia associated with decreased in vitro fluconazole susceptibility: is Candida speciation predictive of the susceptibility pattern? J Antimicrob Chemother. 2010;65:7.
23. Ben-Ami R, Rahav G, Elinav H, Kassis I, Shalit I, Gottesman T, et al. Distribution of fluconazole-resistant Candida bloodstream isolates among hospitals and inpatient services in Israel. Clin Microbiol Infect. 2013;19:8.
24. Grim SA, Berger K, Teng C, Gupta S, Layden JE, Janda WM, et al. Timing of susceptibility-based antifungal drug administration in patients with Candida bloodstream infection: correlation with outcomes. J Antimicrob Chemother. 2012;67:3.
25. Chen SY, Tsai CL, Lin CH, Lee CC, Chiang WC, Wang JL, et al. Impact of liver cirrhosis on mortality in patients with community-acquired bacteremia. Diagn Microbiol Infect Dis. 2009;64:2.
26. Bartoletti M, Giannella M, Caraceni P, Domenicali M, Ambretti S, Tedeschi S, et al. Epidemiology and outcomes of bloodstream infection in patients with cirrhosis. J Hepatol. 2014;61:1.
27. Bonnel AR, Bunchorntavakul C, Reddy KR. Immune dysfunction and infections in patients with cirrhosis. Clin Gastroenterol Hepatol. 2011;9:9.
28. Bellot P, Frances R, Such J. Pathological bacterial translocation in cirrhosis: pathophysiology, diagnosis and clinical implications. Liv Int. 2013;33:1.
29. Uzun O, Ascioglu S, Anaissie EJ, Rex JH. Risk factors and predictors of outcome in patients with cancer and breakthrough candidemia. Clin Infect Dis. 2001;32:12.
30. Anaissie EJ, Rex JH, Uzun O, Vartivarian S. Predictors of adverse outcome in cancer patients with candidemia. Am J Med. 1998;104:3.
31. Rex JH, Bennett JE, Sugar AM, Pappas PG, Serody J, Edwards JE, et al. Intravascular catheter exchange and duration of candidemia. NIAID Mycoses Study Group and the Candidemia Study Group. Clin Infect Dis. 1995;21:4.
32. Nucci M, Anaissie E, Betts RF, Dupont BF, Wu C, Buell DN, et al. Early removal of central venous catheter in patients with candidemia does not improve outcome: analysis of 842 patients from 2 randomized clinical trials. Clin Infect Dis. 2010;51:3.
33. Andes DR, Safdar N, Baddley JW, Playford G, Reboli AC, Rex JH, et al. Impact of treatment strategy on outcomes in patients with candidemia and other forms of invasive candidiasis: a patient-level quantitative review of randomized trials. Clin Infect Dis. 2012;54:8.
34. Garey KW, Rege M, Pai MP, Mingo DE, Suda KJ, Turpin RS, et al. Time to initiation of fluconazole therapy impacts mortality in patients with candidemia: a multi-institutional study. Clin Infect Dis. 2006;43:1.
35. Kollef M, Micek S, Hampton N, Doherty JA, Kumar A. Septic shock attributed to Candida infection: importance of empiric therapy and source control. Clin Infect Dis. 2012;54:12.
36. Pfaller MA, Diekema DJ, Gibbs DL, Newell VA, Ellis D, Tullio V, et al. Results from the ARTEMIS DISK global antifungal surveillance study, 1997 to 2007: a 10.5-year analysis of susceptibilities of Candida species to fluconazole and voriconazole as determined by CLSI standardized disk diffusion. J Clin Microbiol. 2010;48:4.
37. Pfaller MA, Messer SA, Woosley LN, Jones RN, Castanheira M. Echinocandin and triazole antifungal susceptibility profiles for clinical opportunistic yeast and mold isolates collected from 2010 to 2011: application of new CLSI clinical breakpoints and epidemiological cutoff values for characterization of geographic and temporal trends of antifungal resistance. J Clin Microbiol. 2013;51:8.
38. Marcos-Zambrano LJ, Escribano P, Sanchez C, Munoz P, Bouza E, Guinea J. Antifungal resistance to fluconazole and echinocandins is not emerging in yeast isolates causing fungemia in a Spanish tertiary care center. Antimicrob Agents Chemother. 2014;58:8.
39. Won EJ, Shin JH, Choi MJ, Lee WG, Park YJ, Uh Y, et al. Antifungal susceptibilities of bloodstream isolates of Candida species from nine hospitals in Korea: application of new antifungal breakpoints and relationship to antifungal usage. PLoS One. 2015;10:2.
40. Posteraro B, Spanu T, Fiori B, De Maio F, De Carolis E, Giaquinto A, et al. Antifungal susceptibility profiles of bloodstream yeast isolates by Sensititre YeastOne over nine years at a large Italian teaching hospital. Antimicrob Agents Chemother. 2015;59:7.
41. Vallabhaneni S, Cleveland AA, Farley MM, Harrison LH, Schaffner W, Beldavs ZG, et al. Epidemiology and risk factors for Echinocandin nonsusceptible Candida Glabrata bloodstream infections: data from a large multisite population-based Candidemia surveillance program, 2008-2014. Open Forum Infect Dis. 2015;2:4.
42. Pfaller MA, Diekema DJ, Procop GW, Wiederhold NP. Multicenter evaluation of the new Vitek 2 yeast susceptibility test using new CLSI clinical breakpoints for fluconazole. J Clin Microbiol. 2014;52:6.

27

Bacterial bloodstream infections in a tertiary infectious diseases hospital in Northern Vietnam: aetiology, drug resistance, and treatment outcome

Vu Quoc Dat[1,2,3*], Hieu Ngoc Vu[1], Hung Nguyen The[1], Hoa Thi Nguyen[1], Long Bao Hoang[3], Dung Vu Tien Viet[3], Chi Linh Bui[1], Kinh Van Nguyen[2], Trung Vu Nguyen[1,2], Dao Tuyet Trinh[2], Alessandro Torre[3], H. Rogier van Doorn[3,4], Behzad Nadjm[3,4] and Heiman F.L. Wertheim[3,4,5]

Abstract

Background: Bloodstream infections (BSIs) are associated with high morbidity and mortality worldwide. However their aetiology, antimicrobial susceptibilities and associated outcomes differ between developed and developing countries. Systematic data from Vietnam are scarce. Here we present aetiologic data on BSI in adults admitted to a large tertiary referral hospital for infectious diseases in Hanoi, Vietnam.

Methods: A retrospective study was conducted at the National Hospital for Tropical Diseases between January 2011 and December 2013. Cases of BSI were determined from records in the microbiology department. Case records were obtained where possible and clinical findings, treatment and outcome were recorded. BSI were classified as community acquired if the blood sample was drawn ≤48 h after hospitalization or hospital acquired if >48 h.

Results: A total of 738 patients with BSI were included for microbiological analysis. The predominant pathogens were: *Klebsiella pneumoniae* (17.5%), *Escherichia coli* (17.3%), *Staphylococcus aureus* (14.9%), *Stenotrophomonas maltophilia* (9.6%) and *Streptococcus suis* (7.6%). The overall proportion of extended spectrum beta-lactamase (ESBL) production among *Enterobacteriaceae* was 25.1% (67/267 isolates) and of methicillin-resistance in *S. aureus* (MRSA) 37% (40/108). Clinical data was retrieved for 477 (64.6%) patients; median age was 48 years (IQR 36–60) with 27.7% female. The overall case fatality rate was 28.9% and the highest case fatality was associated with *Enterobacteriaceae* BSI (34.7%) which accounted for 61.6% of all BSI fatalities.

Conclusions: *Enterobacteriaceae* (predominantly *K. pneumoniae* and *E. coli*) are the most common cause of both community and hospital acquired bloodstream infections in a tertiary referral clinic in northern Vietnam.

Keywords: bacteremia, bloodstream infection, Vietnam, sepsis, drug resistance, bacterial, Gram-negative bacteria, *Streptococcus suis*, *Burkholderia pseudomallei*

* Correspondence: datvq@hmu.edu.vn; quocdat181@yahoo.com
[1]Department of Infectious Diseases, Hanoi Medical University, Hanoi, Vietnam
[2]National Hospital for Tropical Diseases, Hanoi, Vietnam
Full list of author information is available at the end of the article

Background

Bloodstream infections (BSIs) are an important cause of sepsis-related morbidity and mortality worldwide [1]. A systematic review of BSI burden in population based studies estimated the annual numbers of BSI episodes ranged from 575.462–677.389 in North America and 1,213,460–1,381,590 in Europe with the annual numbers of BSI associated deaths were 79,466–93,655 and 57,750–276,318 respectively [2]. In developed setting, the BSI and BSI associated septic shock still accounted for 6% and 3% of all admission to ICUs with the in-hospital mortality rates of 40% and 49% respectively [3]. Additionally, BSIs are associated with long-term risk of mortality among survivors [4]. In a population based study in Denmark, while the incidence of community and hospital acquired BSIs annually decreased 3.7% and 4.2% respectively between 1998 to 2008, the incidence rate of healthcare-associated bloodstream infection BSI remained unchanged [4]. Data from low and middle income countries (LMIC) on the causes of bloodstream infection are limited [5], but crucial for enabling clinicians to direct antimicrobial therapy appropriately and for the design of preventive measures. Useful lessons can be learned from analysing the bacterial aetiology of BSIs as most cases reflect severe illness and bacteria detected are usually directly responsible for disease [6, 7]. The causative agent will be affected by a number of factors, particularly the focus of infection, comorbidities like immunodeficiency, chronic renal and liver disease, in addition to socio-economic, climatic and other geographical factors [8]. The level of economic development can also impact aetiology distribution through changing exposure to environmental organisms associated with urbanisation, changing farming and food consumption practices, vaccination and comorbidities associated with increased wealth and improved life expectancy [9]. Consequently, data from tropical emerging economies are important to understanding and updating worldwide trends of the aetiology of severe bacterial disease in the tropics.

Vietnam is a low middle income country (LMIC), an emerging economy and a hotspot for emerging infectious diseases [10]. Levels of antibiotic resistance, an important cause of treatment failure and subsequent mortality are also high in Vietnam [11, 12]. In the Asian Network for Surveillance of Resistant Pathogens with 11 participating countries in 2001, Vietnam had a highest prevalence of pneumococcal multidrug resistance (defined as resistance to at least three classes of antibiotics) (71.4%) which much higher than the second and third highest countries and territories of Korea (54.8%) and Hong Kong (43.2%) [12]. In another study in 20 hospitals in 5 Asia-Pacific countries, the prevalence of carbapenem non-susceptible Gram-negative pathogens was highest at 35.0% in Vietnam, in which the prevalence of carbapenem non-susceptiblity among *Pseudomonas aeruginosa, Enterobacteriaceae* and *Acinetobacter baumannii* were 46.7%, 5.6% and 89.5% respectively [11].

In-hospital mortality among patients with sepsis is reduced by early initiation of adequate empiric antibiotic therapy [13, 14] and strategies to promote appropriate antibiotic use may help to prevent antimicrobial resistance and optimise use of hospital resources. However, the epidemiology of BSI in Vietnamese adults and associated treatment outcomes are not well studied. An understanding of BSI in Vietnam, its resistance patterns and their impact on patient's outcomes is important to guide clinical management and appropriate antibiotic use. This article reports on a retrospective analysis of three years of BSI data at the National Hospital for Tropical Diseases (NHTD), a large tertiary referral hospital for infectious diseases in Hanoi, Vietnam.

Methods

Study design and data collection

This is a retrospective, cohort study of patients with bacterial bloodstream infection (BSI) admitted to the National Hospital for Tropical Diseases (NHTD) between January 1st, 2011 and December 31st, 2013. NHTD is a 300-bed tertiary teaching hospital that provides care to individuals suspected of an infectious disease living within its catchment area. NHTD is also a referral hospital assigned to all provincial hospitals in the north of Vietnam for infectious diseases that cannot be managed locally. As a result the hospital receives patients both directly from the community and transferred from hospitals in the region. The study included all positive blood cultures with recognized bacterial pathogens among patients who were hospitalized during the study period and additional clinical information from a subgroup of patients whose patient records were available to the investigators. A standard data collection form was created to extract demographic & clinical data, microbiology and outcome information from routine patient and microbiology records. Where patients had been transferred from another hospital, the transfer letter was examined for any record of antibiotic therapy having been provided at the referring hospital.

Study definitions

A recognised bacterial pathogen identified as an organism which is not on the CDC's National Healthcare Safety Network (NHSN) common commensal list unless there were 2 bottles from the same set were positive for the same organism or a single positive bottle plus an evident focus of infection (abscess or valvular vegetation). An episode of BSI was defined as the isolation of the organism(s) from one or more positive blood bottles which were explainable by a common source of infection and the time between two isolations was not interrupted by an asymptomatic period. When the clinical information was not available for judgment, the same organism(s) isolated within 48 h of another positive culture was considered as the same episode [15].

A case of community-acquired BSI (CABSI) was defined as a patient with a positive blood culture from a blood sample drawn ≤48 h after hospitalization at any health care facility (to ensure correct categorisation of patients referred from another hospital) for the current illness. Hospital-acquired BSI (HABSI) cases were defined as patients with >48 h between admission at any health care facility and the blood being drawn using the referring letter when applicable [16, 17]. These data were only available from patients whose clinical records were available. Any BSI caused by *Streptococcus suis* or *Burkholderia pseudomallei*, was classified as CABSI regardless of when samples were taken with the assumption that the acquisition of those infection due to occupational exposure to pigs and environmental exposure to contaminated environment are unlikely in the hospital setting respectively [18, 19].

Blood for culture, approximately 5–10 mL of blood, was collected in a single commercially sourced aerobic bottle and incubated in an automated system (Bactec, Becton Dickinson, USA) for five days (5–10 mL blood). Bottles that flagged positive were Gram-stained, subcultured and identified using standard microbiological techniques, including VITEK and API testing (bioMérieux, France). Antibiotic susceptibilities were performed using CLSI guidelines with breakpoints from 2013 [20]. For *S. suis*, the susceptibility was evaluated using CLSI breakpoints for *Streptococcus viridans* group [21].

Fatal cases were defined as patients who died in hospital or were discharged with diagnosis of brain death and the expectation that they will die imminently within hours or days (palliative discharge to die at home, a common practice in Vietnam).

Data entry and statistical analysis

Data were entered in Epidata (EpiData Association, Odense, Denmark) and analysed using SPSS 22.0.0 (IBM Co., Armonk, NY, USA). Standard descriptive statistics were calculated for categorical (in percentage) and continuous variables (median and interquartile, IQR). Bivariate analyses were performed using Pearson's chi-squared test or Fisher's Exact Test for categorical variables as appropriate. The possible selection bias was assessed by chi-square and t-test analyses to compare gender and age differences between those with and without clinical outcomes, respectively. Cox proportional-hazards regression was used to identify variables that predict clinical outcomes. Cox's proportional hazards regression was performed to analyse factors associated with all-cause in-hospital mortality. BSI episodes of polymicrobial infection and *S. maltophilia* infections were excluded from regression analysis due to a small number and an uncertain pathogenicity respectively. In cases where there were multiple blood cultures positive, we only included the first positive blood culture. All tests were two-tailed and differences were considered statistically significant at p values ≤0.05.

Results

Study population's demographics

There were 894 positive blood cultures corresponding to 835 BSI episodes in 825 patients recorded between January 2011 and December 2013. Notes from 543/825 (65.8%) patients could be retrieved to collect clinical details of individual patients while 282 (34.2%) were not available (Fig. 1). Sensitivity analysis of age and gender showed no differences between cases with and without clinical outcome (chi-square test, p = 0.664 and t-test, p = 0.053 respectively). Among collected records, sixty-six cases (12.2%, 66/543) were subsequently classified by cultured organism as having a pseudo-bacteremia due to contamination, including 16 cases with *Burkholderia cepacia*, 19 cases with *Alcaligenes species*, 5 cases with *Ralstonia pickettii* and 4 cases with *Pseudomonas species* (2 *P. putida* and 2 *P. stutzeri*). There were 3 cases with *Serratia marcescens*, 3 *S. maltophilia*, 1 *K. pneumoniae* and 1 *E. coli* which were classified as contaminants by treating doctors at the time of results return, based on patient's survival and recovery without antibiotic treatment for bacterial disease and with an alternative possible viral diagnosis. Other contaminated cultures were 3 cases with *Ochrobactrum anthropi*, 1 case with *Chryseobacterium indologenes*, 1 case with *Chryseomonas luteola*, 1 case with (non-diphtheroid) *Corynebacterium spp.*, 1 case with *Staphylococcus spp.* and 7 cases with single culture of viridans group streptococci without an endovascular or other focus. As a result, 477 cases were included for the clinical analysis.

The median age of the group of 477 patients with BSI was 48 years (IQR 36–60), 27.7% of patients were female (132/477), 14 (10.6%) of whom were pregnant). Common co-morbidities were chronic hepatitis or cirrhosis (14.3%, 68/477), diabetes mellitus (7.1%, 34/477) and HIV infection (6.3%, 30/477) (Table 1).

In patients with CABSIs, 12.5% (50/400) had multiple positive blood cultures with either *S. aureus* or *K. pneumoniae*. Whilst most patients with CABSI were admitted directly from the community, 153/400 patients (38.3%) were transferred from other hospitals within 48 h, with 62/153 patients (40.5%) recorded as

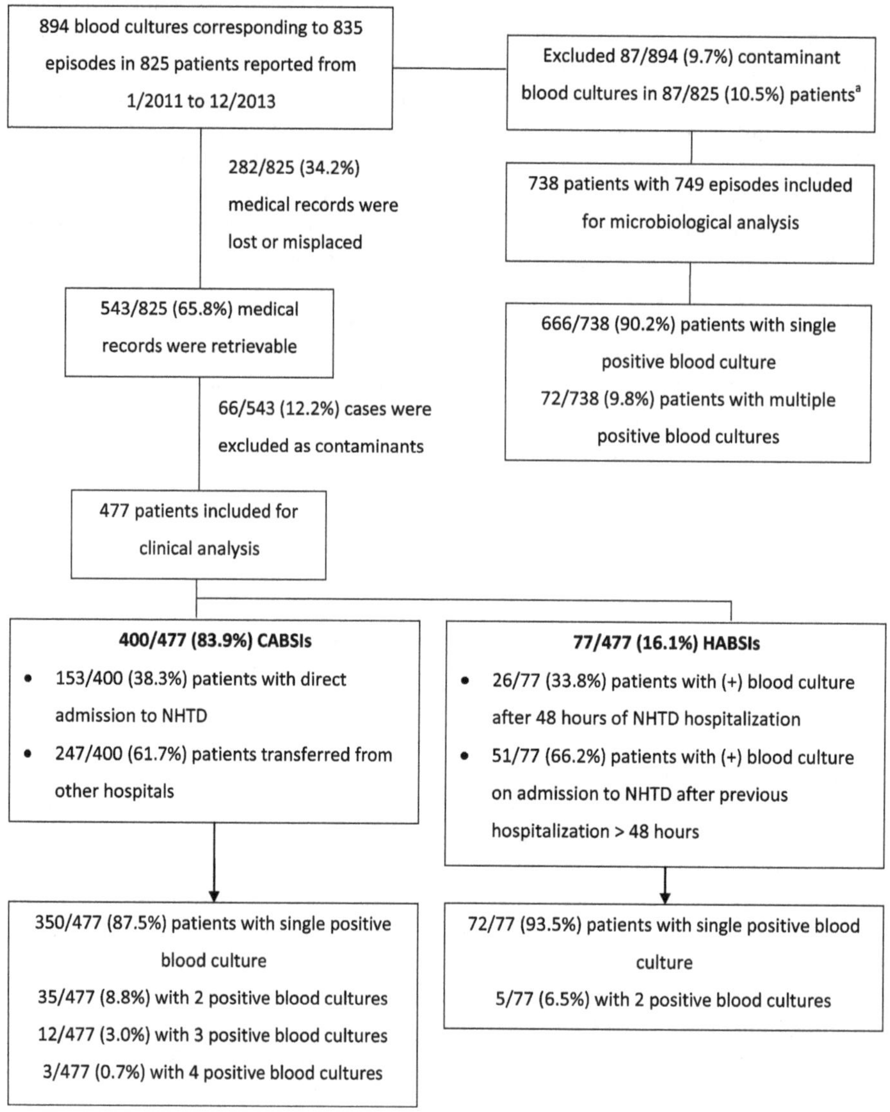

Fig. 1 Flowchart of BSI episodes and classification of BSI by location of acquisition. Classification based on the first isolate during hospitalization. HABSI: Hospital-acquired bloodstream infection; CABSI: Community-acquired bloodstream infection. **a** Contaminant episodes included 22 episodes of *B. cepacia*, 25 episodes of *Alcaligenes spp.*, 7 episodes of viridans group streptococci, 8 episodes of *Ralstonia picketii*, 6 episodes of Pseudomonas species (*P. fluorescens*, *P. putida* and *P. stutzeri*) 4 episodes of *Chryseobacterium spp., 3 episodes of S. maltophilia, 3 episodes of Serratia marcescens*, 3 episodes of *Ochrobactrum antrhopi*, 2 episodes of *Sphingomonas paucimobilis*, 1 episode of each *E. coli, K. pneumonia, Corynebacterium spp.* and *Chryseomonas luteola*

having received antibiotics before admission to the study hospital.

Aetiology of bloodstream infections

Analysis of microbiological dataset

During the 3 year period, a total of 738 BSI patients were identified with 67.9% (501/738) with Gram-negative bacteria isolated, 31% (229/738) Gram-positive bacteria, and 1.1% (8/738) had two pathogens isolated in the same culture bottle (n = 8). *Enterobacteriaceae* were the most frequently isolated group of organisms among patients with BSI (46.7%, 345/738) with the predominant *Enterobacteriaceae* being *K. pneumoniae* (37.4%, 129/345) and *E. coli* (37.1%, 128/345), followed by *Salmonella* enterica (13.0% or 45/345) (Table 2).

Among Gram-positive isolates, *S. aureus* was the leading pathogen (48% or 110/229), followed by *S. suis* (24.5% or 56/229) and other *Streptococcus* species (16.2% or 37/229). Non- *Enterobacteriaceae* Gram-negative bacteria were identified in 156 cases (21.1%), of which *S. maltophilia* accounted for 45.5% (71/156).

The overall proportion of extended spectrum beta-lactamases (ESBL) production among *Enterobacteriaceae* was 25.1% (67/267 isolates, 78 missing result). Tables 3 and 4 display the antibiotic resistance of *K. pneumoniae* and *E. coli*. The prevalence of ESBL production among

Table 1 Characteristics of the clinical study population

	Total	Community acquired BSI	Hospital acquired BSI
	N = 477	N = 400	N = 77
		n (%)	n (%)
Age – median (IQR)	48 (36–60)	48 (36–60)	50 (32–60)
Female sex	132 (27.7%)	122 (30.6%)	10 (13%)
Any ICU admission during NHTD hospitalisation	245 (51.4%)	190 (47.5%)	55 (71.4%)
Any history of medical condition	142 (29.8%)	109 (27.3%)	33 (42.9%)
Liver disease	68 (14.3%)	54 (13.5%)	14 (18.2)
Diabetes	34 (7.1%)	25 (6.3%)	9 (11.7%)
Moderate or severe renal disease	9 (1.9%)	6 (1.5%)	3(3.9%)
HIV infection	30 (6.3%)	21 (5.3%)	9 (11.7%)
Other morbidity	10 (2.1%)	8 (2%)	2 (2.6%)
Long-term corticosteroid use	8 (1.7%)	7 (1.8%)	1 (1.3%)
Self-report alcoholism	67(14%)	56 (14%)	11 (14.3%)
Intravenous drug use	23 (4.8%)	17 (4.3%)	6 (7.8%)

[a]Liver disease was defined in a patient with chronic hepatitis and/or cirrhosis
[b]Moderate or severe renal disease was defined in a patient with baseline creatinine >3 mg% (265 umol/l), dialysis or kidney transplantation

E. coli isolates was significantly higher than in *K. pneumoniae* (45%, 50/111 vs 12.3%,15/122, p < 0.001). Among Gram-positive bacteria, 97.4% (38/39) of *S. suis* isolates were susceptible to penicillin with penicillin MIC median of 0.032 (IQR 0.023–0.032) and only 1 case was intermediate susceptible to penicillin with an MIC of 0.23, though no confirmatory testing was performed. Methicillin resistance was observed in 37% (40/108) of *S. aureus* isolates and all 29 MRSA isolates tested with vancomycin E-test were susceptible. Among 67 *S. aureus* isolates tested for vancomycin by E-test, 62.7% (42/67) of isolates had vancomycin MIC ≤1 μg/ml and 37.3% (25/67) 1.5–2 μg/ml (Table 5).

Analysis of the clinical dataset

The proportions of CABSI and HABSI caused by *Enterobacteriaceae* were not statistically different (55.1%, 203/397 vs 58.4%, 45/77, p = 0.24), similar for for non-enterobacteriaceae Gram-negative bacteria (19.6%, 78/397 vs 27.3%, 21/77, p = 0.132). In contrast, Gram-positive bacteria were more frequently identified in CABSI (29.2%, 116/397 vs 14.3%, 11/77, p = 0.011) and *Acinetobacter* species were more common in HABSI (Table 2).

There was no difference in the proportion of ESBL production in community versus hospital setting among *E. coli* isolates (53.8%, 28/52 vs 55.6%, 5/9, p = 1.0). In *K. pneumoniae* isolates, the proportion of ESBL production were higher in HABSI (21.1%, 4/19 vs 6.1%, 5/82 vs, p = 0.039). Compared with *K. pneumoniae*, *E. coli* isolates were also more frequently resistant to aminoglycosides (23.3%, 30/129 vs 13.0%, 17/131, p = 0.031) and fluoroquinolones (31.8%, 41/128, vs 8.4%, 11/131, p < 0.001).

K. pneumoniae isolates associated with HABSI more frequently showed antibiotic resistance compared to CABSI isolates, though statistical significance was only reached for quinolones, while the pattern of resistance among *E. coli* isolates did not differ between the hospital and community (Tables 3 and 4). MRSA rates differed between community (38.7%, 12/31) and hospital settings (0/7), though this did not reach statistical significance (p = 0.074). Case notes were not retrievable in 69/110 (62.7%) cases of *S. aureus* bacteremia.

Case fatality of bloodstream infection

Case fatality was assessed in the clinical dataset only. The overall in-hospital case fatality rate among patients was 138/477 (28.9%). Overall case fatality rates among patients infected with *Enterobacteriaceae*, non-*Enterobacteriaceae* and Gram-positive bacteria were 34.7% (85/245), 29.3% (29/99) and 19% (24/126), respectively (Fig. 2). There was no case of death among patients with mix infections (0/7). Case fatality rate in CABSI (27.5%, 110/400) was lower, but not statistically different from HABSI (36.4%, 28/77) (p = 0.131). In the most frequent isolates of *E. coli*, *K. pneumoniae*, *S. aureus*, *S. maltophilia* and *S. suis*, case-fatality rates were 35.6% (26/73), 35.5% (39/110), 26.8% (11/41), 17.0% (8/39) and 9.3% (4/39).

Multivariate Cox proportional hazard regression analysis was used to measure the effect of demographics, acquisition of infection, co-morbidities, previous hospital referring factors and bacterial species. Independent factors associated with case fatality were *Enterobacteriaceae*

Table 2 Aetiology of bloodstream infections

Pathogen	All patients	Sampled clinical cases			
		Total	CABSI	HABSI	p[g]
	N = 738	N = 477	N = 400	N = 77	
Enterobacteriaceae	345 (46.7%)	245 (51.4%)	200 (50%)	45 (58.4%)	0.213
Klebsiella pneumoniae	129 (17.5%)	110 (23.1%)	88 (22%)	22 (28.6%)	0.237[d]
Escherichia coli	128 (17.3%)	73 (15.3%)	64 (16%)	9 (11.7%)	0.391
Salmonella enterica	45 (6.1%)	30 (6.3%)	24 (6%)	6 (7.8%)	0.606
serovar Typhi	10 (1.4%)	4 (0.8%)	4 (1.00%)	0	1
non-typhi Salmonella	35 (4.7%)	26 (5.5%)	20 (5%)	6 (7.8%)	0.407
Serratia marcescens	16 (2.2%)	12 (2.5%)	9 (2.3%)	3 (3.9%)	0.421
Enterobacter species	16 (2.2%)	12 (2.5%)	8 (2.0%)	4 (5.2%)	0.112
Other *Enterobacteriaceae* species[a]	11 (1.5%)	8 (1.7%)	7 (1.8%)	1 (1.3%)	1
Non-Enterobacteriacae	156 (21.1%)	99 (20.8%)	78 (19.5%)	21 (27.3%)	0.127
Stenotrophomonas maltophilia	71 (9.6%)	47 (9.9%)	39 (9.8%)	8 (10.4%)	0.836
Aeromonas species	34 (4.6%)	14 (2.9%)	12 (3.0%)	2 (2.6%)	1
Burkholderia pseudomallei	15 (2.0%)	13 (2.7%)	13 (3.3%)	0	
Pseudomonas aeruginosa	16 (2.2%)	13 (2.7%)	9 (2.3%)	4 (5.2%)	0.240
Acinetobacter species[b]	16 (2.2%)	10 (2.1%)	3 (0.8%)	7 (9.1%)	<0.001
Other gram-negative bacteria[c]	4 (0.5%)	2 (0.4%)	2 (0.5%)	0	1
Gram-positive isolates	229 (31.0%)	126 (26.4%)	115 (28.8%)	11 (14.3%)	0.007
Staphylococcus aureus	110 (14.9%)	41 (8.6%)	34 (8.5%)	7 (9.1%)	0.826
Streptococcus suis	56 (7.6%)	43 (9.0%)	43 (10.8%)	0	-
Streptococcus species	37 (4.9%)	23 (4.8%)	21 (5.3%)	2 (2.6%)	0.559
S. pneumoniae	7 (0.9%)	5 (1.0%)	4 (1.0%)	1 (1.3%)	0.587
S. viridans group[d]	21 (2.8%)	11 (2.3%)[b]	10 (2.5%)	1 (1.3%)	1
Beta-hemolytic streptococci	9 (1.2%)	7 (1.5%)	7 (1.8%)	0	0.604
Enterococcus species	14 (1.9%)	12 (2.5%)	10 (2.5%)	2 (2.6%)	1
Other gram-positive bacteria[e]	12 (1.6%)	7 (1.5%)	7 (1.8%)	0	0.604
Polymicrobial[f]	8 (1.1%)	7 (1.5%)	7 (1.8%)	0	0.604

[a]Including 3 cases with *Klebsiella oxytoca*, 3 cases with *Proteus mirabilis*, 2 cases with *Escherichia hermannii*, 1 case with *Citrobacter freundii*, 1 case with *Morganella morganii and 1 case with Vibrio vulnificus*

[b]Including 12 cases with *A. baumannii*, 3 cases with *A. lwoffii* and 1 case with *A. junii*

[c]Including 1 case for *Elizabethkingia meningosepticum, Haemophilus influenzae, Pasteurella multocida* and *Neisseria meningitidis,*

[d]Cases with viridans group infection had at least two positive blood culture or single positive blood culture plus vegetation on echocardiography

[e]Including 4 cases with *Rhodococcus equi*, 3 cases with *Listeria monocytogenes*, 2 cases with *Aerococcus viridians*, 2 cases with *Listeria spp.* and 1 case with *Listeria innocua*

[f]In 8 dual infection cases, 3 HIV infected cases had co-infection with *Talaromyces marneffei* and *S. aureus, Escherichia hermannii* or *Salmonella group D;* 1 case with *S. aureus* and *K. pneumoniae*, 1 case with *Enterococcus faecalis* and viridans streptococci, 1 case with *E. coli* and *K. pneumoniae* and 1 case with *S. aureus* and *E. coli* co-infection

[g]*p* values were calculated using Chi-square test or Fisher's Exact test as appropriate

and non-*Enterobacteriaceae* infection (HR 2.485, 95%CI 1.546–3.994 and HR 1.931, 95% CI 1.063–3.50, respectively), co-morbidities (HR 1.467, 95% CI 1.017–2.114) and referring from other hospital (HR 2.049, 95% CI 1.411–2.975) (Table 6).

Discussion

This retrospective study includes 3-years of complete microbiological data on aetiology of BSI for 738 patients and almost two thirds (64.6%, 477/738) of these patients for clinical outcome analysis in a tertiary hospital in the north of Vietnam.

Our study shows the important role of pathogenic Gram-negative bacteria with a high proportion of cephalosporin-resistant *E. coli* and *K. pneumoniae* isolates and high prevalence of MRSA in CABSI. Our study shows the high contribution of *Enterobacteriaceae* BSI to mortality among adults admitted to our hospital in Vietnam, with over 60% of deaths associated with this group of bacteria. This study supports the observed shift

Table 3 Resistance among *K. pneumoniae* from BSI

Resistance	All isolates	Sampled clinical cases			
		Total	CABSI	HABSI	*P* value [a]
Any extended spectrum cephalosporin	19/133 (14.3%)	13/112 (11.6%)	8/90 (8.9%)	5/22 (22.7%)	0.128
ESBL production	15/122 (12.3%)	9/101 (8.9%)	5/82 (6.1%)	4/19 (21.1%)	0.062
Others	4/133 (3.0%)	4/112 (3.6%)	3/90 (3.3%)	1/22 (4.5%)	1
Any carbapenem	1/131 (0.8%)	1/109 (0.9%)	0/89 (0%)	1/20 (5%)	0.183
Any aminoglycoside	17/131 (13.0%)	13/109 (11.9%)	9/89 (10.1%)	4/20 (20%)	0.252
Any fluoroquinolone	11/131 (8.4%)	8/109 (7.3%)	4/89 (4.5%)	4/20 (20%)	0.036
Co-trimoxazole	24/124 (19.4%)	19/102 (18.6%)	14/84 (16.7%)	5/18 (27.8%)	0.318

[a]*p* values were calculated using Fisher's Exact Test

within *Enterobacteriaceae* organisms from typhoidal and non-typhoidal *Salmonella* to *K. pneumoniae* and *E. coli*, the current leading causes of community acquired blood stream infections.

In Vietnam, *Salmonella enterica* serovar Typhi was reported to be the major cause of BSI, accounting for up to 74% of isolates from blood in the 1990s but gradually declined to 6% by 2008 [22]. With the recent emergence of *K. pneumoniae* and *E.coli*, we observed the high prevalence of extended spectrum Beta-lactamase (ESBL) production in these pathogens, especially in the hospital setting. In surveillance data from five Asia-Pacific countries in 2010, Vietnam reported the highest rate of ESBL positive *Enterobacteriaceae* isolates with an overall prevalence of 55.1% and 80.1% in ICU patients [11]. The high prevalence of antibiotic resistance in Vietnam may be attributed to multiple factors, such as dispensing practices in the community, lack of enforcement of regulation, limited resources for microbiological diagnostics, injudicious use of antibiotics in hospital, community and agriculture and insufficient antibiotic resistance surveillance and infection control [23].

In our study, ESBL production was detected among 6.1% *K. pneumoniae* from CABSI, which is consistent with the low ESBL prevalence of 4.1% among *K. pneumoniae* oropharyngeal carriers reported previously from northern Vietnam [24]. The rate of ESBL-production in *E. coli*(45%) was higher than in Thailand (CABSI, 11.8%) and Korea (31.3% in HABSI and 8.8% in CABSI) and comparable to the prevalence of ESBL among *E. coli* isolates in BSI in Cambodia (47.7%), [15, 17, 25]. The high rate of ESBL carriage in *E. coli* from CABSI is deeply worrying and likely reflects extensive overuse of oral cephalosporins in the community, their use in agriculture or other environmental sources [26, 27]. *S. suis* is a well-recognized zoonotic pathogen associated with bacterial meningitis and BSI among adults in Vietnam [10] and was noted as an important Gram-positive pathogen cultured from blood with high levels of susceptibility to penicillin.

Our study showed a higher case-fatality rate (110/400 or 27.5%) among community-acquired bacterial bloodstream infections than the rate of 9% reported in a review from 1990 to 2010 in south and southeast Asia and the rate of 18.1% among patients with CABSI in a meta-analysis in Africa from 1984 to 2006 [28, 29]. This difference is likely related to the changes in spectrum of aetiology with higher prevalence of *Salmonella spp.* (53.2% of *Enterobacteriaceae* isolates) in the past [28], the emergence of high levels of antibiotic resistance in Vietnam and the tertiary referral nature of the study hospital. The overall mortality in our study was slightly higher than the overall mortality of 22.5% in Cambodia

Table 4 Resistance among *E. coli* from BSI

Resistance	All isolates	Sampled clinical cases			
		Total	CABSI	HABSI	*P* value[a]
Any extended spectrum cephalosporin	72/131 (55.0%)	45/74 (60.8%)	39/65 (60%)	6/9 (66.7%)	1
ESBL production	50/111 (45%)	33/61 (54.1%)	28/52 (53.8%)	5/9 (55.6%)	1
Others	22/131 (16.8%)	12/74 (16.2%)	11/65 (16.9%)	1/9 (11.1%)	1
Any carbapenem	1/130 (0.8%)	0/73 (0.0%)	0/64 (0.0%)	0/9 (0.0%)	-
Any aminoglycoside	30/129 (23.3%)	15/73 (20.5%)	14/64 (21.9%)	1/9 (11.1%)	0.675
Any fluoroquinolone	41/129 (31.8%)	26/72 (36.1%)	22/63 (34.9%)	4/9 (44.4%)	0.714
Cotrimoxazole	62/90 (68.9%)	27/38 (71.1%)	24/33 (72.7%)	3/5 (60.0%)	0.615
Fosfomycin	1/52 (1.9%)	1/44 (2.3%)	1/38 (2.6%)	0/6 (0%)	-

[a]*p* values were calculated using Fisher's Exact Test

Table 5 Resistance among *S. aureus* from BSI

Susceptibility	All isolates	Sampled clinical cases			
		Total	CABSI	HABSI	*P* value [a]
Methicillin (MRSA)	40/108 (37%)	12/38 (31.6%)	12/31 (38.7%)	0/7 (0%)	0.074
Erythromycin	39/72 (54.2%)	11/23 (47.8%)	10/18 (55.6%)	1/5 (20%)	0.317
Clindamycin	56/109 (51.4%)	21/40 (52.5%)	18/23 (54.5%)	3/7 (42.9%)	0.689
Chloramphenicol	35/105 (33.3%)	14/38 (36.8%)	11/31 (35.5%)	3/7 (42.9%)	1
Gentamicin	18/76 (23.7%)	9/26 (34.6%)	7/21 (33.3%)	2/5 (40%)	1
Ciprofloxacin	19/99 (19.2%)	7/33 (21.2%)	6/28 (21.4%)	1/5(20%)	1
Levofloxacin	18/103 (17.5%)	9/40 (22.5%)	6/13 (18.2%)	3/7 (42.9%)	0.316
Co-trimoxazole	8/62 (12.9%)	5/28(17.9%)	4/21 (19%)	1/7 (14.3%)	1
Rifampicin	10/95 (10.5%)	6/33 (18.2%)	5/27 (18.5%)	1/6 (16.7%)	1
Vancomycin[b]	0/63 (0%)	-	-	-	-

[a] *p* values were calculated using Fisher's Exact Test
[b] The vancomycin susceptibility and the MRSA rate were defined by Minimum Inhibitory Concentrations (MICs) using E-test

where the epidemiology and pattern of resistance are similar [15]. We reported a high mortality of 35.6% among E. coli BSI, which is higher than mortality of 18.2% and 8% and in a large surveillance in England and in a population-based study in Finland [30, 31]. It is not clear about the reasons of the differences, but it may relate to pneumonia focus, severity of infection, antibiotic susceptibilities and seasonal variation [31]. As NHTD is a tertiary referral hospital, potentially more severe cases or cases that have failed therapy elsewhere may have been referred as compared to the hospitals included in other studies, leading to higher resistance and case fatality rates.

In North America and Europe, the nosocomial BSI case fatality rate ranges from 12 to 32% [2]. Changes in the aetiology of HABSI began in the 1960s–1970s in the United States of America (US) with replacement of Gram-negative by Gram-positive organisms, such that 65% of BSIs were *S. aureus*, the most common nosocomial pathogen [32]. However, a Vietnamese population based study indicated *S. aureus* nasopharyngeal carriage proportion (33.8%, CI 29.4–38.8) was higher than in European regions and the States [33], and *S. aureus* BSI is still mainly community-acquired in Vietnam [34]. In Vietnam the proportion of BSI attributable to *S. aureus* did not change during the 15-years from 1994 to 2008 [22]. Gram-negative bacilli are still recognized as the most frequent nosocomial isolates in developing countries [35]. In a multicenter surveillance study in Thailand, Gram-negative bacteria accounted for 67.6% of HABSI, of which *Acinetobacter spp.* (16.2%) was detected most frequently, followed by *K. pneumoniae* (13.9%) and *S. aureus* (13.9%) and the in-hospital mortality was 26.6% [36]. The overall case fatality rate of 36.4% among HABSI in our study population was higher than seen in North America and Europe. This may be related to higher levels of antibiotic resistance, differences in the availability of resources or the nature of admissions to NHTD, as described earlier.

Table 6 Cox proportional hazards model of factors associated with all-cause in-hospital case fatality among patients with bloodstream infections due to a single organism in clinical dataset

Variable	Hazard ratio (95% CI)[a]	*P*-value[b]
Gender (male/female)	1.347 (.857–2.115)	0.196
Age (1-yr. increment)	1.008 (0.998–1.01)	0.118
Aetiology of BSI (gram-positive bacterial infection as reference)		
Enterobacteriaceae infections	2.485 (1.546–3.994)	<0.001
Non *Enterobacteriaceae* Gram-negative infections	1.931 (1.063–3.50)	0.031
Acquisition of infection (CABSI as reference)	1.006 (0.633–0.399)	0.053
Any co-morbidities	1.467 (1.017–2.114)	0.040
Referring from another hospital	2.049 (1.411–2.975)	<0.001

[a] Cases with *S. maltophilia* infection were excluded from analysis
[b] Hazard ratios and *P*-values were calculated using Cox proportional hazards model

We observed a predominance of males among patients with BSI (72.3%). This phenomenon was similar as in the cause of death reports in another tertiary hospital in the north of Vietnam where the top three of causes of death were septic shock, intracerebral haemorrhage and pneumonia. The proportion of males in this report was higher than females (1577/2340 or 67.4%) [37].

Among common isolates causing BSI, we reported the high prevalence of *S. maltophilia* (9.6%. 71/738) which is only rarely considered a pathogen, particularly from the community [32]. Whilst *S. maltophilia* was described as a recognised cause of CABSI among patients with

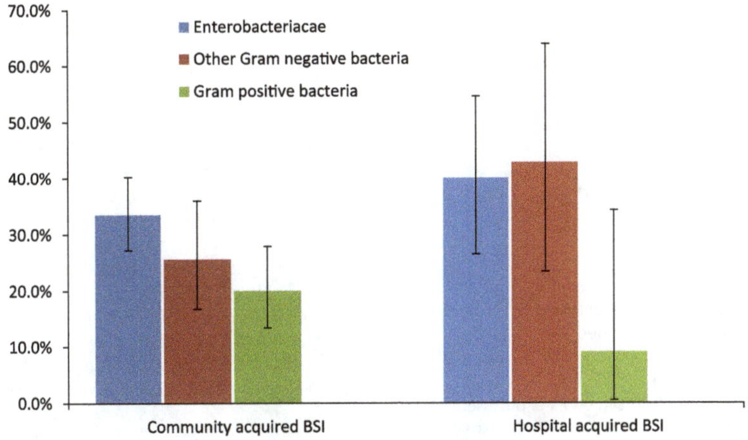

Fig. 2 Case-fatality by etiology of bloodstream infection (BSI). Error bars represent the 95% confidence interval (CI) for case mortality proportions

comorbidities in a systematic review [38] and a recent publication from Taiwan [39], another publication describes contamination of blood culture bottles with *S. maltophilia* due to growth of the bacteria in disinfectant [40]. Furthermore, we have observed pseudoepidemics of *S. maltophilia* in this hospital (multiple patients from geographically disparate sites with different infection syndromes, newly admitted on the same ward with *S. maltophilia* cultured from blood at the same time). The retrospective nature of this study makes it difficult to define whether these isolates were true pathogens or represented contamination. Given how frequently this organism was isolated, further prospective investigation is required.

Our study has some important limitations. Firstly, NHTD is a tertiary referral hospital and specializes in infectious diseases. Therefore, the pattern of aetiology, resistance and spectrum of clinical disease is different from that seen in district and provincial level hospitals due to referral of certain syndromes, more severe and non-responsive cases.

Secondly, during the study period, only a single blood culture was routine collected and as a cost saving technique, routine laboratory practice was that cultures showing obvious contamination (multiple organisms, skin flora etc.) were discarded before full work up without recording this finding. This will have lowered estimations of blood culture sensitivity, which can be improved with more blood cultures and higher volumes of blood [41, 42]. Additionally, although the isolates of Enterobacteriaceae members are almost always interpreted as true bloodstream infections, single blood culture practice may underestimate the roles of fastidious pathogens in the era of increased catheters and prosthetic devices-related bloodstream infections [43].

In our study hospital acquired BSI was defined as cases with positive blood culture after any hospitalization for more than 48 h. Thus, patients who in reality had CABSI but with persistent bacteraemia, who were transferred after an inpatient stay at another hospital may have been misclassified as HABSI. The significance and role of certain bacteria, such as *S. maltophilia* or *Aeromonas* species, which have been associated with both pseudo-bacteraemia and real infection was not easy to establish because of a lack of repeat sampling in most of patients and the retrospective nature of the study. Lastly, clinical outcome analysis was only applied for 64.6% (477/738) of patients during the study period because the remaining patient's notes could not be retrieved. This has resulted in significant gaps in the data and may have introduced bias if the sample was not random.

Conclusions

Gram-negative bacteria are the most common cause of both community and hospital acquired blood stream infection in adults presenting to our tertiary referral hospital, with high associated mortality. The extended spectrum beta-lactamase (ESBL)-producing *Enterobacteriaceae* are prevalent in both community and health care setting. Our findings further support the need, as described in the GARP situation analysis [44] and the 2013 Vietnamese National Action Plan for AMR [45], for establishment of a comprehensive microbiological and antibiotic susceptibility surveillance system in Vietnam, with representation of the different levels of healthcare and to inform treatment guidelines and other public health measures.

Abbreviations

BSIs: Bloodstream infections; CABSI: Community-acquired bloodstream infections; ESBL: Extended Spectrum Beta-Lactamases; HABSI: Hospital-acquired bloodstream infections; IQR: Interquartile range; LMIC: Low and middle income countries; MICs: Minimum Inhibitory Concentrations; MRSA: Methicillin-resistant *Staphylococcus aureus*; NHTD: National Hospital for Tropical Diseases

Acknowledgements
We gratefully acknowledge the bacteriology laboratory and General Planning Department in National Hospital for Tropical Diseases for providing the list of bacterial isolates, susceptibility results and for providing the list of medical records.

Funding
This study was funded by the Wellcome Trust Major Overseas Programme Vietnam.

Authors' contributions
DVQ designed the study, collected & analysed the data and wrote the first & final draft; HNV, HNT, HTN, LBH, CLB collected, entered data, drafted sections of the manuscript; DVTV was responsible for cleaning data, analysis and drafted sections of the manuscript; KVN, TVN, DTT contributed to study design and were responsible for laboratory and clinical care, provided revisions of the manuscript edited the final draft; AT and HRvD helped with interpretation of the data, revision of the manuscript and edited the final draft; BN & HFLW helped design the study, interpreted the data, revised the manuscript and edited the final draft. All authors approved of the final draft.

Consent for publication
Not applicable.

Competing interests
HRvD is a member of the editorial board (Associate Editor) of the BMC Infectious Diseases. The authors otherwise declare that they have no competing interests.

Author details
[1]Department of Infectious Diseases, Hanoi Medical University, Hanoi, Vietnam. [2]National Hospital for Tropical Diseases, Hanoi, Vietnam. [3]Wellcome Trust Major Overseas Programme, Oxford University Clinical Research Unit, Hanoi, Vietnam. [4]Nuffield Department of Clinical Medicine, Centre for Tropical Medicine, University of Oxford, Oxford, UK. [5]Department of Medical Microbiology, Radboudumc, Nijmegen, Netherlands.

References
1. Mortality GBD, Causes of Death C. Global, regional, and national age-sex specific all-cause and cause-specific mortality for 240 causes of death, 1990–2013: a systematic analysis for the Global Burden of Disease Study 2013. Lancet. 2015;385:117–71.
2. Goto M, Al-Hasan MN. Overall burden of bloodstream infection and nosocomial bloodstream infection in North America and Europe. Clin Microbiol Infect. 2013;19:501–9.
3. Laupland KB, Davies HD, Church DL, Louie TJ, Dool JS, Zygun DA, Doig CJ. Bloodstream infection-associated sepsis and septic shock in critically ill adults: a population-based study. Infection. 2004;32:59–64.
4. Nielsen SL. The incidence and prognosis of patients with bacteremia. Dan Med J. 2015;62.
5. Southeast Asia Infectious Disease Clinical Research Network. Causes and outcomes of sepsis in Southeast Asia: a multinational multicentre cross-sectional study. Lancet Glob Health. 2017;5:e157–67.
6. Melamed A, Sorvillo FJ. The burden of sepsis-associated mortality in the United States from 1999 to 2005: an analysis of multiple-cause-of-death data. Crit Care. 2009;13:R28.
7. Sogaard M, Norgaard M, Dethlefsen C, Schonheyder HC. Temporal changes in the incidence and 30-day mortality associated with bacteremia in hospitalized patients from 1992 through 2006: a population-based cohort study. Clin Infect Dis. 2011;52:61–9.
8. Mayr FB, Yende S, Angus DC. Epidemiology of severe sepsis. Virulence. 2014;5:4–11.
9. Cohen ML. Changing patterns of infectious disease. Nature. 2000;406:762–7.
10. Wertheim HF, Nghia HD, Taylor W, Schultsz C. Streptococcus suis: an emerging human pathogen. Clin Infect Dis. 2009;48:617–25.
11. Kiratisin P, Chongthaleong A, Tan TY, Lagamayo E, Roberts S, Garcia J, Davies T. Comparative in vitro activity of carbapenems against major Gram-negative pathogens: results of Asia-Pacific surveillance from the COMPACT II study. Int J Antimicrob Agents. 2012;39:311–6.
12. Song JH, Jung SI, Ko KS, Kim NY, Son JS, Chang HH, Ki HK, Oh WS, Suh JY, Peck KR, et al. High prevalence of antimicrobial resistance among clinical Streptococcus pneumoniae isolates in Asia (an ANSORP study). Antimicrob Agents Chemother. 2004;48:2101–7.
13. Ferrer R, Martin-Loeches I, Phillips G, Osborn TM, Townsend S, Dellinger RP, Artigas A, Schorr C, Levy MM. Empiric antibiotic treatment reduces mortality in severe sepsis and septic shock from the first hour: results from a guideline-based performance improvement program. Crit Care Med. 2014;42:1749–55.
14. Paul M, Shani V, Muchtar E, Kariv G, Robenshtok E, Leibovici L. Systematic review and meta-analysis of the efficacy of appropriate empiric antibiotic therapy for sepsis. Antimicrob Agents Chemother. 2010;54:4851–63.
15. Vlieghe ER, Phe T, De Smet B, Veng HC, Kham C, Lim K, Koole O, Lynen L, Peetermans WE, Jacobs JA. Bloodstream infection among adults in Phnom Penh, Cambodia: key pathogens and resistance patterns. PLoS One. 2013;8:e59775.
16. Siegman-Igra Y, Fourer B, Orni-Wasserlauf R, Golan Y, Noy A, Schwartz D, Giladi M. Reappraisal of community-acquired bacteremia: a proposal of a new classification for the spectrum of acquisition of bacteremia. Clin Infect Dis. 2002;34:1431–9.
17. Kanoksil M, Jatapai A, Peacock SJ, Limmathurotsakul D. Epidemiology, microbiology and mortality associated with community-acquired bacteremia in northeast Thailand: a multicenter surveillance study. PLoS One. 2013;8:e54714.
18. Huong VTL, Ha N, Huy NT, Horby P, Nghia HDT, Thiem VD, Zhu X, Hoa NT, Hien TT, Zamora J, et al. Epidemiology, Clinical Manifestations, and Outcomes of Streptococcus suis Infection in Humans. Emerg Infect Dis. 2014;20:1105–14.
19. Cheng AC, Currie BJ. Melioidosis: epidemiology, pathophysiology, and management. Clin Microbiol Rev. 2005;18:383–416.
20. Clinical and Laboratory Standards Institute. Performance Standards for Antimicrobial Susceptibility Testing; Twenty-Third Informational Supplement. CLSI document M100-S23. Wayne: Clinical and Laboratory Standards Institute; 2013.
21. Hoa NT, Chieu TT, Nghia HD, Mai NT, Anh PH, Wolbers M, Baker S, Campbell JI, Chau NV, Hien TT, et al. The antimicrobial resistance patterns and associated determinants in Streptococcus suis isolated from humans in southern Vietnam, 1997–2008. BMC Infect Dis. 2011;11:6.
22. Nga TV, Parry CM, Le T, Lan NP, Diep TS, Campbell JI, Hoang NV, Dung le T, Wain J, Dolecek C, et al. The decline of typhoid and the rise of non-typhoid salmonellae and fungal infections in a changing HIV landscape: bloodstream infection trends over 15 years in southern Vietnam. Trans R Soc Trop Med Hyg. 2012;106:26–34.
23. Nguyen KV, Thi Do NT, Chandna A, Nguyen TV, Pham CV, Doan PM, Nguyen AQ, Thi Nguyen CK, Larsson M, Escalante S, et al. Antibiotic use and resistance in emerging economies: a situation analysis for Viet Nam. BMC Public Health. 2013;13:1158.
24. Dao TT, Liebenthal D, Tran TK, Ngoc Thi Vu B, Ngoc Thi Nguyen D, Thi Tran HK, Thi Nguyen CK, Thi Vu HL, Fox A, Horby P, et al. Klebsiella pneumoniae oropharyngeal carriage in rural and urban Vietnam and the effect of alcohol consumption. PLoS One. 2014;9:e91999.
25. Moon HW, Ko YJ, Park S, Hur M, Yun YM. Analysis of community- and hospital-acquired bacteraemia during a recent 5-year period. J Med Microbiol. 2014;63:421–6.
26. Nakayama T, Ueda S, Huong BT, Tuyen le D, Komalamisra C, Kusolsuk T, Hirai I, Yamamoto Y. Wide dissemination of extended-spectrum beta-lactamase-producing Escherichia coli in community residents in the Indochinese peninsula. Infect Drug Resist. 2015;8:1–5.
27. Nguyen VT, Carrique-Mas JJ, Ngo TH, Ho HM, Ha TT, Campbell JI, Nguyen TN, Hoang NN, Pham VM, Wagenaar JA, et al. Prevalence and risk factors for carriage of antimicrobial-resistant Escherichia coli on household and small-scale chicken farms in the Mekong Delta of Vietnam. J Antimicrob Chemother. 2015;70:2144–52.
28. Deen J, von Seidlein L, Andersen F, Elle N, White NJ, Lubell Y. Community-acquired bacterial bloodstream infections in developing countries in south and southeast Asia: a systematic review. Lancet Infect Dis. 2012;12:480–7.

29. Reddy EA, Shaw AV, Crump JA. Community-acquired bloodstream infections in Africa: a systematic review and meta-analysis. Lancet Infect Dis. 2010;10:417–32.
30. Skogberg K, Lyytikainen O, Ollgren J, Nuorti JP, Ruutu P. Population-based burden of bloodstream infections in Finland. Clin Microbiol Infect. 2012;18: E170–6.
31. Abernethy JK, Johnson AP, Guy R, Hinton N, Sheridan EA, Hope RJ. Thirty day all-cause mortality in patients with Escherichia coli bacteraemia in England. Clin Microbiol Infect. 2015;21:251.e251–8.
32. Anderson DJ, Moehring RW, Sloane R, Schmader KE, Weber DJ, Fowler VG Jr, Smathers E, Sexton DJ. Bloodstream infections in community hospitals in the 21st century: a multicenter cohort study. PLoS One. 2014;9:e91713.
33. Van Nguyen K, Zhang T, Thi Vu BN, Dao TT, Tran TK, Thi Nguyen DN, Thi Tran HK, Thi Nguyen CK, Fox A, Horby P, Wertheim H. Staphylococcus aureus nasopharyngeal carriage in rural and urban northern Vietnam. Trans R Soc Trop Med Hyg. 2014;108:783–90.
34. Thwaites GE. The management of Staphylococcus aureus bacteremia in the United Kingdom and Vietnam: a multi-centre evaluation. PLoS One. 2010;5:e14170.
35. Allegranzi B, Bagheri Nejad S, Combescure C, Graafmans W, Attar H, Donaldson L, Pittet D. Burden of endemic health-care-associated infection in developing countries: systematic review and meta-analysis. Lancet. 2011;377:228–41.
36. Hongsuwan M, Srisamang P, Kanoksil M, Luangasanatip N, Jatapai A, Day NP, Peacock SJ, Cooper BS, Limmathurotsakul D. Increasing incidence of hospital-acquired and healthcare-associated bacteremia in northeast Thailand: a multicenter surveillance study. PLoS One. 2014;9:e109324.
37. Walton M, Harrison R, Chevalier A, Esguerra E, Van Duong D, Chinh ND, Giang H. Improving hospital death certification in Viet Nam: results of a pilot study implementing an adapted WHO hospital death report form in two national hospitals. BMJ Global Health. 2016;1
38. Falagas ME, Kastoris AC, Vouloumanou EK, Dimopoulos G. Community-acquired Stenotrophomonas maltophilia infections: a systematic review. Eur J Clin Microbiol Infect Dis. 2009;28:719–30.
39. Chang YT, Lin CY, Lu PL, Lai CC, Chen TC, Chen CY, Wu DC, Wang TP, Lin CM, Lin WR, Chen YH. Stenotrophomonas maltophilia bloodstream infection: comparison between community-onset and hospital-acquired infections. J Microbiol Immunol Infect. 2014;47:28–35.
40. Siebor E, Llanes C, Lafon I, Ogier-Desserrey A, Duez JM, Pechinot A, Caillot D, Grandjean M, Sixt N, Neuwirth C. Presumed pseudobacteremia outbreak resulting from contamination of proportional disinfectant dispenser. Eur J Clin Microbiol Infect Dis. 2007;26:195–8.
41. Lee A, Mirrett S, Reller LB, Weinstein MP. Detection of bloodstream infections in adults: how many blood cultures are needed? J Clin Microbiol. 2007;45:3546–8.
42. Lin HH, Liu YF, Tien N, Ho CM, Hsu LN, Lu JJ. Evaluation of the blood volume effect on the diagnosis of bacteremia in automated blood culture systems. J Microbiol Immunol Infect. 2013;46:48–52.
43. Weinstein MP. Blood culture contamination: persisting problems and partial progress. J Clin Microbiol. 2003;41:2275–8.
44. The GARP Vietnam National Working Group. Situation Analysis Reports: Antibiotic use and resistance in Vietnam. Washington (District of Columbia): Center for Disease Dynamics, Economics and Policy; 2010.
45. Liew Kong Cheng. State of Play of Antimicrobial Resistance Research and Surveillance in Southeast Asia. SEA-EU-NET II. 2016.

28

Clinical characteristics, organ failure, inflammatory markers and prediction of mortality in patients with community acquired bloodstream infection

Vu Quoc Dat[1,2,3*], Nguyen Thanh Long[1], Vu Ngoc Hieu[4], Nguyen Dinh Hong Phuc[1], Nguyen Van Kinh[3], Nguyen Vu Trung[3,4], H. Rogier van Doorn[2,5], Ana Bonell[2] and Behzad Nadjm[2,5]

Abstract

Background: Community acquired bloodstream infection (CABSI) in low- and middle income countries is associated with a high mortality. This study describes the clinical manifestations, laboratory findings and correlation of SOFA and qSOFA with mortality in patients with CABSI in northern Vietnam.

Methods: This was a retrospective study of 393 patients with at least one positive blood culture with not more than one bacterium taken within 48 h of hospitalisation. Clinical characteristic and laboratory results from the first 24 h in hospital were collected. SOFA and qSOFA scores were calculated and their validity in this setting was evaluated.

Results: Among 393 patients with bacterial CABSI, approximately 80% (307/393) of patients had dysfunction of one or more organ on admission to the study hospital with the most common being that of coagulation (57.1% or 226/393). SOFA performed well in prediction of mortality in those patients initially admitted to the critical care unit (AUC 0.858, 95%CI 0.793–0.922) but poor in those admitted to medical wards (AUC 0.667, 95%CI 0.577–0.758). In contrast qSOFA had poor predictive validity in both settings (AUC 0.692, 95%CI 0.605–0.780 and AUC 0.527, 95%CI 0.424–0.630, respectively). The overall case fatality rate was 28%. HIV infection (HR = 3.145, $p = 0.001$), neutropenia (HR = 2.442, $p = 0.002$), SOFA score 1-point increment (HR = 1.19, $p < 0.001$) and infection with Enterobacteriaceae (HR = 1.722, $p = 0.037$) were independent risk factors for in-hospital mortality.

Conclusions: Organ dysfunction was common among Vietnamese patients with CABSI and associated with high case fatality. SOFA and qSOFA both need to be further validated in this setting.

Keywords: Bloodstream infection, Organ failure, Sequential organ failure assessment score, SOFA, qSOFA, Inflammatory markers, Procalcitonin, C-reactive protein

Background

Bloodstream infection (BSI) is a common cause of sepsis and is associated with significant morbidity and in-hospital mortality worldwide [1]. It is ranked the 11th leading cause of death among adults in USA in 2014, with an age-adjusted death rate of 10.7 per 100,000 standard population [2]. In South and Southeast Asia, the incidence rate of community-acquired BSI in the period of 2004–2010 increased from 16.7 to 38.1 per 100,000 people per year and the 30 days mortality rate can reach up to 37.5% [3].

In patients with BSI, an increasing number of organs with dysfunction is correlated with increased morbidity and mortality [4]. Multiple organ dysfunction is a leading cause of morbidity and mortality in patients admitted to intensive care units (ICUs) in Europe, with an in-hospital mortality of 34.2% [5]. Sequential organ failure assessment (SOFA) score, and the related qSOFA (quickSOFA) score have been recently recommended for

* Correspondence: datvq@hmu.edu.vn; quocdat181@yahoo.com
[1]Department of Infectious Diseases, Hanoi Medical University, no 1 Ton That Tung street, Dong Da district, Hanoi, Vietnam
[2]Wellcome Trust Major Overseas Programme, Oxford University Clinical Research Unit, Hanoi, 78 Giai Phong street, Dong Da district, Hanoi, Vietnam
Full list of author information is available at the end of the article

identifying sepsis and predicting outcome by the Third International Consensus Definitions for Sepsis and Septic Shock (Sepsis-3) [6]. qSOFA was originally designed for use outside the ICU, but it's simplicity, brevity and lack of laboratory results, make it compelling for use in emergency departments and resource-constrained setting. However the validation of qSOFA is not consistent among studies quantifying the risk of death in those presenting with suspected infection in critical care [6–9]. Development and validation of these scores were mostly carried out in high income countries, with limited data on their validity in low- and middle income countries (LMICs) [7, 8, 10]. Additionally there have been few studies looking specifically at patients with BSI, a population with an associated increase in mortality.

This study aims to describe the clinical manifestations and associated organ dysfunctions as described by Sequential [Sepsis-related] Organ Failure Assessment (SOFA) scores and its correlation with mortality in patients with community acquired bloodstream infection at the time of presenting to a large teaching hospital in Vietnam, and their associated mortality.

Methods

Study design

This was a retrospective, cohort study of patients hospitalised at the National Hospital for Tropical Diseases (NHTD) (a tertiary referral infectious disease hospital) in northern Vietnam between January 2011 and December 2013. As a referral centre, this hospital often receives patients with specific infections (eg. central nervous system infections), complicated infections and those with severe infections who have failed on treatment elsewhere. Additionally, at the time of the study, the hospital had not establish a separate emergency department and intensive care unit (ICU), therefore we refer to the critical care unit (CCU) for the unit with both ventilated and unventilated beds, available haemodynamic support and renal replacement therapy. A convenience sampling method was used to select medical notes from the list of all hospitalised patients with positive bacterial blood cultures during the study period. The inclusion criteria were having a blood culture, taken within 48 h of hospitalisation (to any institution) for the current admission, positive for a recognised pathogen according to the US CDC's National Healthcare Safety Network (NHSN) list [11]. Patients with infection with more than one bacterium were excluded, as were cases considered to be pseudobacteraemia [12].

Data collection

Data was extracted from patients' medical notes using a case-report form that captured patient demographics, reported history of prior medical illness, clinical manifestations, laboratory results, inflammatory markers within the first 24 h of admission to the study hospital and outcome at hospital discharge.

BSI with concurrent meningitis was defined in bacteremic patients who had cerebrospinal fluid examination within 24 h of blood drawn for microorganism isolation showing at least one of the following criteria: (1) turbid appearance; (2) leukocytosis (> 100 cells/mm3) or (3) leukocytosis from 10 to 100 cells/ mm3) and either an elevated protein (> 100 mg/dl) or decreased glucose (< 40 mg/dl) [13]. BSI with concurrent pneumonia was confirmed by radiology within 24 h of blood drawn for microorganism isolation. Gastrointestinal tract infection and urine tract infection were defined by the CDC/NHSN Surveillance Definitions for Specific Types of Infections [14]. Sequential [Sepsis-related] Organ Failure Assessment (SOFA) score, and quick SOFA (qSOFA) score were calculated using the worst parameters recorded within the first 24 h of admission to the study hospital and missing values were considered to be normal [6]. Organ dysfunction was defined by organ-specific SOFA scores ≥1. Failure of kidney function was further evaluated using the RIFLE criteria with RIFLE-F (Failure) defined as patients with a serum creatinine greater than three times the age adjusted upper limit of serum creatinine [15]. Neutropenia was defined as an absolute neutrophil count < 1500 cells/mm^3, severe anemia as hemoglobin concentration was < 80 g/L and thrombocytopenia as a platelet count below 100 × 10^3 cells/mm^3.

The outcome at hospital discharge was defined as death for those who died in hospital or were palliatively discharged (discharged home for palliative care with the expectation of an early death, as per common practice in Vietnam) and 'survived' in all other cases.

Data analysis

Data was analysed using IBM SPSS Statistics for Windows (IBM Corp., Armonk, NY). Depending on the distribution, continuous data were presented as mean (95% confidence interval) or median (interquartile range) and categorical data as number (percentage). To evaluate the predictive value of SOFA, qSOFA score, white blood cell counts, C-Reactive Protein (CRP) and procalcitonin levels, a receiver operating characteristic (ROC) curve and the area under the curve (AUC) were calculated along with the sensitivity, specificity, positive and negative predictive values, positive and negative likelihood ratios associated with the cut-off value that gave the highest difference between sensitivity and (1-specificity) (Youden index). Since procalcitonin level was obtained by a semi-quantitative test that was only quantitatively measured for levels under 100 ng/mL, the result of "above 100 ng/mL" was considered as 100 ng/mL. The Mann Whitney U test and Kruskal Wallis test were used to analyze continuous variables and the Chi-square and Fisher's exact were used for bivariate analyses as appropriated. Logistic regression models were used to calculate unadjusted odds ratios (ORs) and 95% confidence intervals (CIs) for associations between clinical, laboratory characteristics and case fatality rate. Comparison of AUC between different ROC curves was performed using a nonparametric approach [16]. Cox proportional hazards regression was used to identify variables that predicted clinical outcomes. Variables for inclusion were selected by review of the literature (age, HIV infection status, neutropenia, SOFA score and aetiology of CABSI). All tests were two-tailed and differences were considered statistically significant at p values ≤0.05.

Results

Among 400 patients with community acquired bloodstream infections (CABSI) there were 393 patients with infection with one bacterium included in this analysis, 7 dual infection cases were excluded (including 3 HIV infected cases with co-infection of *T. marneffei* and *S. aureus*, *Escherichia hermannii* or *Salmonella group D*; 1 case with *S. aureus* and *K. pneumoniae*, 1 case with *Enterococcus faecalis* and viridans streptococci, 1 case with *E. coli* and *K. pneumoniae* and 1 case with *S. aureus* and *E. coli* co-infection). Gram-negative bacteria dominated (70.7%, 278/393), comprising *Enterobacteriaceae* (50.9%, 200/393) and non-*Enterobacteriaceae* Gram-negative bacteria (19.8%, 78/393) followed by Gram-positive bacteria 29.3% (115/393).

Clinical characteristics, aetiology of CABSI and organ failure

The median age of patients included was 48 years (IQR 36–60), with 271 males and a male to female ratio of 2.2:1. There was a history of chronic disease in 27% of patients, with the highest prevalence in patients with *Enterobacteriaceae* BSI, 34% (38/200). Thirty-eight percent (150/393) of patients were transferred from another hospital (< 48 h) for the current illness episode. The median time from onset of illness to hospitalisation at the study site was 5 days and 36.9% (145/393) were admitted directly to critical care.

Concurrent meningitis was confirmed in 18.3% (72/393) and pneumonia in 24.9% (98/393) of patients, with both conditions occurring in 2.8% (11/393) of patients with CABSI. Gram-positive organisms were isolated from 72.2% (52/72) of those with meningitis, *Enterobacteriaceae* in 18.1% (13/72) and non-*Enterobacteriaceae* Gram-negative bacteria in 9.7% (7/72), see Table 1 for details. Concurrent meningitis was found in 6.5% (13/200) patients with *Enterobacteriaceae* BSI, 9.0% (7/71) patients with non-*Enterobacteriaceae* Gram-negative bacteria BSI and 45.2% (52/115) patients with gram positive BSI. In the 98 cases of pneumonia the causative pathogens isolated from blood were *Enterobacteriaceae* (46.9%, 46/98), non-*Enterobacteriaceae* Gram-negative bacteria (25.5%, 25/98) and Gram-positive bacteria (27.6%, 27/98) (see Additional file 1: Table S1).

A further 8.4% (33/393) of patients presented with or developed at least one abscess, of which 2 patients (6.1%) had 2 abscess foci and 1 patient (3.0%) had 3 abscess foci in different locations. The locations were 16/37 (43.2%) liver, 8 (21%) skin, 4 (10.8%) muscle, 3 (8.1%) brain, 3 (8.1%) spleen, 2 (5.4%) lung, 1 (2.7%) eyelid. Endocarditis was confirmed by echocardiography in 4.1% (16/393) patients. These were due to *Staphylococcus aureus* (7/16, 43.8%), viridans group *streptococci* (4/16, 28.6%), *Enterococcus* species (3/16, 18.8%), *Klebsiella pneumoniae* (1/16, 6.25%) and *Pseudomonas aeruginosa* (1/16, 6.25%). The distribution of aetiology by the foci of infection is presented in Additional file 1: Table S1.

On the day of admission to the study hospital, BSI patients had a median SOFA score of 3 (IQR 1–7) and 78.1% (307/393) of patients had dysfunction of at least one organ. The SOFA score differed significantly between patients admitted direct to CCU (median of 7, IQR 4–12) and medical wards (median of 2, IQR 0–4) ($p < 0.001$). *Enterobacteriaceae* BSIs accounted for most cases with SOFA score above 12 (74% or 28/38, vs. 48% (172/355) in patients with SOFA score ≤ 12, $p = 0.003$) or more than 3 organ dysfunctions (60% or 47/78, vs. 49% or 153/315 in patients with ≤3 organ dysfunctions, $p = 0.065$). qSOFA score was ≥2 in 28.6% (71/248) of patients that were initially admitted to medical wards. The unadjusted associations between clinical factors and case fatality are presented in Table 1.

Laboratory results and inflammatory markers

The proportions of patients with white blood cells count $< 4 \times 10^9$/l, $4–12 \times 10^9$/l and $> 12 \times 10^9$/l were 11.8% (46/389), 47% (183/389) and 41.1% (160/389) respectively. Neutropenia, severe anaemia and thrombocytopenia was presented in 7.2% (28/388), 8% (31/389) and 43.4% (169/389) patients with BSI on admission to the study hospital, respectively. The proportion of patients with RIFLE-F, increased lactate, procalcitonin or CRP were not significantly different when classified by bacterial aetiology (*Enterobacteriaceae*, non-*Enterobacteriaceae* and Gram-positive). Lactate levels were only available for 73 patients and 52/73 (69.9%) patients had lactate level ≥ 2 mmol/L on admission. The median lactate level increased significantly with increasing SOFA score; from 1.23 mmol/L (IQR: 0.99–2.04 mmol/L) in those with a SOFA score < 6, to 7.89 mmol/L (IQR: 3.7–10.38) in those with a SOFA score > 12 ($p < 0.001$, Kruskal Wallis test). There was no significant difference between median lactate levels in those with qSOFA < 2 and qSOFA≥2 ($p = 0.055$, Mann-Whitney U test). Laboratory factors associated with case mortality was showed in

Table 1 Clinical characteristic on admission of patients with bloodstream infection

Factor	Proportion	Case fatality rate	Unadjusted odds ratios (95%CI) for case fatality	P values
Age (yrs)				
≤ 40 years old	122/393 (31%)	27 (22.1%)	1	
41–55 years old	152/393 (38.7%)	46 (30.3%)	1.527 (0.881–2.646)	0.131
≥ 56 years old	119/393 (30.3%)	37 (31.1%)_	1.588 (0.891–2.828)	0.117
Male sex (%)	271/393 (69.0%)	84 (31.0%)	1.659 (1.002–2.746)	0.049
Any previous hospitalisation (%)	150/393 (38.2%)	62 (41.3%)	2.862 (1.819–4.503)	< 0.001
Any antibiotic prior to NHTD hospitalisation (%)	50/150 (33.3%)	23 (46.0%)	1.332 (0.671–2.646)	0.412
Time from onset to current hospitalisation < 5 days	217/393 (55.2%)	57 (26.3%)	0.827 (0.532–1.286)	0.399
Direct ICU admission	145/393 (36.9%)	68 (46.9%)	4.331 (2.720–6.898)	< 0.001
Any history of medical disease	106/393 (27.0%)	44 (41.5%)	2.376 (1.479–3.818)	< 0.001
HIV	19/393 (4.8%)	10 (52.6%)	3.044 (1.202–7.710)	0.019
Moderate or severe liver disease	53/393 (13.5%)	25 (47.2%)	2.679 (1.481–4.844)	0.001
Diabetes	25/393 (6.4%)	7 (28.0%)	1.001 (0.406–2.466)	0.999
Concurrent foci of infection				
Radiology-confirmed pneumonia on admission	98/393 (24.9%)[a]	29 (29.6%)	1.11 (0.671–1.837)	0.684
Lumbar puncture confirmed meningitis on admission	72/393 (18.3%)[b]	19 (26.4%)	0.906 (0.509–1.614)	0.738
Heart valve vegetations during hospitalisation	16/393 (4.1%)	4 (25.0%)	0.852 (0.269–2.701)	0.786
Any abscess during hospitalisation	33/393 (8.4%)[c]	6 (18.2%)	0.547 (0.219–1.364)	0.196
Organ dysfunction on admission				
Cardiovascular	65/393 (16.5%)	52 (80.0%)	18.621 (9.522–36.415)	< 0.001
Respiratory	87/393 (22.1%)	53 (60.9%)	6.81 (4.057–11.431)	< 0.001
CNS	105/393 (26.7%)	55 (52.4%)	4.66 (2.876–7.551)	< 0.001
Hepatic	146/393 (37.2%)	57 (39.0%)	2.344 (1.494–3.678)	< 0.001
Renal	153/393 (38.9%)	66 (43.1%)	3.379 (2.139–5.339)	< 0.001
Coagulation	226/393 (57.5%)	85 (37.6%)	3.424 (2.070–5.663)	< 0.001

[a]Isolates from blood in patients with pneumonia were *K. pneumoniae* (22.4%, 22/98), *E. coli* (16.3%, 16/98), *S. maltophilia* (11.2%, 11/98), *Burkholderia pseudomallei* (8.2%, 8/98), *S. aureus* (7.1%, 7/98) and *S. suis* (7.1%, 7/98) and other pathogens (23.5%, 27/98)
[b]Isolates from blood in patients with meningitis were *S. suis* (40/72, 55.6%), *K. pneumoniae* (8/72, 11.1%), *Stenotrophomonas maltophilia* (7/72, 9.7%), *S. aureus* (5/72, 6.9%). *Enterococcus* species (2/72, 2.8%), *Listeria* species (2/72, 2.8%), *E. coli* (2/72, 2,8%), *Salmonella enterica (2/72,2.8%)* and each of *S. pneumoniae*, beta hemolytic *Streptococcus*, *viridans* group *Streptococcus* and *Enterobacter* species (1/72, 1.4%)
[c]There were 16 cases with liver abscess with isolates from blood were *K. pneumoniae* (8/16 or 50%), *E. coli* and *Salmonella enterica* (2/16 of each, or 12.5%), *Aeromonas* species, *Enterobacter* species, *S. suis* and *viridans* group *streptococci* (1/16 of each, 6.3%)

Table 2. There was no unadjusted associated between procalcitonin and CRP levels with case fatality rates.

Mortality and associated factors

The overall case-fatality of CABSI was 28% (110/393), of which 71.8% (79/110) occurred within 7 days of admission to the study hospital. Case fatality rates in patients with CABSI due to *Enterobacteriaceae*, non-*Enterobacteriaceae* Gram-negative bacteria and Gram-positive bacteria were 33.5%, 25.6% and 20%, respectively. Among the most common isolates, the case fatality was 35.2% (31/88) in *K. pneumoniae*, 32.8% (21/64) in *Escherichia coli*, 9.3% (4/43) in *Streptococcus suis*, 15.4% (6/39) in *Stenotrophomonas maltophilia* and 32.4% (11/34) in *S. aureus*. The case-fatality in patients directly admitted to CCU was 46.9% (68/145).

Organ dysfunction was associated with higher risk of in-hospital mortality (33.2% patients with at least one organ dysfunction on admission to the study hospital vs 9.3% patients without, $p < 0.001$). Case fatality rate increased with increasing SOFA score (Fig. 1). The mortality in patients with 1, 2, 3 and more than 4 organs dysfunction was 17% (17/100), 19.5% (16/82), 31.9% (15/47) and 69.2% (54/78), respectively. The highest case fatality rates were observed in patients with cardiovascular, respiratory and central nervous system (CNS) dysfunction, 80% (52/65), 60.9% (53/87), 52.4% (55/105), respectively. qSOFA < 2 was associated with lower mortality compared with qSOFA ≥2, 18.8% (26/138) vs 40.6% (63/155), $p < 0.001$. Among patients admitted directly to CCU, SOFA performed well at predicting in-hospital mortality (AUC 0.858, 95%CI 0.793–0.922)

Table 2 Laboratory characteristics on admission

	Proportion	Case fatality	Unadjusted odds ratios (95%CI) for case fatality	*P* values
Neutropenia (< 1500 cell/mm^3) (%)	28/388 (7.2%)	22 (78.6%)	11.682 (4.588–29.746)	< 0.001
Hemoglobin< 80 g/L	31/389 (8.0%)	11 (35.5%)	1.459 (0.675–3.156)	0.337
RIFLE criteria				
No renal dysfunction	283/386 (73.3%)	56 (19.8%)	1	
RIFLE-risk	50/386 (13.0%)	16 (32.0%)	1.908 (0.984–3.699)	0.056
RIFLE-failure	52/386 (13.5%)	35 (67.3%)	8.346 (4.361–15.971)	< 0.001
Hypoalbuminemia (albumin ≤30 g/L)	72/245 (29.4%)	39 (54.2%)	3.263 (1.839–5.789)	< 0.001
Aspartate Aminotransferase (AST) ≥ 2 ULN	153/379 (40.4%)	65 (42.5%)	3.435 (2.150–5.487)	< 0.001
Alanine aminotransferase (ALT) ≥ 2 ULN	109/378 (28.8%)	45 (41.3%)	2.449 (1.520–3.947)	< 0.001
Platelet < 100 × 10^3/mm^3	169/389 (43.4%)	70 (41.4%)	3.282 (2.068–5.208)	< 0.001
Procalcitonin				
PCT ≤ 0.005 ng/mL (%)	6/239 (2.5%)	2 (33.3%)	1	
PCT > 0.005–2 ng/mL (%)	83/239 (34.7%)	11 (13.3%)	0.306 (0.050–1.871)	0.2
PCT > 2–10 ng/mL (%)	59/239 (24.7%)	20 (33.9%)	1.026 (0.173–6.087)	0.978
PCT > 10–100 ng/mL (%)	69/239 (28.9%)	29 (42.0%)	1.45 (0.249–8.457)	0.68
PCT > 100 ng/mL (%)	22/239 (9.2%)	14 (63.6%)	3.5 (0.520–23.559)	0.198
C-reactive protein (CRP) (median, IQR) (mg/L)				
CRP less than 5 mg/L (%)	14/341 (4.1%)	4 (28.6%)	1	
CRP from 5.01 to 20 mg/L (%)	26/341 (7.6%)	4 (15.4%)	0.455 (0.094–2.195)	0.326
CRP from 20.001 to 100 mg/L (%)	112/341 (32.8%)	29 (25.9%)	0.873 (0.254–3.001)	0.83
CRP more than 100 mg/L (%)	189/341 (55.4%)	56 (29.6%)	1.053 (0.317–3.498)	0.933

ULN upper limit of normal; *RIFLE* Risk, Injury, Failure, Loss of kidney function, and End-stage kidney disease

while qSOFA was a poor predictor (AUC 0.692, 95%CI 0.605–0.780) in this population. However, outside of CCU, regardless of eventual CCU admission, both SOFA and qSOFA had poor predictive validity (AUC 0.667, 95%CI 0.577–0.758 and AUC 0.527, 95%CI 0.424–0.630, respectively).

Table 3 shows the prognostic validity of the Youden index of SOFA, qSOFA, WBC, CRP and PCT on admission to NHTD in all patients. The SOFA score was more accurate than qSOFA in predicting mortality (AUC = 0.795 vs 0.658, $p < 0.001$); PCT (AUC = 0.703), and WBC (AUC = 0.642) was more accurate than CRP (AUC =

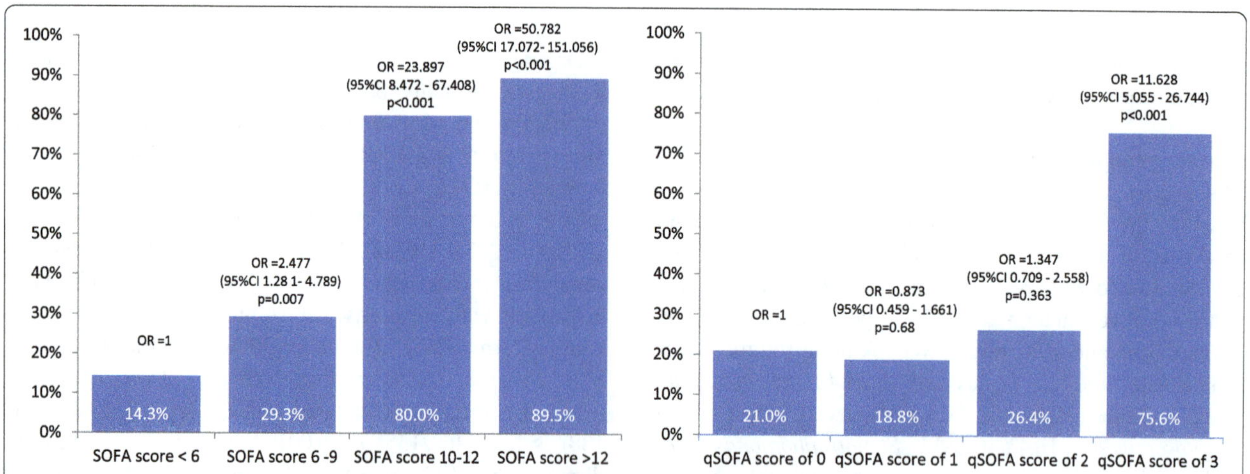

Fig. 1 Case fatality rate by the SOFA and qSOFA scores within the first 24 h of admission

Table 3 Performance of initial SOFA score, qSOFA score, white blood cells, C-reactive protein and procalcitonin, in prediction of in-hospital mortality

	SOFA ($n = 393$)	qSOFA ($n = 393$)	WBC ($n = 389$)	CRP ($n = 341$)	Procalcitonin ($n = 239$)
AUC (95% CI)	0.795 (0.741–0.850)	0.658 (0.595–0.721)	0.642 (0.576–0.708)	0.561 (0.492–0.630)	0.703 (0.629–0.776)
Cut-off value	≥ 9	≥ 3	≤ 7.39	≥ 210	≥ 5.49
Sensitivity	53.6%	30.9%	77.9%	35.5%	69.7%
Specificity	94.7%	96.1%	49.5%	75.8%	63.2%
Positive predictive value	79.7%	75.6%	79.9%	35.5%	46.9%
Negative predictive value	84.0%	78.2%	46.6%	75.8%	81.8%
Positive likelihood ratio	10.1194	7.9521	1.5430	1.4667	1.8945
Negative likelihood ratio	0.4896	0.7189	0.4470	0.8511	0.4789

SOFA Sequential Organ Failure Assessment, *qSOFA* quick Sequential Organ Failure Assessment, *WBC* white blood cell, *CRP* C-reactive protein

0.561) in predicting mortality ($P < 0.001$ and $P = 0.0498$ respectively).

In unadjusted association analysis, higher mortality was associated with male sex, any previous hospitalisation, direct CCU admission, history of HIV infection, moderate severe liver diseases and. Analysis, male sex, previous hospitalisation prior to NHTD admission, any history of chronic disease, history of moderate or severe liver diseases, HIV infection, organ dysfunctions on admission, neutropenia, haemoglobin < 80 g/L, RIFLE failure (RIFLE-F), hypoalbuminemia (< 30 g/L), elevated liver enzymes (> 2 times the upper limit of normal), thrombocytopenia ($< 100 \times 10^3/mm^3$) and were associated with increased in-hospital mortality (p values < 0.05). In Cox regression proportional hazards model, HIV infection (HR = 3.145, $p = 0.001$), neutropenia (HR = 2.442, $p = 0.002$), SOFA score 1-point increment (HR = 1.19, $p < 0.001$) and infection with *Enterobacteriaceae* (HR = 1.722, $p = 0.037$) were significant risk factors for in-hospital mortality (Table 4).

Discussion

This retrospective study describes the clinical characteristics and outcomes in this high-risk group of patients with community acquired BSI. Multi-organ dysfunction and case-fatality rates were high in all aetiological bacterial groups. SOFA score on CCU admission had good prognostic accuracy for in-hospital mortality whilst qSOFA, WBC, CRP and PCT did not.

BSI patients admitted directly to CCU in our study had a median SOFA score of 7 (IQR 4–12), comparable with large-scale validation studies of Sepsis-3 criteria in the US (median of 6, IQR 3–9) [10] and Australia and New Zealand (median of 5, IQR 3–8) [7]. The proportion of bacteraemic patients with qSOFA of 2 or above in our study (39.4%) was also higher than in studies of sepsis conducted in high income countries (10–27%) [8, 10]. The percentage of patients with pneumonia in our CABSI cohort (24.9%) was lower than or similar to other studies on CABSI (24–38%) [17–19]. *K. pneumoniae* was the most common pathogen isolated from bacteremic patients with pneumonia in our study, reflecting its role here as an important cause of community acquired pneumonia [20]. We also confirmed the role of *S. suis* as the leading pathogen causing BSI associated with meningitis in Viet Nam [21]. Our findings further confirmed the reduction of *Neisseria meningitidis* in Viet Nam which was reported in 0.5% of blood isolates [22] and around 4.4% of cerebral spinal fluid (CSF) isolates before 2005 [23]. We also report the high prevalence of *Enterobacteriacaea* (18.1% or 13/72) as a cause of meningitis in adult BSI patients compared to previous studies from Viet Nam (13.5% or 30/222 of CSF isolates from 1996 and 2005) [23], Iceland (11.3% or 12/106

Table 4 Cox proportional hazards model of factors associated with all-cause in-hospital case fatality

Variable	Hazard ratio (95% CI)	*P*-value
Age (each increase of 1 year)	1.006 (0.994–1.019)	0.321
HIV infection	3.145 (1.569–6.305)	0.001
Absolute neutrophil count < 1500 cells/mm^3	2.442 (1.381–4.319)	0.002
SOFA score (each increase of 1 point)	1.190 (1.146–1.235)	< 0.001
Aetiology of CABSI (gram-positive bacterial infection as reference)		
Enterobacteriaceae infections	1.722 (1.034–2.869)	0.037
Non *Enterobacteriaceae* Gram-negative infections	1.528 (0.824–2.834)	0.178

of positive CSF cultures during 1995–2010) [24] and Denmark (6.1% or 88/1437 during 1991–2000) [25]. The high prevalence of meningitis associated with *Enterobacteriaceae* in this setting may be related to *Strongyloides* hyperinfection, given the evidence for high seroprevalence of *Strongyloides* infection in this population [26].

A review of CABSI in south and Southeast Asia from 1990 to 2010 showed the most frequent isolates in adult patients were *Salmonella enterica* (37.8%), *S. aureus* (12.6%) and *E. coli* (12%) with an overall case fatality rate of 9% [27]. In North America and Europe, there was a significant increase in bloodstream infection caused by Gram-negative bacteria, and case fatality rates in the period 1992–2008 were 13–20.6% in patients with CABSI [1]. The overall case fatality of 28% in our CABSI patients was lower than in a study in Thailand [3] from 2004 and 2010 (37.5%) where the most common pathogens were *E. coli* (23.1%), *Burkholderia pseudomallei* (19.3%), and *S. aureus* (8.2%) but higher than in Cambodia (22.1%) where there was a predominance of *E. coli* (29.7%), *Salmonella* spp. (14.4%) and *B. pseudomallei* (12.6%) in the period of 2007–2010) [28]. The higher case fatality in Thailand and our study may relate to the shift in the aetiology of CABSI from *Salmonella* to other Gram-negative bacteria observed since the last decade.

Organ dysfunction is strongly associated with in-hospital mortality. In a multicentre study of severe sepsis in Spain, case fatality in patients with more than 4 organs with dysfunction was 78.4% [29]. From a large prospective European study, case fatality in patients with more than 3 organs with dysfunction was 58% and the, highest in-hospital mortality rates were observed in patients with coagulation failure (45%) [5]. In high income settings, among ICU patients with suspected infection, the predictive accuracy for in-hospital mortality is higher using SOFA than qSOFA (AUC = 0.74; 95% CI, 0.73–0.76; vs AUC = 0.66; 95% CI, 0.64–0.68) whilst outside of ICU, the predictive validity of qSOFA (AUC = 0.81; 95% CI, 0.80–0.82) was better than SOFA (AUC = 0.79; 95% CI, 0.78–0.80; $P < 0.001$) [10]. In a prospective study of patients with suspected infection admitted to an emergency department in Norway, the qSOFA had poor performance to predict 7-day and 30-day mortality with AUCs < 0.6 in both multiple imputation and complete case analysis [30]. The usefulness of qSOFA in low- and middle income countries has not been well established. Procalcitonin levels can serve as a useful marker to rule out sepsis and discriminate contamination from true bloodstream infection [31, 32]. Our study shows a poor prediction of initial PCT and CRP in prediction of mortality.

Our study has some major limitations. Firstly, as the study site is a referral hospital specialising in infectious diseases, the aetiologies, clinical manifestations, severity and response to the treatment may be different from those presenting to a general hospital. Secondly, SOFA and qSOFA was calculated based on the worst parameters within 24 h of admission to the study hospital which may not accurately present the severity of infection at arrival. Thirdly, due to the retrospective design, the data collection was incomplete and unbalanced distribution of missing data can be a bias in the prediction models The utilisation of SOFA and qSOFA needs to be validated prospectively in other setting at different time points of assessment.

Conclusions

In conclusion, community acquired BSI has a high rate of organ dysfunction and mortality in this setting. SOFA performed well at predicting those at risk of death admitted directly to CCU, whilst qSOFA performed poorly. Further prospective validation in low- and middle income settings is needed.

Abbreviations

AUC: Area under the curve; BSI: Bloodstream infection; CABSI: Community acquired bloodstream infection; CCU: Critical care unit; CI: Confidence interval; CNS: Central nervous system; CRP: C-reactive protein; CSF: Cerebral spinal fluid; HR: Hazard ratio; ICU: Intensive care unit; IQR: Interquartile range; LMICs: Low- and middle income countries; NHSN: National Healthcare Safety Network; NHTD: National Hospital for Tropical Diseases; OR: Odds ratio; PCT: Procalcitonin; qSOFA: Quick sequential organ failure assessment; ROC: Receiver operating characteristic; SOFA: Sequential organ failure assessment

Acknowledgments

We gratefully acknowledge the General Planning Department in National Hospital for Tropical Diseases for providing the list of medical records. We also thank Nguyen The Hung, Nguyen Thi Hoa, Bui Linh Chi and Hoang Bao Long for their assistance with data collection.

Funding

This study was funded by the Wellcome Trust of Great Britain.

Authors' contributions

VQD designed the study, collected & analysed the data and wrote the first & final draft; NTL, VNH, NDHP collected, entered data, drafted sections of the manuscript; NTL was responsible for cleaning data, analysis and drafted sections of the manuscript; NVT, NVK contributed to study design and were responsible for laboratory and clinical care, provided revisions of the manuscript edited the final draft; HRvD and AB helped with interpretation of the data, revision of the manuscript and edited the final draft; BN involved to design the study, interpreted the data, revised the manuscript and edited the final draft. All authors approved of the final draft.

Consent for publication

Not applicable.

Competing interests

HRvD is a member of the editorial board (Associate Editor) of the BMC Infectious Diseases. The authors otherwise declare that they have no competing interests.

Author details
[1]Department of Infectious Diseases, Hanoi Medical University, no 1 Ton That Tung street, Dong Da district, Hanoi, Vietnam. [2]Wellcome Trust Major Overseas Programme, Oxford University Clinical Research Unit, Hanoi, 78 Giai Phong street, Dong Da district, Hanoi, Vietnam. [3]National Hospital for Tropical Diseases, 78 Giai Phong street, Dong Da district, Hanoi, Vietnam. [4]Department of Microbiology, Hanoi Medical University, no 1 Ton That Tung street, Dong Da district, Hanoi, Vietnam. [5]Nuffield Department of Clinical Medicine, Centre for Tropical Medicine, University of Oxford, Oxford, UK.

References

1. Goto M, Al-Hasan MN. Overall burden of bloodstream infection and nosocomial bloodstream infection in North America and Europe. Clin Microbiol infect off Publ Eur Soc Clin Microbiol. Infect Dis. 2013;19:501–9.
2. Kochanek KD, Murphy SL, Xu J, Deaths T-VB. Final data for 2014. Natl vital stat rep cent dis control Prev Natl cent health stat Natl vital stat. Syst. 2016; 65:1–122.
3. Kanoksil M, Jatapai A, Peacock SJ, Limmathurotsakul D. Epidemiology, Microbiology and mortality associated with community-acquired bacteremia in Northeast Thailand: a multicenter surveillance study. PLoS One. 2013;8:e54714.
4. El-Menyar A, Thani HA, Zakaria ER, Zarour A, Tuma M, AbdulRahman H, et al. Multiple organ dysfunction syndrome (MODS): is it preventable or inevitable? Int J Clin Med. 2013;03:722.
5. Sakr Y, Lobo SM, Moreno RP, Gerlach H, Ranieri VM, Michalopoulos A, et al. Patterns and early evolution of organ failure in the intensive care unit and their relation to outcome. Crit Care Lond Engl. 2012;16:R222.
6. Singer M, Deutschman CS, Seymour CW, Shankar-Hari M, Annane D, Bauer M, et al. The third international consensus definitions for Sepsis and septic shock (Sepsis-3). JAMA. 2016;315:801.
7. Raith EP, Udy AA, Bailey M, McGloughlin S, MacIsaac C, Bellomo R, et al. Prognostic accuracy of the SOFA score, SIRS criteria, and qSOFA score for in-hospital mortality among adults with suspected infection admitted to the intensive care unit. JAMA. 2017;317:290–300.
8. Freund Y, Lemachatti N, Krastinova E, Van Laer M, Claessens Y-E, Avondo A, et al. Prognostic accuracy of Sepsis-3 criteria for in-hospital mortality among patients with suspected infection presenting to the emergency department. JAMA. 2017;317:301–8.
9. Churpek MM, Snyder A, Han X, Sokol S, Pettit N, Howell MD, et al. Quick Sepsis-related organ failure assessment, systemic inflammatory response syndrome, and early warning scores for detecting clinical deterioration in infected patients outside the intensive care unit. Am J Respir Crit Care Med. 2017;195:906–11.
10. Seymour CW, Liu VX, Iwashyna TJ, Brunkhorst FM, Rea TD, Scherag A, et al. Assessment of clinical criteria for Sepsis: for the third international consensus definitions for Sepsis and septic shock (Sepsis-3). JAMA. 2016;315: 762–74.
11. Centers for Disease Control and Prevention. NHSN Organism List. 2017. https://www.cdc.gov/nhsn/xls/master-organism-com-commensals-lists.xlsx. Accessed 7 Oct 2017.
12. Dat VQ, Vu HN. Nguyen the H, Nguyen HT, Hoang LB, vu Tien Viet D, et al. bacterial bloodstream infections in a tertiary infectious diseases hospital in northern Vietnam: aetiology, drug resistance, and treatment outcome. BMC Infect Dis. 2017;17:493.
13. World Health Organization. Invasive Bacterial Vaccine Preventable Diseases (IB-VPD) Surveillance Network Case definitions. 2012. http://www.who.int/immunization/monitoring_surveillance/resources/IB-VPD_Case_Defs.pdf. Accessed 7 Oct 2017.
14. Centers for Disease Control and Prevention. CDC/NHSN Surveillance Definitions for Specific Types of Infections. 2018. https://www.cdc.gov/nhsn/pdfs/pscmanual/17pscnosinfdef_current.pdf. Accessed 29 Aug 2018.
15. Uchino S, Bellomo R, Goldsmith D, Bates S, Ronco C. An assessment of the RIFLE criteria for acute renal failure in hospitalized patients. Crit Care Med. 2006;34:1913–7.
16. DeLong ER, DeLong DM, Clarke-Pearson DL. Comparing the areas under two or more correlated receiver operating characteristic curves: a nonparametric approach. Biometrics. 1988;44:837–45.
17. Zahar J-R, Timsit J-F, Garrouste-Orgeas M, Français A, Vesin A, Vesim A, et al. Outcomes in severe sepsis and patients with septic shock: pathogen species and infection sites are not associated with mortality. Crit Care Med. 2011;39:1886–95.
18. Park HK, Kim WY, Kim MC, Jung W, Ko BS. Quick sequential organ failure assessment compared to systemic inflammatory response syndrome for predicting sepsis in emergency department. J Crit Care. 2017;42:12–7.
19. Artero A, Zaragoza R, Camarena JJ, Sancho S, González R, Nogueira JM. Prognostic factors of mortality in patients with community-acquired bloodstream infection with severe sepsis and septic shock. J Crit Care. 2010; 25:276–81.
20. Peto L, Nadjm B, Horby P, Ngan TTD, van Doorn R, Kinh NV, et al. The bacterial aetiology of adult community-acquired pneumonia in Asia: a systematic review. Trans R Soc Trop Med Hyg. 2014;108:326–37.
21. Huong V, Ha N, Huy N, Peter H, Nghia H, Thiem V, et al. Epidemiology, clinical manifestations, and outcomes of Streptococcus suis infection in humans. Emerg Infect Dis. 2014;20:1105–14.
22. Hoa NT, Diep TS, Wain J, Parry CM, Hien TT, Smith MD, et al. Community-acquired septicaemia in southern Viet Nam: the importance of multidrug-resistant Salmonella typhi. Trans R Soc Trop Med Hyg. 1998;92:503–8.
23. Mai NTH, Chau TTH, Thwaites G, Chuong LV, Sinh DX, Nghia HDT, et al. Dexamethasone in Vietnamese adolescents and adults with bacterial meningitis. N Engl J Med. 2007;357:2431–40.
24. Thornórðardóttir A, Erlendsdóttir H, Sigurðardóttir B, Harðardóttir H, Reynisson IK, Gottfreðsson M, et al. Bacterial meningitis in adults in Iceland, 1995-2010. Scand J Infect Dis. 2014;46:354–60.
25. Meyer CN, Samuelsson IS, Galle M, Bangsborg JM. Adult bacterial meningitis: aetiology, penicillin susceptibility, risk factors, prognostic factors and guidelines for empirical antibiotic treatment. Clin Microbiol Infect. 2004;10: 709–17.
26. Diep NTN, Thai PQ, Trang NNM, Jager J, Fox A, Horby P, et al. Strongyloides stercoralis seroprevalence in Vietnam. Epidemiol Infect. 2017;145(15):3214–8.
27. Deen J, von Seidlein L, Andersen F, Elle N, White NJ, Lubell Y. Community-acquired bacterial bloodstream infections in developing countries in south and Southeast Asia: a systematic review. Lancet Infect Dis. 2012;12:480–7.
28. Vlieghe ER, Phe T, Smet BD, Veng HC, Kham C, Lim K, et al. Bloodstream infection among adults in Phnom Penh, Cambodia: key pathogens and resistance patterns. PLoS One. 2013;8:e59775.
29. Blanco J, Muriel-Bombín A, Sagredo V, Taboada F, Gandía F, Tamayo L, et al. Incidence, organ dysfunction and mortality in severe sepsis: a Spanish multicentre study. Crit Care. 2008;12:R158.
30. Askim Å, Moser F, Gustad LT, Stene H, Gundersen M, Åsvold BO, et al. Poor performance of quick-SOFA (qSOFA) score in predicting severe sepsis and mortality – a prospective study of patients admitted with infection to the emergency department. Scand J Trauma Resusc Emerg Med. 2017;25:56.
31. Riedel S, Melendez JH, An AT, Rosenbaum JE, Zenilman JM. Procalcitonin as a marker for the detection of bacteremia and Sepsis in the emergency department. Am J Clin Pathol. 2011;135:182–9.
32. Schuetz P, Mueller B, Trampuz A. Serum Procalcitonin for discrimination of blood contamination from bloodstream infection due to coagulase-negative staphylococci. Infection. 2007;35:352.

Permissions

All chapters in this book were first published in ID, by BioMed Central; hereby published with permission under the Creative Commons Attribution License or equivalent. Every chapter published in this book has been scrutinized by our experts. Their significance has been extensively debated. The topics covered herein carry significant findings which will fuel the growth of the discipline. They may even be implemented as practical applications or may be referred to as a beginning point for another development.

The contributors of this book come from diverse backgrounds, making this book a truly international effort. This book will bring forth new frontiers with its revolutionizing research information and detailed analysis of the nascent developments around the world.

We would like to thank all the contributing authors for lending their expertise to make the book truly unique. They have played a crucial role in the development of this book. Without their invaluable contributions this book wouldn't have been possible. They have made vital efforts to compile up to date information on the varied aspects of this subject to make this book a valuable addition to the collection of many professionals and students.

This book was conceptualized with the vision of imparting up-to-date information and advanced data in this field. To ensure the same, a matchless editorial board was set up. Every individual on the board went through rigorous rounds of assessment to prove their worth. After which they invested a large part of their time researching and compiling the most relevant data for our readers.

The editorial board has been involved in producing this book since its inception. They have spent rigorous hours researching and exploring the diverse topics which have resulted in the successful publishing of this book. They have passed on their knowledge of decades through this book. To expedite this challenging task, the publisher supported the team at every step. A small team of assistant editors was also appointed to further simplify the editing procedure and attain best results for the readers.

Apart from the editorial board, the designing team has also invested a significant amount of their time in understanding the subject and creating the most relevant covers. They scrutinized every image to scout for the most suitable representation of the subject and create an appropriate cover for the book.

The publishing team has been an ardent support to the editorial, designing and production team. Their endless efforts to recruit the best for this project, has resulted in the accomplishment of this book. They are a veteran in the field of academics and their pool of knowledge is as vast as their experience in printing. Their expertise and guidance has proved useful at every step. Their uncompromising quality standards have made this book an exceptional effort. Their encouragement from time to time has been an inspiration for everyone.

The publisher and the editorial board hope that this book will prove to be a valuable piece of knowledge for researchers, students, practitioners and scholars across the globe.

List of Contributors

Sung-Yeon Cho, Su-Mi Choi, Jae-Ki Choi, Hyo-Jin Lee, Sun Hee Park, Jung-Hyun Choi and Jin-Hong Yoo
Division of Infectious Diseases, Department of Internal Medicine, College of Medicine, The Catholic University of Korea, St. Mary's Hospital, 222, Banpo-daero, Seocho-gu, Seoul, Republic of Korea
Vaccine Bio Research Institute, College of Medicine, The Catholic University of Korea, St. Mary's Hospital, 222, Banpo-daero, Seocho-gu, Seoul, Republic of Korea

Chulmin Park and Hye-Sun Chun
Vaccine Bio Research Institute, College of Medicine, The Catholic University of Korea, St. Mary's Hospital, 222, Banpo-daero, Seocho-gu, Seoul, Republic of Korea

Dong-Gun Lee
Division of Infectious Diseases, Department of Internal Medicine, College of Medicine, The Catholic University of Korea, St. Mary's Hospital, 222, Banpo-daero, Seocho-gu, Seoul, Republic of Korea
Vaccine Bio Research Institute, College of Medicine, The Catholic University of Korea, St. Mary's Hospital, 222, Banpo-daero, Seocho-gu, Seoul, Republic of Korea
The Catholic Blood and Marrow Transplantation Center, College of Medicine, The Catholic University of Korea, St. Mary's Hospital, 222, Banpo-daero, Seocho-gu, Seoul, Republic of Korea

Yeon-Joon Park
Department of Laboratory Medicine, College of Medicine, The Catholic University of Korea, St. Mary's Hospital, 222, Banpo-daero, Seocho-gu, Seoul, Republic of Korea

Sainan Bian, Yueqiu Zhang and Xiaochun Shi
Department of Infectious Diseases, Peking Union Medical College Hospital, Peking Union Medical College, Chinese Academy of Medical Sciences, No.1 Shuaifuyuan, Dongcheng District, Beijing 100730, China

Xiaoqing Liu and Lifan Zhang
Department of Infectious Diseases, Peking Union Medical College Hospital, Peking Union Medical College, Chinese Academy of Medical Sciences, No.1 Shuaifuyuan, Dongcheng District, Beijing 100730, China
Clinical Epidemiology Unit, International Epidemiology Network, Peking Union Medical College, No.1 Shuaifuyuan, Dongcheng District, Beijing 100730, China

Yao Zhang
Clinical Epidemiology Unit, International Epidemiology Network, Peking Union Medical College, No.1 Shuaifuyuan, Dongcheng District, Beijing 100730, China

Qiwen Yang, Peng Wang and Yingchun Xu
Laboratory Department, Peking Union Medical College Hospital, Liu et al. BMC Infectious Diseases (2016) 16:750 Page 5 of 6 Peking Union Medical College, Chinese Academy of Medical Sciences, No.1 Shuaifuyuan, Dongcheng District, Beijing 100730, China

Roy F. Chemaly
Department of Infectious Diseases, Infection Control and Employee Health, Unit 1460, The University of Texas MD Anderson Cancer Center, 1515 Holcombe Blvd, Houston, TX 77030, USA

Tran Thi Thu Hien, Tran Thi Thanh Huyen, Dao Thanh Quyen and Phan Quoc Hoan
Department of Molecular Biology, 108 Military Central Hospital, Hanoi, Vietnam

Le Huu Song
Department of Molecular Biology, 108 Military Central Hospital, Hanoi, Vietnam
Institute of Clinical Infectious Diseases, 108 Military Central Hospital, Hanoi, Vietnam
Vietnamese - German Centre for Medical Research (VG-CARE), Hanoi, Vietnam

Trinh Van Son
Institute of Clinical Infectious Diseases, 108 Military Central Hospital, Hanoi, Vietnam
Vietnamese - German Centre for Medical Research (VG-CARE), Hanoi, Vietnam

Nguyen Thi Kim Phuong
Department of Clinical Microbiology, 108 Military Central Hospital, Hanoi, Vietnam

Tran Thi Lien
Faculty of Infectious Diseases, Hai Phong Medical University, Hai Phong, Vietnam

Mai Thanh Binh
Department of Gastroenterology, 108 Military Central Hospital, Hanoi, Vietnam
Vietnamese - German Centre for Medical Research (VG-CARE), Hanoi, Vietnam

Hoang Van Tong, Christian G. Meyer and Thirumalaisamy P. Velavan
Institute of Tropical Medicine, University of Tübingen, Tübingen, Germany
Vietnamese - German Centre for Medical Research (VG-CARE), Hanoi, Vietnam

Ngo Tat Trung
Department of Molecular Biology, 108 Military Central Hospital, Hanoi, Vietnam
Vietnamese - German Centre for Medical Research (VG-CARE), Hanoi, Vietnam

Fabianne Carlesse and Antonio Sérgio Petrilli
Institute of Paediatric Oncology, Universidade Federal de São Paulo, Rua Botucatu 743, São Paulo 04037020, Brazil

Paola Cappellano, Milene Gonçalves Quiles, Liana Carballo Menezes and Antonio Carlos Pignatari
Infectious Diseases Division, Universidade Federal de São Paulo, São Paulo, Brazil

Heloise Buys
Department of Paediatrics and Child Health, Red Cross War Memorial Children's Hospital, Klipfontein Road, Cape Town, Rondebosch 7700, South Africa
University of Cape Town, Cape Town, South Africa
Ambulatory and Emergency Paediatrics, Red Cross War Memorial Children's Hospital, Klipfontein Road, Cape Town, Rondebosch 7700, South Africa

Rudzani Muloiwa and Brian Eley
Department of Paediatrics and Child Health, Red Cross War Memorial Children's Hospital, Klipfontein Road, Cape Town, Rondebosch 7700, South Africa
University of Cape Town, Cape Town, South Africa

Colleen Bamford
University of Cape Town, Cape Town, South Africa
National Health Laboratory Service (Groote Schuur Hospital), Cape Town, South Africa

Dayana Fram, Meiry Fernanda Pinto Okuno, Cibele Grothe, Angélica Belasco and Dulce Barbosa
School of Nursing, Paulista School of Nursing, Universidade Federal de São Paulo (Federal University of São Paulo - EPE/UNIFESP), R. Napoleão de Barros 754, São Paulo 04024-002, Brazil

Mônica Taminato
School of Nursing, Paulista School of Nursing, Universidade Federal de São Paulo (Federal University of São Paulo - EPE/UNIFESP), R. Napoleão de Barros 754, São Paulo 04024-002, Brazil
Infection Control Unit, Children's Institute and Institute for the Treatment of Childhood Cancer, School of Medicine, Universidade de São Paulo (University of São Paulo - ITACI/FMUSP), Av. Dr. Enéas Carvalho de Aguiar 647, São Paulo 05403-000, Brazil

Vinicius Ponzio
Division of Infectious Diseases, Escola Paulista de Medicina, Universidade Federal de São Paulo (Paulista School of Medicine, Federal University of São Paulo - EPM/ UNIFESP), R. Napoleão de Barros, 715, 7° andar, São Paulo 04024-002, Brazil

Silvia Regina Manfredi
Division of Dialysis, Hospital do Rim e Hipertensão, Fundação Oswaldo Ramos, (Kidney and Hypertension Hospital, Foundation Oswaldo Ramos - HRIM/FOR), R. Pedro de Toledo 282, São Paulo 04039-030, Brazil

Ricardo Sesso
Division of Nephrology, Paulista School of Medicine, Universidade Federal de São Paulo
(Federal University of São Paulo - EPM/UNIFESP), R. Botucatu 740, São Paulo 04023-900, Brazil

Kristine Hofseth and Leif Kibsgaard
Department of Orthopedic Surgery, Levanger Hospital, Nord-Trøndelag Hospital Trust, Levanger, Norway

Håvard Dalen
Department of Medicine, Levanger Hospital, Nord-Trøndelag Hospital Trust, Levanger, Norway
Cardiac Exercise Research Group, Department of Circulation and Medical Imaging, Norwegian University of Science and Technology (NTNU), Trondheim, Norway
Department of Cardiology, St. Olavs University Hospital, Trondheim, Norway

Solrun Nebb and Angela Kümmel
Department of Laboratory Medicine, Levanger Hospital, Nord-Trøndelag Hospital Trust, Levanger, Norway

Arne Mehl
Department of Medicine, Levanger Hospital, Nord-Trøndelag Hospital Trust, Levanger, Norway
Mid-Norway Sepsis Research Group, Norwegian University of Science and Technology, Trondheim, Norway

Appiah-Korang Labi
Department of Microbiology, Korle-Bu Teaching Hospital, Accra, Republic of Ghana

Noah Obeng-Nkrumah
Microbiology Department, School of Biomedical and Allied Health Sciences, College of Health Sciences, University of Ghana, Accra, Republic of Ghana

Stephanie Bjerrum
Department of Infectious Diseases, Institute of Clinical Research, Odense University Hospital, Sdr. Boulevard 29, Odense C, 5000 Odense, Denmark

Christabel Enweronu-Laryea
Department of Child Health, School of Medicine and Dentistry, College of Health Sciences, University of Ghana, Republic of Ghana

Mercy Jemima Newman
Department of Medical Microbiology, School of Biomedical and Allied Health Sciences, University of Ghana, Accra, Republic of Ghana

Arne Mehl
Department of Medicine, Levanger Hospital, Nord-Trøndelag Hospital Trust, Levanger N-7601, Norway
Unit for Applied Clinical Research, Department of Cancer Research and Molecular Medicine, NTNU, Norwegian University of Science and Technology, Trondheim, Norway
Mid-Norway Sepsis Research Group, Faculty of Medicine, NTNU, Norwegian University of Science and Technology, Trondheim, Norway

Bjørn Olav Åsvold
Mid-Norway Sepsis Research Group, Faculty of Medicine, NTNU, Norwegian University of Science and Technology, Trondheim, Norway
Department of Public Health, NTNU, Norwegian University of Science and Technology, Trondheim, Norway
Department of Endocrinology, St Olavs Hospital, Trondheim University Hospital, Trondheim, Norway

Angela Kümmel
Department of Laboratory Medicine, Levanger Hospital, Nord-Trøndelag Hospital Trust, Levanger, Norway

Stian Lydersen
Regional Centre for Child and Youth Mental Health and Child Welfare - Central Norway, NTNU, Norwegian University of Science and Technology, Trondheim, Norway

Julie Paulsen
Department of Medicine, Levanger Hospital, Nord-Trøndelag Hospital Trust, Levanger N-7601, Norway
Mid-Norway Sepsis Research Group, Faculty of Medicine, NTNU, Norwegian University of Science and Technology, Trondheim, Norway
Centre of Molecular Inflammation Research, Department of Cancer Research and Molecular Medicine, NTNU, Norwegian University of Science and Technology, Trondheim, Norway

Ingvild Haugan
Department of Medical Microbiology, St Olavs Hospital, Trondheim University Hospital, Trondheim, Norway

Erik Solligård
Mid-Norway Sepsis Research Group, Faculty of Medicine, NTNU, Norwegian University of Science and Technology, Trondheim, Norway
Clinic of Anesthesia and Intensive Care, St Olavs Hospital, Trondheim University Hospital, Trondheim, Norway
Department of Circulation and Medical Imaging, NTNU, Norwegian
University of Science and Technology, Trondheim, Norway

Jan Kristian Damås
Mid-Norway Sepsis Research Group, Faculty of Medicine, NTNU, Norwegian University of Science and Technology, Trondheim, Norway
Centre of Molecular Inflammation Research, Department of Cancer Research and Molecular Medicine, NTNU, Norwegian University of Science and Technology, Trondheim, Norway
Department of Infectious Diseases, St Olav's Hospital, Trondheim University Hospital, Trondheim, Norway

Stig Harthug
Department of Research and Development, Haukeland University Hospital, Bergen, Norwa
Department of Clinical Science, University of Bergen, Bergen, Norway

Tom-Harald Edna
Unit for Applied Clinical Research, Department of Cancer Research and Molecular Medicine, NTNU, Norwegian University of Science and Technology, Trondheim, Norway
Department of Surgery, Levanger Hospital, Nord-Trøndelag Hospital Trust, Levanger, Norway

R. P. Schade
Department of Medical Microbiology and Infection control, VU University Medical Center, Amsterdam, The Netherlands

P. H. M. Savelkoul
Department of Medical Microbiology and Infection control, VU University Medical Center, Amsterdam, The Netherlands
Department of Medical Microbiology, Maastricht University Medical Center, Maastricht, The Netherlands

A. Beishuizen
Department of Intensive Care Medicine, VU University Medical Center, Amsterdam, The Netherlands
Department of Intensive Care, Medisch Spectrum Twente, Enschede, The Netherlands

B. Henrich, B. Lamik and C. R. MacKenzie
Institute of Medical Microbiology and Hospital Hygiene, University Clinic of Heinrich-Heine University Düsseldorf, Düsseldorf, Germany

D. Kindgen-Milles
Department of Anesthesiology, University Clinic of Heinrich-Heine University Düsseldorf, Düsseldorf, Germany

A. Helmers and C. Diaz
Department of Microbiology, Merheim Zentrallabor, MVZ synlab Leverkusen GmbH, Leverkusen, Germany

S. G. Sakka
Department of Anesthesiology and Intensive Care Medicine, Medical Center Cologne-Merheim, University Witten/Herdecke, Cologne, Germany

A. E. Nieman
Department of Medical Microbiology and Infection control, VU University Medical Center, Amsterdam, The Netherlands
Laboratory for Medical Microbiology, Immunology and Infection Control, Elisabeth-Twee Steden Hospital, Tilburg, The Netherlands

Håvard Aamodt, Nina Langeland and Bjørn Blomberg
Department of Clinical Science, University of Bergen, Bergen, Norway
Center for Tropical Infectious Diseases, Department of Medicine, Haukeland University Hospital, Bergen, Norway

Stein Christian Mohn
Center for Tropical Infectious Diseases, Department of Medicine, Haukeland University Hospital, Bergen, Norway

Samuel Maselle
Department of Microbiology and Immunology, Muhimbili University of Health and Allied Sciences, Dar es Salaam, Tanzania

Karim P Manji
Department of Pediatrics and Child Health, Muhimbili University of Health and Allied Sciences, Dar es Salaam, Tanzania

Rob Willems
Department of Medical Microbiology, University Medical Center Utrecht, Utrecht, Netherlands

Roland Jureen
National University Health System, Singapore City, Singapore

Pankaj G. Vashi, Natasha Virginkar, Brenten Popiel, Persis Edwin and Digant Gupta
Cancer Treatment Centers of America (CTCA) at Midwestern Regional Medical Center, 2520 Elisha Ave, Zion, Illinois 60099, USA

Francesco Barchiesi and Elena Orsetti
Clinica Malattie Infettive; Università Politecnica delle Marche, Azienda Ospedaliero-Universitaria, Ospedali Riuniti Umberto I°- G.M. Lancisi - G. Salesi, Ancona, Italy

Carlo Catassi
Clinica Pediatrica; Università Politecnica delle Marche, Azienda Ospedaliero-Universitaria, Ospedali Riuniti Umberto I°- G.M. Lancisi - G. Salesi, Ancona, Italy

Patrizia Osimani
Pediatria, Azienda Ospedaliero-Universitaria, Ospedali Riuniti Umberto I°- G.M. Lancisi - G. Salesi, Ancona, Italy

Fabio Santelli
Anestesia e Rianimazione Pediatrica, Azienda Ospedaliero-Universitaria, Ospedali Riuniti Umberto I°- G.M. Lancisi - G. Salesi, Ancona, Italy

Esther Manso
Laboratorio di Microbiologia, Azienda Ospedaliero-Universitaria, Ospedali Riuniti Umberto I°- G.M. Lancisi - G. Salesi, Ancona, Italy

Mei-Yin Lai, Ming-Chou Chiang, Reyin Lien, Ren-Huei Fu and Hsuan-Rong Huang
Division of Pediatric Neonatology, Department of Pediatrics, Chang Gung Memorial Hospital, Taoyuan, Taiwan
College of Medicine, Chang Gung University, Taoyuan, Taiwan

Ming-Horng Tsai
Division of Neonatology and Pediatric Hematology/ Oncology, Department of Pediatrics, Chang Gung Memorial Hospital, Yunlin, Taiwan
College of Medicine, Chang Gung University, Taoyuan, Taiwan

Shih-Ming Chu and Jen-Fu Hsu
Division of Pediatric Neonatology, Department of Pediatrics, Chang Gung Memorial Hospital, Taoyuan, Taiwan
College of Medicine, Chang Gung University, Taoyuan, Taiwan
Linkou Chang Gung Memorial Hospital, No. 5, Fu-Shin Rd., Kwei-Shan, Taoyuan, Taiwan

Chiang-Wen Lee
Department of Nursing, Division of Basic Medical Sciences and Chronic Diseases and Health Promotion Research Center, Chang Gung University of Science and Technology, Chia-Yi, Taiwan
Research Center for Industry of Human Ecology, Chang Gung University of Science and Technology, Taoyuan, Taiwan

Elisabetta Venturini, Carlotta Montagnani, Alessandra Benni, Sabrina Becciani, Elena Chiappini and Maurizio de Martino
Department of Health Sciences, University of Florence, Meyer Children's University Hospital, Florence, Italy

Klaus Peter Biermann and Salvatore De Masi
Meyer Children's Hospital Healthcare Associated Infection Control Committee, Florence, Italy

Luisa Galli
Department of Health Sciences, University of Florence, Meyer Children's University Hospital, Florence, Italy
Meyer Children's Hospital Healthcare Associated Infection Control Committee, Florence, Italy
Pediatric Infectious Diseases Division, Department of Pediatric Medicine, Meyer Children's University Hospital, viale Pieraccini 24, I-50139 Florence, Italy

Cristiano Alicino, Andrea Orsi, Federico Tassinari, Cecilia Trucchi and Giancarlo Icardi
Department of Health Sciences, University of Genoa and Hygiene and Infection Control Unit, IRCCS AOU San Martino-IST teaching Hospital, Genoa, Italy

Daniele Roberto Giacobbe, Giovanni Sarteschi, Valerio Del Bono and Claudio Viscoli
Department of Health Sciences, University of Genoa and Infectious Diseases Unit, IRCCS AOU San Martino-IST teaching Hospital, L.go R. Benzi, 10-16132 Genoa, Italy

Francesco Copello
Occupational Medicine Unit, IRCCS AOU San Martino-IST teaching Hospital, Genoa, Italy

Itaru Nakamura and Shinji Fukushima
Department of Infection Prevention and Control, Tokyo Medical University Hospital, 6-7-1 Nishishinjuku, Shinjuku-ku, Tokyo 160-0023, Japan

Akihiro Sato
Department of Infection Prevention and Control, Tokyo Medical University Hospital, 6-7-1 Nishishinjuku, Shinjuku-ku, Tokyo 160-0023, Japan
Department of Infection Prevention and Control, Tokyo Medical University Hachioji Medical Center, 1163 Tatemachi, Hachioujishi, Tokyo 193-0998, Japan

Hiroaki Fujita, Ayaka Tsukimori and Takehito Kobayashi
Department of Infection Prevention and Control, Tokyo Medical University Hospital, 6-7-1 Nishishinjuku, Shinjuku-ku, Tokyo 160-0023, Japan
Department of Microbiology, Tokyo Medical University, 6-1-1 Shinjuku, Shinjuku-ku, Tokyo 160-8402, Japan

Takeshi Fujii
Department of Infection Prevention and Control, Tokyo Medical University Hachioji Medical Center, 1163 Tatemachi, Hachioujishi, Tokyo 193-0998, Japan

Tetsuya Matsumoto
Department of Microbiology, Tokyo Medical University, 6-1-1 Shinjuku, Shinjuku-ku, Tokyo 160-8402, Japan

Ye Zhang, Ling-Yun Guo and Gang Liu
Department of Infectious Disease, Beijing Children's Hospital, Capital Medical University, No. 56 Nanlishi Road, Xi Cheng District, Beijing 100045, People's Republic of China

Wen-Qi Song, Yan Wang and Fang Dong
Department of Laboratory Medicine, Beijing Children's Hospital, Capital Medical University, No. 56 Nanlishi Road, Xi Cheng District, Beijing 100045, People's Republic of China

Jun Suzuki, Masaki Toshima and Yuji Morisawa
Division of Infectious Diseases, Jichi Medical University Hospital, 3311-1 Yakushiji, Shimotsuke, Tochigi 329-0498, Japan

Teppei Sasahara
Division of Infectious Diseases, Jichi Medical University Hospital, 3311-1 Yakushiji, Shimotsuke, Tochigi 329-0498, Japan
Department of Infection and Immunity, School of Medicine, Jichi Medical
University, 3311-1 Yakushiji, Shimotsuke, Tochigi 329-0498, Japan

Harsha Lochan, Vashini Pillay, James Nuttall and Brian Eley
Paediatric Infectious Diseases Unit, Red Cross War Memorial Children's Hospital and the Department of Paediatrics and Child Health, University of Cape Town, Cape Town, South Africa

Colleen Bamford
Division of Medical Microbiology, University of Cape Town and the National Health Laboratory Service, Groote Schuur Hospital, Cape Town, South Africa

Tatiana Aporta Marins
Hospital Israelita Albert Einstein, São Paulo, Brazil

Paula Kiyomi Onaga Yokota and Marcelino Souza Durão Junior
Division of Medical Practice, Hospital Israelita Albert Einstein, São Paulo, Brazil

Alexandre R. Marra
Division of Medical Practice, Hospital Israelita Albert Einstein, São Paulo, Brazil
Office of Clinical Quality, Safety and Performance Improvement, University of Iowa Hospitals and Clinics, Iowa City, IA, USA

Michael B. Edmond
Office of Clinical Quality, Safety and Performance Improvement, University of Iowa Hospitals and Clinics, Iowa City, IA, USA
Division of Infectious Diseases, Department of Internal Medicine, University of Iowa Carver College of Medicine, Iowa City, IA, USA

Marines Dalla Valle Martino
Clinical Laboratory, Hospital Israelita Albert Einstein, São Paulo, Brazil

Ana Carolina Cintra Nunes Mafra
Instituto Israelita de Ensino e Pesquisa Albert Einstein, Hospital Israelita Albert Einstein, São Paulo, Brazil

Dmitriy M. Martirosov, Monique R. Bidell, Manjunath P. Pai, Corey Faragon, M. Malik and Thomas P. Lodise
Albany College of Pharmacy and Health Sciences, Albany, NY 12208-3492, USA

Marc H. Scheetz
Midwestern University Chicago College of Pharmacy, Downers Grove, IL, USA
Northwestern Medicine, Chicago, IL, USA

Susan L. Rosenkranz
Harvard School of Public Health, Boston, MA, USA

R. E. Mendes and R. N. Jones
JMI Laboratories, North Liberty, IA, USA

Louise-Anne McNutt
University at Albany, State University of New York, Albany, NY, USA

Dominic Wichmann, Timo Kock and Stefan Kluge
Department of Intensive Care Medicine, University Medical Center Hamburg-Eppendorf, Martinistrasse 52, 20246 Hamburg, Germany

Cristina E. Belmar Campos and Holger Rohde
Institute for Medical Microbiology, Virology and Hygiene, University Medical Center Hamburg-Eppendorf, Martinistrasse 52, 20246 Hamburg, Germany

Stephan Ehrhardt
Department of Epidemiology, Johns Hopkins Bloomberg School of Public Health, 615 North Wolfe Street, Baltimore, MD 21205, USA

Claudia Weber
Schoen-Klinik Hamburg Eilbek, Dehnhaide 120, 22081 Hamburg, Germany

Elina Fechtner, Sven Poppert and Norbert Georg Schwarz
Infectious Disease Epidemiology, Bernhard Nocht Institute for Tropical Medicine (BNITM), Bernhard-Nocht-Str. 74, D-20359 Hamburg, Germany

Denise Dekker, Ralf Krumkamp, Daniel Eibach and Jürgen May
Infectious Disease Epidemiology, Bernhard Nocht Institute for Tropical Medicine (BNITM), Bernhard-Nocht-Str. 74, D-20359 Hamburg, Germany
German Center for Infection Research (DZIF), Hamburg-Borstel, Lübeck, Germany

Nimako Sarpong, Kennedy Gyau Boahen, Michael Frimpong and Ellis Owusu-Dabo
Kumasi Centre for Collaborative Research in Tropical Medicine (KCCR), Kumasi,
Ghana

Ralf Matthias Hagen
Bundeswehr Hospital of Hamburg, Germany, Department of Tropical Medicine at the Bernhard Nocht Institute, Bernhard-Nocht-Str. 74, D-20359 Hamburg, Germany

Yaw Adu-Sarkodie
Kwame Nkrumah University of Science and Technology (KNUST), Kumasi, Ghana

Justin Im
Epidemiology Unit, International Vaccine Institute (IVI), Seoul, Republic of Korea

Florian Marks
Epidemiology Unit, International Vaccine Institute (IVI), Seoul, Republic of Korea
The Department of Medicine, The University of Cambridge, Cambridge, UK

Hagen Frickmann
Bundeswehr Hospital of Hamburg, Germany, Department of Tropical Medicine at the Bernhard Nocht Institute, Bernhard-Nocht-Str. 74, D-20359 Hamburg, Germany
Institute for Medical Microbiology, Virology and Hygiene, University Medicine Rostock, Schillingallee 70, 18055 Rostock, Germany

Min Xu
Key Laboratory of Clinical In Vitro Diagnostic Techniques of Zhejiang Province, Center of Clinical Laboratory, The First Affiliated Hospital, College of Medicine, Zhejiang University, Hangzhou, China

Yu Chen
Key Laboratory of Clinical In Vitro Diagnostic Techniques of Zhejiang Province, Center of Clinical Laboratory, The First Affiliated Hospital, College of Medicine, Zhejiang University, Hangzhou, China
State Key Laboratory for Diagnosis and Treatment of Infectious Diseases, Collaborative Innovation Center for Diagnosis and Treatment of Infectious Diseases, The First Affiliated Hospital, College of Medicine, Zhejiang University, Hangzhou, China

Yiqi Fu
Department of Respiratory Diseases, The First Affiliated Hospital, College of Medicine, Zhejiang University, Hangzhou, China

Haishen Kong, Xiao Chen, Lanjuan Li and Qing Yang
State Key Laboratory for Diagnosis and Treatment of Infectious Diseases, Collaborative Innovation Center for Diagnosis and Treatment of Infectious Diseases, The First Affiliated Hospital, College of Medicine, Zhejiang University, Hangzhou, China

María Fernanda González-Lara, Pedro Torres-González, Areli Martinez-Gamboa, Andrea Rangel-Cordero, Miriam Bobadilla-del-Valle and Alfredo Ponce-de-León
Department of Infectious Diseases, Instituto Nacional de Ciencias Médicas y Nutrición Salvador Zubirán, Vasco de Quiroga 15, Belisario Domínguez Sección XVI, Tlalpan, Mexico City, Mexico

Patricia Cornejo-Juárez and Consuelo Velázquez-Acosta
Department of Infectious Diseases, Instituto Nacional de Cancerología, Ave. San Fernando 22, Belisario Dominguez Sección XVI, Mexico City, Mexico

Luis Ostrosky-Zeichner
University of Texas Health Science Center at Houston, 6431 Fannin. MSB 2.112, Houston, TX 77030, USA

José Sifuentes-Osornio
Department of Medicine, Instituto Nacional de Ciencias Médicas y Nutrición Salvador Zubirán, Vasco de Quiroga 15, Belisario Domínguez Sección XVI, Tlalpan, Zip Code 14080 Mexico City, Mexico

Hieu Ngoc Vu, Hung Nguyen The, Hoa Thi Nguyen and Chi Linh Bui
Department of Infectious Diseases, Hanoi Medical University, Hanoi, Vietnam

Vu Quoc Dat
Department of Infectious Diseases, Hanoi Medical University, Hanoi, Vietnam
National Hospital for Tropical Diseases, Hanoi, Vietnam
Wellcome Trust Major Overseas Programme, Oxford University Clinical Research Unit, Hanoi, Vietnam

Trung Vu Nguyen
Department of Infectious Diseases, Hanoi Medical University, Hanoi, Vietnam
National Hospital for Tropical Diseases, Hanoi, Vietnam

Kinh Van Nguyen and Dao Tuyet Trinh
National Hospital for Tropical Diseases, Hanoi, Vietnam
Dung Vu Tien Viet, Long Bao Hoang and Alessandro Torre
Wellcome Trust Major Overseas Programme, Oxford University Clinical Research Unit, Hanoi, Vietnam

H. Rogier van Doorn and Behzad Nadjm
Wellcome Trust Major Overseas Programme, Oxford University Clinical Research Unit, Hanoi, Vietnam
Nuffield Department of Clinical Medicine, Centre for Tropical Medicine, University of Oxford, Oxford, UK

Heiman F.L. Wertheim
Wellcome Trust Major Overseas Programme, Oxford University Clinical Research Unit, Hanoi, Vietnam
Nuffield Department of Clinical Medicine, Centre for Tropical Medicine, University of Oxford, Oxford, UK
Department of Medical Microbiology, Radboudumc, Nijmegen, Netherlands

Nguyen Thanh Long and Nguyen Dinh Hong Phuc
Department of Infectious Diseases, Hanoi Medical University, no 1 Ton That Tung street, Dong Da district, Hanoi, Vietnam

Vu Quoc Dat
Department of Infectious Diseases, Hanoi Medical University, no 1 Ton That Tung street, Dong Da district, Hanoi, Vietnam
Wellcome Trust Major Overseas Programme, Oxford University Clinical Research Unit, Hanoi, 78 Giai Phong street, Dong Da district, Hanoi, Vietnam
National Hospital for Tropical Diseases, 78 Giai Phong street, Dong Da district, Hanoi, Vietnam

H. Rogier van Doorn and Behzad Nadjm
Wellcome Trust Major Overseas Programme, Oxford University Clinical Research Unit, Hanoi, 78 Giai Phong street, Dong Da district, Hanoi, Vietnam
Nuffield Department of Clinical Medicine, Centre for Tropical Medicine, University of Oxford, Oxford, UK

Ana Bonell
Wellcome Trust Major Overseas Programme, Oxford University Clinical Research Unit, Hanoi, 78 Giai Phong street, Dong Da district, Hanoi, Vietnam

Nguyen Vu Trung
National Hospital for Tropical Diseases, 78 Giai Phong street, Dong Da district, Hanoi, Vietnam
Department of Microbiology, Hanoi Medical University, no 1 Ton That Tung street, Dong Da district, Hanoi, Vietnam

Nguyen Van Kinh
National Hospital for Tropical Diseases, 78 Giai Phong street, Dong Da district, Hanoi, Vietnam

Vu Ngoc Hieu
Department of Microbiology, Hanoi Medical University, no 1 Ton That Tung street, Dong Da district, Hanoi, Vietnam
Nuffield Department of Clinical Medicine, Centre for Tropical Medicine, University of Oxford, Oxford, UK

Index

www.ingramcontent.com/pod-product-compliance
Lightning Source LLC
LaVergne TN
LVHW080914210926
848485LV00004B/651